Textbook of
Educational Technology/Nursing Education

Textbook of Educational Technology/Nursing Education

As per the Revised Nursing Syllabus

I Clement

PhD (Nursing) Doctor of Science (DSc) MSc (N) Medical Surgical Nursing
MBA (Education) (Madras University) MA (Sociology)
MSc (Psychology) MA (Child Care and Education) MSW (Master of Social Work) (TNOU)

Working at
Professor and Principal, Sparsh College of Nursing
Former Professor and Head, Department of Research and Development
RV College of Nursing
Former Principal and Professor
Columbia College of Nursing and VSS College of Nursing, Bengaluru, Karnataka, India

Professional Life Member
PhD Society of India, Chennai, Tamil Nadu
Nursing Research Society of India, New Delhi
Trained Nurses Association of India, New Delhi
Christian Medical Association of India, New Delhi
Indian Society of Psychiatric Nursing, Bengaluru
Medical Surgical Nursing Society of India, Chennai
Indian Society of Neuroscience Nursing, New Delhi
Asian Association of Cardiac Nurses, Kolkata

Health Organization Member
Indian Red Cross Society, Bengaluru
St. Johns Ambulance Association, Bengaluru
General Secretary—Indian Society of Medical Surgical Nurses

Assignments and Examiner
PhD-Guide, Co-Guide and Examiner-INC, RGUHS and other Indian Nursing Universities
Faculty of Nursing, RGUHS, Bengaluru, Karnataka, India
LIC Inspector, Chief Squad, Observer
UG and PG-Examiner, Paper-setter, Valuator for many Nursing Universities in India

Professional Activity and Editorial
Chief Editor-RJNS-RGUHS, Bengaluru
Indian Journal of Practical Nursing
National Editorial Advisory Board, New Delhi
Nurses of India (*former*), Bengaluru
Chairman-Souvenir Committee, Florence Nightingale Awards-2012

Winner
Florence Nightingale Awards-2013
Rajiv Gandhi Education Excellence Award
National Mahila Rattan Gold Medal Award, New Delhi

ELNEC (End of Life Nursing Education Council, USA)-Award of Excellence (2021) for Outstanding Commitment to Promote Excellent Palliative Care
Research Excellence Award in International conference for award winners of Engineers, Science and Medicine, organized by Award by INSO

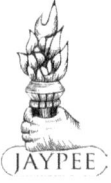

JAYPEE BROTHERS MEDICAL PUBLISHERS

The Health Sciences Publisher

New Delhi | London

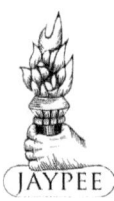

Jaypee Brothers Medical Publishers (P) Ltd

Headquarters
Jaypee Brothers Medical Publishers (P) Ltd
EMCA House, 23/23-B
Ansari Road, Daryaganj
New Delhi 110 002, India
Landline: +91-11-23272143, +91-11-23272703
+91-11-23282021, +91-11-23245672
Email: jaypee@jaypeebrothers.com

Overseas Office
J.P. Medical Ltd
83 Victoria Street, London
SW1H 0HW (UK)
Phone: +44 20 3170 8910
Email: info@jpmedpub.com

Corporate Office
Jaypee Brothers Medical Publishers (P) Ltd
4838/24, Ansari Road, Daryaganj
New Delhi 110 002, India
Phone: +91-11-43574357
Fax: +91-11-43574314
Email: jaypee@jaypeebrothers.com

EU GPSR Authorised Representative
Logos Europe, 9 rue Nicolas Poussin
17000, La Rochelle, France
Phone: +33 (0) 6 67 93 73 78
E-mail: Contact@logoseurope.eu

Website: www.jaypeebrothers.com
Website: www.jaypeedigital.com

© 2024, Jaypee Brothers Medical Publishers

The views and opinions expressed in this book are solely those of the original contributor(s)/author(s) and do not necessarily represent those of editor(s) and publisher of the book.

All rights reserved. No part of this publication may be reproduced, stored or transmitted in any form or by any means, electronic, mechanical, photocopying, recording or otherwise, without the prior permission in writing of the publishers.

All brand names and product names used in this book are trade names, service marks, trademarks or registered trademarks of their respective owners. The publisher is not associated with any product or vendor mentioned in this book.

Medical knowledge and practice change constantly. This book is designed to provide accurate, authoritative information about the subject matter in question. However, readers are advised to check the most current information available on procedures included and check information from the manufacturer of each product to be administered, to verify the recommended dose, formula, method and duration of administration, adverse effects and contraindications. It is the responsibility of the practitioner to take all appropriate safety precautions. Neither the publisher nor the author(s)/editor(s) assume any liability for any injury and/or damage to persons or property arising from or related to use of material in this book.

This book is sold on the understanding that the publisher is not engaged in providing professional medical services. If such advice or services are required, the services of a competent medical professional should be sought.

Every effort has been made where necessary to contact holders of copyright to obtain permission to reproduce copyright material. If any have been inadvertently overlooked, the publisher will be pleased to make the necessary arrangements at the first opportunity.

Inquiries for bulk sales may be solicited at: jaypee@jaypeebrothers.com

Textbook of Educational Technology/Nursing Education

First Edition: **2024**

ISBN: 978-93-5696-383-2

Dedicated to

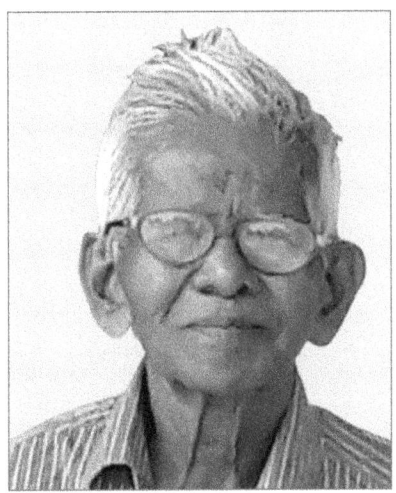

My Beloved Father

Late **A Irudayanathan**

Preface

It gives me immense pleasure and privilege to draft *Textbook of Educational Technology/Nursing Education* dedicated to all nursing students. First and foremost, I thank my Lord Almighty for his wonderful blessing that has given me strength to complete this book in time. Educational Technology is the field of study that investigates the process of analyzing, designing, developing, implementing, and evaluating the instructional environment, learning materials, learners and learning process in order to improve teaching and learning.

Nursing is a noble profession. It encompasses a comprehensive approach toward health care. Today's health care demands a multitasking and dynamic healthcare professional who can keep pace with growing science and technology. Today's nursing demands quality care that requires great preparation from student period. As a nurse educator, my contribution to the nursing society is to present this textbook to the nursing community that will help every nursing personnel to nourish themselves with knowledge on nursing management and become a good nursing leader to lead future nursing community.

Teaching skills are critical to nursing profession, and use of educational technology becomes an important medium to impart the skills. It also promotes students' learning. On the other hand, innovations that suit learners are essential to enhance and sustain the students' interest and understanding. This book contain 8 units with keywords and 21 chapters based on the revised syllabus recommended by Indian Nursing Council. Each chapter has valid diagrams, tables, adequate illustration of the content in par with the syllabus designed from the examination point of view, and also has review questions include long and short questions. Every part of the content has been narrated in simple lucid English that helps every student to prepare for the examination well as per the new syllabus.

I wish the entire nursing community to cherish this book.

I Clement

Acknowledgments

I am thankful to the Lord Almighty, who strengthens me with his abundant blessings through innumerable means, helping me in all my accomplishments. Fistful thanks to all the contributors and reviewers for their active participation. My heartfelt thanks to Shri V Sommanna, Ex-housing Minister of Karnataka and Chairman of VSS Group of Institutions, Bengaluru, Karnataka, India, for his constant support and encouragement.

I extend sincere gratitude to Dr Sharan Shivraj Patil, MBBS, MS (Orth), MCh (Orth), Liverpool, FRCS (England), Chairman and Chief Orthopedic Surgeon, SPARSH Group of Hospitals, Bengaluru. I also express my sincere thanks to my guru BT Basavanthappa, *Former* Principal, Rajarajeshweri College of Nursing, Bengaluru, and PV Ramachandran, *Former* Chairman, College of Nursing, Sri Ramachandra University, Chennai—a great philosopher and an internationally renowned teacher of nursing who helped me in discovering the world of knowledge. I am also grateful to Dr BC Bhagavan, Professor, Department of Surgery, Kempegowda Institute of Medical Sciences, Bengaluru.

I extend my special thanks to Dr TV Ramakrishnan, Professor of Anesthesiology and Head of Clinical Services, Department of Accident and Emergency Medicine, Sri Ramachandra University, Chennai. Dr Jeyaseelan Manickam Devadasan, Dean; Dr Tamilmani, Principal; Professor (Mrs) Jessie Sudarsanam, HOD, Department of Medical Surgical Nursing, Annai JKK Sampoorani Ammal College of Nursing, Tamil Nadu, and all my teachers and students deserve my gratitude. I convey my sincere thanks to my beloved parents, brothers, sisters and my wife Dr Nisha Clement for her continuous support and constant encouragement in each step of my life. I take this opportunity to thank my children—Cibin John, Cynthia Elizabeth, and Cavin Jacob.

I am very grateful to the whole team of M/s Jaypee Brothers Medical Publishers (P) Ltd, New Delhi, India, who helped and guided me, Shri Jitendar P Vij (Group Chairman), Mr Ankit Vij (Managing Director), Mr MS Mani (Group President), Dr Madhu Choudhary (Director-Educational Publishing), Ms Pooja Bhandari [Director-Production (Books and Journals)], Ms Sunita Katla (Executive Assistant to Group Chairman and Publishing Manager), Mr Ajay Kumar Sharma [DGM-Production (Books and Journals)], Ms Samina Khan (Executive Assistant to Director-Educational Publishing), Ms Alisha Talwar (Team Lead–Nursing), Mr Rajesh Sharma (Production Coordinator), Ms Seema Dogra (Cover Visualizer), Ms Neelam Kakriya (Proofreader), Mr Kuldeep Dobriyal (Typesetter), Mr Satender Singh (Graphic Designer) and their team members for all their support to work in this project and make it a success. Without their cooperation, we could not have completed this project.

I would also like to thank Mr Venugopal V (Associate Director-South), Mr Santhosh Kumar (Author Coordinator, Bengaluru), and other staff members of M/s Jaypee Brothers Medical Publishers (P) Ltd, Bengaluru Branch.

Contents

Unit 1: Introduction and Theoretical Principles: Teaching and Teaching Technology

1. **Teaching Methods in Education** 3
   - Importance of Education 3
   - Characteristics of Education 4
   - Types of Education 4
   - Goals and Purpose 5
   - Type of Education 6
   - Educational Institutions 7
   - Scope of Education 8
   - Features of Education 8

2. **Education and Educational Technology** 11
   - Importance of Educational Technology 11
   - Educational Technology Goals 12
   - Revolutions and Developments in Educational Technology 13
   - Characteristics of Teaching Technology 13
   - Necessity and Importance of Education Technology 13
   - Fields of Application Pedagogical Technology 14
   - Approaches to Educational Technology 14
   - Modern Approach to Education 16
   - Transformational Education 17
   - Relationship-based Education 21
   - Competency-based Education 21

3. **Educational Philosophy** 26
   - The Relationship between Philosophy and Philosophy Education 26
   - Objectives of Philosophy of Education Studies 27
   - Branches of Philosophy 27
   - Meaning of Philosophy 27
   - Science and Philosophy 28
   - Philosophy and Education 28
   - Important Philosophies 28
   - Nursing Philosophy 29
   - Pedagogical Application of Philosophy 30
   - Naturalism 30
   - Realism 31
   - Idealism 33
   - Pragmatism 34
   - Progressivism 35
   - Reconstructionism 36
   - Eclecticism 38
   - Perennialism 39
   - Existentialism 40
   - Philosophy of Mahatma Gandhiji 42
   - Tagore's Philosophy of Education 44
   - John Dewey's Philosophy of Education 46
   - Learning by Practice Limitations 48

4. **Teaching-Learning Process** 50
   - Teaching-Learning Process 50
   - Importance of Teaching in the Learning Process 51
   - Nature and Components of Teaching and Learning Processes 52
   - Principles of Teaching and Learning 52
   - Teaching-Learning Strategies 54
   - Teaching and Learning Barriers 54
   - Learning Theory 55
   - Modern Learning Approaches 60

Unit 2: Assessment of Teacher and Learner

5. **Assessment of Teacher and Learner** 75
   - Teacher Evaluation 76
   - Essential Characteristics of Teachers 78
   - Teaching Styles—Formal Authority Demonstrator Facilitator Delegator 79
   - Learner Assessment 80
   - Learning Types 81
   - Determinants of Learning 81
   - Today's Generation of Learners and their Skills and Characteristics 83
   - Motivational Factors—Personal Factors, Environmental Factors and Support Systems 86

6. **Curriculum Planning** 89
   - Curriculum Types 89
   - Curriculum Objectives 90
   - Factors Influences Curriculum Development 90
   - Curriculum Features 91
   - Principles of Curriculum 91
   - Curriculum Types 92
   - Core Curriculum 93

- Curriculum Design—Component Approach *94*
- Curriculum Planning and Development *95*
- Stages of Curriculum Planning *96*
- Level of Curriculum Planning *97*
- Curriculum Management *97*
- Curriculum Process *98*
- Writing Learning Outcomes/Behavioral Objectives *99*
- Subject Classification *100*
- Lesson Planning *102*
- Course Planning *103*
- Unit Planning *105*

Unit 3: Teaching in Classroom and Skill Lab

7. **Teaching Methods in Education** 111
   - Importance of Educational Methods *112*
   - Teaching Objectives *112*
   - Types of Teaching Methods *113*
   - Classification of Teaching Methodology *113*
   - Factors that Determine the Choice of Teaching Method *113*
   - Characteristics of Teaching Methods *114*
   - The Benefits of Choosing the Right Teaching Method *115*
   - Classroom Management *115*
   - Educational Management Strategies *120*
   - Communication in the Classroom *121*
   - Classroom Communication Facilitator *123*
   - Communication Barriers in the Classroom *125*
   - Information Communication Technology *126*
   - Classroom Teaching Method *128*
   - Lecture Method *128*
   - Group Discussion *130*
   - Microteaching *132*
   - Simulation *135*
   - Demonstration Methods *137*
   - Re-Demonstration *139*
   - Symposium *139*
   - Chairman Qualities *140*
   - Panel Discussion *140*
   - Seminar *141*
   - Workshop *143*
   - Exhibition *144*
   - Role Play *145*
   - Project Law *147*
   - Excursion/Fieldtrip *149*
- Self-Directed Learning *152*
- Computer-Assisted Learning *153*
- One-to-One Lessons *155*
- Active Learning Strategies *156*
- Team-based Learning *156*
- Problem-based Learning *158*
- Peer Sharing *161*
- Case Study Analysis *163*
- Journaling *163*
- Debate *167*
- Gaming *169*
- Interprofessional Education *172*
- Programmed Lessons *174*

Unit 4: Clinical Teaching Methods

8. **Teaching in the Clinical Setting** 181
   - Meaning of Clinical Teaching *182*
   - Objectives of Clinical Education *182*
   - Use of Clinical Education *182*
   - Clinical Learning Environment *182*
   - Factors Influences Clinical Learning Experience Selection *183*
   - Teaching Models in Clinical Use *184*
   - Description of Clinical Learning Outcomes/ Practical Skills *185*
   - Clinical Instructor *186*
   - Applying Clinical Teaching Methods in Education *187*
   - Clinical Education Issues *187*
   - Clinical Teaching Skills *188*
   - Clinical Teaching Challenges *188*
   - Clinical Teaching Strategies *189*
   - Patient Order/Assignment *190*
   - Clinical Meetings: Individual and Group *193*
   - Group Conference *194*
   - Clinical Presentation/Bedside Clinic *196*
   - Bed Side Clinic/Bed Side Teaching *199*
   - Case Studies/Care Studies *199*
   - Case Presentation *201*
   - Case Studies *202*
   - Care Plan *203*
   - Nursing Rounds *206*
   - Concept Mapping *207*
   - Project *210*
   - Debate *211*
   - Game *212*

- Roleplay *212*
- Problem-based Learning *214*
- Ask/Questioning *216*
- Written Assignment *216*
- Process Recording Teaching *218*

Unit 5: Educational/Teaching Media

9. **Educational/Teaching Media** 225
   - Brief History of AV-Aids Use *226*
   - Importance of Audiovisual Aids *227*
   - Categories of Educational Media *227*
   - Important Values of AV Resources *227*
   - Teaching Aid/Materials *228*
   - Teaching Aid Issues *230*
   - Classifications of Teaching Aids *231*
   - Cone of Experience *232*
   - The Importance of AV Aids in Educational Communication *232*
   - The Role of Educational Media in Teaching *233*
   - Psychological Basis for AV-Aids *233*

10. **Still Visuals** 235
    - Benefits of Still Images *235*
    - Visual Learning Strategies *235*
    - Non-projection Media *236*
    - Chart *236*
    - Graph *239*
    - Poster *240*
    - Cartoon *241*
    - Blackboard/Whiteboard *242*
    - Bulletin Board *243*
    - Flannel Sheet *245*
    - Flipcharts *245*
    - Flashcards *247*
    - Still Image/Photo *247*
    - Print Materials *248*
    - Handouts *249*
    - Newspaper *250*
    - Magazines *250*
    - Projected Aids *250*
    - Filmstrip Principles *251*
    - Microscope *252*
    - Powerpoint Slide *252*
    - Overhead Projector *253*
    - Opaque Projector *254*
    - LCD Panels *255*
    - The Slide Projector *256*
    - Slide *256*

11. **Moving Visuals and Audio Aids** 258
    - Moving Visuals/Moving Images *258*
    - Video Learning Tools *261*
    - Video Cassettes/Videotapes *262*
    - DVD (Digital Versatile Disk) *264*
    - Blu-Ray *264*
    - USB *265*
    - Realia and Models/Three-Dimensional Aids *266*
    - Puppets *267*
    - Models *269*
    - Mockups *269*
    - Object and Specimen *270*
    - Moulage *270*
    - Diorama *271*
    - Audio Aids/Audio Media *272*
    - Compact Disk *273*
    - Public Address System *273*
    - Digital Audio *275*

12. **Electronic and Telecommunication** 278
    - Electronic Media *278*
    - Telecommunications *278*
    - Computer *279*
    - Internet *281*
    - Web-based Video Conferencing *284*
    - E-Learning *286*
    - Smart Classroom *289*
    - Cable TV *291*
    - Types of Educational Television Programs *292*
    - Satellite Transmission *292*
    - Video Conferencing *293*
    - Telehealth *294*
    - Telenursing *296*
    - Mobile Technologies *297*

Unit 6: Assessment/Evaluation Methods

13. **Assessment/Evaluation Methods/Strategies** 305
    - Purpose of Assessment *306*
    - Evaluation Principles *307*
    - Scope of Assessment and Scope Assessment *307*
    - Rating Type *307*
    - Evaluation Steps *307*
    - Rating Features *308*

- Teaching Measurements Function *308*
- Evaluation Tools *309*
- Assessment Methods *310*
- Choosing an Assessment Method *311*
- Types of Tools used in the Evaluation *312*
- Evaluation Methods *313*
- Case Study *314*
- Assessment Issues *314*
- Achievement Tests *314*
- Standardized Tests *315*
- School Performance Test *315*
- Interpretation Items *316*

14. Assessment of Knowledge 318
- Essay Type Test *318*
- Short Answer Questions *320*
- Multiple Choice Questions *322*
- Objective Tests *323*
- Matching Type *325*

15. Assessment of Skills 328
- Clinical Evaluation *328*
- Objective Structured Clinical Examination *331*
- Observation *332*
- Checklists *333*
- Rating Scale *333*
- Videotape *335*
- Written Communication *336*
- Progress Notes *336*
- Care Plan *337*
- Process Record *338*
- Written Assignments *340*
- Oral Test (Viva) *340*
- Practical Exam *341*
- Simulation *341*
- Objectively Structured Clinical Examinations *343*
- Anecdotal Notes *345*
- Performance Evaluation in Nursing *345*
- Self-Assessment *348*
- Clinical Portfolio *349*
- Clinical Log *350*

16. Assessment of Attitude and Higher-Learning 353
- Attitude Component *353*
- Bogardus Social Distance Scale *353*
- Higher Education Assessment Test *354*
- Interpretive Questions *357*
- Hotspot Questions *358*
- Drag-and-Drop Questions *359*

Unit 7: Guidance/Academic Advising, Counseling and Discipline Guidance

17. Guidance and Counseling 363
- Guidance and Advice Objectives *364*
- Need for Guidance and Advice *365*
- Difference between Accompany and Advice *365*
- Scope of Guidance and Advice in Education *366*
- Principles of Leadership and Counseling *366*
- Effective Leadership and the Benefits of Effective Leadership Advice *367*
- Leadership and Leadership Role Advice *367*
- Instructions and Instructions Advisory: Program Component *368*
- Comprehensive Instruction and Counseling Plan *368*
- Guidance Counselor Responsibilities *368*
- Guidance and Advice for Nurses *369*
- Nurse Manager's Role in Guidance and Guidance Consult *369*

18. Counseling 371
- Counseling Meaning *371*
- Definition of Counseling *372*
- Counseling Objectives *372*
- Counseling Goals *372*
- Purpose of Counseling *372*
- Need Advice/Counseling *373*
- Scope of Counseling *373*
- Advisory Staff *374*
- Consultation Procedure *374*
- Counseling Features *375*
- Core Principles of Counseling *375*
- Consulting Skills *376*
- Counseling Ethics *377*
- Types of Advice *377*
- Benefits of Counseling *378*
- Organization of Counseling Services *378*
- Counseling Rules and Roles *380*
- Advice Compared to Other Terms *380*
- Counseling Approach *380*
- Counseling Techniques *381*
- Policy Counseling *382*
- Non-policy Consulting *382*
- Eclectic Counseling *383*
- Counselor Qualities *384*
- Counselor Duties *384*
- Advisor Characteristics or Qualifications *385*
- Objectives of Student Counseling *385*

19. Guidance/Academic Advising 388
- Leadership Concepts *388*
- Definition of Leadership *388*
- Objectives of Instruction *389*
- Leadership Principles *389*
- Pipe Element *389*
- Leadership Characteristics *390*
- Basic Assumptions of the Guide *390*
- Need Advice *390*
- Types of Counseling *390*
- Organizing Counseling Services *391*
- Individual Counseling Services *392*
- Personal Counseling Needs *392*
- Individual Counseling Procedures *393*
- Educational Counseling *394*
- Career Advice *396*

20. Discipline and Grievance 399
- Discipline Means *399*
- Discipline Purpose *399*
- Nature of Discipline *400*
- Discipline Components *400*
- Disciplinary Characteristics *400*
- Principles for Maintaining Discipline *401*
- Disciplinary Matters *401*
- Disciplinary Matters Management *402*
- Complaints *402*
- Complaints Committee *404*

Unit 8: Teaching (EBT) in Nursing Education

21. Teaching (EBT) in Nursing Education 409
- VBE Meaning *410*
- VBE Purpose *410*
- Ethics Review *411*
- Nurses and People *411*
- Important for Values-based Education *412*
- Values Education *412*
- Values Education in Schools *414*
- Values-based Nursing Education *415*
- Value Development Strategies *415*
- Approaches to Values Education *417*
- Ethical Decision-making *417*
- Student Ethical Standards *418*
- Student-Faculty Relationship *419*
- Responsibilities for Student-Teacher Relationships *420*
- Evidence-based Teaching *420*
- Evidence-based Teaching Strategies *421*
- Using Evidence-based Instruction in the Classroom *422*
- Care Education Applications *422*

Multiple Choice Questions 425

Index 439

Syllabus

Placement: V Semester
Theory: 2 Credits (40 hours)
Practicum: Lab/Practical: 1 Credit (40 hours)

Description

This course is designed to help the students to develop knowledge, attitude and beginning competencies essential for applying basic principles of teaching and learning among individuals and groups both in educational and clinical settings. It also introduces basics of curriculum planning and organization. It further enables students to participate actively in team and collaborative learning.

Competencies

On completion of the course, the students will be competent to:
- Develop basic understanding of theoretical foundations and principles of teaching and learning.
- Identify the latest approaches to education and learning.
- Initiate self-assessment to identify one's own learning styles.
- Demonstrate understanding of various teaching styles that can be used, based on the learners' readiness and generational needs.
- Develop understanding of basics of curriculum planning and organizing.
- Analyze and use different teaching methods effectively that are relevant to student population and settings.
- Make appropriate decisions in selection of teaching-learning activities integrating basic principles.
- Utilize active learning strategies that enhance critical thinking, team learning and collaboration.
- Engage in team learning and collaboration through interprofessional education.
- Integrate the principles of teaching and learning in selection and use of educational media/technology.
- Apply the principles of assessment in selection and use of assessment and evaluation strategies.
- Construct simple assessment tools/tests integrating cognitive, psychomotor and affective domains of learning that can measure knowledge and competence of students.
- Develop basic understanding of student guidance through mentoring and academic advising.
- Identify difficult situations, crisis and disciplinary/grievance issues experienced by students and provide appropriate counseling.
- Engage in ethical practice in educational as well as clinical settings based on values, principles and ethical standards.
- Develop basic understanding of evidence-based teaching practices.

COURSE OUTLINE

T: Theory, P: Practical (Laboratory)

Unit	Time (hours) T	Time (hours) P	Learning outcomes	Content	Teaching/Learning activities	Assessment methods

I	6	3	Explain the definition, aims, types, approaches and scope of educational technology.	**Introduction and theoretical foundations**
				Education and educational technology
				• Definition, aims
				• Approaches and scope of educational technology
				• Latest approaches to education:
				  ▪ Transformational education
				  ▪ Relationship-based education
				  ▪ Competency-based education
					Lecture cum discussion	Quiz

			Compare and contrast the various educational philosophies.	*Educational philosophy* • Definition of philosophy, education and philosophy • Comparison of educational philosophies • Philosophy of nursing education		

			Explain the teaching-learning process, nature, characteristics and principles.	*Teaching-learning process*
				• Definitions
				• Teaching-learning as a process
				• Nature and characteristics of teaching and learning
				• Principles of teaching and learning
				• Barriers to teaching and learning
				• Learning theories
				• Latest approaches to learning
				  ▪ Experiential learning
				  ▪ Reflective learning
				  ▪ Scenario-based learning
				  ▪ Simulation-based learning
				  ▪ Blended learning
					Group exercise: Create/discuss scenario-based exercise	**Assessment of assignment:** Learning theories—analysis of any one

II	6	6	• Identify essential qualities/attributes of a teacher. • Describe the teaching styles of faculty. • Explain the determinants of learning and initiates self-assessment to identify own learning style. • Identify the factors that motivate the learner. • Define curriculum and classify types. • Identify the factors influencing curriculum development. • Develop skill in writing learning outcomes, and lesson plan.	**Assessment and planning** *Assessment of teacher* • Essential qualities of a teacher • Teaching styles: Formal authority, demonstrator, facilitator, delegator *Assessment of learner* • Types of learners • Determinants of learning—learning needs, readiness to learn, learning styles • Today's generation of learners and their skills and attributes • Emotional intelligence of the learner • Motivational factors—personal factors, environmental factors and support system **Curriculum planning** • Curriculum—definition, types • Curriculum design—components, approaches • Curriculum development—factors influencing curriculum development, facilitators and barriers • Writing learning outcomes/behavioral objectives • Basic principles of writing course plan, unit plan and lesson plan	Lecture cum discussion **Self-assessment exercise:** • Identify your learning style using any learning style inventory (e.g., Kolb's learning style inventory) • Lecture cum discussion **Individual/group exercise:** • Writing, learning outcomes • Preparation of a lesson plan	• Short answer • Objective type **Assessment of assignment:** Individual/group

Syllabus **xix**

Unit	Time (hours) T	Time (hours) P	Learning outcomes	Content	Teaching/Learning activities	Assessment methods

III	8	15	Explain the principles and strategies of classroom management.
			
			Describe different methods/strategies of teaching and develop beginning skill in using various teaching methods.
			
			Explain active learning strategies and participate actively in team and collaborative learning.
				Implementation
				Teaching in classroom and skill lab—teaching methods
				• Classroom management—principles and strategies
				• Classroom communication
				  ▪ Facilitators and barriers to classroom communication
				  ▪ Information communication technology (ICT)—ICT used in education
				Teaching methods—features, advantages and disadvantages
				• Lecture, group discussion, microteaching
				• Skill lab—simulations, demonstration and re-demonstration
				• Symposium, panel discussion, seminar, scientific workshop, exhibitions
				• Role play, project
				• Field trips
				• Self-directed learning (SDL)
				• Computer-assisted learning
				• One-to-one instruction
				Active learning strategies
				• Team-based learning
				• Problem-based learning
				• Peer sharing
				• Case study analysis
				• Journaling
				• Debate
				• Gaming
				• Interprofessional education
					• Lecture cum discussion
					• Practice teaching/microteaching
					• Exercise (peer teaching)
					• Patient-teaching session
					• Construction of game—puzzle
					• Teaching in groups—interdisciplinary
						• Short answer
						• Objective type
						• Assessment of microteaching

IV	3	3	Enumerate the factors influencing selection of clinical learning experiences. Develop skill in using different clinical teaching strategies.	**Teaching in the clinical setting—teaching methods** • Clinical learning environment • Factors influencing selection of clinical learning experiences • Practice model • Characteristics of effective clinical teacher • Writing clinical learning outcomes/practice competencies • Clinical teaching strategies—patient assignment—clinical conference, clinical presentation/bedside clinic, case study/care study, nursing rounds, concept mapping, project, debate, game, roleplay, PBL, questioning, written assignment, process recording	• Lecture cum discussion • Writing clinical outcomes—assignments in pairs	• Short answer • Assessment of written assignment

Unit	Time (hours) T	Time (hours) P	Learning outcomes	Content	Teaching/learning activities	Assessment methods
V	5	5	Explain the purpose, principles and steps in the use of media. Categorize the different types of media and describe its advantages and disadvantages. Develop skill in preparing and using media.	**Educational/teaching media** • Media use: Purpose, components, principles and steps • Types of media *Still visuals* • Non-projected—drawings and diagrams, charts, graphs, posters, cartoons, board devices (chalk/whiteboard, bulletin board, flannel board, flip charts, flash cards, still pictures/photographs, printed materials-handout, leaflet, brochure, flyer • Projected—film stripes, microscope, power point slides, overhead projector *Moving visuals* • Video learning resources—videotapes and DVD, blu-ray, USB flash drive • Motion pictures/films *Realia and models* Real objects and models *Audio aids/audio media* • Audiotapes/compact discs • Radio and tape recorder • Public address system • Digital audio *Electronic media/computer learning resources* • Computers • Web-based videoconferencing • E-learning, Smart classroom *Telecommunication (Distance education)* • Cable TV, satellite broadcasting, videoconferencing telephones—telehealth/telenursing *Mobile technology*	• Lecture cum discussion • Preparation of different teaching aids—(integrate with practice teaching sessions)	• Short answer • Objective type • Assessment of the teaching media prepared
VI	5	3	Describe the purpose, scope, principles in selection of evaluation methods and barriers to evaluation. Explain the guidelines to develop assessment tests. Develop skill in construction of different tests. Identify various clinical evaluation tools and demonstrate skill in selected tests.	**Assessment/evaluation methods/strategies** • Purposes, scope and principles in selection of assessment methods and types • Barriers to evaluation • Guidelines to develop assessment tests *Assessment of knowledge* • Essay type questions • Short answer questions (SAQ) • Multiple choice questions (MCQ—single response and multiple response) *Assessment of skills* • Clinical evaluation • Observation (checklist, rating scales, videotapes) • Written communication—progress notes, nursing care plans, process recording, written assignments • Verbal communication (oral examination) • Simulation • Objective Structured Clinical Examination (OSCE) • Self-evaluation • Clinical portfolio, clinical logs	• Lecture cum discussion • Exercise on constructing assessment tool/s	• Short answer • Objective type • Assessment of tool/s prepared

Unit	Time (hours) T	Time (hours) P	Learning Outcomes	Content	Teaching/learning activities	Assessment Methods
				Assessment of attitude Attitude scales *Assessment tests for higher learning* Interpretive questions, hotspot questions, drag and drop and ordered response questions		
VII	3	3	Explain the scope, purpose and principles of guidance. Differentiate between guidance and counseling. Describe the principles, types, and counseling process. Develop basic skill of counseling and guidance. Recognize the importance of preventive counseling and develop skill to respond to disciplinary problems and grievance among students.	**Guidance/academic advising, counseling and discipline** *Guidance* • Definition, objectives, scope, purpose and principles • Roles of academic advisor/faculty in guidance *Counseling* • Difference between guidance and counseling • Definition, objectives, scope, principles, types, process and steps of counseling • Counseling skills/techniques—basics • Roles of counselor • Organization of counseling services • Issues for counseling in nursing students *Discipline and grievance in students* • Managing disciplinary/grievance problems— preventive guidance and counseling • Role of students' grievance redressal cell/committee	• Lecture cum discussion • Role play on student counseling in different situations • Assignment on identifying situations requiring counseling	• Assessment of performance in role play scenario • Evaluation of assignment
VIII	4	2	Recognize the importance of value-based education. Develop skill in ethical decision making and maintain ethical standards for students. Introduce knowledge of EBT and its application in nursing education.	**Ethics and evidence based teaching (EBT) in nursing education** *Ethics—review* • Definition of terms • Value based education in nursing • Value development strategies • Ethical decision making • Ethical standards for students • Student-faculty relationship *Evidence based teaching—introduction* Evidence based education process and its application to nursing education	• Value clarification exercise • Case study analysis (student encountered scenarios) and suggest ethical decision-making steps • Lecture cum discussion	• Short answer • Evaluation of case study analysis • Quiz – MCQ

Unit 1
Introduction and Theoretical Principles: Teaching and Teaching Technology

Chapters

1. Teaching Methods in Education
2. Education and Educational Technology
3. Educational Philosophy
4. Teaching-Learning Process

KEYWORDS

Achievement test: A test designed to discover how well the targets of a learning program has been reached.
Aptitude testing: Testing the ability to learn a subject.
Audio-visual aid: Any chart, diagram, object, video sequence or audio recording, etc., used in a classroom.
Bloom's taxonomy: A way of categorizing and describing educational objectives in terms of the cognitive difficulty of tasks.
Classroom climate: The intellectual, social, emotional, and physical environments in which students learn.
Student-centered teaching: Instructor-center teaching refers to instructors teaching content solely through a passive approach such as lecturing while students listen and take notes with minimal interaction with other students.
Synchronous instruction: Synchronous instruction is the idea that students learn material at the same time.
Summative assessment: Summative assessment is the process of measuring a student's learning at the conclusion of a course (or a portion of the course).
Scaffolding: A process by which instructors build on a student's previous experience or knowledge by adding in specific timely support structures in the form of activities or assignments for students to master new knowledge or skills and achieve learning goals.
Retrieval practice: Retrieval practice involves retrieving new knowledge from memory in order for durable retention in long-term memory.
Project-based learning: A form of student-centered teaching that engages students with course content as they work through a complex project.

Problem-based learning: A form of student-centered teaching that focuses on having students work through open-ended problems to explore course material.

Pedagogy: Pedagogy is the method, practice and study of effective teaching. In order to be effective, instructors must have both subject-based knowledge and pedagogic knowledge and skills.

Learning management system (LMS): Learning management system is a platform that enables instructors to organize and distribute course materials in a digital format.

Augmented reality (AR): An interactive experience of a real-world environment where objects are augmented with overlaid sensory information generated by a computer.

Assessment: A measureable way of identifying a learner's knowledge and skills in regards to certain course content.

Blended learning: Combines classroom (or face-to-face learning) learning with online learning to increase interactivity while still providing purpose and structure.

Chunk: A short piece of content within a larger unit designed to combat content overload and help increase retention.

Computer-based training (CBT): An interactive instructional approach where education and training are done on a computer.

Distance education/learning: Distance learning represents education away from the traditional classroom.

Gamification: Applying game-design elements and game principles to education to improve engagement, learning, and ease of use while adding a sense of accomplishment with rewards like badges or points.

Hybrid learning: Similar to blended learning, except hybrid learning incorporates any combination of learning methods that best suits the individual learner (rather than only classroom and online).

Informal learning: Any learning that is not formal or non-formal, such as learning from experience or self-directed learning.

Learning management system (LMS): A software application designed for creating and delivering educational courses and training programs.

Microlearning: A learner-centered model that delivers information in bite-sized chunks to reduce cognitive load, combat information overload, and improve retention.

Personalized learning: An educational approach that focuses on individual learners and customizes learning plans based on the strengths, needs, skills, and interests of each learner.

Social media learning: A form of collaborative learning based on the use of social media tools and technology.

Virtual classroom: A virtual classroom allows learners to work in groups to interact and engage with resources in a collaborative, virtual way.

Virtual reality (VR): An interactive, simulated environment. In EdTech, VR is useful for training simulations and learning that would be dangerous or difficult in non-virtual settings.

Axiology is the branch of philosophy that considers the study of fundamental principles.

Classical conditioning is another term for conditioned behavior, a behavior that responds to a stimulus that does not normally cause that reflexive response.

Cognitive psychology, also known as constructivism, is the perspective that students "build" their knowledge as new experiences are linked to previous experiences.

Deductive reasoning is reasoning that allows a person to think from general principles to a specific event.

Essentialism is a philosophy of education that consists of core knowledge in reading, writing, math, science, history, foreign language, and technology.

Idealism is a major school of thought in educational philosophy, of which the underlying principle is that reality is mostly spiritual. It is the belief that physical things exist only in the mind.

Teaching Methods in Education

Chapter 1

Learning Objectives
- Importance of Education
- Characteristics of Education
- Types of Education
- Educational Institutions
- Scope of Education
- Features of Education

INTRODUCTION

In literary sense, education owes its origin to the two Latin words: 'Educate means to nurture, to educate. To educate means to bring forth, draw out. Educatum means the act of education and training. The word education comes from the Latin word educare, which means to lead. This derivation means growth from within. Therefore, the basic meaning of education can be given as a manifestation of the child's inherent potential. The idea of education is not only to equip students with the knowledge of some subjects, but also to develop habits and attitudes that will enable them to face the future successfully. Education is the process of helping children adapt to this changing world. Parenting exposes children to specific experiences aimed at modifying behavior in order to achieve appropriate adaptation to changing environments. Rather, education is the foundation of life for a goal-oriented and ideal life.

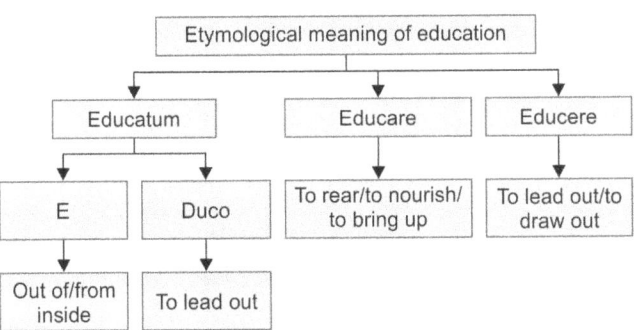

Fig. 1.1: Etymological meaning of education.

DEFINITION

- Swami Vivekananda regarded education as "an expression of the divine perfection already present in man". Education means expressing the full personality of a human being.
- Education, according to John Dewey, is the development of all the capacities of an individual to help him control his environment and realize his potential.
- Education, says Aristotle, "is the keeping of a sound mind in a sound body." It develops human faculties, especially the mind, so that it can take pleasure in contemplating the supreme truth, goodness and beauty that essentially constitute perfect happiness.
- T Raymont defines education as "the developmental process from infancy to adulthood, the process of gradual adaptation in various ways to the physical and mental environment". Education is the ability to feel joy and pain at the right moment. It unfolds in the body and soul of the student all the beauty and perfection he is capable of.

IMPORTANCE OF EDUCATION

- Education changes behavior. It makes changes in the child's behavior for their own benefit. In the old days, raising children meant filling their minds with knowledge.
- Modern education aims at the harmonious development of the child's personality. Schools and teachers need to

create conditions in which individuality can develop freely and fully.
- Education is a social process. Their main concern is behavioral change. Educational psychology thus examines human behavior as influenced by social educational processes.
- Also examines and explores the processes that lead to an understanding of how behavior can be modified through education.

CHARACTERISTICS OF EDUCATION

- Education is the process of continually restructuring experience. Education has a wide range of characteristics, the most important of which are: As we know, experience is the most important part of education and is a social process because it can only be perceived in a social environment.
- **Life and education links:** Various situations and strange events that occur in our lives and education have a great impact on our lives. Therefore, life can be called education and education life.

Characteristics of education
- Education is purposive
- Drawing out or bringing up process
- Knowledge as well as experience
- For the good of the individual and the welfare of the society
- Liberal and vocational
- Stabilizer, conservator and reconstruction
- Education is deliberate
- Education is planned
- Education is life long
- Education is influence exerted
- Education is bipolar and tripolar
- Education is psychological and social
- Education is growth

Fig. 1.2: Characteristics of education.

- **Education is development:** Education directly or indirectly contributes to the overall development of the child. The goal of education is the full development of the child. So education is development and development itself is life.
- **Education is the source of creativity:** Education provides individuals with new experiences and helps them create new things.
- Education is the reconstruction of experience, and people acquire different experiences in different situations. Over time, some of these were left out, others changed, and new experiences filled the empty spaces. In human life, this transformation and reconstruction of experience is called formation.
- **Education plays an important role in the maintenance of a society:** Every society has its own rituals, ethics, morals, language, culture, beliefs, etc. Education helps society maintain it.
- **Education is an art:** Like art, it beautifully develops a child's natural qualities. Teaching is also an art. Thus, the teacher, under his guidance, promotes good and healthy character in his pupils.
- **Education is a process of socialization:** Every society has its own set of moral values. With the help of education, people can develop these moral values. Therefore, it is called the socialization process.
- **Education brings about positive changes in behavior:** Education brings about positive changes in people's behavior. Good and ethical behavior makes us good people and contributes to our development.
- **Education is the power to adapt to new situations:** Education gives us the power to solve the difficult problems we face in life.

TYPES OF EDUCATION

Formal

Preplanned, directly organized and delivered in a particular educational institution such as a school or college. It has a well-defined curriculum that is limited to a specific period of time. Delivered by qualified and trained teachers. Formal education is subject to strict discipline. This also includes any form of vocational or general education provided by a teacher or mother at home or by a teacher in or out of school. While churches and temples consciously try to instill values and standards of behavior, states enact laws to dictate the conduct of their citizens.

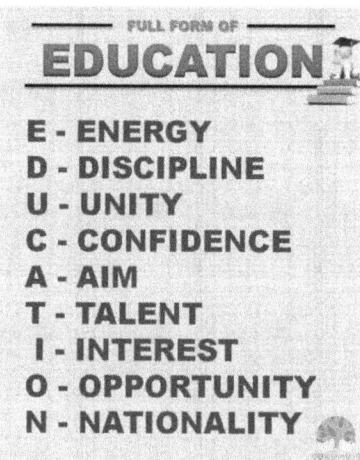

Fig. 1.3: Forms of education.

Formal education is the form of education provided by a particular institution such as a school, college or university. Formal education is designed with fixed goals and objectives and delivered according to a curriculum. We have a regular review system and discipline. This is provided in accordance with the rules and regulations of the relevant schools and colleges. Features include:
- It is predetermined and preplanned
- Time limited and regulated by routine
- Space bound or institutional
- Due to aging
- Follows a structured curriculum
- Taught by a qualified teacher
- Observe strict discipline
- Methodical in nature.

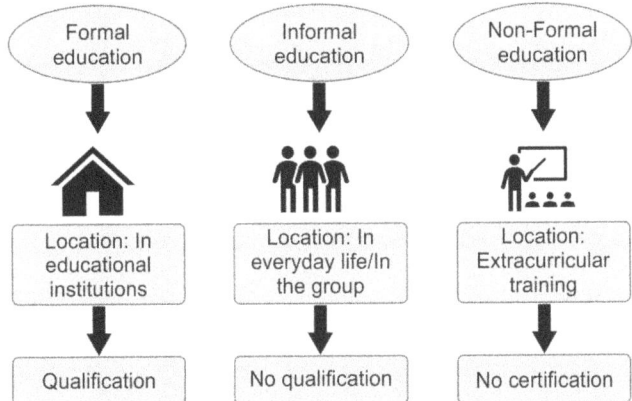

Fig. 1.4: Classification of education.

Informal Education

No plans. It is a type of education that children receive while traveling and living with other people. He/she will pick up on and adopt the behaviors and habits of adult members of his/her community. Informal education is indirectly contingent and voluntary. There are no special institutions or institutions like schools that provide this kind of education. There is no set timetable or curriculum, no formal goals or objectives. Informal education does not require qualified or trained teachers and does not require syllabus exams.

Informal or incidental education is education that occurs automatically during the course of life. It is received by those who live with other people, such as cycling, horseback riding, fishing. Families are one of the most important institutions of informal education because they learn a lot from their members. The main features of non-formal education are:
- Casual and spontaneous
- Unplanned and intentional
- It is not tied to any institution
- No prescribed curriculum and schedule
- Not bound by time or age
- There are many institutions of informal education
- Also called extracurricular education.

Non-formal Education

Receive formal and non-formal education. Informal education is deliberately random and takes place outside the formal system. It is consciously planned, organized and consistently implemented.

Non-formal education is organized and systematic educational activity conducted outside the framework of the established formal system. Non-formal education is provided at appropriate times and levels of understanding or intellectual development for children and adults.

Key features include:
- Non-formal education is structured and planned, but outside the scope of formal education
- Consciously and intentionally organized and implemented
- Service demanding programmed
- Flexible in curriculum design, processes and assessment
- In non-formal education, the relationship between teachers and students is very close
- Participation in non-formal education is voluntary
- Many students are employed in non-formal education.

GOALS AND PURPOSE

John Dewey said, "A purposeful activity is anything that is done intelligently." A goal is a given goal that inspires an individual to achieve it through appropriate activity. Likewise, a meaningful activity without a purpose or goal has no real power to direct and give meaning to it.
- Education is a deliberate and organized activity that consciously seeks to change the behavior of educated people.
- Intentional action accompanies intelligent action. Goals enable meaningful action.
- Goals help measure success and failure.
- Educational goals guide both teachers and scholars on the right path.

Determining Factors
- **Philosophy:** Philosophy determines the educational goals.
- Human factors are always taken into account when determining educational goals.
- **Religious factors:** Buddhism emphasized the inculcation of its religious ideals.

- **Political ideology:** The educational goals of democratic political regimes can be very different from those of autocratic political regimes.
- Socio-economic factors and issues of the country.
- **Cultural factors:** A country's socio-cultural heritage has a significant impact on its educational goals.
- **Seeking knowledge:** Today's education is science-oriented and technology-based.

Educational Goals Related to Time and Space

Educational goals are not fixed in every time and place:
- Education is not an activity with a single goal.
- Human nature is diverse and has diverse needs.
- Educational goals relate to ideas about life.

Individual Training Goals

Training should be aimed at individual training and development.

Individual educational goals are emphasized for the following reasons:
- **Biological:** Every child born into this world is a new and unique product, an experiment in life. Biologists believe that everyone is different.
- **Naturalistic perspective:** According to naturalists, the central goal of education is the independent development of the individual. Education must therefore correspond to the qualities that make an individual what he or she should be.
- **Psychological perspective:** Psychologists believe that education is an individual process. No two children of hers have the exact same intellectual abilities and emotional tendencies.
- **Spiritual or moral perspective:** Since human spiritual development is individual, the human function of education should lead the individual towards self-actualization and the realization of higher life values.
- **Progressive perspective:** Progressives believe that human progress and progress are due to great figures born in different eras of history. These include great scientists, inventors, researchers, religious leaders, social reformers, philosophers, and more.

Importance of Educational Goals

- Education is a purposeful, useful, planned activity.
- Achieving clearly defined life goals is done by educators (teachers) and educators (children).
- A goal-oriented action cannot be achieved without a goal. Lack of goals makes activities haphazard, confusing, and chaotic.
- Without goals, no individual or organization can realize its educational potential.

Educational Goals

- Any activity that has a beginning and an end and a process of discussion between them can be described as a goal.
- John Dewey defined goals to mean ordered and orderly activities, where the order is the gradual completion of a process.
- A consists of a system of activities and a sense of order in activities. So, simply put, a goal is a predictable purpose that gives direction to an activity.

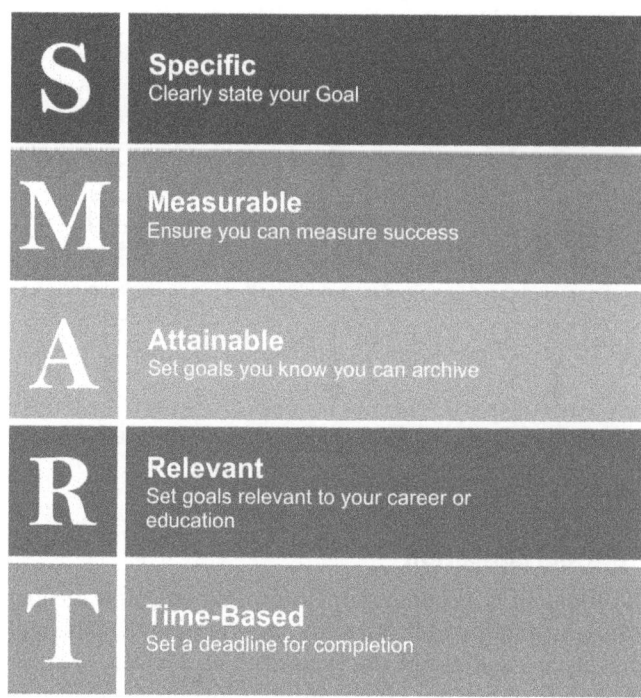

Fig. 1.5: Educational goals.

Benefits of Educational Goals

- Educational goals orient children towards achieving their goals in life.
- Gives you the foresight to train for effective planning.
- Inspire both teachers and educators to know what the outcome will be before the activity is completed.
- Guide each child to act meaningfully and intelligently.
- Guide both teachers and scholars on the right path.

TYPE OF EDUCATION

- **Educational goals are never fixed:** Education is not a single activity goal. It has many goals. It is not limited to any particular stage in an individual's life. It is for different levels, it is for different levels. When developing educational goals, educators should take into consideration the special needs and intellectual development of individual children. Example: Primary level education goals are not the same as secondary or college level education goals.

- **Human needs are multifaceted and multiple needs:** No single educational goal can meet the needs of the multifaceted nature of humans. Example: A teacher cannot take care of the body without neglecting the mind and soul. Similarly, we cannot afford to train an amoral profession. He should follow an educational program that can meet the diverse needs of children.

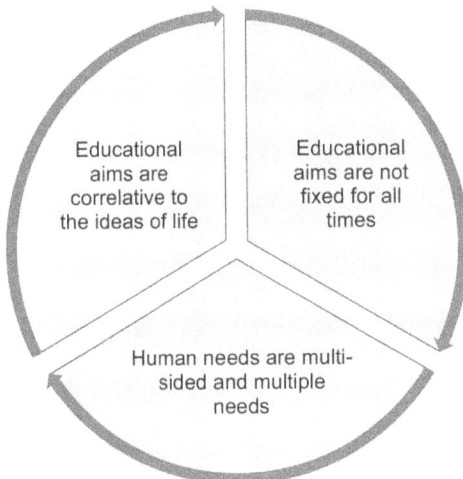

Fig. 1.6: The nature of education.

- **Educational goals are interrelated with the concept of life:** The concept of life changes with time and country in response to changing political, social, economic and physical conditions. Changes depending on educational goals also change according to different directions of philosophical, religious, social and scientific influences. The Secondary School Commission's report clearly states that as the political, social and economic conditions change, new problems arise. At each stage, the goals that education should aim for should be thoroughly reviewed and articulated.

EDUCATIONAL INSTITUTIONS

Society depends on education for the development of communities and the advancement of their physical and social lives. Each generation must pass on to the next generation its own experiences, habits, thoughts and values as well as those inherited from the previous generation. You cannot succeed without an education. Therefore, all societies must maintain and develop institutions to pass on their rich cultural heritage to the next generation. Such institutions are called educational institutions.

Type of Institution

Educational institutions can be described as formal and informal on the one hand and active on the other.

- **Official agencies:** Official agencies are scientifically developed official agencies for the sole purpose of providing education. They are consciously and purposefully planned programs. The procedures and conduct of their activities are fixed and precisely defined. These providers include schools, churches and government leisure facilities. They have a direct and significant educational impact on members. Such institutions are called informal institutions. Family reunion playgroups, etc.

- **Active agencies:** Agencies that provide education through the interaction of people are called active agencies. Education is a two-way process. Here there is an interaction between educators and educators, individuals and groups. They aim to control and direct social processes. House churches, schools, sports clubs and social welfare agencies are some of these agencies.

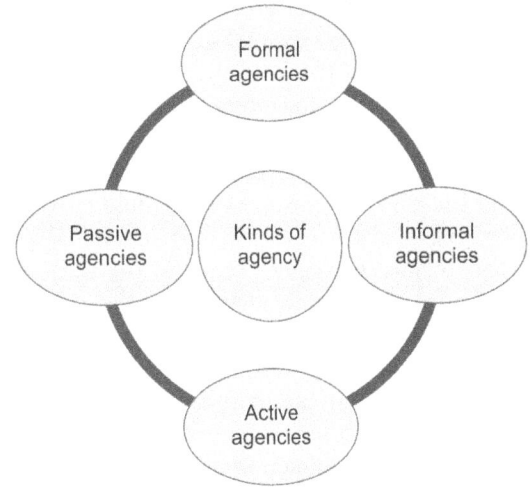

Fig. 1.7: Types of institutions.

- **Passive institutions:** Passive institutions are meant to be a one-way process. Individually influenced, but not influenced by him. However, they are subject to public scrutiny, public taste, and government censorship. For example, cinema, radio, press, television, etc.

SCOPE OF EDUCATION

Scope means the scope, outlook or opportunity of activity, operation and application. Education has a broader meaning and application. Aspects of the field of education are: Relations with other subjects areas of education and types of education.

Relations with Other Subjects

- **Pedagogy and philosophy:** Philosophy of education includes educational goals, types of education importance of education and functions of education. It is very old and an integral part of education.
- **Education and psychology:** The primary goal of education is child development. Psychology helps us better understand children and their development in terms of physical, mental, emotional, social adjustment, individual differences, personality, thinking, reasoning, and problem-solving.
- **Education and sociology:** Children live in society, so it is important to know about society. Types of society, the interdependence of cultures and societies.
- **Education and history:** Background origin development It is also important to know the development and subject aspects. Also teaching methods of ancient, medieval, British and modern educational systems.
- **Education and economics:** For the growth of the enterprise and the market, first-class economic education is important and important for everyone.
- **Education and politics:** Political institutions have influenced the theory and practice of education from the beginning. The influence of politics has helped educate people to stand against exploitation and injustice and uphold their human rights as individual citizens and consumers.
- **Education and census:** A view on the undesirable increase in population awareness is provided by population education.
- **Education and environmental studies:** Ecological accounting is the focus of today's intelligentsia. Therefore, it is very important to consider environmental issues in environmental education research.

Research Areas of Education

- **Philosophy of education:** Philosophy is an integral part of our lives. Philosophy provides basic principles and education implements these principles in the field of educational philosophy.
- **The sociology of education:** Schools are small societies. Teachers are social engineers, trying to make a difference in society through their students and their parents. Through the sociology of education, we can understand how public institutions and individual experiences influence education and its outcomes. It mainly deals with the public school system of modern industrial society, including the extension and further education of the upper adulthood.
- **Educational psychology:** Educational psychology is the branch of psychology that deals with the scientific study of human learning.
- **Teaching:** In the past, students were passive and good listeners, but now they are actively participating with their teachers in the educational process. Therefore, it is necessary to develop skills and competencies in different teaching methods.
- **History of education:** Records the stages of development of education in relation to various aspects and the role of revolutionary teachers and philosophers who helped shape educational systems around the world.
- **Comparative education:** To compare educational systems and policies in different countries with a view to facilitating educational comparisons of structures, operational goals, methods and practices in different countries.
- **Educational management:** Educational management refers to the management of the education system by which the group combines human and material resources to oversee the planning, strategy, and implementation of the organization to implement the education system. increase.
- **Educational technology:** Educational technology is the use of both physical hardware software and educational theory to create and manage appropriate technical processes and resources to facilitate learning and improve performance.

FEATURES OF EDUCATION

The following are the features of education:

- **Completion of the socialization process:** One of the most important social goals of education is the completion of the socialization process. The advent of the nuclear family has greatly increased the role of schools and other institutions in the socialization process. At school, children are trained to develop sincere consideration for others and the ability to distinguish between right and wrong. The process of socialization also enables children to cooperate with other people, respect the laws established by society, and grow up to be good citizens. Accomplished through textbooks and learning experiences.

- **Transmission of cultural heritage:** All societies take pride in preserving or enhancing their cultural heritage, ensuring that culture is preserved and passed on to future generations through social institutions. Education and educational institutions of all kinds must seriously perform their cultural mediation function by imparting elements of culture such as literary history, art philosophy, and so on.
- **Social personality formation:** The personalities of individual members of society share some common traits of culture. In addition to the mediation process of culture, education also contributes to the formation of social personality. The formation of a social personality helps people adapt to their environment and thrive in cooperation with others.

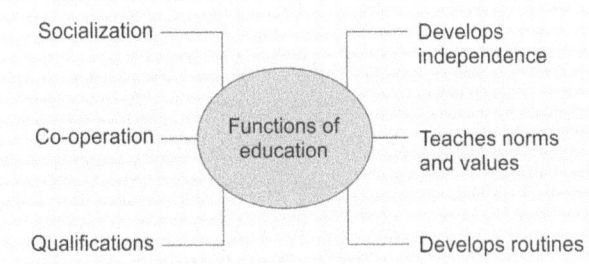

Fig. 1.8: Functions of education.

- **Behavioral reforms:** Children's developmental processes may incorporate unwanted behaviors such as beliefs and mistrust, prejudice, jealousy and hatred. The task of education is to improve unwanted behaviors and other negative aspects by removing false beliefs, illogical prejudices and irrational places from children's minds. A concerted effort by schools and families will have a dramatic effect on changing attitudes.
- **Education for placement—means of livelihood:** Today, this is recognized by many as the first and most important task of education. This function is related to the practical goals of education and receives more attention due to the different needs of society. Education must prepare students not only to predict their future professional status, but to achieve it in an impressive way.
- **Status conferment:** It is understood that an individual's status in society is determined by the amount and type or kind of education received. In the current situation, the type of knowledge acquisition is more important than the quantity. For example, registered nurses compared to those with PhDs be successful anywhere in the world with traditional themes.
- **Education promotes a spirit of competition:** Healthy competition is essential to the growth of democratic societies. Healthy competition can take the form of quality products and services. From the school level, students should be aware of the need to participate in healthy competition in order to have a better life.
- **Education develops the skills necessary for business:** For example, business and education are always bilateral. The number of functioning hospitals is directly related to the number of qualified and qualified nurses leaving nursing facilities. More patients are admitted to hospitals that provide quality care. This will lead to more financial transactions and ultimately economic development in the area surrounding the hospital.
- **Promote participatory democracy:** In participatory democracy, citizens are aware of their rights and responsibilities and actively participate in the democratic process. Literacy is essential to fostering participatory democracy, and literature is the product of education. Education therefore promotes participatory democracy.
- **Education conveys values:** Education helps students to recognize the role of values in a good life as a social being. Through various activities, education conveys values such as cooperation, team spirit and obedience. Generally speaking, students learn social skills from educational institutions. Through education, India teaches the concept of "Unity in Diversity" as part of developing this integrative capacity.
- **Occupational values and orientations are also conveyed through training:** This function deals mainly with professional training. For example, in nursing schools, nursing students are specially trained to meet the health needs of society.

REVIEW QUESTIONS

Long Essays
1. Define education, explain the importance of education.
2. Describe the types of education, explain the formal education in detail.
3. Differentiate between informal and non-formal education.
4. Define educational institution, explain the types of educational institutions.

Short Essays
1. Characteristics of education.
2. Determing factors of education.
3. Individual training goals.
4. Benifits of educational goals.
5. Scope of education.
6. Features of education.

Short Answers
1. Educational goals.
2. Behavioral reforms.
3. Status conferment.
4. Pedagogy.
5. Philosophy.
6. Education.
7. Teaching.
8. Educational technology.
9. Cultural heritage.

Chapter 2

Education and Educational Technology

Learning Objectives

- Importance of Educational Technology
- Educational Technology Goals
- Revolutions and Developments in Educational Technology
- Characteristics of Teaching Technology
- Necessity and Importance of Education Technology
- Fields of Application Pedagogical Technology
- Approaches to Educational Technology
- Modern Approach to Education
- Transformational Education
- Relationship-Based Education
- Competency-Based Education

INTRODUCTION

The word "technology" comes from two Greek words "technology" and "logic". "Technique" means "art" or "skill". "Logia" means "science or research". So the simple meaning of 'technology' is 'science for the study of an art or craft'. The term technology in education is a service concept such as technology to agriculture by farmers or science to mankind. Refers to the use of equipment or machines for educational purposes. This includes the use of various audiovisual hardware and advanced electronic devices such as movie projectors, radios, televisions, tape recorders, educational machines and computers. As mentioned earlier, educational technology is a broader term than technology in education. This includes hardware, software and system approaches.

DEFINITION

- "Educational technology can be defined as the application of scientific and technological laws and recent discoveries to educational processes." —**SS Kulkarni**
- "It's about adapting to human learning conditions." —**Robert A Cox**
- "Pedagogical technology is the application of scientific knowledge about learning to real learning situations." —**J Bloomer**
- The human learning condition of the scientific process called Notes Educational Technology. —**Robert A Cox**
- It is a detailed application of the psychology of learning to real classroom problems. —**Dececco**
- Pedagogical technology can be understood as a means of developing a set of systematic techniques, accompanied by practical knowledge of test design and test operation. Schools as Educational Systems. —**Robert M Gagne**

IMPORTANCE OF EDUCATIONAL TECHNOLOGY

Educational technology is the process of analyzing, designing, developing, implementing and evaluating classroom environments, learning materials, learners and learning processes to enhance teaching and learning. It is a research field that studies pedagogical technology in education is important because it helps today's teachers integrate new technologies and tools into the classroom. Teachers can improve and improve learner orientation in the classroom. This allows teachers to engage students in unique, innovative and equitable ways. Teachers can also expand their network and connect with other teachers and educators nationally and internationally.

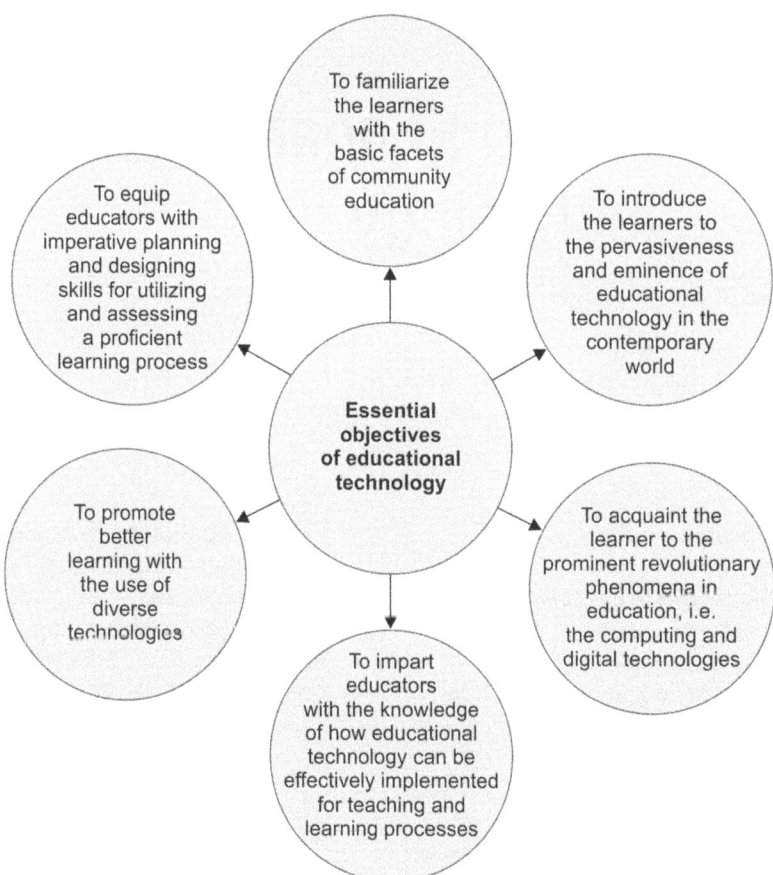

Fig. 2.1: Objectives of educational technology.

EDUCATIONAL TECHNOLOGY GOALS

Macro Level

Given the growing importance of technology in education, there are different goals that this phenomenon meets at the macro level.

- Identify community educational needs and desires.
- Understand the structure of the school board strategy and its goals.
- Design and develop curricula that incorporate art and human values.
- Support strategy and human and material resources to achieve set goals.
- Create appropriate tools and means to support educational objectives.
- Developing educational technology models to improve existing teaching and learning processes.
- Identify and find solutions to address key environmental issues.
- Expand and support educational opportunities for people around the world, especially those in disadvantaged parts of society.
- Management of the entire educational system from planning to implementation, and evaluation.

Micro Level

- Discover and analyze characteristics and educational needs of each student.
- Determine and state specific behavioral goals for the classroom.
- Understand class content and organize it in the correct order.
- Review existing teaching/learning resources and materials.
- Identify the nature of interaction of subsystems such as teacher, student, classroom material content, and various methods.
- Plan instructional strategies and use human and material resources to achieve specific instructional goals.
- Evaluate behavioral change and performance of each student to determine the effectiveness of classroom instruction.
- Provide teachers and students with the feedback necessary to change teaching and learning practices.

REVOLUTIONS AND DEVELOPMENTS IN EDUCATIONAL TECHNOLOGY

Erich Ashley (1967) identified his four revolutions in education.
- **First revolution:** A revolution that shifts the education of adolescents from parents to teachers and from homes to schools.
- **The second revolution:** A revolution in the acceptance of written language as a means of education.
- **The third revolution:** The revolution caused by the invention of the printing press and the availability of books and other educational materials.
- **The fourth revolution:** A revolution brought about by the development of electronics centered on radios, televisions, cassette recorders, and computers, and the development of system concepts.

CHARACTERISTICS OF TEACHING TECHNOLOGY

- ET has contributed to the development of various methods. Microteaching methods, interaction analysis audiovisual materials and programmed learning methods.
- AV aids and machines are used in the fields of ET psychology, science and technology, and system art.
- Based on the application of scientific knowledge.
- It helps to keep educational process focused, clear, interesting and scientific
- Continuous dynamic technology.
- An important medium of communication.
- Desirable changes in teacher and student behavior are possible.

NECESSITY AND IMPORTANCE OF EDUCATION TECHNOLOGY

- **Population explosion:** The population of Asian countries is growing rapidly and using teachers in class rooms alone will not educate all these people.
- **Rapid generation of new knowledge:** New knowledge spreads very rapidly, nearly doubled in just three years. Teachers should not impart this amount of knowledge in tutorials or face-to-face classes. ET can perform this function very easily.
- **Developing new strategies microteaching**
  - Teaching techniques to teachers
  - Programmatic teaching (creating materials in written or CAI forms for individualized study).
  - Teaching analysis (analysis of material into practical parts that are presented to students one by one) and the use of hardware technology in teaching, etc.
- **Controlled atmosphere:** The whole process of teaching objectively has become clear, scientific and interesting. Teachers control the classroom environment to their advantage, but at the same time use tests to assess performance.
- **Importance of the teacher's role:** Emphasize theory and knowledge. The principle of teaching rather than the principle of learning. Thus, many of ETs shortcomings have been eliminated and given importance and advantages. Teacher relevance within the class.

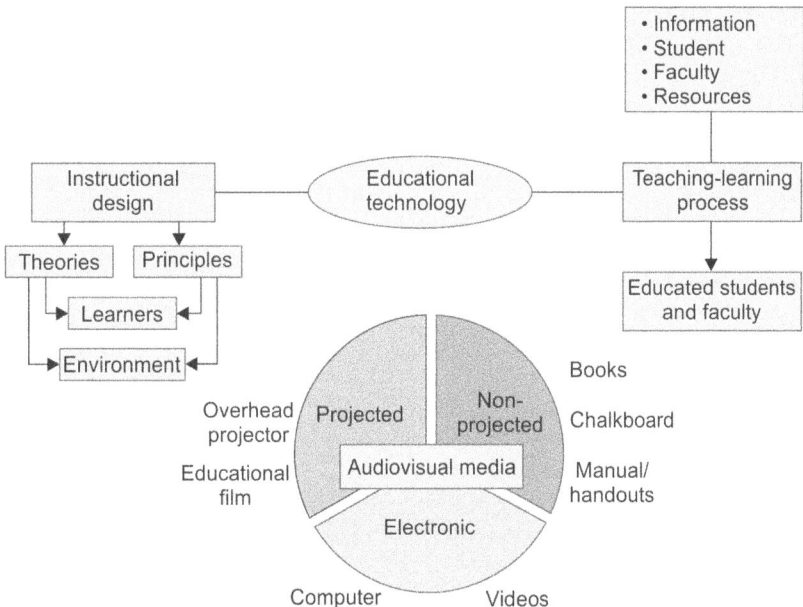

Fig. 2.2: Scope of educational technology.

- **Mass expansion of model instructions:** Radio and TV installations are now available on a large scale. By demonstrating the effective teaching of these media renowned teachers, together we can benefit millions of students can benefit from these demonstrations improve their teaching.
- **Benefits for private students:** Many universities allow students to take private exams even in higher education. These students are not attending class. The use of ET is becoming necessary to maintain educational standards in higher education.
- **Advantages for teacher training colleges:** Teacher training colleges cannot train good teachers without using ET, that's why. This educational stream focuses on changing teacher behavior. We can use (for example) microteaching techniques to develop your students› teaching skills.
- **Improvement of school management:** ET analyzes school management problems scientifically and helps to improve the system. This is done by using different combinations of inputs or by adopting other school system approaches.
- **Knowledge storage:** Using hardware technology, knowledge can be stored on audiocassettes, videocassettes, CDs and Floppy disk (pen drive).
- **Developing an educational model:** Where a particular combination of inputs and strategies yields repeatably good results in a variety of educational situations. Converts into a universally applicable educational model. Also leads to the development of educational theory.
- **Creating interesting learning situations:** ET can transform the teaching and learning process from stress to joy. Example: Using materials in the classroom increases student interest.

FIELDS OF APPLICATION PEDAGOGICAL TECHNOLOGY

The aim of pedagogical technology is process-oriented. The use of educational technology is not confined to teaching and learning methods and theories, but can serve to thoroughly support personal development. Below is a list of a wide range of educational technologies.
- Educational technology makes teaching and learning processes more efficient and process-oriented.
- Mechanical and electronic devices can be readily used for educational purposes
- Educational technology has improved the learning process of students with the help of educational materials and programmed materials. Computers can be used to provide distance and distance learning.
- The advancement of the Internet has made education very easy to spread around the world.
- Technology-enabled feedback mechanisms improve the quality of teacher education in academic institutions.
- Innovative, technology-driven analytical tools and tools help solve educational management problems.
- Educational technology is used to develop and understand the structure and nature of education.
- Optimal use of educational technology supports scientific foundations and new discoveries.

APPROACHES TO EDUCATIONAL TECHNOLOGY

Scientific research in technological development has impacted every area of human life. The educational process is immune to these advances. The field of education is becoming increasingly mechanized. This has led to the introduction of technology in education. Various technical approaches can be used to support and enhance learning. Different approaches to educational technology provide different types of content and serve different purposes in the classroom. Each approach to technology can play a different role in student learning.

Hardware Approach

It is based on the application of engineering principles to the development of electromechanical devices such as motion picture films, tape recorders, educational machines, computers, videotapes and video surveillance. Technology is a byproduct of 20th century scientific and technological development.

Today's educational technology strains modern audiovisual equipment with this hardware approach. A hardware approach mechanizes the teaching process, enabling teachers to educate more students with less effort.

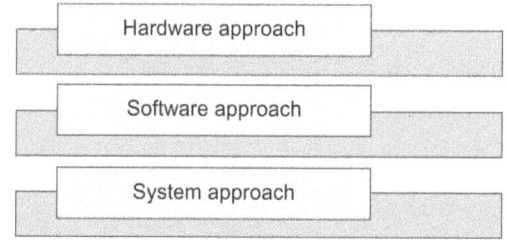

Fig. 2.3: System approach.

Fundamentals of the Hardware Approach

- The hardware approach is based on science and applied engineering.
- A hardware approach has mechanized the entire teaching and learning process.

- Hardware approach takes a product-centric approach.
- A hardware approach has the potential to bring the benefits of education to the masses more easily and cheaply.

Characteristics of the Hardware Approach

- Silverman called this type of instructional technology Relative Technology. It is based on the field approach of physics and applied engineering. The concept of the hardware approach comes from the application of "physics" to education.
- New mechanisms of teaching and learning based on improved technology. Proposing a myriad of new ways for teachers in the classroom
- A teacher's job and duties are likely to change in many ways as we deal with many new devices for teaching and learning.
- Engineering principles are used in the development of this type of technical equipment. Teachers can use these 'mechanical devices' or 'machines' to accommodate larger groups of students.
- Teachers can use this "mechanical device" or "machine" to handle larger groups of students, thus reducing costs and saving finances.

Software Approach

Using principles of psychology for the purpose of behavior modification. It stems from the pioneering work of Skinner and other behaviorists. The programs produced by such technologies are often referred to as "software". Newspapers, books, magazines, program learning, micro-his lessons, team-his lessons, and other educational games can also be part of the software. The software approach is characterized by task analysis that writes out precise goals, selection of appropriate learning strategies, immediate reinforcement of answers, and constant assessment.

The so-called software and hardware approaches cannot be separated from each other. Both are connected in some way to the educational technology plants and seeds.

Fundamentals of the Software Approach

- In the software approach, behavioral science and learning psychology are the foundations of all thinking and working.
- A software approach uses principles of psychology for the purpose of behavior change.
- Teachers with additional knowledge of software approaches can use films, flashcards, tapes, etc., for a variety of purposes.
- Teachers can plan better lessons that lead to better learning. His thoughts are not finished.

Characteristics of Software Approaches

- This view of educational technology is closely related to modern principles of programmed learning, including task analysis, the creation of precise goals, the selection of appropriate learning strategies, and the reinforcement of correct answers, and characterized by continuous learning.
- Silverman called this pedagogical technique "a constructive pedagogical technique." Also known as "managerial technology".
- A modern approach to educational administration and organization. It has brought a scientific approach to education management to solve the problems of education management.
- The origin of the software approach lies in the application of "behavioral science" to education. It refers to the application of teaching and learning principles in the design of behavior.
- Its application in describing behavioral goals selection of appropriate teaching strategies reinforcement to correct answers, etc.

Use of Hardware and Software Teaching: Learning Experiences

- Pedagogical technology includes the entire process of testing methods and materials on the one hand and the evaluation of the system as an integrated whole on the other.
- Educational technology uses a variety of technological devices, from blackboards to computers.
- These are books, paper and pencil, maps, globes, movie projectors, slide projectors, language labs, tape recorders, radios, televisions, video recorders, computers.

System Approach

A system approach is a systematic attempt to coordinate all aspects of a problem toward a specific goal. Webster's dictionary defines a system as "a group of regularly interacting or independent elements that form a unified whole." The features of the digestive system can be illustrated with an example. The various parts of the digestive system can be called components of the digestive system. Each component of the digestive system helps support the functioning of the entire digestive system.

Developing Specific Learning Goals to be Achieved and Defining Learning Goals

- Selecting appropriate media to achieve those goals
- Defining learner characteristics and requirements

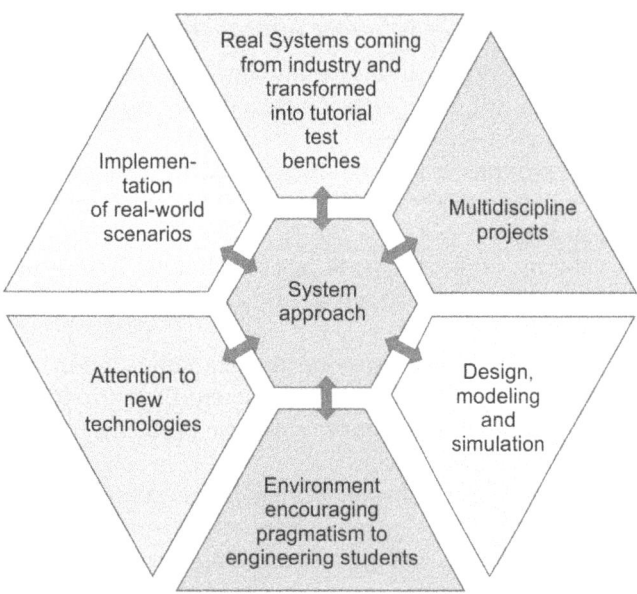

Fig. 2.4: System approach.

- Effective choosing the right method for learning
- Choosing the right learning experience from available alternatives
- Selection of appropriate teaching materials and necessary tools
- Allocation of appropriate personal roles for teachers, students and support staff
- Program implementation
- Systems for improving student learning
- Efficiency improvement revisions.

Benefits of the System Approach

- The system approach helps identify the adequacy of resource material to achieve a particular goal.
- Technological advances can be used to integrate machines, media, and humans to achieve defined goals.
- Helps assess resource needs, their sources, and facilities in terms of volume, time, and other factors.
- Allows for the orderly introduction of the components shown to be necessary for the system's success with respect to student learning.
- Rigidity in action plans is avoided because continuous evaluation allows for desirable and beneficial changes.

Limitations of the System Approach

- **Resistance to change:** The old ways are hard to get rid of. There is always resistance to new methods and approaches.
- **It also includes hard work:** A systematic approach requires hard and continuous work by school staff. Some are not prepared for the additional workload.
- **Incomprehensible:** Teachers and administrators are still new to the systems approach. It has been successfully implemented in industry, but has yet to make progress in education.

MODERN APPROACH TO EDUCATION

- **Diversity from the ground up:** The late Sir Ken Robinson championed educational transformation by writing, advising and teaching. He believes that education needs to change because it is an outdated environment where most students are not actually learning what they should or want to learn. is born. People, students and teachers, not administrators and leaders, make the difference.
- **Leading students out of stagnant** learning and into other realms means merging traditional education with modern communication. Many educators see this as a way to get their students to learn all the basic skills they need.
- **Competency-based learning:** Competency-based learning is an educational approach that focuses on demonstrating desired learning outcomes for students.
- **Underground education:** According to John Taylor Gut, teachers should prioritize the real world over the classroom. Students do not learn to live or survive in the classroom. As they are learning to survive in the real world, the concept of underground education challenges educators of all walks of life, giving students the tools to live and breathe in the world around them. If you need to teach, teach them and think about who they will become.
- **Navdanya:** Dr Mission Vadhana Shiva lives and breathes Navdanya, an organization that promotes self-reliance and global democracy. Organizational leaders are women who find strength in the women's movement and give women a voice. Global democracy evolved from the idea of seed preservation to help communities become self-reliant.
- **Social status:** Social status, which is more important to learning than assets, is the presence of a small or large group of people, whether it is a national agenda or a trade in a particular region or community. It plays a fundamental role in education in this country. In other words, if a community values education as a benefit, students and people in that community will strive to achieve this in order to improve their status in the community.
- **Instructional study:** Apply instructional study originated in Japan to teaching style. Conceptually, instructional studies promote the idea that teachers are constantly improving and changing their teaching styles based on student performance and reactions to them. It sounds like

what we are already doing, but it is not exactly. As with change, collaboration among teachers is paramount. The combination of these two factors and constant change ensures that students never stop learning.

- **Constructive combat:** Another Japanese form of education is to enable students to combat through lessons under the guidance of a teacher.
- **In other words, students should not be ashamed** of their first, second, and third failures. Teachers really need to encourage students to learn from this mistake.
- **Problem-based learning:** When it comes to higher education, problem-based learning is growing in popularity in Australia. Students are presented with real-world problems and collaborate to find solutions. In Australia, nursing programs are beginning to incorporate this style of teaching and learning to make students work as if they are dealing with real problems they encounter in the workplace. Teachers find it invaluable because they learn about
- **Technology-enabled learning:** Another view around the world concerns the use of technology as a key to enforcing the rules of learning and student 'marketability' and adaptation.
- **Constructivist learning:** This concept is based on the idea that students create their own learning environment and actively participate in the knowledge they absorb. Creating your own learning requires making mistakes without a predetermined agenda. Constructive learning is not stable and many educational systems reject it.
- **Competency-based education:** In competency-based education, students complete a course based on what they already know, no matter how long it takes them to complete the course. The only factor that determines how or when a student completes a course is their proficiency in knowledge within the subject.
- **Mobile education:** We operate as a global society, so we carry our smartphones with us everywhere. In between conversations, we look down and tap into whatever our hearts need or find interesting. It goes with us on our journeys, whims, detours, and desires. According to the theory of mobile education, when you take your laptop around the world, your education goes along with it.
- **Vocational training:** Whether students seek higher professional education or specific skills to advance their career paths, vocational training is a common vehicle and perspective on education in general. It is becoming more and more popular. It is commonly used by governments to train displaced persons and can be a valuable source of learning for various types of medical technicians and those wishing to specialize in areas such as graphics.

- **Gamification:** The concept of gamification in learning is to add game-like mechanics to non-game ideas and practices. The term gamification was coined by British programmer Nick Pelling in 2004. Adding games to education means that users are rewarded for completing specific tasks, similar to video games.
- **Blended learning:** The combination of learning and technology gives students an advantage over others. One is to move at your own pace. Learning at your own pace is another. Teachers don't have to blow on students' necks. Guiding students is often enough.
- **Group education:** Individuals recede into the background when it comes to the idea of group education. Students learn better and more effectively in groups and especially with each other than alone. This does not mean ignoring individual online learners, but online learners, when exposed to groups of like-minded learners who provide insight and questions about the learning process of a particular topic.
- **Personalized education:** Ironically, personalized education is more valuable than ever. The difference is that individualized education does not mean that there is no group education. It means that education should care about the needs and desires of the individual, and that the individual should be important in the collective forum. Value should be addressed. Flexible learning provides students with convenient choices and a personalized approach to studying specific subjects. As we are individuals, learning and teaching should include some degree of flexibility in the area of standardization.
- **Flipped learning:** "The flipped classroom" means, as frankly as possible, flipping learning. Turn the learning environment upside down so that students do the essential thing of studying with teachers and professors instead of studying alone in a dark room. The fun part happens at home with short articles or links to videos. The hard part happens at school and teachers can help students fill in the blanks.
- **Expeditionary learning:** Expeditionary Learning takes learning out into the world and accelerates the need to learn more than is confined to the walls of the classroom, but it also increases the need to use the world for learning, Students feel engaged in learning while achieving their goals.

TRANSFORMATIONAL EDUCATION

Transformational Education moves from mechanical to ecological paradigms in healthcare to enable happy, healthy learners to make informed decisions and decisions at the individual, community and global levels. It encompasses teaching and learning designed to motivate and empower you to take action. Transformational learning involves deep structural changes in fundamental aspects of thinking, feeling and behavior. Such changes are related to ourselves and our place in the world, our relationships with other people, and our understanding of the natural world. increase the importance of transformational education.

Transformational education is about motivating and empowering happy, healthy learners to make informed decisions and actions at the individual, community and global levels. Designed for teaching and learning. The purpose of transformational education is to empower learners to see the social world differently through an ethical lens so that they can challenge and transform the status quo as agents of change.

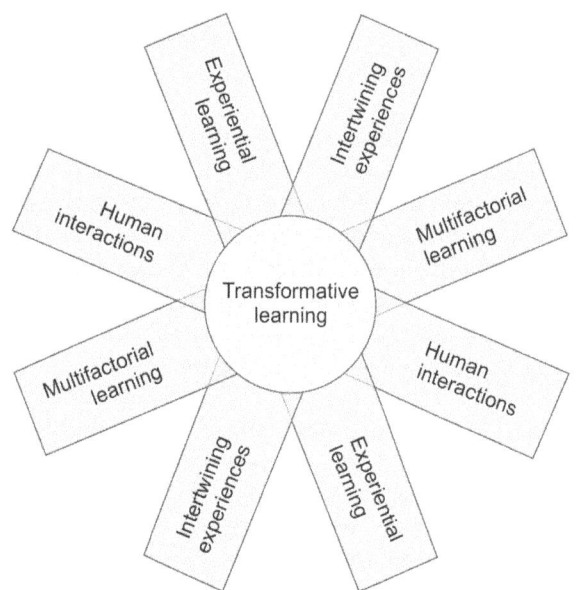

Fig. 2.5: Transformative learning.

Vision of Transformational Education

Peace education, non-violence/prevention of violence education; education for conflict resolution and mediation
- Human rights education
- Education for international understanding internationality
- Multicultural education
- Education for sustainable development (ESD), climate change education biodiversity education
- Global citizenship education development (GCED), citizenship education, comprehensive sex education
- Life skills education
- Sex education
- Ethical, moral or value-based education.

Need for Transformative Education

According to UNESCO, transformative education is needed: Learning through connection with other people and nature together, we transform the communities, environments and societies in which they live, as responsible global citizens, we make people and the planet better ensure teachers' commitment and motivation for educational reform and ensure that the teaching methods and materials teachers use are meaningful and relevant to the specific situations in which they work.

Transformative Education Principles

The first five principles of his listed are the core principles of transformative education. The following seven principles are the more concrete elements essential to the concept of Transformational Education as pedagogically practiced. These 12 principles of transformational education are designed to create sustainable, diverse and conscientious global citizens who can solve complex problems for better, fairer and more sustainable solutions. Designed to help define an educational system that "transforms" old, outdated models of human learning to solve the world.

- **Principle 1—human rights:** Transformational education should promote and uphold the universal declaration of human rights to promote the full development of the human personality and to strengthen respect for human rights and fundamental freedoms. Transformational education recognizes the right of all people of all nations, races, ages and economic status, especially girls and women of all nations, to a transformative education equal to that of men.
- **Principle 2—sustainability:** Transformational education should promote and support sustainable development practices that combine economic growth, respect and protection of the environment with social justice and well-being. Humans have the right to live a healthy and productive life in harmony with nature.
- **Principle 3—the importance of value systems:** Morality, Ethics, and Spirit: Transformational education must embrace ethical, moral, and spiritual values that are recognized around the world of all life. Transformational education focuses on empathy and compassion to become more conscientious global citizens, understanding that science, technology, engineering and mathematics are meaningless without the underlying values of sustainability. Designed to connect earth and mankind.
- **Principle 4—diversity:** Transformational education promotes the value of diversity, embraces cultural differences, recognizes heterogeneity as a gift of strength

and adaptability, and sustains itself in a diverse and complex world. It should be recognized as a key concept in developing viable solutions for possibilities.
- **Principle 5—economic and social justice/justice:** Transformational education should encourage and support the special circumstances and needs of developing countries, especially least developed countries and the most environmentally vulnerable countries I have. Transformative education should also address the interests and needs of all countries including developed countries where poverty and racial and economic inequities still exist and thereby contribute to the prevention and reduction of economic global inequality.
- **Principle 6—peace education and conflict resolution:** Transformative education shall promote and teach the tools of peaceful conflict resolution including alternative dispute resolution which is defined as any process or collection of processes established to resolve disputes without trial or violence.
- **Principle 7—holistic education:** Transformative education shall be holistic and aim at education of the whole person – mind body and animating spirit including their emotional social and physical development as well as valued multiple divergent and creative/artistic intelligences important to problem-solving in a complex world.
- **Principle 8—community-based learning and indigenous wisdom:** Transformative education shall be community-based and take local needs into account as well as value indigenous wisdom and their contexts while promoting service learning including an ability to identify community needs and the skills to address them.
- **Principle 9—simulation/experiential learning:** Transformative education shall encourage and promote the use of simulation and experiential learning programs such as Model United Nations Model Governments and Model Corporations to build dynamism active complex problemsolving emotional social and cultural intelligences and other core elements of human capacity.
- **Principle 10—embedding new neuroscience and critical thinking skills:** Transformational education includes integrative neurophysiology and educational learning theories about how the integrated brain actually learns best. It is intended to support the application and integration of new educational neuroscience. Transformational education is designed to encourage and incorporate transformative educational practices that develop critical thinking and emotional skills and abilities throughout the brain.
- **Principle 11—use technology to connect, not alienate:** Transformational education uses technology in ways that enhance rather than hinder a child's education, providing a transformative education that cannot otherwise be delivered. Should allow to aware that US politics has a strong push for science, technology and mathematics (STEM). Instead, TEF-US takes the above principles further, transforming its focus into "STEM +" and emphasizing such a STEM focus on the necessary values, ethics, morals, and sustainability of the arts. We would like to encourage you to investigate.
- **Principle 12—the sanctity of human learning and life:** The learning environment must be sacred. Trust the wisdom of the imagination. Let all the diverse and precious species of this earth and each other live.

Essential Elements of Transformational Learning Theory

- **Critical reflection:** Individuals need to think critically about their experiences, which leads to a change of perspective. This process increases self-confidence and promotes a deeper self-understanding.
- **Rational disclosure:** This component of transformative learning theory relates to experiences that can produce

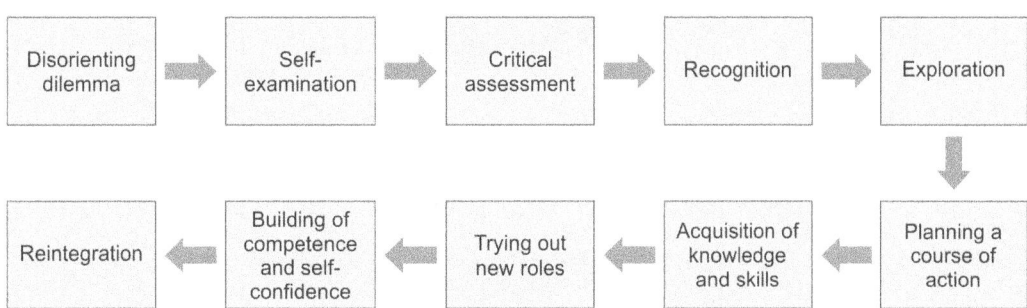

Fig. 2.6: Steps of the transformative learning.

transformative learning. Essentially, theoretically, it is presented in the form of discussions with others focused on personal and societal beliefs and assumptions, and finds congruence in existing blind spots or prejudices, logical and rational.

- **Centrality of experience:** The final component of Mezirow's theory of transformational learning states that such experiences include. It includes what you do, what you believe, what you can endure, how you react to certain situations, and what you are willing to suffer. What they willingly suffer, as well as the desires of perspective dreams and beliefs.

Principles of Transformation Theory

This theory contains four general scientific laws.

- **Instrumental:** Individuals tasked with identifying the cause or effect of a particular event or situation.
- **Communication skills:** Individuals acquire communication skills and learn to express their desires, feelings and emotions.

Reflecting on the process or premise of the content changes the semantic structure. Learning may involve learning new schemas, changing perspectives, or giving meaning to existing plans and programs.

Benefits of Transformational Learning

- Improving problem solving applications
- Changing habitual perspectives
- Suffering from developmental and cyclic transition problems
- Work and workplace coordination
- Social education projects
- Critical reflection
- Reasonable disclosure
- Centrality of experience.

Challenges

- **Transitioning from vision to reality:** Many impediments to implementation are not unique to Transformational Education, but rather major reforms, various laws and departmental policies, and multiple coherent policies.
- Embedding transformational education young people's interest in active citizenship is often the greatest, and the pressure to prepare for difficult exams collides with the

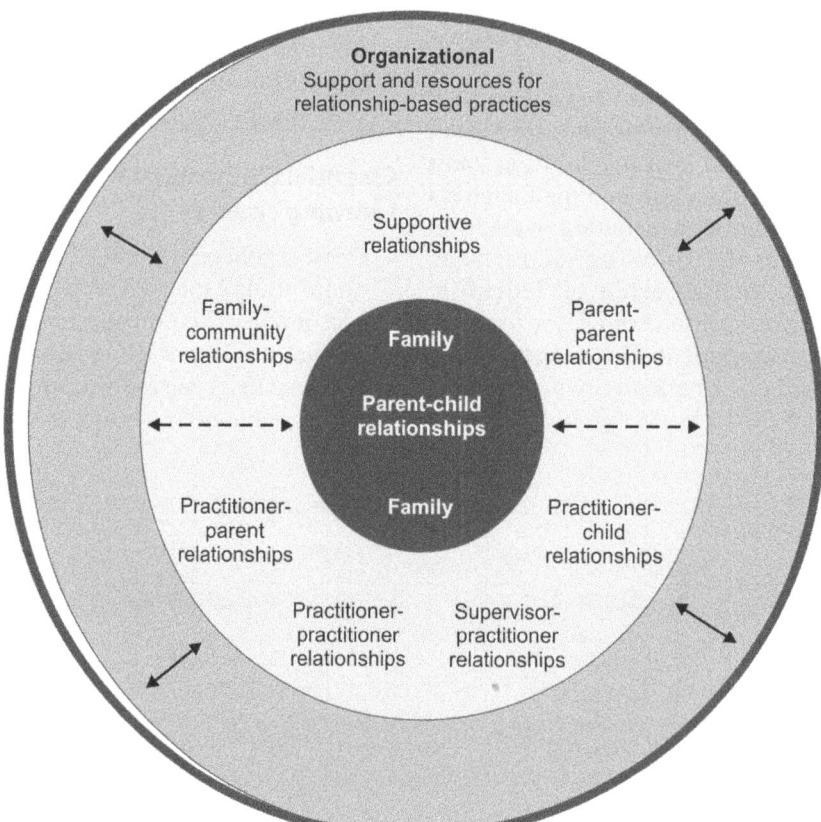

Fig. 2.7: Principles of transformation theory.

late few longitudinal studies assess the sustainability of transitions to secondary education into adulthood.

RELATIONSHIP-BASED EDUCATION

Relationship-based education is an academic setting that focuses primarily on existing relationships. Rather than being tied to the specific outcomes of every student, relational education takes a more holistic view by viewing each student as an individual learner. This difference in individual child priorities has important implications.
- In practice, this means that teachers are often more concerned with the respect, integrity, concern, appreciation, ambition, and enjoyment of learning than with specific academic instruction.
- This means that teachers use real assessments that more accurately reflect a student's knowledge and abilities than standardized exams.
- This means that children can be good at math and basketball at the same time and give equal importance to both.
- This means that children are not categorized based on 'behavior' or 'gifted status'.
- In short, the relationship-based model enables students to succeed in all aspects of life.

Importance of Relationship-Based Education

Education relationships can be didactically supportive, supportive, or advisory. They tend to evolve from didactic to advisory over time, and higher levels may contain elements of the base level. Roles within individual relationships may vary, but the nature of the content remains relatively constant. Understanding the teaching relationship helps improve the education of clinical teachers.

Principles

Relationship-based learning through coaching includes the following principles:
- Partnerships are based on respect.
- Positive and active communication is used.
- Collaboration is a core component of any coaching program.
- Partnerships embrace a common vision and common goals by sharing power, authority and decision-making.

Features

Positive communication is essential for relationship learning.
- Positive language, paraverbal and non-verbal language should always be used.
- The "moments of communication" are often as important as the words of a conversation.
- Clarity is an essential strategy for positive communication.
- In other words, it is a preventive strategy.
- "Collective understanding" must be achieved at the moment of communication.
- The final strategy for positive communication is summarizing.

Tutoring

- Tutoring is a proactive approach to a student's learning needs. All students in a given classroom receive standard curriculum content, but the way that content is delivered is personalized based on the student's learning style and personal preferences.
- While working on a writing task in the classroom, for example, a student who needs additional handwriting practice may do so by handwriting, while another student may be doing it by hand in a particular language, such as: Due to the differences, we use dictation software to perform the same tasks.
- This means that while one student is reading a fantasy novel on his own, has a learning disability, or has an external or interventional. It could also mean that you need a base educational service.

Empowered Learners

- Empowered Learners are students and teachers who are confident, capable and cooperative.
- Effective learners have a solid knowledge base in key content areas and a rich toolkit of learning strategies. But more importantly, empowered learners are those who can confidently explore new concepts and content with or without the help of others.
- Any learner can receive information, but effective learners seek out new information, ask meaningful and thoughtful questions, and think critically about the answers and information they receive.
- Students graduating from Venn Academy will excel in future academic environments, whether highly structured, minimally structured, entry-level or advanced. You have to feel like you can.
- Students must be personally and professionally supported to achieve this.
- You have to build trust. To do this, you need to engage in carefully selected, challenging and engaging activities.

COMPETENCY-BASED EDUCATION

Competency-based education (CBE) is an approach to teaching learning and assessment that focuses on students demonstrating learning outcomes and proficiency in specific competencies in each subject. Teaching using the CBE methodology empowers students and provides them with a meaningful and positive learning experience. Focus on learners and actively involve them in the learning process. It emphasizes the practical application of knowledge and skills and the authenticity of the learning experience.

Definition

- Competency-based education focuses on learning outcomes. CBE is concerned with what learners are expected to do, not what they expect to learn."
- Harness the power of technology in teaching and learning.
- Substantially change the role of departments.

Concepts of Competency-Based Education

- Students progress according to their demonstrated proficiency. The transition to proficiency may allow students to spend more time in areas that are more challenging to them. Some areas even progress beyond the grade level in some areas, while spending more time in the more difficult areas. You can focus your support where your students need it most, while ensuring that they can learn.
- Competencies include tangible, measurable and transferable learning outcomes that empower students. Greater transparency in learning goals gives students more ownership over their education and gives them more choice in how they learn and how they present what they learn. In this process, teachers also collaborate more with their students as their intentions increase in what they want their students to know and be able to do.
- Assessment is meaningful and a positive learning experience for students. Formative assessment is emphasized to help teachers understand where students are misunderstanding and provide the necessary feedback for students to improve.
- Students receive timely and differentiated support based on their individual learning needs. Students have flextime available during the day to provide additional educational support and expedite any misunderstandings. For example, if a student fails to complete a course, they will focus on the specific skills they need to develop rather than repeating the entire course.
- Students develop and apply a wide range of skills and dispositions. Students will learn and actively apply critical thinking and problem-solving skills, as well as develop "important communication and collaboration skills and cultural responsiveness that will help them work in an ever-changing and diverse workplace."

Characteristics of Competency-Based Education

- Ensure equal opportunity for all students, regardless of educational background.
- We offer different levels of support depending on the needs of each student.
- Student progress is measured solely by the skills and knowledge acquired.

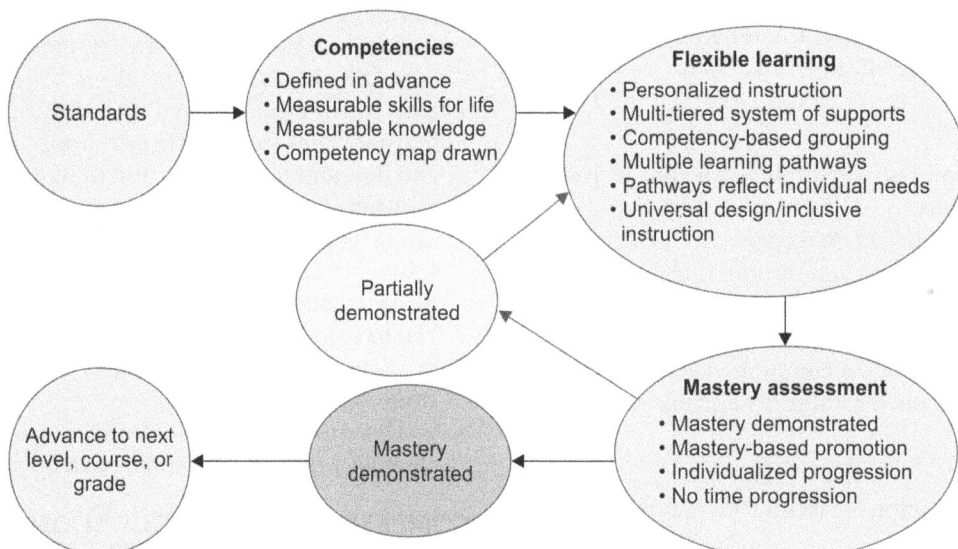

Fig. 2.8: Concepts of competency-based education (CBE).

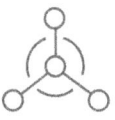 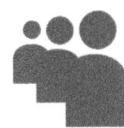 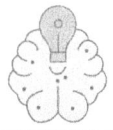 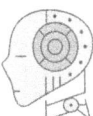

Structure	Culture	Teaching	Learning
Assessment system	Institutional mission	Teachers as facilitators/coaches	Student ownership of learning
Seat time	Knowledgeable staff	Personalized learning	Student voice
Learning management system	Culture of innovation	Tools/Resources for teaching	Lead learner
Scheduling	Engaged parents/families	Content expertise	Learning anytime, anywhere
Standard/Defined competencies	Engaged stakeholders	Curriculum design	
Professional development	Effective communications	Assessment design and use	
Physical infrastructure	Culture of relevance		

Fig. 2.9: Competency-based education (CBE) mastery framework.

- Students are encouraged to evaluate themselves and understand their progress and shortcomings in order to take responsibility for their results.

Steps in Competency-Based Curriculum Development

- Develop or identify general competencies.
- Divide competencies into specific topics.
- Set performance standards.
- Create a learning experience.
- Competence assessment.
- Evaluation of curriculum effectiveness.

Objectives of Competency

Based education it may help you become more effective in your success.

- **Enhanced teaching and learning:** Learning experiences are designed to enable learning, with clear consistency and transparency. Between what students should learn and how to get there.
- **individual student progress:** Students learn at their own pace and progress as they demonstrate their mastery.
- **Student ownership and investment:** Learning goals are transparent and students are self-directed in their learning. Reaches the next course or evaluates based on demonstration of skills and expertise.
- **Pace:** "Students progress at different rates in different areas rather than on a teacher driven classwide schedule." is not about giving every student the same as every other student. Instead, it means giving each student what they need to achieve the same end goal.
- Classes emphasize measurable competencies that help build skills over a lifetime. Competencies should be predefined and set as learning goals for each student.
- **Transparency helps students take responsibility:** The learning goals set for the class (and the school as a whole) should be clear to both students and parents.
- **Students receive the individualized support they need:** Competencies indicate how long students need to work on a problem before asking for help and when to approach them during class to contact the teacher. You should have a framework for understanding what to do.
- **Teachers assess growth and proficiency:** Assessments come in many shapes and sizes.
- **Students progress while demonstrating mastery:** By incorporating regular assessments and data-driven progress reports, teachers can understand where each individual student is in the learning process.

Below are three of her assessments that are particularly useful for competency-based teaching.

1. **Formative assessment:** These assessments help teachers determine where each student is in the learning process and adjust teaching as needed.
2. **Authentic assessment:** Having students apply their knowledge to real-world situations is another great way to demonstrate student proficiency. It also allows students to develop the skills they will need in the future.

3. **Digital content assessment:** Using technology in the classroom makes assessment much easier. Many classroom software include assessment and progress reports that help teachers know exactly where each student is in the learning process.

Benefits of Competency-Based Education

CBE integrates higher order thinking skills, interdisciplinary approaches, and problem solving. They are essential for the modern world and the workplace. In addition to developing social and emotional skills and developing global literacy and citizenship, this approach enables learners to become competent not only in domestic settings but also in the international job market.

- Competency-based education programs enhance the student experience.
- Competency-based education programs welcome non-traditional learners.
- Competence-based educational programs offer flexibility of time and place.
- Competency-based education programs help students save time and money.
- Competency-based education programs can increase student productivity.
- Competency-based educational programs aim at proficiency.
- Competence-based educational programs produce more capable graduates.
- Competency-based education gives students the confidence that comes with mastering a skill.

Pros and Cons of Competency-Based Education

Using a competency-based education system in schools has both pros and cons.

Pros

- Offers flexibility for all types of students, regardless of background knowledge or literacy level.
- Prejudice is removed and justice is achieved.
- Students do better learn and take responsibility for education.

Cons

- Key competencies need to be identified and defined for each class, which is difficult.
- Assessment should be more meaningful and creative.
- Teachers should always monitor student progress must be aware of students who are not.

Difference between outcome-based education (OBE) vs competency-based education (CBE)

- **Developing competency:** The students are encouraged to develop logical thinking rather than mugging up the theoretical knowledge.
- **Skills-based assessments:** The assessments are designed to measure the skills of students. It can be achieved with competency-based tools.
- **Fair mindset:** The students that learn by the CBE method are encouraged to have a fair mindset and perform their work with ethical means.
- **Life-long learner:** A fair attitude and logical thinking helps students overcome any problem later in their life and not just restricted to a career.
- **Various faculties:** Various faculties like healthcare, nursing, etc., can reap the benefits of CBE-based learning.

CONCLUSION

Educational technology is the field of study that investigates the process of analyzing, designing, developing, implementing, and evaluating the instructional environment, learning materials, learners, and the learning process in order to improve teaching and learning. Educational technology in education is important because it helps today's teachers to integrate new technologies and tools into their classroom. Teachers are able to upgrade and improve the learner-centeredness of their classroom. It enables teachers to engage their students in unique, innovative, and equitable ways. Teachers are also able to expand their network and connect with other teachers and educators nationally and globally.

REVIEW QUESTIONS

Long Essays
1. Define educational technology, explain the goals and importance of educational technology.
2. Explain the approaches to educational technology.
3. Define system approach, explain the benefits and limitations of system approach.
4. Discuss the modern approach to education.
5. Define transformational education, explain the need and principles of transformative learning.
6. Define relationship-based education, explain the importance and principles of relationship-based education.
7. Define competency-based education, explain the objectives and characteristics of competency-based education.

Short Essays
1. Explain macro level and micro level in education.
2. Revolutions and developments in educational technology.
3. Necessity and importance of education technology.
4. Describe the fields of application pedagogical technology.
5. Characteristics of software approaches.
6. Essential elements of transformational learning theory.
7. Steps of the transformative learning.
8. Principles of transformation theory.
9. Benefits of transformational learning.
10. Empowered learners.
11. Benefits of competency-based education.

Short Answers
1. Characteristics of teaching technology.
2. Hardware approach.
3. System approach.
4. Competency-based learning.
5. Instructional study.
6. Problem-based learning.
7. Technology-enabled learning.
8. Constructivist learning.
9. Competency-based education.
10. Mobile education.
11. Vocational training.
12. Gamification.
13. Blended learning.
14. Expeditionary learning.
15. Vision of transformational education.
16. Steps in competency-based curriculum development.
17. Pros and cons of competency-based education.

Chapter 3

Educational Philosophy

Learning Objectives

- Relationship between Philosophy and Philosophy Education
- Objectives of Philosophy of Education Studies
- Science and Philosophy
- Philosophy and Education
- Important Philosophies
- Nursing Philosophy
- Pedagogical Application of Philosophy
- Naturalism
- Realism
- Idealism
- Pragmatism
- Progressivism
- Reconstructionism
- Eclecticism
- Perennialism
- Existentialism
- Philosophy of Mahatma Gandhi
- Tagore's Philosophy of Education
- John Dewey's Philosophy of Education
- Learning by Practice Limitations

INTRODUCTION

According to plate knowledge of the eternal nature of things which is infant knowledge of the true nature of different things is philosophy. The word philosophy combined from two Latin word Philos and Sofia. Philos means love and Sofia means wisdom (or) knowledge. Thus, philosophy means love for knowledge or passion for learning.

According to Henderson philosophy is an attempt to conceive and present the inclusive and systematic view of the universe and its main place in it. An institution's department or program philosophy is a statement of a belief system that guides a particular group of individuals in achieving their goals. It should be a statement you can make to explain why things are done the way they are.

DEFINITION

Philosophy has been defined differently by scholars and thinkers:

- **Aristotle:** "Philosophy is the science which seeks the essence of existence itself."
- **Breitman:** "Philosophy can be defined as really considering the human experience as a whole and trying to make our overall experience comprehensible."
- **Marcus Tullius Cicero (106-43 BC):** Philosophy is the mother of all arts and the true medicine of the mind.
- **Dr Radhakrishnan (1888-1975):** Philosophy is the logical study of the nature of reality.
- **Henderson (1947):** Philosophy is the search for a comprehensive view of nature and an attempt to universally explain the nature of things.
- **Herbert Spencer:** Philosophy as a universal science deal with everything.
- **Huxley Aldous (1984-1963):** Politicians live according to their philosophy of life, their worldview.

THE RELATIONSHIP BETWEEN PHILOSOPHY AND PHILOSOPHY EDUCATION

- Philosophy and education are closely related and interdependent. Philosophy shows the way and education follows. Without philosophy, education is a

blind endeavor, and without education philosophy will not work.
- **Ross:** Philosophy and education are two sides of the same coin. The former is the meditative side, the latter is the active side. Education is the process, philosophy is the product. In other words, the application of philosophical principles in the field of education to solve various educational problems is regarded as educational theory at its most general stage.
- **Fichte's view:** The art of education can never achieve perfect clarity without philosophy'.
- **The gentile view:** Education without philosophy means not understanding the precise nature of education.
- **John Adams:** Education is a dynamic aspect of philosophy.
- **TP Nunn:** Educational goals correlate with outlook on life.
- **Dewey:** Education is the laboratory where philosophical directions are identified and tested.

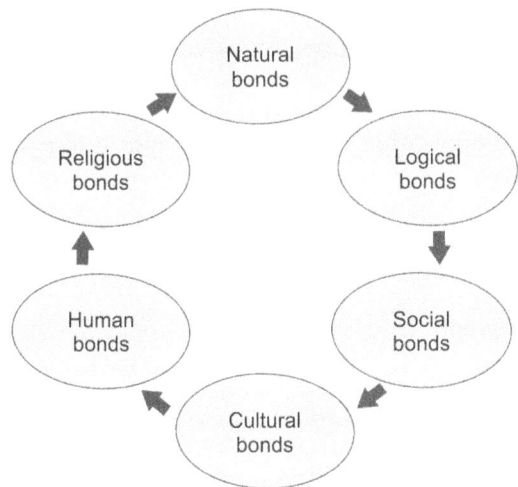

Fig. 3.1: Relationship between philosophy and education.

OBJECTIVES OF PHILOSOPHY OF EDUCATION STUDIES

Philosophy deals with the most fundamental problems that people face. Philosophical content is seen as asking questions rather than giving answers. You could even say that philosophy is the study of problems.
- To find out the solution for various educational issues.
- The purpose of studying educational philosophy is to make education according to the need-based life and society.
- To determine the aim of human life aim of survival.
- Create better citizens by promoting democratic action.
- Make the teaching and learning process more effective and engaging according to the needs, interests and abilities of children.
- Recognize different philosophies and choose one to live a fruitful life in society.
- Expand our knowledge and experience and incorporate it into our educational practice.
- Emphasizes the child's overall personal development and prepares them to stand on their own two feet.
- Make education flexible to achieve the goals of cross-border integration, international understanding and globalization.
- To develop education as a powerful tool for bringing about social, cultural, political and economic change in society.

BRANCHES OF PHILOSOPHY

S. No.	Branches	Description
1.	Metaphysics	Study of the fundamental nature of reality and existence general theory of reality.
2.	Ontology	Study of theory of being
3.	Cosmology	Study of physical universe
4.	Epistemology	Study of knowledge (ways of thinking, nature of truth, and relationship between knowledge and belief
5.	Logic	Study of principles and methods of reasoning (interference and arguments)
6.	Ethics (axiology)	Study of nature of values; right and wrong (moral philosophy)
7.	Aesthetics	Study of appreciation of the arts or things beautiful.
8.	Philosophy of science	Study of science and scientific practices
9.	Political philosophy	Study of citizen and state

MEANING OF PHILOSOPHY

Philosophy combined with two Latin words philos and sofia. Philos means love and Sophia means wisdom or knowledge. Philosophy therefore means a love of knowledge or a passion for learning. Philosophy means loving or seeking wisdom.

The aim of philosophy is to examine the totality of things independently of the nexus that makes them specific or transitory. A thing, not a specific one. Not a single phenomenon, but the universe as a whole. The content of philosophy is not a temporary relationship, but an eternal and unchanging relationship between things and the universe.

SCIENCE AND PHILOSOPHY

Science deals with causality (cause and effect). A scientific approach to understanding reality is characterized by observational verifiability and experience. Hypothesis testing and experimentation are considered scientific methods. In contrast, philosophy deals with the purpose of human life, the nature and reality of existence, and theories and limits of knowledge, intuition, introspection, and reasoning are examples of philosophical methods.

S. No.	Methodology	Description
1.	Socratic	Know thyself
2.	Realism	Be thyself
3.	Humanism	Give thyself
4.	Rationalism	Understand thyself
5.	Naturalism	Describe thyself
6.	Pragmatism	Prove thyself
7.	Idealism	Imagine thyself
8.	Existentialism	Choose thyself

PHILOSOPHY AND EDUCATION

In many cases these definitions are quite incomplete often including only the aim or only the process of education. It is difficult to give a adequate definition of education since the subject of education is the human who is complex in his makeup and is gifted with a free will. Since the human is the subject of education the underlying concept of the origin the nature and destiny of man will greatly influence the concept of education and its function that is held by the individual educator.

Education is the deliberate and systematic influence extorted by the mature person upon the immature through instruction discipline and the harmonious development of all the powers of the human being physical, social intellectual, aesthetic and spiritual according to their essential hierarchy by and for their individual and social use and directed toward the union of the education with his creator as the final end. Philosophy and education are so closely connected that one without the other is meaning. Many ties link education and philosophy.

A brief description of some of these relationships will help illustrate the close relationship between philosophy and education.

- **Natural connection:** A natural connection between two or more things or processes. There is a natural link between spiritual life and education and the ideals and cultural norms of the adult generation.
- **Logical bonds:** The heart or core of any educational system lies in the ideals it seeks to achieve. These ideals are determined by philosophy. It is logical to say that once an ideal is established, an educational system should be put in place to perpetuate it.
- **Social ties:** Education aims to maintain a social system based on the philosophy of life and social processes. History is a surefire way of recording human activity and the progress of human societies for posterity.
- **Cultural connections:** Culture is not only the sum of people's achievements, but also the ideals and virtues they aspire to. Therefore, there is a cultural link between philosophy and education.
- **Human bonds:** Psychology, or the treatment of human relationships, is the foundation of education. A recognized educational goal is to develop the personality of the student. This is done by knowing the individual student and the best ideal model for that student's training.
- **Religious ties:** Philosophy and education are linked by religious ties in addition to the ties already mentioned. In religious instruction one acquires not only the usual philosophy of life, but also a philosophy inspired by the above.

IMPORTANT PHILOSOPHIES

S. No.	Concept	Description
1.	Idealism	Idealism idolizes **mind and self**. Idealism believes in universal mind. Idealism regards man as a spiritual being. The world of ideas and values are more important than the world of matter. Real knowledge is perceived in mind.
2.	Naturalism	Naturalism believes that education should be according to the **nature** of the child. Naturalism advocates the creation of conditions in which the natural development of a child can take place in a natural way. The different forms of naturalism are physical naturalism, mechanical naturalism and biological naturalism.
3.	Pragmatism	The term pragmatism derives its origin from a Greek word meaning to do, to make, to accomplish. **Experience** is central here; everything is tested on the touchstone of experience. The basis of all teaching is the activity of the child.

Contd...

Contd...

S. No.	Concept	Description
4.	Existentialism	According to existentialism, the primary aim of education is making of a human person as one who lives and makes decisions.
5.	Realism	Realism is concerned with the study of the world we live in. Realism believes that all knowledge is derived from experience. The realist believes that everything that exists in the universe is matter or energy or matter of motion.
6.	Humanism	Humanism is a movement to gain for man a proper recognition in the universe. Man is a free agent.
7.	Humanistic existentialism	Humanistic existentialism is the youngest philosophy. Existentialism may be described as a modern philosophy which is primarily upon the work of the scholars of the twentieth century.
8.	Experimentalism	Experimentalism is unreservedly a philosophy of change and of process. It teaches that everything is changing continually—man, morality, democracy and education; experience is the only reality.
9.	Neorealism	Neorealism is a theory which excludes philosophy and theology as source of knowledge and truth; it looks to science as its primary source.
10.	Eclectic tendency in education	It is a process of putting together the common view of different philosophies, into one comprehensive whole is eclectic tendency in education. It is the fusion or synthesis of different philosophies of education, is known as eclectic tendency in education. According to Munroe, the eclectic tendency is that which seeks the harmonization on principles, underlying various tendencies and rationalization of educational practices.
11.	Progressivism	The term progressivism in education is an American philosophy, which is a revolt against the formal, conventional and traditional system of education. The progressivism in education advocates that the education of the child should be for the present life itself and not for a future life.
12.	Reconstrutionism	Reconstructionism has its origin in Plato; his republic is his vision of an ideal society. Reconstruction is of two forms; total change or desirable change. The present educational system does not represent Indian cultures and traditions. The primary aim of education is an all round development of personality.

Contd...

Contd...

S. No.	Concept	Description
13.	Eclecticism	The dictionary meaning of the word eclectic means selecting or borrowing the best out of everything. According to eclectic tendency in education, modern education wants to synthesis the brief form of all the past movements into new structure.
14.	Perennialism	Perennialism is a very constructive and inflexible philosophy of education. It is based on the view that reality comes from fundamental fixed truths, especially related to God. It believes that people find truth through reasoning and revelation and that goodness is found in rational thinking.
15.	Existentialism	Existentialism is an attitude and outlook that stress human existence that is the distinctive qualities of individual persons rather than man in abstract on nature and the world in general. It is a type of philosophy which endeavors to analyze the basic structure of human existence in its essential freedom.

NURSING PHILOSOPHY

Nursing philosophy is the motivation for becoming a nursing profession and a nurse. A mission statement outlining nurses' values, beliefs, and personal and professional ethics as they relate to this statement allows consideration of the undergraduate nurse's personal approach to patient care and career goals as a nurse. Nursing theory and nursing philosophy are related because they directly influence each other. A nurse's nursing philosophy determines the types of models or theories she uses, as the nursing theories used help develop her personal philosophy. In a way, nursing theory and philosophy are the same in that they provide a way for nurses to approach their day-to-day practice and individual patients in ways that provide the best possible care.

General Philosophical Concepts

- People are unique individuals with biopsychosocial and spiritual needs.
- People have the right to receive what is best for them, regardless of their race, religion or social status.
- People are responsible for maintaining good health and participating in personal healthcare.
- Nursing is dynamically evolving from changes in healthcare and medical science and technology advice.

Individual Nursing Philosophy Components

Nursing philosophy has multiple components, but important components of nursing philosophy are role, knowledge, values and processes.

Below is a brief description of all the factors to consider when formulating a personal care philosophy.
- **Role:** Role refers to the relationship between the provider or manager of care and the nursing profession. This role emphasizes the nurse's responsibility to the patient and the profession in the delivery and management of patient care.
- **Knowledge:** Knowledge deals with the academic and clinical experiences of nurses and how these experiences contribute to their role.
- **Values:** Values are beliefs that guide caregiver attitudes and moral judgments. Values are personal or professional. They are shaped by cultural and social influences, individual needs, and relationships. Other professional values influence the way nurses act in relation to nursing practice.
- **Processes:** Processes are the systems nurses use to implement and, if necessary, modify nursing interventions. The nursing philosophy process recognizes the caregiver's responsibility for continuously applying the nursing process to promote positive patient outcomes.
- **Nursing philosophy in transition:** The past four decades have been characterized by a wealth of nursing literature and the development of nursing theory. While each theory approaches the question of what nursing is from different perspectives and arrives at different answers, there are commonalities.

Importance of Nursing Care Philosophy

There are several reasons why a personal care philosophy is important. **Here are seven reasons why every nurse should consider developing a nursing philosophy.**
1. A personal philosophy of care guides the caregiver to live up to the standards they set for themselves.
2. A personal philosophy of care can improve interactions with patients, their families and peers.
3. Personal nursing philosophies help guide ethical competent evidence-based and science-driven nursing practice.
4. Personal nursing philosophies can keep you motivated when faced with a professional challenge.
5. If you have a personal nursing philosophy you may be better prepared to answer nursing interview questions than nurses who do not have a personal philosophy.
6. According to American Nurse which is the official journal of the American Nurses Association a nursing philosophy helps nurses identify theories and beliefs necessary for everyday choices.
7. The nursing philosophy is a means by which you capture your innermost beliefs and goals and identify ways to demonstrate them. A personal care philosophy helps you take responsibility.

PEDAGOGICAL APPLICATION OF PHILOSOPHY

- Educational Philosophy can be a reference in curriculum development, an expert and an expert in charting and creating guidelines.
- Educational philosophers can give tips for shaping politics.
- As collaborators, educational philosophers can collect and summarize different findings from different projects in different fields.
- Pedagogical Philosophy Helps Class Teachers Philosophy and pedagogy are also so closely related that they are meaningless without the other.

NATURALISM

The philosophically used term naturalism is most contrasted with the terms supernaturalism and other secularism. In the history of educational philosophy, naturalism is as old as idealism. The term naturalism, in its usual sense, refers to doctrines that place emphasis on nature in all areas of education. Thus, the philosopher of science derives from nature the aims and ideals of educational methods, the principles of curriculum and school leadership.

Definition

- Naturalism is the doctrine which separates nature from God, subordinates mind to matter, and establishes immutable laws as supreme —**James Wards**
- Naturalism is not science, it is a statement about science. More specifically, the claim that scientific knowledge is final and leaves no room for additional scientific or philosophical knowledge —**RB Perry**
- Naturalism is a philosophical position adopted by those who approach philosophy from a purely scientific point of view —**Rusk**
- Naturalism is a system whose distinguishing feature is our natural philosophy and exclusion from human spiritual or transcendent experience —**George Hayward Joyce**

Characteristics of Naturalism

- **Faith in nature:** Naturalism as opposed to Idealism Naturalism means faith in and return to nature. These people think that everything does not exist. I believe that everything that is natural does not exist.

- **Belief in science:** Naturalists claim that scientific knowledge is fried. They also emphasize that science evolves over time, and that even the underlying concepts can change. Naturalism is simply a philosophical generation of science.
- **Don't believe in souls:** Naturalists don't believe in spirits, souls, or God. Human life should be interpreted materially. Beyond that, there is nothing like spirit. The mind leaves the brain, which is essentially matter.
- **Genetics and environment:** According to naturalists, both heredity and environment influence a person's personality. There are two types of her in this environment: physical or geographical or material and psychological. It is the psychological environment that is the more useful environment and that humans have to adapt to.

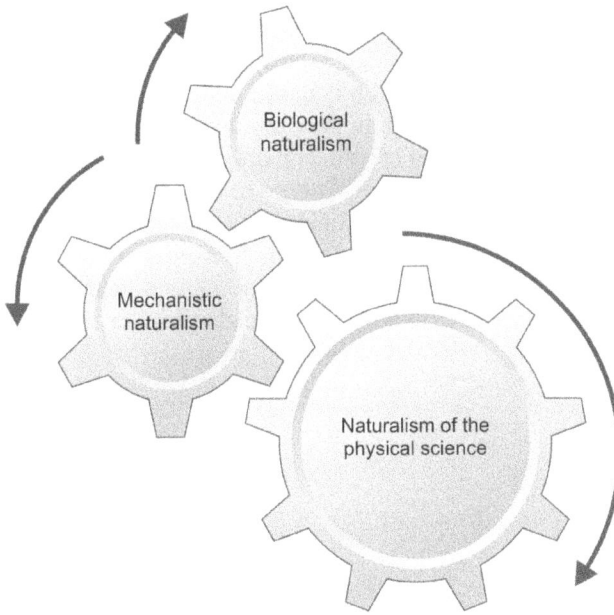

Fig. 3.2: Forms of naturalism.

Principles of Naturalism
- Education should be child-centered.
- Education is the natural development of a child's strengths and abilities.
- Education should be based on the origin of the child.
- Education should be planned according to the psychology of the child.

Forms of Naturalism
- **Scientific naturalism:** This kind of naturalism puts humans in the background and contributes little to education, which is a purely or deeply rooted human activity.
- **Mechanistic naturalism:** The universe he regards as one great machine. Beautifully placed by director RL Ahuja, it rounded up perfectly like a clock in an unknown age. It is now flowing down within the universe. Its laws of motion are also mechanical organisms are too small mechanical complexes of atoms and molecules. Humans are also mechanical beings. He has no creativity, no purpose, no direction.
- **Biological naturalism:** This type of naturalism is also known as Darwinian naturalism. It is based on evolutionary theory. We (humans) evolved from animals. Human nature is first animal, second believes in survival of the fittest, the weak die.

Naturalistic Goals
- Enable individuals to survive
- Self-expression
- Sublimation of instinct
- Adjust.

Criticism of Naturalism
- The spiritual element is ignored
- I cannot see the goal
- No moral value
- Overemphasis on genetics
- Look back.

According to naturalism, fathers and mothers, nurses and educators, and public schooltrained teachers are the most important players in education. Naturalism emphasizes direct experience of things.

REALISM

It is allowed to be true and real in everyday life. The implication of not being able to see the physical foundation and feel the reality is impermissible and unreal. This is the point of view of realism. Realism is as old as ancient Greek naturalism and materialism. Realism is education as a result of an emphasis on abstract literal and verbal knowledge and sophistication.

Meaning of Realism

The term realism means dealing with what actually exists. The development of the mind is part of the progress of world development. In fact, realism is the result of scientific development when something turns out to be true based on observational experiments and investigations. Only then can realism directly relate to humans and society.

The American educator Franklin Bobbitt classified human responsibilities and duties in the development of education as:

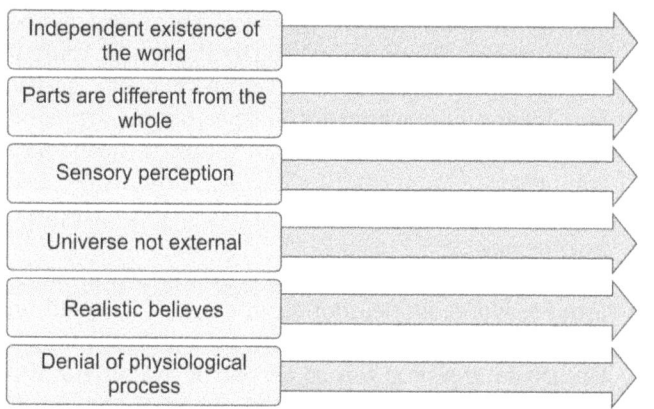

Fig. 3.3: Aims of education according to realism.

- Activities dealing with language
- Hygiene related activities
- Civic activities
- Normal social activities
- Recreational activities
- Breed conservation activities
- Mental health activities
- Religious activity
- Professional conduct activities.

Principles of Realism

- **Independent existence of the world:** Realism is basically the philosophical doctrine that the material world has an independent and objective existence. Its existence and nature do not depend on intelligence. This philosophy is not very different from the view of ordinary people. This could be a form of materialism.
- **The parts are different from the whole:** Be realistic about the parts being independent of the whole, giving them more importance.
- **Sensations:** Realistic disregard for high mental abilities and abilities at first. Sensory perception is paramount to them.
- **The universe is not external:** The realistic belief that the universe is not external, that there are laws that govern it, and that those laws, order, and cohesion prevail.
- **Realist belief:** Realism believes in examining things individually. Realism is the result of scientific thinking in the 16th century and his 17th century when humans began to examine things individually arose as a result.
- **The denial of physiological processes:** the reality that what is presented to us is not physiological in us.

Forms of Realism

- **Humanistic realism:** Developed in the 15th century after the end of the European Renaissance. Humanistic realism believes:
  - Simply interpret knowledge
  - Direct study of people and things
  - This realistic ideal and real man.
- **Social realism:** The term social realism is used to denote the views of an early century educator that became generally accepted in the 17th and his 18th centuries. This realism is a rebellion against the outdated life of man. All learning should be done with others.
- **Erotic realism:** Also known as Scientific Realism, its origins date back to the 17th century. Many scientific discoveries have been made, all of which emphasize the fact that the senses are the gateway to knowledge. The term sensory realism thus derives from the fundamental belief that knowledge arises primarily through the senses, that education is based on training in sensory perception rather than pure memory activity, and then on different types of subject matter.
- **Scholastic realism:** This type of realism involves the study of eternal truths held about objects in the world around us. Academic realists therefore believe that education leads to salvation and view religion as the primary source of ethics and social normalcy.

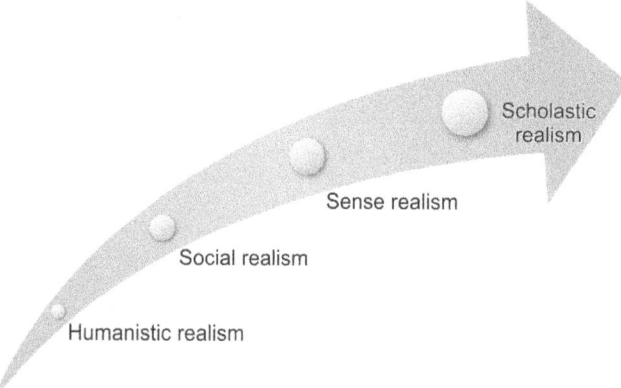

Fig. 3.4: Forms of realism.

Contributions of Realism to Education

- Realist philosophers are influencing practical education Technical and professional education has become a hallmark of education.
  Therefore, the education plan of every country in the world today is based on the needs of such individuals and is the development of the nation.

- **Practice oriented:** Modern education is empirical, experimental and hands-on, with a realistic assertion of the practical nature of education.
- **Practical goal:** Emphasize the development of the country in which we live.

IDEALISM

Idealism is a very old philosophical thought and it was exercised a great and potent influence on man and his mind. Even today idealism has certain attracting and we Indian have cherished those and a living with those ideas. If we look into history it was found that right advocate like Socrates Froebel and WE Hocking then in India idealism was reached by Gurdev and Rabindarnath Tagore which has something meaning and associated with other currents. Man is also spirit or mind he is more important in the world. Idealism drives the importance of matter and mechanism. The idealist does not accept the biological account man in terms of his evolution. Idealism is entirely different from naturalism because it denies the existence of the nature and accepts of existence of conscious.

Meanings of Idealism

- One who accepts and lives by lofty moral aesthetic and religious standards.
- Who can imagine a game or program that does not exist yet, and who will support it? For example, social reform.
- Dreamer ignores the practical conditions of the situation.
- Who can compliment it? Example: Mr and Mrs So-and-so are idealists who refer to their own attitudes.

The Philosophical Significance of Idealism

According to Mahatma Gandhi, idealism forms the core of Gandhian philosophy in his education. That is not reflected in his ultimate educational goal, which is nothing but self-actualization.

According to Titus, it was derived from the "concept" of the ideal world of the time. Idealism arose from the fact that ideas come from the mind. So, idealism means that reality is made up of ideas, thoughts, minds, or selves, no different than material forces.

Principles of Idealism

- Mind and mind constitute reality
- A spiritual person is the highest creature
- God is the source of all knowledge
- Values are absolute and immutable
- It is not the object itself that becomes reality in the end, but the idea behind it
- Humans are not creators of value.

Idealistic Claims

- **Ideas are final:** An idea, mind, thought, or ideal is the ultimate reality. Idealism emphasizes the spirit and also some senses—more than matter. The spirit and ideas are real. Matter is subordinate.
- **Faith in the universal heart:** It means that God is present everywhere in the human mind. A universal mind environment of its kind:
  - Intellectual
  - Emotional
  - Willing.
- **Human image:** The idealist human image is completely different. Humans are not animals, they can live and die, but the body perishes, but they believe that the body underlies the spirit.
- **Idealism and knowledge:** At attaché's great importance to the knowledge which serves as model activities. It is a secondary phase; knowledge is gained through the senses.

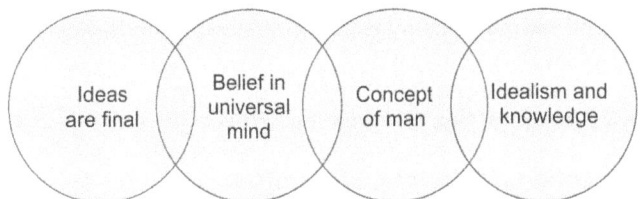

Fig. 3.5: Philosophical significance of idealism.

Types of Idealism

According to plate knot Hegel briefly mention three types of idealism:

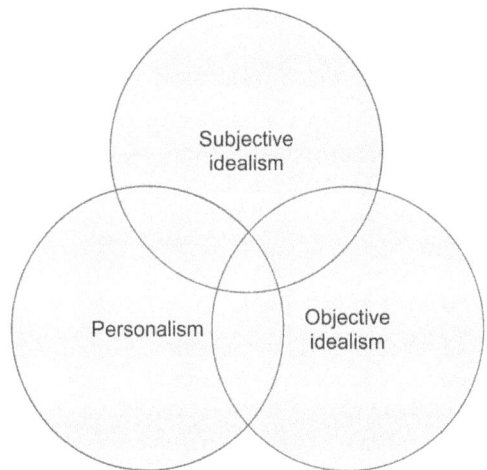

Fig. 3.6: Types of idealism.

1. **Subjective idealism:** It is called metalism or phenol mentalism. Yours Goerge Babkelry 1685–1753 is the best representative of idealism. Here subjective ideals capture the mind, spirit and perception.
2. **Objective idealism:** The second form of idealism represented by Pratt and Hegel. It's the outside world. It feels artificial. They do not determine existence or objective reality.
3. **Individualism:** Man as a gift from God. Reality is the nature of a conscious personality. Human freedom with values that are more important than life. Here, the personal idealist is interested in one or the other. Low interest is logical.

General Characteristics of Idealism

- Creation has a purpose
- Not only in the physical world
- The universe is not without purpose
- Nature is not an independent existence
- The universe is an expression of the mind, a perceptual consciousness
- The ultimate reality is consciousness (mind), and the world is carved by it
- Consciousness is also the basis of matter
- Harmony reigns in nature and man.

Educational Principles of Idealism

Idealism emphasized the essential need for moral education in all nations. It can also develop the personality of teachers and students.
- Education should be universal.
- Education requires both individual welfare and social welfare.
- Education is preservation and transmission.
- Education is the realization of national unity.

Importance of Idealism in Nursing

- Nursing education helps young men grow and is conditioned by supernatural motives.
- Helps in integrated personality.
- Idealism helps you to have intellectual and moral judgment.

Disadvantages of Idealism

- Easy to preach difficult to practice.
- Idealism is a dogmatic philosophy.
- It ignores psychology—it ignores child psychology.
- No contributions to teaching methods.
- Idealists of external values.
- Science and technology are not given much importance.
- Nobody practices strict discipline.

PRAGMATISM

A philosopher is a person who likes all kinds of knowledge, is curious about learning, and is never satisfied. Different thinkers have tried to interpret man in their own way. Pragmatism is considered a modern teaching philosophy and trust works.

History of Pragmatism

Pragmatism is a distinctive American philosophy that began in the 19th century. American partisan settlers faced many problems in building their own civilization in these new environments. There were no readymade solutions to these problems. Old ideas will not help. So they experimented with new ideas and adopted ideas that they found useful in solving everyday problems. As a result, they build a philosophy of life based on their own experiments and experiences. Old traditions and ideas seemed incomplete to them. Whatever problems they had, they were solved by these new ideas. These ideas were the doctrines of experimentalism or pragmatism. These teachings may not have changed the foundations of human life, but they have influenced their philosophies.

Definition

William James defines pragmatism as an attitude of looking away from the first things, principles, categories, and perceived necessities, to the facts that bear fruit in the end. Rusk defines pragmatism simply as the development of a new idealism that justifies reality.

Meaning of Pragmatism

Pragmatism is understood as an important modern educational philosophy, but its origins lie in ancient Greece. The Greek word pragma itself means action, from which comes the words practice and practice.

Principles of Pragmatism

- **Pluralism:** Philosophically speaking, pragmatism is pluralism, where everyone seeks truth and purpose in life according to their experience. Truth depends on different spatio-temporal situations.
- **Emphasis on change:** Pragmatism emphasizes change. Truth is always present. The world is progressing and evolving. That is why everything is changing here.
- **Utilitarianism:** Pragmatists are utilitarians utilitarianism is the test of all truth and reality. A useful principle is truth. Utility means the fulfillment of a human purpose. Outcomes determine the right or wrong of all ideas, beliefs, and theories dictated by circumstances. Utility means meeting human needs.

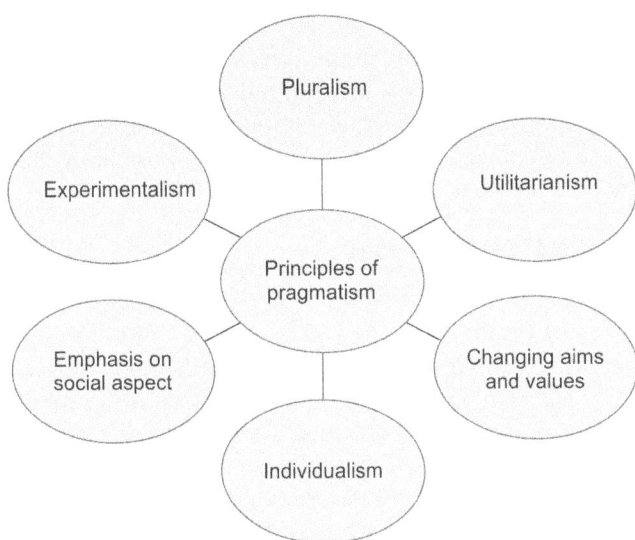

Fig. 3.7: Principles of pragmatism.

Forms of Pragmatism

- **Humanistic pragmatism:** This form of pragmatism is found especially in the social sciences. After satisfying humanity is the standard of utility. All truths are human truths.
- **Experimental pragmatism:** Modern science is based on experimental methods. A fact that can be proven by experiment is true. The real world is true for any job. The truth of a theory in science can be established by its practicability. Pragmatists apply this standard of truth to all areas of life. The field of experimentation is the broadest in the realm of science. In science, experiments are only the basis for reaching conclusions about controversial issues.

PROGRESSIVISM

The term progressivism in education is an American psychology that describes a formally traditional and rebellion against the traditional educational system. Progressive education was first recognized in 1919 when the Association for Progressive Education was founded in Washington, DC. Already used. The underlying principles of progressive education have greatly influenced contemporary educational theory and practice around the world.

Meaning

- Progressivism in education advocates that a child's education should be for the present life itself, not for the future life.
- Arguing that individual and social development is possible only if education supports the development of children at every stage.

Progressive Principles

The progressive education association (PEA) consists of the following principles:
- Freedom to grow naturally.
- Interest in work motivation.
- Teachers are guides, not taste masters.
- Scientific research on student development.
- Paying more attention to everyone affects a child's physical development.
- Coordinating school and home to meet the needs of children's lives.
- Progressive schools are at the forefront of the education movement.

Progressive Goals in Education

To develop individuality by providing a democratic environment in educational institutions.
- Cooperative social participation.
- General development of the child.
- Education of the whole person or personality, including physical, emotional, social and intellectual aspects of the individual.

Types of Education

Progressivism recognizes the child as a fully dynamic, living organism. Therefore, any kind of education is always necessary.
- Education should address the needs of all stages of development and tap into all aspects of development, including experience. This is what we see in dynamic cultures where individual lives are seen.
- Progressive education represents emotional and emotional education as important to them as intellectual education.
- The importance of social pedagogy is also recognized by progressive educators.
- Consider also that your child acquires skills for both financial and non-financial purposes in life.
- Training in recreational and leisure activities, developing hobbies and maintaining aesthetic interest are considered very important.
- Progressivism in education stands for functional activity rather than passive acceptability.
- It is not intended to provide students with objective information only. It also aims to provide opportunities for all types of experiences.

Progressivism and Teaching Methods

- Progressivism advocates a project approach in which students actively participate in learning.
- Emphasis on socialized methods.
- Efforts will be made to involve all individuals in group systems of interaction, meetings, consultation, planning and participation.
- Students are given a variety of opportunities to experience situations of an emotional, social, aesthetic and practical nature.
- Progressive the underlying principle method is that active participation in a variety of life activities can develop an important integrated personality.
- Totality of methods is the basis of progressive learning because progressive education considers learning as a whole experience in which a single thing branches off and grows.
- Progressive educators embrace the principles of motivation and gratitude.
- Progressivism requires teachers to know their students well in order to guide their independent learning process. He must know the values students seek, the problems they face, and the interests that motivate them to act.
- Critics of progressive teaching methods say that progressively taught students lack discipline. This criticism may be justified when teachers give liberty instead of liberty and encourage students' whims and whims instead of their active goals and interests. It is a voluntary activity and is only encouraged by well-trained schools.

Progressive Benefits

- It emphasizes the importance of human individuality.
- The school could focus primarily on the development of the child as a whole, both as an individual and as a member of society.
- Progressives view emotions as aspects of various biochemical and biophysical processes in an organism. Emotional education is therefore the same as mental and physical education, and all three are interdependent.
- Progressive refers to the child's acquisition of skills for both money-making and non-money-making life purposes.
- It is not intended to provide students with objective information only. It also aims to provide opportunities for all types of experiences.

Disadvantages of Progressivism

- Progressives oppose a predetermined, literal curriculum.
- Progressive education does not promote school organization with clearly segregated classes.
- Those who criticize progressive teaching say that progressive teaching students lack discipline.

Progressivism has influenced education around the world. She has helped me focus primarily on the development of the child as a whole, both as an individual and as a member of society.

RECONSTRUCTIONISM

Recovery is future-oriented. It is a gift to progressivism. It has its origins in Plato and is pushed out of modern tradition with Western thought. The difference between early utopianism and more recent reconstructions is that the latter is based on empirical scientific discoveries and the former is purely speculative. From a physical point of view, reconstruction is later shared with progressivism directed at nature and experience. Experience shows that reconstruction emphasizes a world in which it affects individuals. Reconstructionism as a complement to Progressivism, missing certain elements that Progressivism lacks. Reconstructionism has its roots in Plato. His Republic is his vision of an ideal society. Karl Marx Bernad Shaw and Karl Mannheim are his Reconstionism belonging to the great past. They want to quickly and directly transform not only education, but also large institutions. Theodore Brameld is a major proponent of Reconstructionism. Paulo Freire's educational philosophy has strong elements of Reconstructionist thought.

- Comprehensive human resource development is necessary. But in our country educated people are proud to show off their knowledge of foreign cultures and traditions. This shows ignorance of the country's culture and philosophy.

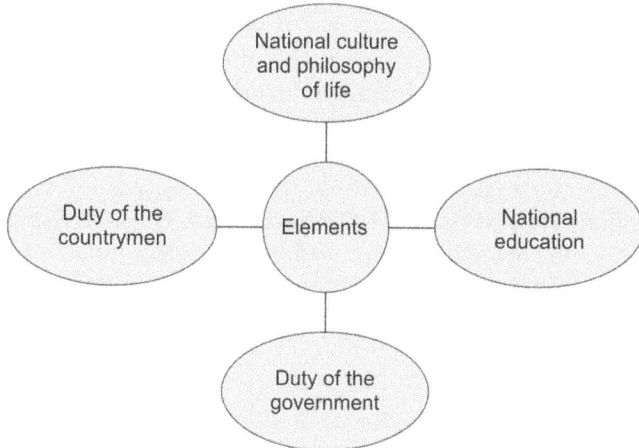

Fig. 3.8: Elements of reconstructionism.

- **National education:** In education, there must be a national perspective, drawing on the knowledge experiences and scientific successes of other countries, which will be adapted according to the changing national needs. The goal of education should be the development of the mind and character that makes a person grow.
- **Government obligation:** Reconstruction requires a lot of money. The government should take an interest in revivalism. Ignoring all aspects is a disservice to the country.
- **Obligations of compatriots:** Together with the government, compatriots have a certain responsibility for the reconstruction of education. Each field signifies sociopolitical and educational activity.

Forms of Reconstructionism

Reconstructionism has two forms. Overall change or desired change. The current education system is not representative of Indian culture and traditions and is a complete change or reform. A complete transformation is a difficult task and requires intensive thought, funding and research, so the more convenient and better way to achieve the desired transformation is. But whether it is a gross change or a step-by-step reform, our education system must be grounded in Indian culture and traditions, yet viable.

Reconstructionist Goals

The primary goal of education is comprehensive personal development. It mainly includes physical and mental morality and spiritual development. Along with this, logical thinking and intelligence must also be developed. The country now adopts a democratic system. The purpose of education should therefore be to foster confidence in democratic principles. Instilling in students a sense of social service should also be an educational goal, as should instilling in students the ability to adapt to their environment and earn a living.

Emotional integration with people from other states should also be developed. People should be taught the ability to use their free time in constructive activities. In this way, people can use their free time to protect themselves from unwanted influences. These things need to be taken into account when building education. The ability to control partisan tendencies such as communicative caste, regionalism, etc. to produce national unity should also be the goal of educational reconstructionism.

Other Aspects of Reconstructionism

- **Curriculum:** A curriculum should be established based on and to achieve the above objectives. Curriculum should be determined according to age, social status, environment and geographical conditions.
- **Freedom:** Education should be completely free to some extent and these costs should be borne by the state. I wish all secondary education was free. We need to adopt democratic principles in curricula and in the administration of institutions. General technical and vocational education should be provided, and desirable changes should be made in primary and higher education.
- **Educational method:** The goal of the educational method is not only to pass exams, but also to develop the necessary qualities and skills, education should be action-oriented. Teaching methods should be organized in a way that allows students to become independent.
- **Discipline:** Teaching should be organized and conducted in such a way that there is no problem of lack of discipline in the institution. Tolerance and discretion can be developed in students because of qualities such as libertarianism.
- **Competent teachers:** Education is nothing without a competent teacher. Appropriate arrangements should therefore be made for the training of teachers. This work requires a necessary change in the perspective of educational institutions.
- **Testing:** The general testing system is inadequate because it does not adequately assess the abilities of the students. Therefore, such changes must be made in order for a student's competence to be properly assessed. The exam should be based on the work of the entire session. We have to eliminate the shortcomings of the thesis exam.
- **Parents:** The cooperation of teachers and parents should be considered in restoring education as children spend time in the company of both. In this regard, there is also a need for training for parents to understand their duties.
- **Health environment:** The work of educational reform is facilitated when schools are set up in a health environment. Therefore, it is necessary to have a good school environment, high aspirations, and ideal traditions.

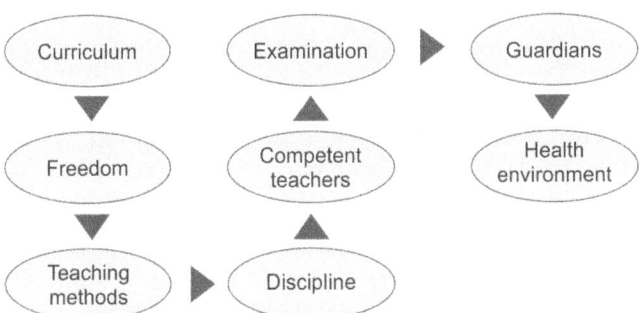

Fig. 3.9: Other aspects of reconstructionism.

ECLECTICISM

Eclecticism is the term given to a group of ancient philosophers who chose from existing philosophical beliefs the most rational doctrines and tried to construct new systems. The first use of this name is in his 1st century AD. Desperate to focus on absolute truth, eclecticism sought the highest possible odds through choice.

The dictionary meaning of the word eclectic is to select or borrow the best of everything. Wide as opposed to exclusive. An eclectic is someone who chooses opinions from different systems, especially in philosophy. According to the eclectic trend in education, modern education wants to integrate the short forms of all past movements into new structures. We aim to create resonance between all principles. Psychology and the social sciences have largely influenced teaching methods. Material educational goals and school administration have influenced every movement and have affected not only all areas of education, but all areas of life.

Key Elements of Eclectic Trends in Education

- The modern trend in education is to eliminate existing differences in persistent ideologies.
- Eclecticism embraces common principles in educational theory and practice.
- There are some commonalities of a highly eclectic nature regarding the child's individual development, physical environment, and social goals.
- Eclecticism does not take into account the need to dogmatically follow a particular theoretical idea or philosophy or to advocate for an idea in the field of education.
- All philosophies are free.
- Contemporary eclectic trends in education reflect the aims, methods, and techniques of education through the accumulated experience of mankind.
- A harmonious mixture of different philosophies is called an eclectic trend.
- No educational thinker is only an idealist, a naturalist, or a pragmatist.

Eclecticism and the Role of Education

Eclecticism is evident in today's teaching profession. In the past, he was primarily concerned with mediation. Today, his work is extremely challenging, delicate and complex. He is expected to have some knowledge in various fields. Today's situation in philosophy and psychology places high demands on teachers. Therefore, teachers should be careful in their approach. No profession is more morally demanding than teaching.

According to eclecticism, an ideal educational system should be idealistic in its purpose, naturalistic in its setting, and practical in its methods and program of work. One philosophy should not be emphasized at the expense of the other. All philosophies should be transformed into unity. The method of education should be to draw inspiration from the collective experience of an entire race, rather than from a generation preaching a particular ideology. It is called eclecticism.

Similarities between different philosophies and their influence on education:

Different philosophies meet at a certain point.
These are areas of agreement and influence on education.

- **Value:** All philosophies emphasize using the curriculum and classroom facilities in a way that works for the student. This practical value has always been accepted by all philosophies.
- **Spiritual goal:** It is accepted by all philosophies. That is, the goal of cognition. All philosophies strive to know Lended.
- **Student respect:** Individual dignity is accepted by all. It offers a certain degree of freedom as it guarantees student value.

Educational Impact

- **Goals:** All philosophies have goals, but they may differ. All philosophies emphasize fundamental processes such as talking about health and family life, civic and professional relationships. They differ only in the way they help.
- **Syllabus:** All philosophies agree that experience teaches everyone. For example, history, grammar, logic, race sciences and natural sciences all must be learned to a large extent.
- **Methods:** All philosophies agree that there are methods of teaching, selection and application of which will depend on the circumstances, local conditions, or facilities.
- **Motivation:** All philosophies believe in the principles of motivation and education.
- **Individual differences:** Individual differences are accepted by any philosophy.

Finally, all philosophies embrace educational science. They recognize the contributions of psychology. All encourage the student union to run the school. All philosophies believe in excellent material protection and healthcare for students.

PERENNIALISM

Perennialism attaches great importance to the value of education. It is modified from realism. Philosophers believe that there are some eternal values to which we must return and which must be brought to the attention of all the young people of the school.

- Logic is essential to the study of ideas. Ideas are verbalized and interrelated.
- **Good people:** Aristotle's attention is primarily directed to good people and good condition. His ethical theory dealt with the attainment of ends. The ultimate human goal is goodness and happiness, which can only be achieved by reason. Good conditions are created by people. A nation exists for a specific purpose. In other words, it exists for faster moral and intellectual achievement.
- In science, Aristotle believed that abstract ideas transcend experiential knowledge.

Definition of Perennialism

Perennialism is a very constructive and inflexible educational philosophy. It is based on the view that reality arises from basic and established truths that relate specifically to God. People find truth through reasoning and revelation, and believe that goodness lies in rational thinking.

General Principles

- Persistence is more real than change.
- Human nature is essentially unchanged.
- The good life, the life worth living for people, remains above all else.
- Moral principles remain essentially the same.
- Therefore, the education men receive should remain essentially the same.

Pedagogical Application of Perennial Studies

- Humans are essentially the same, so education should be essentially the same for everyone. The functioning of a citizen can vary greatly from society to society, but the functioning of a human being as a human being is the same in every era and society, as it arises from his nature as a human being.
- Because human nature is constant: Men are the same everywhere, so education should be basically the same for all men. This means that children are rational and not plastic personalities shaped by the whims of their teachers. Solving problems is a waste of time for students. Why spend hours discovering facts and principles when students can be taught in minutes. Repetition and memorization of exercises is very important to the learning process.
- Man's highest nature, that which distinguishes him from the lower life forms, is his foundation, and he must use it to guide his life and control his instincts. It won't work. Men are free and indecisive. You are responsible for his actions. You cannot allow your child's behavior because of environmental (or) personal problems. Humans are rational, so we must live rationally. Therefore, children must adhere to the standards of reason, and this is a function of parenting.
- Education should adapt people to external truths. Although the modern world is not. Education requires teaching. Teaching means knowledge. Knowledge is truth. The truth is the same everywhere. Therefore, education should be the same everywhere.
- Education should be for the long term, not for fads. It is not the school's job to communicate current issues of social reform and political action. Providing education is the school's job, on which diplomas can initiate efforts to bring about meaningful social reform and political action.

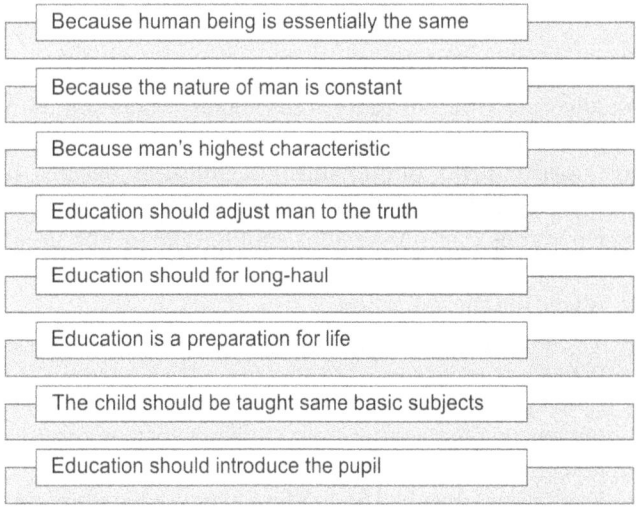

Fig. 3.10: Educational applications of perennialism.

- Education is preparation for life, not imitation of life. It's not life itself, as progressive claims.
- A child should be taught the same basic subjects that accustom him to the constancy of the world. A child must learn to read, write, speak and listen. He is a social creature and lives in a male community. Therefore, he must use his reason and rational powers to communicate with other people.
- Education aims to introduce students to the universal interests of mankind through the study of the great works of literature, philosophy, history and science.

Perennialism and Education

Perennialism has two main divisions.

Durability Overtime

Durability over time emphasizes the importance of reasoning. Their precise and independent thinking is the biggest difference between developed and undeveloped minds. It should be the primary goal of education. An advocate of teaching reasoning through targeted reading lists of the great Western books. Complemented by minimal guided discussion using the Socratic method. Secular perennialism also advocates the use of translated original works rather than textbooks.

Religious Perennialism

Religious Perennialism was developed by Thomas Aquinas in his 13th century. It also focuses on the personal growth of the student, as Christianity is about love (ideal of full blood, not sex). He argued against two errors. First, he argued that not all learning comes from within, because it must always serve as a felt sign for the learner to perceive.

Perennialism Key Ideas

- Advocate a true educational community where common goals should be true.
- Consistent with utilitarianism in education because it signifies the worship of technology and materialism.
- He argues that universities should take up the great books, the great ideas of mankind, the liberal arts.
- Attack the specialization.
- She sees her vision of one world established by cultivating reason.
- Emphasizes the need for modern man to have the broad perspective that comes from studying ancient cultures and civilizations.
- Emphasizes the need for modern man to have a broader perspective resulting from the study of ancient cultures and civilizations.
- Education means knowledge. Knowledge is truth. The truth is the same everywhere. Therefore, education should be the same everywhere.
- Human nature is the same. The history of the human species reveals the same role of humans in all ages.
- A true educator does not blame others. He tries to overcome difficulties.
- Education is life. It is not preparation for life.
- School is only a place of education. A place to introduce children to real-life situations and truths of eternal value.
- A teacher is a disciplined, benevolent master of work. A perfect school is not the result of a good method as much as a good teacher. Teachers must possess moral virtues. He must have a pure and divine love for youth. They must have the real interests of their family and country in mind.
- The longtime favorite believes in methods of mental education of children. Lecture method is preferable.
- Discipline is maintained by the moral foundations of the school environment.

Criticisms of Perennialism

- The absoluteness of truth is challenged by scientific attitudes.
- Pluralism has been denounced as the aristocracy of intelligence and intellectual luxury.
- Perennialism relies too heavily on rigorous student training, which can hinder student initiative and creativity.
- The overemphasis on intellectual training is an end in itself and seems unreasonable to some educators.

EXISTENTIALISM

Existentialism is an attitude and view that emphasizes individual, rather than human, characteristics in abstract terms about human existence, nature and the world in general. Presence comes first. It means an inner direct experience of self-awareness.

Definition of Existentialism

Attempts have been made to trace the beginnings of existentialism in Greek philosophy.

According to Ternand's existentialism, it is a philosophy that seeks to analyze the basic structure of human existence in essential freedom.

According to Dr Radhakrishnan existentialism is the new name for old method.

Features of Existentialism

- **Criticism of idealism:** Existentialism arose and developed as an interaction with idealism. Existentialist philosophers are highly critical of idealism and conceptualism. According to idealism, human beings are basically expressions of an underlying spiritual or spiritual element that has a universal character. It is a shared personality that really defines a man. Human freedom is therefore subject to the interests of humanity in general.

- **Criticism of naturalism:** Existentialist philosophers are also critical of naturalistic philosophy. According to naturalists, life is governed by universal causality. According to the law of causality, everything has a cause before it and nothing happens suddenly. Therefore, if the law of cause and effect is universal, there can be no human subject. Human behavior is as mechanical as animal behavior.
- **Critique of the philosophy of science:** Existentialist philosophers criticize not only idealism and naturalism, but also scientific acceptance. Scientific abstractions from direct data bring them under universal laws or general rules, but according to existentialists all abstractions are false realities that exist only in direct data.
- **The value of the human person:** For existentialists, the human being is the center of the universe, unrivaled. Even the Bralman God Universe is subordinate to humans. A fundamental characteristic of the human staff is this unfiltered, unrestricted freedom. Society and social institutions serve human interests and are not universal as idealists and others believe. There is a general will that the individual will follow. If basic social law restricts human freedom, it is invalid and unjust. Anything that hinders personal growth and development must be discarded.
- **No construction of a philosophical system:** The ancient philosophers pondered and pondered such issues as God, soul, space, time, the physical world, their origin and development. They have attempted to present a philosophy that encompasses all these issues and have developed a system of theories. Existentialists distrust building and theorizing systems. In their opinion, the real goal of philosophy is action, not theory. That's why they don't think about traditional issues.
- **Existential harmony:** True harmony is not harmony of ideas and thoughts, but harmony of desires. True philosophy is not the philosophy of reality, but the philosophy of reality, the philosophy of direct experience. The true way of the nature of this philosophy does not consider not participating in that movement whose existence is a duty. Existentialist philosophy has no specific goal. Because it is impossible to tie life to a specific goal, because life is a movement and life is creative progress, not just mechanical change, because it is impossible to tie life to a specific goal.

Existentialism and Educational Goals

- Existentialism embraces the psychological view that each individual is unique. Education must promote the growth of human uniqueness. Since existentialists are not interested in universal human beings, this should be the primary goal of education. You are interested in unique people made of concrete. Education must respond to the needs of individual differences. She must enable students to thrive as individuals.
- Human nature is to be indeterminate in action, and education therefore teaches the student the infinite possibilities of his freedom and the responsibilities of his freedom and the responsibilities he has to bear in life must be recognized. Education must promote self-determination.
- Education must also foster in students a set of values compatible with their absolute freedom. Students must commit to these values and act accordingly. The existentialist message to educational philosophy is to compromise authentic freedom and individual uniqueness.
- Education has no intellectual purpose. From an existentialist perspective, it is more important to develop the effective side of life, the emotional and aesthetic side of human beings, than the rational or cognitive side of life. Again, education should not accept social development as the goal. Because the pursuit of this goal treats the child as a mere (social) group animal.
- Life is viewed as a series of crises. Education must enable students to develop such a level of inner awareness, and education must teach people to accept death with dignity as a natural phenomenon.
- Education should aim at providing individuals with knowledge of human nature, especially from an existential perspective. Education should help people become human.
- The development of reflective skills should also be a goal of education. It is said to foster students' introspection.

Existentialism and Curriculum

Existentialism does not believe in curriculum prescriptions. Subjects should not be imposed on students. Students should choose their own curriculum based on their feelings, needs, abilities, and stage of life. Existentialist thinkers agree to provide some knowledge of the universe in general, but believe that the curriculum should be relevant to the pressing and practical problems individuals have to face. Existentialism emphasized that the curriculum should be appropriate by students, not just by studying for exams to live and experience.

Existentialism and Methodology

- Knowledge through intimate personal contact
- Pay close attention to each person

- Education at home
- No indoctrination
- Creativity education
- No place for group dynamics.

Existentialism and Discipline

A disciplined student is one who has developed a set of values that seeks to act with integrity. Existentialism opposes all kinds of perceptions and sets of rules for children. They also oppose the practice of offering initiative and rewards to students for the purpose of training them. Responsibility for being a disciplined character rests primarily on the student himself.

PHILOSOPHY OF MAHATMA GANDHIJI

Gandhi's educational thought and practice reflects his own educational experiments, his experience in the political, social and economic life of the country, and the low cost of the Western education system. It stems from his perception and reaction to the meaninglessness of limitations. rooted in the country. Gandhiji resembled the American pragmatic educational philosopher John Deway.

Integration of politics and education on a philosophical level Development of Satyagraha as a strategy to resist oppression without hating the oppressor, full commitment to nonviolence as a way of life, a child centered approach to education and craft. The center and medium of the educational experience is a unique contribution from Mahatma Gandhi.

Philosophy of Life

- Gandhi is the greatest in his service to God and mankind. He says the only way to find God is to see him in this creation and become one with it. This can only be done through all services.
- God is truth and man and society can know this truth through Ahimsa. It is love for all and hate for no one. Gandhi believed that God is not found in Hindu temples, Muslim mosques, or Christian churches. He is in the Temple of Humanity.
- Gandhi is very practical. His motto is "One must love his neighbor as oneself" and he believes in freedom and equality for all.
- Gandhi wanted a social order free from exploitation and injustice of any kind. He wanted a class society for workers. He wanted to avoid capitalism. He proposed building an economic and social structure based on decentralized industry and agriculture. He advocates for domestic and village industries.

- Like Rousseau, he wanted to revive society. Indian society can only be regenerated by reviving villages. He wanted to restore the child's rightful place in the education system. He wanted the harmonious development of his four aspects of the human personality: body, mind, spirit and soul.

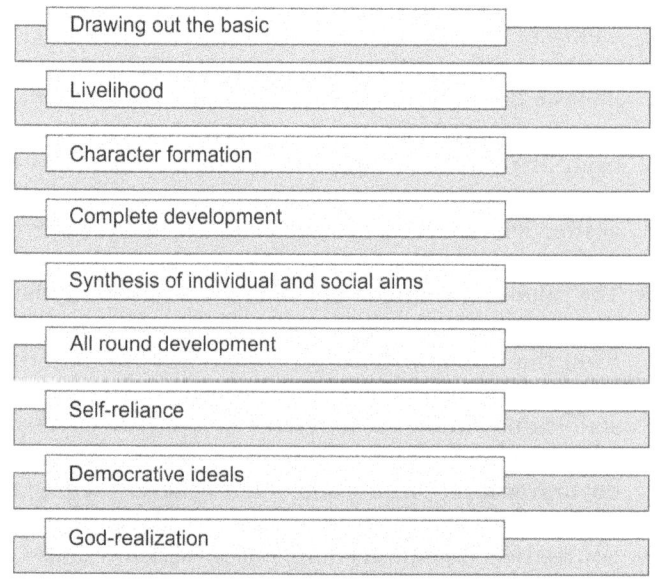

Fig. 3.11: Aims and ideals of education.

Gandhi's Educational Philosophy

Gandhi's educational philosophy has his two basic **principles.**

Educational Goals and Ideals

- **Get the bottom line:** Get his point of view on the goals of education, said Gandhiji. Education means bringing out the best in every aspect of a child's or man's body, mind and soul. Literacy per se is not education.
- **Livelihood:** In his opinion the goal of education is independence and education should enable all girls and boys to develop the ability to rely on themselves. The ability to earn a living is part of his independence from independence.
- **Character education:** Gandhi also believed in child-centered, paid-centered education for centuries. He personified to people that the cultural aspect of education was much more important than the literary one.
- **Full development:** Education must not only lead individuals to self-awareness, but also instill in them all the qualities that make them good and responsible citizens.
- **Integration of individual and social goals:** Gandhiji integrated individual and social goals of education. He

did not limit education to the achievement of a single goal. He reserves the educational process from different perspectives.

- **Overall development:** He wants his child to earn something while studying. He also wanted his child to develop his own personality. In his opinion, the criterion for a person's cultural development is not the breadth of knowledge, but inner growth. He emphasizes physical, spiritual, moral, aesthetic and religious education of all kinds.
- **Independence:** Gandhi seeks independence through education. Thus, he envisioned craft-oriented training. Description of his basic education scheme as insurance against unemployment in India.
- **Democratic ideal:** He aspired to an ideal civic education. In his opinion, education should make children ideal members of a democratic society. According to Gandhi, the school itself is a small democratic society where children are taught democratic values such as foresight, tolerance and love of neighbor. Children learn virtues such as compassion, service, love, brotherhood, equality and freedom.
- **Democratic ideals:** All knowledge is useless without good character. Gandhiji condemned the prevalent disorder among his disciples and called for them to follow the ideals of Brahmacharya.
- **God realization:** The opposite of God realization is the meaning of self-realization. Gandhiji insisted that students should live a *sanyasi* life.

Gandhi's Pedagogical Experiment

Learning is not tied to real situations. I had no vocational training. It could only produce employees. Education classes did not recognize the dignity of work. They were unfit for any living creature.

A child's mind is stuffed with all sorts of information without even thinking about stimulating or growing a human being. True learning could not be conveyed through a foreign language. Gandhiji wanted to educate Indian children through her mother tongue. He wants to educate them through physical labor.

When Gandhiji protested the existing system of parenting, he tried to achieve his goals at home like Pestalozzi. Eight hours were allotted to him for vocational training, and only two hours to him for reading and writing. The occupations I was taught were cooking, digging sandals, carpentry, and cleaning. The curriculum includes Hindi, Tamil, Gujarati and Sanskrit, History, Geography and Mathematics.

Gandhiji's Views on Various Aspects of Education

He published his views in Harijan and many of his books:
- Handicrafts
- Handicraft training
- Read before write
- Play in education
- Education in mother tongue
- **Religious education:** Religious education should be conveyed not through books, but through the lives of teachers and through word of mouth.
- **Job preparation:** Children must learn to work in preparation for their future life
- **Syllabus:** He stated that he would acquire general knowledge of world history, geography, botany, astronomy, arithmetic, geometry and algebra.
- **Independent education:** Education from age 9 must be independent.
- **A teacher of good character:** A teacher cannot have a large saran, but he must give him enough to support himself.
- Cheap school building.
- **Place for english:** English can and should have a place as a language in the curriculum.

Education Type

Gandhi's educational philosophy focused on primary education and child development. Adult Education or Social Pedagogy by Sarvodaya. He made the adult education program a key component of his political campaign. Thousands of volunteers have been trained in adult education at Sabarmati and Sebagram Asham. Spread across thousands of villages and 100 urban areas, they taught adult men and women in night schools. He planned different kinds of education for the country. In addition to primary education, he taught serious peasant education and education for women.

Teaching Methodology

Teachers are exemplary models and central to the Gandhi curriculum. He is not just an intellectual resource like American pragmatism. In this respect, Gandhi is closer to the Indian tradition. But that does not mean that Gandhi took a teacher entered (gurukra) approach to education. Gandhiji was completely child-centered in his approach to parenting. He opposed the bureaucratization of education and industry. He sought to develop a culture of creative discipline through his work. Gandhi was an educational activity done by an educator that also had economic value. Sugandige sought to integrate acquisition and learning into a simultaneous process.

TAGORE'S PHILOSOPHY OF EDUCATION

Tagore wanted to develop the whole human being. For him, the general education system was flawed and inadequate. He couldn't show his personality enough. According to him, the curriculum should be such as to maximize the physical, mental, moral, social and spiritual development of the individual.

Curriculum based on real-life activities and extensive experience where appropriate. This allows the child's personality to fully develop in all aspects.

- Tagore stresses that in addition to the various subjects, various types of extracurricular activities should also be an integral part of the curriculum.
- Their recommended subjects are history, geography, languages, natural history, and scientific activities, and more detailed subjects include music, art, poetry, dance, and drama.
- Music is the essence of life and acting relieves tension and fear in children.
- Tagore's educational philosophy is exactly in line with his general philosophy. He wants to be dissatisfied with the existing education system. Because if we ignore it, our own customer traditions become morals and ideals.
- Removed the Indians from their Altine and Willization. Thus, Tagore saw the educational institution of the time as a noncolorless educational existence, detached from the cosmic context, within the bare white walls starting from the eyeballs of the dead.
- He realized that traditional schools transmit information and knowledge. They emphasized only the intellectual aspect and completely ignored it. They emphasized only the intellectual aspect and ignored other aspects as part of human development.
- On the other hand, Tagore emphasizes the myriad meanings of education, stating: Education is essential to life's adventures. It is not like a painful hospital treatment that cures a student's instincts.

Tagore's Philosophy of Education

- Tagore emphasized the fundamental unity and love between man, nature and international relations. A true education, therefore, should encourage this compassion and sympathy with all that exists.
- He was adamantly opposed to modern education, arguing that education should accustom children to individual voices and missions and international life, and should achieve a harmonious balance of all elements.
- Tagore believed that children should enjoy freedom while receiving an education. He should be free from all restrictions. Like Rousseau, Tagore considered nature to be the most effective and powerful teacher for children. For this, he prescribed the child a natural education.
- He emphasized children's liberty and natural education, but firmly believed that education was a means of social reform. It should serve in many ways as the life-giving current of modern society.
- He believes in international brotherhood. He argued that education should correspond to the realities of life.
- Education disconnected from life is useless. Therefore, any educational plan should incorporate both human nature and needs into a harmonious program.
- Tagore himself wrote—besides nature, children should be exposed to the flow of social behavior.

Principles of Educational Philosophy

Fundamental principles of Tagore's educational philosophy:

- **Freedom:** For Tagore, freedom means the child's own experiences and activities. He wanted the education to be natural in content and quality. The function of education is to bring the child's mind into contact with nature and enable it to learn the books of nature freely and spontaneously.
- **Creative self-expression:** Tagore argues that since the majority of human beings cannot find expression in mere verbal language, more intellectual development is not only a function of education, but of the education of the human being as a whole. I believed it would help me. One's emotions and senses must develop intelligence. The many languages of line and color in his aesthetic applications and creative self-expression. This is the only reason Tagore placed arts and crafts, his drawings in musicals, playwrights, etc. at such an important place in his curriculum. Crafts and art, he said, are a natural outpouring of our deeper nature and spiritual meaning.
- **Positive communication between nature and humans:** Tagore argued that education should take place in an atmosphere of nature with all its beauty, colors, sounds, shapes and other expressions. bottom. In his opinion, education in a natural environment fosters intimacy with the world and the power of communication with nature. In his opinion, naturalism was God's manuscript. He emphasized that education must enable people to recognize a direct relationship with nature. It is intended to bring children closer to nature and closer to God.
- **Internationalism:** Tagore had a deep faith in the unity of people. He loved his faith by expressing it through his international college, Vishwa Bharati. Here he expressed his belief in the mutual communication of hearts and minds as the basis for world harmony. According to

him, Vishwa Bharati recognizes India's right to get the best from others. Here East and West will meet in unity, peace and understanding.
- **Tagore's Shantiniketan:** In 1901, near Calcutta, Tagore established this institution to put his educational ideas into practice. He gave him Shantiniketan or pear abode. Away from the hustle and bustle of city life and surrounded by the surrounding nature. The influence of green trees, fields, seasonal songs, chirping birds and other natural phenomena lifts the spirits of students.

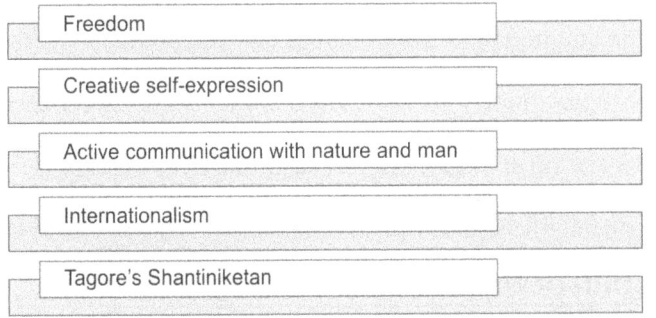

Fig. 3.12: Principles of the educational philosophy.

Principles Involved in Tagore Philosophy

- The medium of instruction must be the mother tongue.
- Children should enjoy complete freedom during their education.
- Children should be given opportunities for self-expression to develop their creativity.
- Children should be raised in the bosom of nature, far from cities.
- Children should be provided with opportunities for social contact during their development in the wild.
- Foreign education is not the basis for nature education.
- Through education, children should become familiar with the ideals and values of natural culture.
- Indian children should have an Indian education.
- Education should harmoniously develop all the abilities of the child.
- Indian philosophy and social ideals should be included in the curriculum.
- National education should be closely linked to national life.
- Children should not be forced to acquire knowledge through books. Instead, we should encourage learning from the original sources.
- Children should be given complete freedom to live in their natural environment and learn through their own experiences.

- Education should not be aimed at training children to be efficient farmers or craftsmen, but to bring them up into full human beings.
- Schools should be reformed.

Tagore's General Philosophy

- **Naturalist and Individualist:** Like Rousseau, Tagore is a naturalist and an individualist. He believes that every individual should be given the freedom to develop in his own way according to his innate abilities. He also believed that each person was different from others and from Enrique. He hypothesized that there was an underlying harmony between life and nature. He believed that the various manifestations of nature represented the Creator, and that through all these things reserved a spiritual bond between man and man, man and nature.
- **Belief in absolute values:** Like all other idealistic philosophers of his time, Tagore believed in absolute values and, like the saints and sages of ancient India, believed in absolute values. Implicitly believed in re-experiencing never believing in absolute values. He should live the truth that will free him from the bondage of death and make him one with the greater. He says he will find God. Let us live for the ultimate truth that frees us from the bondage of dust and enriches us not with things but with light, not with power but with love. He believed that in order to serve God, he needed to serve fellow humans, and that understanding human nature would allow him to reach his ultimate goal in life.
- **Tagore also believed in a universal spirit of humanity** that transcends and influences all individual spirits. Therefore, he believed that human beings encompass a variety of cultural and religious perspectives, policies and political systems. In doing so, he endorsed universalism and breathed the main peculiarities of nationality. He was international, but his internationality was economically or politically sound. It was spiritual. He faced the spiritual shackles of the universe. He imposed a belief in the fundamental unity of mankind and the brotherhood of mankind.
- **Spiritual harmony and salvation:** He has studied Indian philosophy intensively and lived according to it. Therefore, he rejoiced in spiritual harmony and salvation of souls, and pleaded for it according to the teachings of Indian philosophy. Tagore emphasized the spiritual upliftment, development of spiritual powers, and divine potential of man. Books and education should be signposts to the inner path.

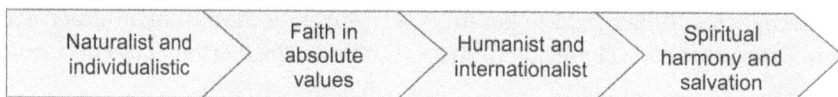

Fig. 3.13: Tagore's general philosophy.

Teaching

- **Teaching while walking:** Tagore believed that classroom-influenced education had no effect on a child's mind and body. He remained passively inert and inactive. Tagore believed that the mind remained alert while walking, and that children could easily grasp knowledge of things through direct contact with them.
- **Discussion and Q and A method:** Real education is not just stuffing books. It should be based on real problems. Therefore, he advocated the question-and-answer method to be very effective. Problems should be presented to children for discussion so that they can think and reason logically. In this way, they can develop their knowledge further and acquire basic knowledge.
- **Active methods:** Vishwa Bharati emphasized active methods as very important because they activate all the faculties of body and mind. He believed in activity methods that allowed physical movement during class and regular study.

Teacher's Role in Education

Only one person can teach another person. He gave teachers a very important place in his educational plan. Therefore, teachers should do the following activities:
- Believing in the purity and innocence of children, teachers should treat them with great love, affection, care and consideration.
- Teachers should provide an environment for children to engage in informative and constructive activities and to learn through their own experiences, rather than emphasizing learning from books.
- Teachers should always be engaged in stimulating children's creativity. To keep them engaged in constructive activities and exercises.

Evaluation of Tagore's Philosophy of Education

In his opinion man and nature have a unique synthesis. He wants to develop the child's natural emotions in a natural atmosphere away from the dirty and immoral atmosphere of the city. He also stressed that the upbringing of the child should meet his needs, but his love of nature should mean that Tagore was a pragmatist naturalist. Viewed nature as a powerful tool for the moral and spiritual development of children.

Tagore's philosophy of life bears the strong impression and influence of the highly religiously educated and philosophical family to which he belonged. He embraced an idealistic philosophy of life and adopted the highest ideals of truth, beauty and goodness as the main goals of education that every person should achieve. He emphasized the adaptation between nature and the human sole. In short, Tagore wanted to inculcate self-respect and dignity into manhood and value his soul. For that, moral and spiritual progress is essential. Therefore, he stressed that education should definitely facilitate his progress. In a nutshell, we can say that naturalism, idealism, humanism and internationalism are the foundations of his philosophy.

JOHN DEWEY'S PHILOSOPHY OF EDUCATION

John Dewey was a famous American philosopher psychologist and educator. He rose from the very beginning that traditional methods of instruction were not at all effective and that contracts of every life provided effective dynamic and unlimited learning situations. These very ideas formed the foundation of two educational theories formulated later by him. This outlook on education reflected the industrial revolution and the development of democracy. He believed in the dynamic nature of things and values. He changed with changing ideas through experience and experimentation, eventually emerging as a pragmatist. Today, he is at the forefront of educators around the world. His educational work is a great source of inspiration and helps us develop our experimental and scientific thinking.

Meaning of Education

Dewey teaches education, he said:
- Education is the holistic process by which communities and social groups, large and small, transmit their acquired power and aspirations to ensure their survival
- Education should help helpless young animals grow into happy, moral and productive human beings.
- Education is not something that is imposed on children and young people from the outside, but is the development of the innate capacities of human beings.
- The result of the educational process is the capacity for further education.
- Social environments are truly educational to the extent that individuals engage in or participate in common activities.

- Education is self-realization.
- All education begins with the participation of the individual in the social consciousness of his race.
- Education is the development of all the abilities that enable an individual to control his environment and realize his potential.
- Education is a life process, not preparation for future life.
- Education is the fundamental method of social progress and reform.
- It is conventional wisdom that character development is the last and most important. Character generally means power, social behavior, and organized social function. It means social performance and social concern or responsiveness.
- Education is the laboratory in which philosophical distinctions are embodied and tested.
- Education is the process of reconstructing experience, giving it more socialized value by increasing its social efficiency.
- It always has an end soon, and as long as the activity is educational it will reach that end.
- Education is a continuous process of adaptation, the goal of which is additional competencies that grow at each stage.

Dewey's Philosophy

Dewey's philosophy is a good combination of naturalism and idealism, and is based on Darwin's conception of evolution and William James' pragmatism. Like Darwin, he believes that the world is still in the process of formation, and that life in this world is a process of constant change and self-renewal. He believed that anything is good and that good things are useful. Truth is also something that works, that satisfies our purpose and satisfies our desires.

- **Dewey's practical philosophy:** According to Dewey, philosophy should not be interpreted in terms of other worldly speculations, but rather a general insight into the process of dynamic adaptation to the environment in which humans find themselves. It is intended to provide. Life is action, movement, and the object of knowledge is the change of the world. Knowledge deals with the constant activities of man in this earthly world.
- **Experimentalism:** Experimentalism is the key word in Dewey's scientific methodological approach. According to him, the core of the experimental method is to determine the meaning of what is observed through the conscious institution of modes of interaction. Dewey's is a company that believes in the universal application of experimental methods developed by modern science.

The new educational philosophy is experimental philosophy. The educator's job is to create experiences that are fun and foster desirable future experiences. A central problem for experiential educators is to select the kind of present experience that will live fruitfully and creatively in later experience. Continuity of experience is a philosophy of educational experience.

Fundamentals of Dewey's Educational Philosophy

- **Education as growth:** Growth is the actual function of education. It should lead to growth. Individuals are changing and growing personalities, and education is designed to foster growth. It is therefore the teacher's duty to awaken the instincts and abilities of children and provide them with appropriate development opportunities by providing them with solutions to problems that stimulate their thinking. In this way the thought grows, and with it the mind, giving it more thinking capacity.
- **Life is the product of activity and education** is born of educational activity. Pupils should be educated to actively participate in school social and community life and to lead cooperative and mutually supportive lives. They are intended to encourage people to face current issues and gain diverse experiences.
- **Education as social efficiency:** Humans are socially normal. He always needs knowledge, experience and attitudes of energy intensity in social systems. As a social being he is a citizen, growing up and thinking in the vast complexity of interactions and relationships. In this sense, education becomes a social process and social efficiency becomes the goal of education.
- **Education as the reconstruction of experience:** According to Dewey, experience is the only source of true knowledge. Experiences lead to further experiences, and each new experience requires modification, modification, or rejection of previous ones. Therefore, we need ongoing experiences that help humans grow physically, mentally, socially and morally. Education must create an environment that fosters continuity of experience. Only through experience can knowledge grow and behavior change occur.

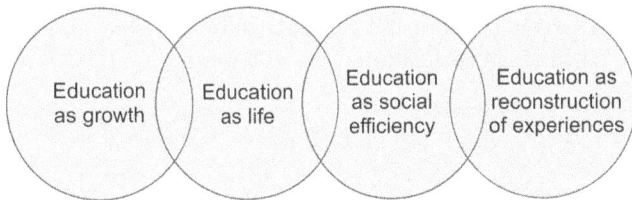

Fig. 3.14: Fundamentals of Dewey's educational philosophy.

Principles of Dewey's Philosophy of Education

- **Usefulness:** Curriculum should be based on the child's interest and initiation at different stages of development. In general the child shows four major interests—the desire to talk and exchange ideas discovery creation and artistic expression. The curriculum should be considered by these four elements and designed to include the teaching of reading and writing counting manual skill, science, music and other arts.
- **Flexibility:** The curriculum should be flexible and not predetermined and rigid. It must be capable of accommodating the change in the child's and inclinations.
- **Experimental:** The curriculum should be relevant to the child's contemporary experience and should double these by presenting different types of problem-solving activities that encourage the child to try solutions, can be strengthened.
- **Completion of life:** Where possible, the syllabus should only include subjects that may be relevant to the child's way of life at each stage of life. Being close to life helps create a unique void in the knowledge given and can create a certain harmony in teaching history, geography, mathematics, language, etc.

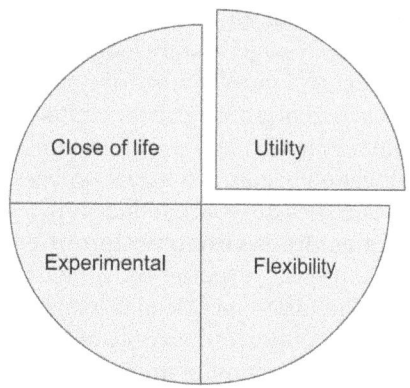

Fig. 3.15: Principles of Dewey's philosophy of education.

Benefits of Dewey's Theory of Education

- Offers a social theory of education rather than emphasizing the individual's isolated self.
- A fervent plea for the widespread use of experimental methods in education.
- There is the concept of democracy as a social psychological theory of progressive expansion.

Flaws in Dewey's Theory of Education

- The richness of the Bible can be confusing.
- Scripture is ambiguous.
- His writings coincide with the rise of so-called progressive education.
- It is very difficult to verify scientific objectivity and reconcile the majority.
- Neglecting religious education can destroy the roots of humanitarian values and social ethics.

Criticism of Dewey's Educational Philosophy

- The difficulty of not accepting the truth as permanent.
- Materialistic prejudices.
- Lack of educational goals.
- Excessive emphasis on individual differences.

LEARNING BY PRACTICE LIMITATIONS

According to RR Rusk one can only thank John Dewey for his great achievement in challenging the old static accumulation of knowledge and adapting education to the realities of modern life. The general principle underlying the developments in his philosophy and his application of these in education appears to be both philosophy and education should reflect the main currents of contemporary thought and incorporate the techniques that have so signally contributed to modern material and social progress.

CONCLUSION

Education is the deliberate and systematic influence exerted by the mature person upon the immature through instruction discipline and harmonious development of all the powers of the human being physical social intellectual aesthetic and spiritual according to their essential hierarchy by and for their individual and social uses and directed towards the union of the educators with his creator as the final end. Since the human is the subject of education the underlying concept of the origin the nature and the destiny of man will greatly influence the concept of education and its function that is held by the individual educator.

REVIEW QUESTIONS

Long Essays
1. Define philosophy, explain the relationship between philosophy and philosophy education.
2. Define nursing philosophy, explain individual nursing philosophy components.
3. Define naturalism, explain the characteristics, principles and forms of naturalism.
4. Define realism, explain the principles and forms of realism.
5. Define idealism, explain principles and characteristics of idealism.
6. Define perennialism, explain pedagogical application of perennial studies.

Short Essays
1. Objectives of philosophy of education studies.
2. Branches of philosophy.
3. Importance of philosophy in education.
4. Importance of nursing care philosophy.
5. Pragmatism: Principles and forms.
6. Progressivism: Types and principles.
7. Progressivism and teaching methods.
8. Elements of eclectic trends in education.
9. Eclecticism and the role of education.
10. Existentialism: Features and educational goals.
11. Gandhi's educational philosophy.
12. Gandhi's pedagogical experiment.
13. Principals involved in Tagore's philosophy.
14. Evaluation of Tagore's philosophy of education.
15. John Dewey's philosophy of education.

Short Answers
1. Meaning of philosophy.
2. Science and philosophy.
3. Philosophy and education.
4. Cultural connections.
5. Human bonds.
6. Naturalistic goals.
7. Contributions of realism to education.
8. Importance of idealism in nursing.
9. Educational principles of idealism.
10. Progressive goals in education.
11. Disadvantages of progressivism.
12. Forms of reconstructionism.
13. Existentialism and curriculum.
14. Tagore's Shantiniketan.
15. Principles of Dewey's philosophy of education.
16. Learning by practice.

Chapter 4

Teaching-Learning Process

Learning Objectives

- Importance of Teaching in the Learning Process
- Nature and Components of Teaching and Learning Processes
- Principles of Teaching and Learning
- Teaching-Learning Strategies
- Teaching and Learning Barriers
- Learning Theory
- Modern Learning Approaches

INTRODUCTION

This is where the teacher assesses comprehension needs, sets specific learning goals, develops teaching and memorization strategies, implements work plans and evaluates lesson results. It is a series of processes that Teaching is the process of listening to and intervening with people's needs, experiences and feelings in order for them to learn specific things. The main function of education is to make learning useful and meaningful. This process is completed as a result of the instructions. So the processes are mostly related to each other. Teaching is the way one person teaches or advises another.

MEANING

Teaching and learning are processes, not deliverables. Learning happens throughout life, including outside of school. Learning is the acquisition of new knowledge that understands skills and behaviors. The role of the education and learning process is very important in modeling young people who will serve the better people in the country, as young people will grow up and lead society. It shows the contact channels for developing the essential ways, skills, competencies, attitudes, integrity and gratitude to survive the times. Teaching and learning thus function as processes by which changes in behavioral structures are produced through development.

DEFINITION

- According to Robert Gagne, learning is "a change in human disposition or ability that persists over time and is not merely a process of development".
- A method of imparting knowledge from a teacher to a student. It can be developed through a variety of systems (e.g. how teachers are the only speakers, circulars where teachers and students contribute to class development).

TEACHING-LEARNING PROCESS

It is a continuous process consisting of various steps.
- **Difficult** to separate steps from each other. According to Wilson and Gallup, the following steps are described in the educational learning process (AIDCAS) as:
  - Attention
  - Interest
  - Desire
  - Conviction
  - Action
  - Satisfaction
- **Interest:** Focused attention enables teachers to address an individual's basic needs and motivations and interest them for further consideration of ideas. Advisory workers demonstrate how new practices contribute to farmers' welfare. The message should be presented attractively.
- **Desire:** Desire refers to the continuation of a farmers' interest in an idea or better practice until the interest

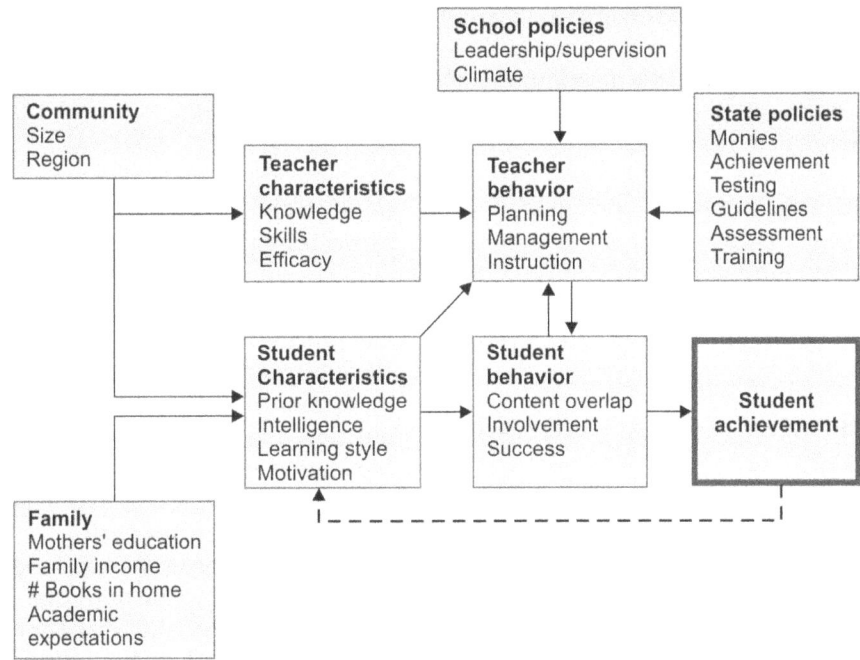

Fig. 4.1: Model of the teaching-learning process.

becomes a desire or motivating force. Advisory workers explain to farmers that the information applies directly to their situation and that this will meet their needs.

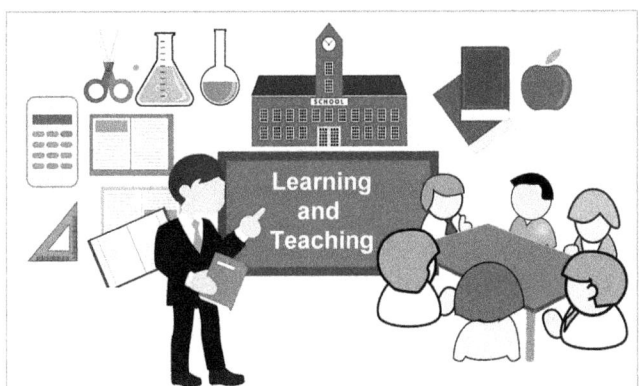

Fig. 4.2: Formal teaching and learning process.

- **Beliefs:** Actions follow people's wants and beliefs and their prospects for satisfaction. In this step, learners will understand what action is required and how to perform that action. Also, make sure the learner visualizes actions in relation to their particular situation and is confident in their ability to do things.,the effort is in vain.
- **Action:** It is the job of the extension worker to make it easy for the farmers to act. If new control measure is action oriented the recommended chemical should be available within the farmers reach. Necessary equipment should also be available. If action does not quickly follow the desire the new idea will fade away. Therefore, this phase should never be neglected.
- **Satisfied:** This is the end result of the process. Advisor follow-up helps farmers assess progress and strengths. Happiness helps you stay happier and stay active. Satisfaction is motivation for further learning. "Satisfied customers are the best publicity" applies to consultants as well. Her six steps above are often confused and lose their distinct identity. Of course, these steps are motivated.

IMPORTANCE OF TEACHING IN THE LEARNING PROCESS

The importance of teaching in the learning process is as follows:
- Learning is very important to education. Teaching is considered ineffective if learners are unable to learn and acquire knowledge. Teaching and learning are therefore processes that cannot exist without the other.
- The teaching and learning process enables teachers to organize and improve teaching skills and techniques for more effective teaching.
- The teaching and learning process allows trainers to refine and clarify their educational goals.
- The teaching and learning process is important to learners. Because it enables learners to acquire new

knowledge, develop responsible personalities, and prepare for the world.
- Learning is the key to education and the most important process for getting an education. The learning process of teaching is very important because there is no learning without teaching.
- The teaching and learning process makes learners aware of their goals and helps them achieve them.
- The process of teaching and learning takes into account the beliefs, ideas, needs and experiences of the individual and makes the individual adaptable to changing circumstances.

NATURE AND COMPONENTS OF TEACHING AND LEARNING PROCESSES

- The nature and components of teaching and learning processes in education are led by a trained individual teacher.
- **Communication:** The teaching and learning process involves a lot of communication and will only be successful if there is good interaction between the learner and the teacher.
- **Interactive process:** Teachers provide information to students and learners collect information. The educational process involves active interaction between learners and teachers.
- **Organized system:** The teaching and learning process takes place in a professional setting and in an organized way.
- **Overall development:** The teaching and learning process contributes to the overall development of the learner.
- **A continuous process:** The process of education and learning is endless, continuing from birth to death. So it is an ongoing process.
- **Non-discrimination:** There is no discrimination against individuals based on race, color, gender, or any other criteria in the teaching and learning process. It is a universal process.

PRINCIPLES OF TEACHING AND LEARNING

- Students' beliefs or perceptions of intelligence and ability influence cognitive function and learning.
- Students already know influences their learning.
- Students' cognitive development and learning are not limited by their general developmental level.
- Because learning is contextual, the generalization of learning to new contexts is not spontaneous and must be facilitated.
- Acquisition of sustainable knowledge and skills is based on practice.
- Clear explanations and timely feedback to students are important for learning.
- Student self-regulation supports learning and can teach self-regulation skills.
- Student creativity is encouraged.
- Students are more likely to enjoy learning and to do better if they have intrinsic motivation rather than extrinsic motivation to achieve something.
- Setting coping goals over performance goals will help students perform better in the face of challenging tasks and process information more intensively.
- What teachers expect of their students influences their motivation and their chances of experiencing learning outcomes.
- Moderately challenging short-term (proximal) specific goals are more motivating than long-term (distal) general and overly challenging goals.
- Learning takes place in several social contexts.
- Interpersonal relationships and communication are essential not only to the social and emotional development of students, but also to the teaching and learning process.
- Emotional well-being influences the development of learning and educational outcomes.
- Expectations for classroom behavior and social interaction are learned and can be taught using proven behavioral principles and effective teaching.
- Effective classroom management is based on (a) setting and communicating high expectations, (b) maintaining positive relationships at all times, and (c) providing a high level of support to students.
- Formative and summative assessments are important and useful, but require different approaches and interpretations.
- Student skills, knowledge and competence are best measured using psychological science-based assessment methods with clearly defined criteria for quality and fairness.
- Evaluation of rating data is dependent on clear, reasonable and fair interpretation.

Principles of effective teaching and learning
- Equips learners for life in its broadest sense
- Engages with valued forms of knowledge
- Recognizes the importance of prior experience and learning
- Requires the tutor to 'scaffold' learning
- Uses assessment as a means of advancing learning
- Promotes the active engagement of the learner
- Fosters both individual and social processes and outcomes
- Recognizes the significance of informal learning
- Depends on and encourages tutors continuing to learn
- Demands consistent policy frameworks with support for teaching and leaning as their primary focus

Principles of Learning

- A student's prior knowledge can either facilitate or hinder learning.
- Students organize their knowledge influences how they learn and apply what they know.
- Student motivation determines what they learn.
- To develop proficiency, students need to acquire component skills, integrate them, and know when to apply what they have learned.
- The combination of targeted practice and targeted feedback improves the quality of student learning.
- A student's current developmental level interacts with the course's social, emotional and intellectual environment to influence learning.
- To become self-motivated learners, students must learn to monitor and adjust their approach to learning.

Teaching Principles

The following principles reflect current research on effective teaching practice.

- Effective teaching involves acquiring relevant knowledge about students and using that knowledge to influence course design and classroom instruction.

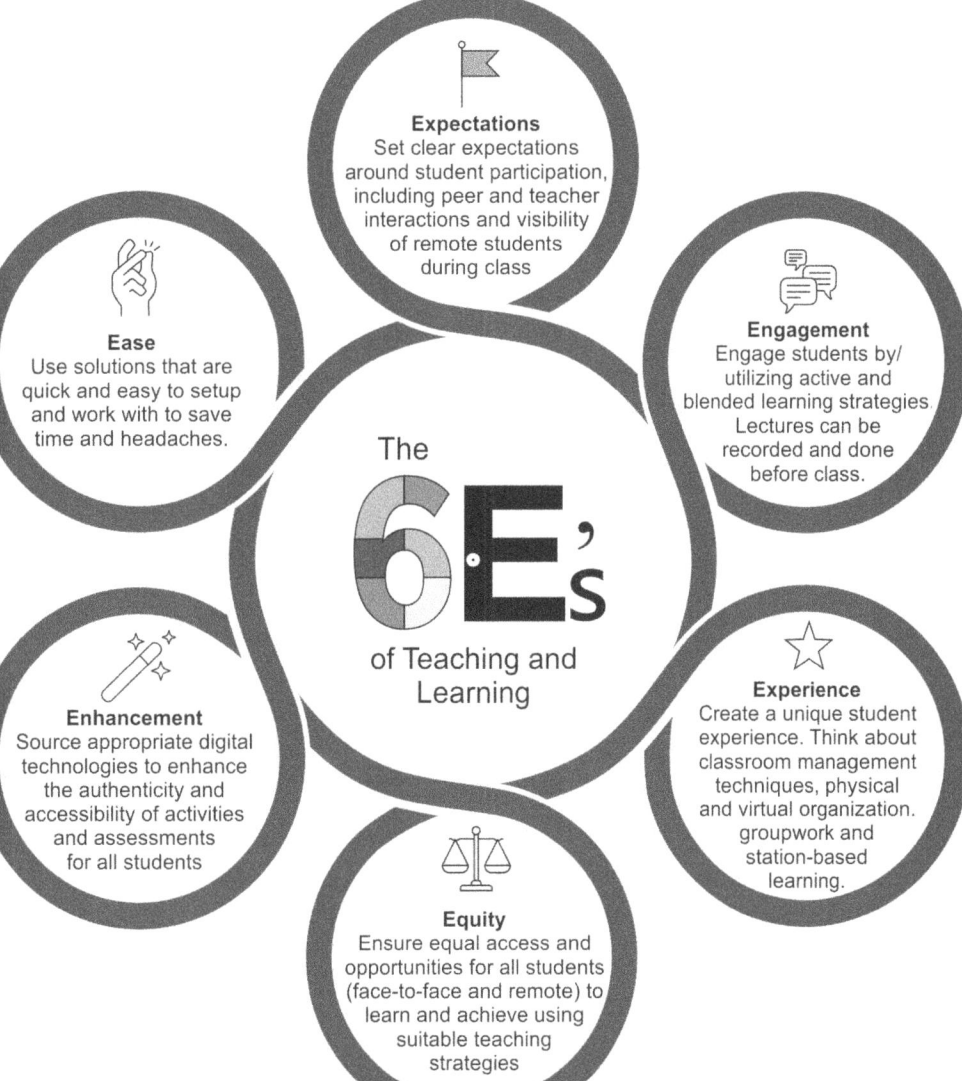

Fig. 4.3: 6E's in teaching and learning.

- Effective teaching involves coordinating the three main components of teaching: assessment of learning outcomes and teaching activities.
- Effective teaching includes setting clear expectations about learning goals and strategies.
- Effective education involves prioritizing knowledge and skills to focus on.
- Effective education involves recognizing and breaking down your blind spots with a professional.
- Effective teaching includes employing appropriate leadership roles that support learning goals.
- Effective teaching involves incremental course improvement based on reflection and feedback.

TEACHING-LEARNING STRATEGIES

Lesson Plan Formats 6E and S (engage, explore, explain, elaborate, evaluate, extend and standards) were developed by teachers in consultation with educators at their institution and are based on constructivist teaching models. The lesson plan is based on the constructivist model of education, where the activities and sections of the plan are designed to allow students to continuously add (or build on) new knowledge to their existing knowledge.

Each of the 6E's represents a learning stage, and each stage begins with the letter 'E'. The 6E's allow students and teachers to experience activities together, build on previous knowledge and experience, construct meaning, and continually assess conceptual understanding.

- **Engagement:** Engagement activities should connect past and current learning experiences. Anticipate activities and direct student thinking to the learning outcomes of the current activity. Students must mentally engage with the conceptual processes or skills they learn. Each lesson plan has a "must-have" question that forms the basis of the survey. The section usually contains a few key questions to guide some of the research in the discovery section.
- **Examine:** Here students explore the topic more thoroughly. It is important to give students the opportunity to 'free move' through the material so that they are not overwhelmed. They need direction and teachers can ask important questions, listen to their interactions, and walk around to keep them on task.
- **Explain:** At this stage, students are able to explain the concepts they have explored, also will have the opportunity to verbalize your conceptual understanding and demonstrate new skills and behaviors. This stage also provides teachers with an opportunity to introduce formal definitions and descriptions of concepts, processes, skills, or behaviors.
- **Elaborate:** Here students are expected to work directly on the given task. An opportunity to demonstrate the application of new information and present your findings and conclusions to others. Now is a good time to submit materials for assessment, make presentations, and complete projects or assignments.
- **Assessment:** Assessment is expected to continue throughout the process, but this is the section where the teacher assesses the learning done. Students usually turn in assignments and homework at this time. At this stage, it is very important that students are encouraged to undertake group assessment self-assessments and develop their own tools for doing so.
- **Extensions:** This section provides some suggestions for getting students out of the classroom. The purpose is to explore how to make your insights available to others or how to apply your understanding to new and unfamiliar situations. This type of activity usually stems from enthusiasm for what has been accomplished. This section is very student-driven, but teachers may wish to gently suggest that students submit their work to contests or display it outside their school.
- **Standards:** Standards are now integrated from lesson plans into lesson plans.

In this area, lessons are compared to state and/or federal standards. This information is primarily for teachers and should provide the information necessary to integrate the lesson into the local school district or school curriculum.

TEACHING AND LEARNING BARRIERS

Learning barriers are anything that interrupts or hinders learning. This hinders how students participate in learning, how they encode information from information stores, and how they recall it during practice. Identifying learning barriers can be difficult as they come in many shapes and sizes and are often unique to each student.

Classroom Barriers

These learning barriers are about the physical structure of the classroom and how you learn in it. This includes:
- Distractions or interruptions that interfere with student concentration.
- Instructional routines that are too demanding or too permissive for students.
- Expectations too high or too low for students to achieve.
- Layouts that do not provide students with adequate space to study most effectively.

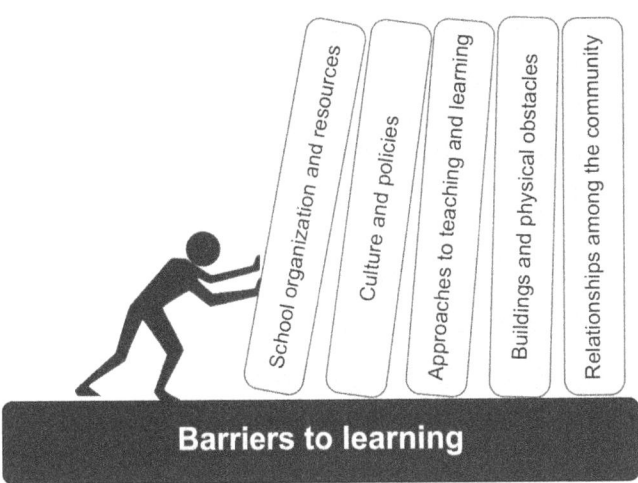

Fig. 4.4: Barriers to learning.

Emotional Barriers

Emotions can affect the enthusiasm students bring to class, the amount of knowledge they absorb, and the effort they put into their work. Some emotions are productive, others inhibit learning.
- Fear of failure can lead to anxiety
- Refusal to learn new things
- Fear of change can make students resist new methods, approaches, or perspectives
- History of struggling to understand and apply certain concepts.

Barriers to Motivation

Learning is not a passive effort. Students have to work on it too. If the students do not want it, the lesson does not work.
- Lessons are not relevant to my interests or life.
- I see no goal, reward, or purpose behind learning what you teach.
- Say nothing about how the learning journey progresses.

Prioritize Barriers

Students have the fewest strengths and weaknesses in how they absorb information and express themselves. Barriers arise here:
- Students are not receiving instruction in a medium or format that is meaningful to them.
- Credits are only accepted in one or two formats and several accepted only at critical points.

Accessibility Barriers

This is a big problem because learning disabilities come in all shapes and sizes. Most of the time they are beyond the control of the student or teacher, but that does not mean they are unresponsive. How technology affects student achievements?

Overcoming Learning Barriers

During education, most learners face a variety of learning barriers. For example, consider a student who left his textbook at home, or an employee who never received the preparation notes for a training workshop. All of these can be considered barriers to learning. If learners cannot fully participate in learning activities, they cannot truly engage in learning. In the adult learning environment, the barriers to learning are varied and totally unpredictable.

LEARNING THEORY

Classical Conditioning

The name of classical conditioning is Ivan P Pavlov (1849–1936). In the late 1890s, this famous Russian physiologist began establishing many of the basic principles of this form of conditioning. Classical conditioning is also known as respondent conditioning or Pavlovian conditioning.

Concepts of Classical Conditioning

- Dogs not only salivated when they actually ate, but they also noticed humans noticed their meals.
- All animals and humans have an innate set of stimulus-response associations that are established at birth before learning occurs.
- Classical conditioning is based on these innate neurological connections.
- Through learning, penetrating neutral stimuli come to assume some of the same properties as unconditioned stimuli. In this case, the previous neutral stimulus is called the conditioned stimulus (cs) and the response it elicits is called the conditioned response (cr).
- Pavlov described the processes by which associations are acquired and the source of more general or complex behaviors, and how learned responses are unlearned or erased, including higher-order conditioning and annihilation.

Principles of Classical Conditioning

- **Acquisition:** The process by which a stimulus triggers a conditioned response. To see how this happens, Pavlov conducted experiments to see if salivation could be generated in response to previously neutral stimuli. This process, which involves the gradual disappearance of the conditioned response to, is called extinction.
- **Stimulus generalization:** Refers to a particular state of learned behavior in which individualized conditions are

created for responses to particular stimuli, resulting in the same responses to other stimuli of a similar nature.
- **Stimulus discrimination:** Stimulus discrimination is the opposite of stimulus generation. Here, subjects learn to react differently in different situations as opposed to reacting in their usual way.
- **Association:** The repetition of the conditioned stimulus following the unconditioned stimulus and the resulting response must occur without exception.
- **Reinforcement:** It is not only the association between two stimuli and responses that is important, but it is the effects of reinforcement that play a role in conditioning. The food that is reinforced in this case reinforces the conditioned stimulus and ties it into the unconditioned response, ultimately turning it into the conditioned response.

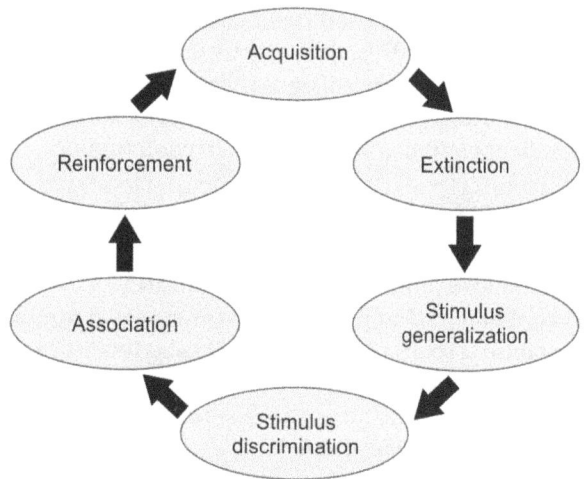

Fig. 4.5: Principles of classical conditioning.

Experiment by Pavlov

- Pavlov began studying this phenomenon, which he called "conditioning." The type of conditioning emphasized is classical and was later renamed classical conditioning because it is quite different from the conditioning emphasized by other psychologists. I left it alone and tried it on the lab bench.
- Observers were kept out of the dog's field of vision, but were able to view the experiment with the help of a set of mirrors.
- Every time you feed your dog and ring the bell, your dog's mouth will automatically salivate. The amount of saliva secreted was measured by repeatedly ringing the bell and offering the food.
- After several attempts, I rang the bell without feeding the dog. Again, the amount of saliva secreted was recorded and measured. They found that ringing a bell (artificial stimulus) caused dogs to salivate (natural response) even without food (natural stimulus).
- Therefore, the above experiments demonstrate four key elements of the conditioning process. They are spontaneous or unconditioned stimuli, unconditioned responses, conditioned stimuli, and conditioned responses.
- Pavlov's theory of conditioning thus views learning as habit formation and is based on the principles of association and substitution.

John Watson's Conditioning Theory

- Watson (1878-1958), the father of behaviorism, supported Pavlov's ideas about conditioned responses. Watson sought to demonstrate the role of conditioning in generating and eliminating emotional responses such as fear.
- When a child gets his or her first injection in the doctor's office, the needle sticks and the child cries. If he received more injections the next day at the same pharmacy from the same doctor, the child would cry when he went to the doctor and even walk past the pharmacy later.
- Most of our attitudes toward people and situations, early verbal responses, many components of complex skills, and a wide variety of emotional responses may be everyday examples of conditioned responses.

Operant Conditioning

Operant conditioning refers to the type of process in which reinforcement makes a response more likely or more frequent.

- Operant conditioning, also known as instrumental conditioning, is a behavior by the learner that results in a change of environment that makes the behavior more likely or more likely to be repeated in the future.
- An environmental event resulting from an instrumental response that increases the likelihood of that response occurring again is called reinforcement.
- Positive reinforcement is a stimulus or event that increases the likelihood that a response will be repeated if the response is dependent.
- Negative reinforcement is an event stimulus that increases the likelihood that a response will occur again or termination is dependent on the response.
- In instrumental or operant conditioning, shaping refers to the process of learning complex responses by first learning a series of simple responses that lead to complex responses.
- Each step is learned using contingent positive reinforcement, each building on the previous step until a complex response occurs and is reinforced.

- In instrumental or operant conditioning, processes that do not reinforce responses are called extinction. After learning, responses are less likely to occur if the reinforcement is response independent.
- In instrumental or operant conditioning, reinforcement that occurs each time a particular response occurs is called continuous reinforcement.
- However, enhancement of operant conditioning is often on a specific schedule and not all responses are enhanced. To illustrate the concept of reinforcement schedules, fixed-ratio (FR), fixed-interval (FI), variable-ratio (VR), and variable-interval (VI) schedules are discussed.

Skinner's Operant Experiments

- Operant conditioning experiments conducted by BF. Skinner used a specially designed box called the Skinner box.
- Inside the box was an iron bar. To get food, the rat had to push down on an iron bar. For each such squeeze, a food pill was thrown from the chute onto the pallet.
- Here, the rat learns to push the bar after following several tracks, then runs to the pallet to secure food.
- If the bar is not pushed, the animal will not gain reinforcement and will not learn the habit. However, the basic elements that work in these two forms of learning are the same.

Difference between Classical and Operant Conditioning

Classical conditioning	Operant conditioning
• It helps in the learning of respondent behavior.	• It helps in the learning of operant behavior.
• It is called type - S conditioning because of the emphasize on the stimulus.	• It is called R conditioning because of the emphasis on the response.
• This beginning is being made with help of specific stimuli that bring certain response.	• Here, beginning is made with the responses as they occur naturally or unnaturally, shaping them into existence.
• Strength of conditioning is usually determined by the magnitude of the condition response.	• Here strength of conditioning is shown by the response rate.

Enhancement Plan

- **Continuous reinforcement schedules:** These are 100% reinforcement schedules, where every correct response of the organism during learning acquisition is assigned to reinforcement or reward.

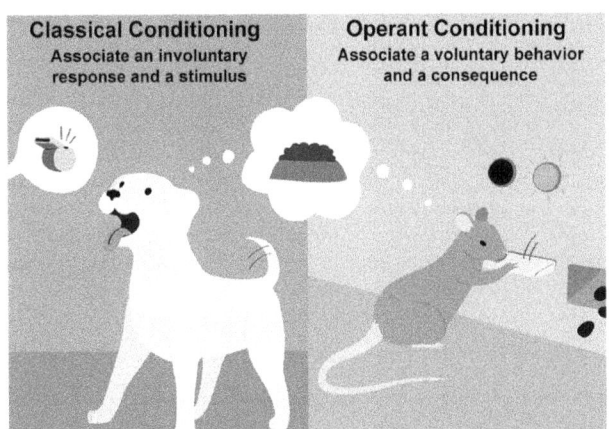

Fig. 4.6: Difference between classical and operant conditioning.

- **Fixed internal schedule:** This schedule will reinforce after a certain number of responses.
- **Variable schedule of reinforcement:** When reinforcement is given after different times or different numbers of responses, it is called variable schedule of reinforcement.

Effects of Operant Conditioning

- The principles of operant conditioning can be successfully applied to behavior modification tasks.
- Human personality development tasks can be successfully manipulated by operant conditioning. According to Skinner, "We are the ones who have been rewarded."
- Operant conditioning theory does not attribute motivation to internal processes of the organism.
- Operant conditioning emphasizes the importance of timing in the process of behavioral reinforcement.
- This theory advocated not learning undesirable behavior and avoiding punishment for shaping desirable behavior.
- At its most effective application, operant conditioning theory has contributed significantly to the development of machine learning and program learning.

Learn Thorndike's Law

- **Law of frequency:** When an activity is repeated several times. It requires a permanently established trend. Repeated answers have power in favor of one or the other.
- **Law of reality:** In a series of activities, the animals at the end of the series are kept fresher in the animal's repertoire, so when placed in similar shows a tendency to respect.
- **Law of effect:** This is perhaps the most important of all laws. It states that responses that give the organism the satisfaction of success are the ones that are most likely to be modified. On the other hand, if you don't get a satisfactory answer, it tends to be discarded.

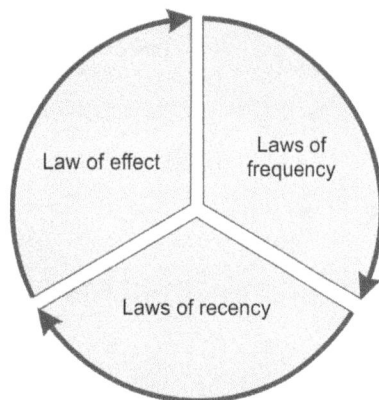

Fig. 4.7: Thorndike's law of learning.

Trial and Error Learning

The theory of trial error learning, popularized by Thorndike, emphasizes that we learn through the mechanism of trial and error. In striving to behave right, people try in so many ways, and they can make so many mistakes before any accidental success occurs. Subsequent trials allow you to avoid the wrong path, repeat the right path, and finally learn the right path.

The Concept of Trial and Error

- When you are put in a new situation or faced with a new problem, you have to look for solutions that you may not understand at first.
- This learning is slow, wasteful and unintelligent. It takes more time and energy than learning higher types.
- Learning involves making new connections between stimuli and responses. These new connections are being created gradually through a process of blind trial and error.
- In this type of learning, which is very common in animals, arbitrary and aimless responses are initially assumed, followed by random correct responses after some time, and finally imprinting on the animal's neuromuscular system.
- At first there are random movements, gradually the number of random movements decreases along with the error, and finally the target is reached. Therefore, improvement comes from repetition.
- The principles involved in the process of how learners stabilize new response patterns provide the key to understanding learning through trial and error.

Thorndike's Trial and Error Experiment

- Thorndike's typical experiment used a puzzle box that could be opened by a mechanical device. Press the button on the bottom.
- If a hungry cat in this puzzle box and place food such as fish outside the box within reach of the animal, the cat will have a very hard time getting out of the box.
- During this process, she performed a series of random activities that did not lead to resolution of the problem.
- She may try to push off the bar, bite, scratch the floor with her nails, or try to walk around. As part of the new reaction pattern, her foot can accidentally fall on the button, causing the door to open.
- Of all the cat's responses, she turned out to be the only one correct. For example, hold the button down with her front paw.
- You will be able to eat strengthening foods that appear immediately after this response. Success on the first trial may be pure coincidence.
- But the next time the animal is placed in the same situation, the random response is greatly reduced, it successfully solves the random response problem, and it takes less time to successfully solve the problem.
- Thus, with practice, mistakes and wrong responses are gradually eliminated and correct responses are strengthened.
- When a person learns to swim or ride a bicycle, the initial pattern of behavior shows a large number of random responses. With practice, all incorrect movements are gradually eliminated.

Thorndike Law Learning: Trial and Error Learning Stage

- **First drive:** In this experiment, it was hunger that intensified at the sight of food put in get out of the box.
- **Lock:** The cat is locked in the box with the door closed.
- **Random movements:** The cat kept trying to get out of the box.
- **Random success:** This tedious random move allowed the cat to accidentally open the door.
- **Choice:** Little by little, the cat learned the correct way to use the handle. It chose the right way to manipulate the bolt from deliberate motion.

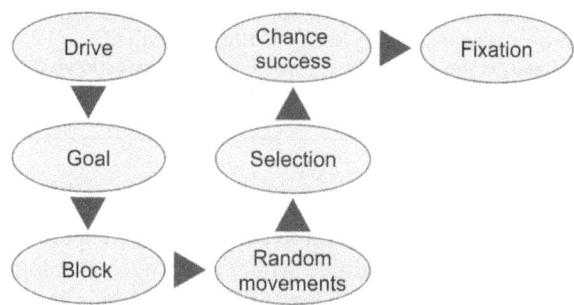

Fig. 4.8: Trial and error learning stages.

- **Fixed:** At least the cat learned to open the door correctly by eliminating all wrong answers and correcting only the correct ones. Now he definitely could open the door or learned how to open it.

Theorist Background
- The eminent psychologist Edward L Thorndike (1874-1949) is known as the founder of the theory of trial-and-error learning.
- Thorndike wrote his learning link. The mind is a relationship system.
- Thorndike called his experimental cat learning trial and error learning. He argued that learning is nothing more than memorizing the correct answers and weeding out the wrong ones by trial and error.

Effects of Trial and Error Learning
- Whatever you want to learn or teach, you must first identify what you should remember and what you should forget.
- Thinking and learning at one point in time must be connected to past experiences and learning on the one hand and to future learning on the other, using associative chains and attachment mechanisms in the learning process.
- Learners seek to understand the similarities and differences between different types of responses to stimuli and use comparisons and contrasts to apply what they have learned in one situation to other similar situations.
- Learners should be encouraged to complete tasks independently. He has to try different solutions to the problem before arriving at the correct one.

Learning by Insight
Gestalt psychologists offer a very different account of the learning process. They do not believe that learning is a process of blind habit formation. According to Kohler, the learning processes studied by Thorndike and behaviorists take place in highly unnatural and restricted situations that deny the animal the possibility of having a clear perception of the overall situation.

Definition
Insight can be defined as the sudden awareness of relationships between various elements that were previously seen independently of each other.

Theorist Background
- Insightful learning introduced by a group of German psychologists called the Gestalt. Wolfgan Kohler, in

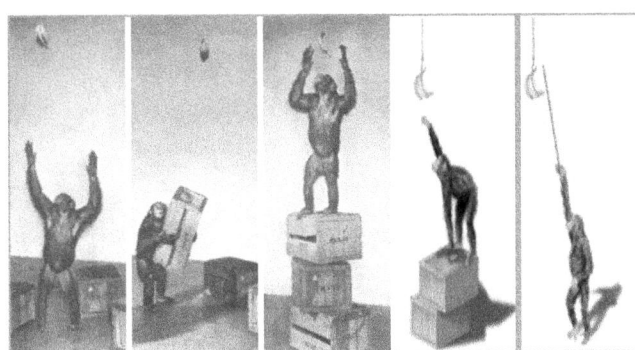

Fig. 4.9: Learning by insight.

particular, developed a theory of learning known as insightful learning.
- The closest English translation of Gestalt is the composition, or, more simply, the organized whole rather than the collection of parts. Gestalt psychologists view the learning process as a Gestalt.
- In a practical sense, Gestalt psychology is primarily concerned with the nature of perception.
- Gestalt psychologists have attempted to interpret learning as a goal-oriented, exploratory and creative endeavor, rather than as trial-and-error or a simple stimulus-response mechanism.

Insight Learning Concepts
- Requires mental exploration and understanding of learning content. It implies some insight, some awareness of the consequences of actions.
- Learners recognize key features of problematic responses or situations and use their intellect to connect appropriate responses to solutions.
- The principles of any learning process depend on the nature of the learning situation.
- In his learning experiments, Kohler presented different kinds of situations and ultimately came to completely different conclusions about the principles of the learning process.
- Insight involves a perceptual reorganization of the elements in your environment so that you suddenly see new relationships between objects and events.
- You are purposeful and focused on problem solving. When an organism finds itself in a problematic situation, it begins to deal with it. Such coping includes recognition of the problem.

Kohler's Insight Learning Experiments
Some of Kohler's famous experiments on chimpanzees were designed as follows:

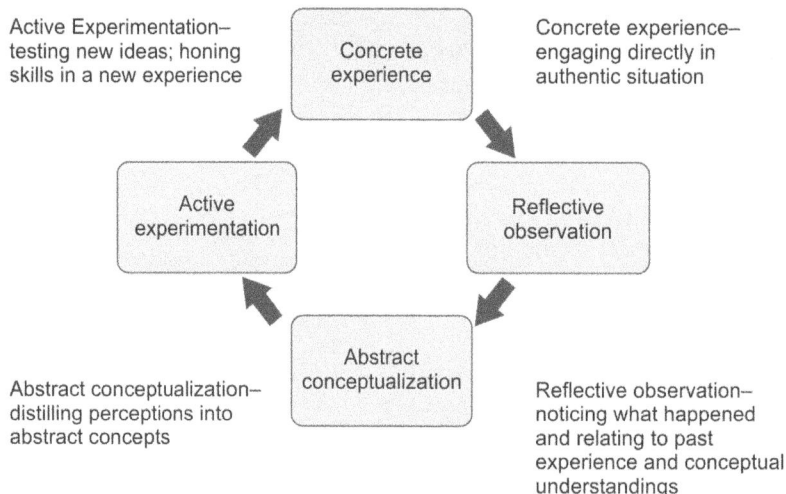

Fig. 4.10: Kolb's cycle of experimental learning.

- We put a hungry chimpanzee in a cage and hung a bunch of bananas from the ceiling.
- Some wooden boxes were lying around. A chimpanzee jumps high to try to reach a banana. When he fails to reach the highest point, he tries to jump off the ceiling.
- When this too proved to be a failure, he gave up the effort for a while. Suddenly the chimpanzee had a new idea and started stacking boxes.
- When I finally reached the top, I managed to grab a banana.
- In the above situation, there was no evidence of blind trial and error resulting in the corrected response over time.

MODERN LEARNING APPROACHES

Experiences Learning

Experiential learning is an active learning process in which students "learn by doing" and reflect on their experiences. Experiential learning activities include handson laboratory experiments, internships, fieldwork, study abroad, undergraduate studies, studio performance, leadership, and other professional and intellectual skills.

History

Experiential learning was developed in his 1980s by David A Kolb with the help of his Ron Fry and other colleagues at the Massachusetts Institute of Technology. The idea behind experiential learning is that what you learn from an educational experience can be applied to what you learn later. In this context, what one knows is what one has done or knows to be true. This is what man does, what he experiences, and what he has to learn.

Elements

- Experiences are carefully selected according to their learning potential (that is, they provide students with opportunities to practice and deepen new skills, or new unpredictable experiences that support new learning). situations, or arise from the natural consequence of mistakes.
- During experiential learning, learners are actively engaged in activities such as asking questions, experimenting, being curious, problem-solving, taking responsibility, being creative, and building meaning. You are asked to be involved, to take the initiative, to make decisions, and to take responsibility result.
- Reflecting on one's own experiential and post-experiential learning is an integral part of the learning process. This reflection leads to analysis, critical thinking and synthesis.
- The learner is intellectually, emotionally, socially and/or physically involved, giving the impression that the learning task is authentic.
- Relationships are developed and nurtured from the learner to the self-learner, to others, and from the learner to the world at large.

Process

Kolb's (1984) learning cycle describes an experiential learning process. This process includes the integration of:
- **Activities:** Application of knowledge to 'real world' environments.
- **Reflection:** Analysis and synthesis of knowledge and activities to create new knowledge.

Principles of Experiential Learning

- Engaged in playing
- This experience is a handson, feel-based dialogue. Experiences can be planned or spontaneous. Little or no tuition is required. Experiences include experiences involving individual or group participation.
- Experience is direct experience with focused reflection and is based on past knowledge and experience. It requires active participation in the construction of meaning and fosters collaboration and exchange of ideas and perspectives among participants.
- Learners actively reflect on this experience through discussion, questioning or journaling in individual thought groups. Engage in group processing and discussion, including debriefing and reflective questions, provided by a facilitator who creates personal meaning for the group and challenges the group to transfer learning into new contexts.

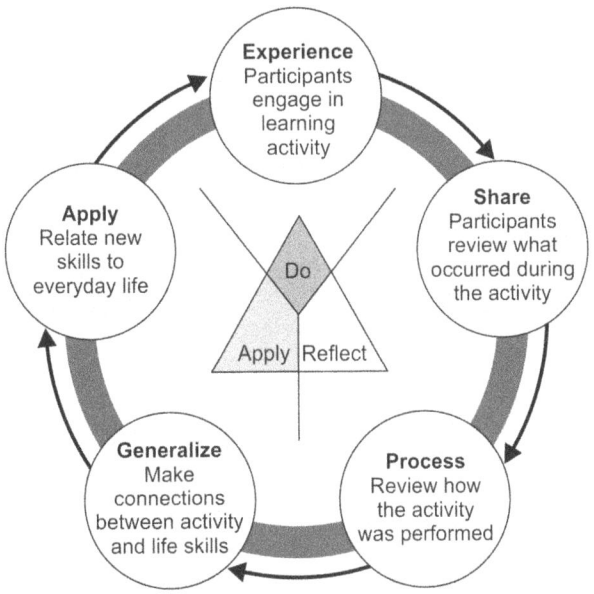

Fig. 4.11: Principles of experiential learning.

- Learning can draw conclusions and make sense of what the learner has experienced. This includes the ability to relate one's own experiences to those of others. Learners can develop theories, models, or concepts about their experiences. Learners can create new questions that lead to the next experience or exploration. Learners can apply their newly learned knowledge to their next experience.

During the experiential learning, the moderator has the following tasks:

- Please select the appropriate experience that meets the above criteria.
- Raise concerns, set limits, support learners, provide appropriate assistance, ensure physical and mental safety, and facilitate the learning process. Recognize and encourage opportunities to deal with situations, experiment (without jeopardizing the well-being of others), and find solutions.
- Helps learners notice the connections between theory and experience from one context to another and encourages this repeated testing.

Forms of Experiential Learning

- **Internship:** A broader term used to describe experiential learning activities, often including other terms such as collaborative learning and field experience. It is often a credible and independent activity in a student's area of interest, unrelated to theoretical research. It is usually assessed by faculty and supervised by a nonfaculty employer. Students can work with Handson professionals, complete projects, attend public events, conduct interviews, and observe constituents and staff. Students may or may not be paid for this experience. When attending facetoface classes, students may volunteer a few hours a week at institutions that support extracurricular activities, track professionals in the field, or observe people in natural settings.
- **Service learning:** This term is used to indicate an optional or mandatory extracurricular experience/project of community service associated with a course, or a separate and credible experience. The location could be the wider community outside the university or a community embedded in cocurricular activities. In these experiences, students participate in organized service activities that meet identified community needs, gain a better understanding of course content, develop a broader understanding of the field and an enhanced sense of civic responsibility. Reflect on your service activities to gain.
- **Coeducation:** Often part of a specialized program, students can gain relevant work experience over several semesters that are steeped in coursework. Students alternate between work and study, typically spending several weeks on campus (usually full-time) and being employed off-campus for several weeks (usually full-time). Alternatively, cooperative education may occur when students attend part-time classes simultaneously and work part-time in consecutive academic years in a deliberately planned and coordinated manner. If the experience meets credit criteria (i.e., faculty supervision, reflective elements, evidence of learning), students receive dual education academic credit. The purpose of

these programs is to develop students' professional skills and knowledge.
- **Clinical training:** This is a more defined internship experience in which students apply the didactic and experiential skills learned most commonly in a medical or legal setting under the supervision of a licensed practitioner. It is often a separate creditable course associated with related theory courses, or an experience culminating after a series of theory courses.
- **Teaching students:** This experience is unique to students in pre-vocational teacher education who have the required and valued experience in supervised instruction.
- **Internships:** A cousin of internships, this form of experiential learning is usually a course or a student exercise that provides Handson experience in a work environment (whether paid or unpaid) and preemployment occupational experience. Provides theoretical studies including supervisory experience as part of training.
- **Undergraduate research experience:** Students act as research assistants and collaborators on faculty projects.
- **Community-based research:** Faculty and students cooperate with local organizations to conduct studies to meet the needs of a particular community. Students gain direct experience in the research process.
- **Field work:** Supervised student research or practice carried out away from the institution and in direct contact with the people natural phenomena or other entities being studied. Fieldwork is particularly common in fields such as anthropology, archaeology, sociology, social work, geosciences, and environmental studies.
- **Study abroad:** Usually students complete a course at a university in another country. A component of experiential learning is cultural immersion, offering new challenges for navigating life in a new place. Coursework related to study abroad may also include internships and service learning experiences.

Importance: The experiential educational opportunities they have:
- Better understanding of course materials
- Broader view of the world and appreciation of community
- Personal skills, Insights into interests, passions and values
- Opportunities to work with different organizations and people
- Positive professional practice and skills
- Satisfaction in helping meet community needs
- Confidence and leadership skills.

Experiential Learning Styles

Experiencing: Experiencing styles connect warmly and intuitively, characterized by your ability to work in teams and build trust with others and also used to expressing emotions.
- **Imagining:** When using the imagining style, one is sensitive and creatively attentive to trust. They exhibit confidence and empathy for others. I am comfortable with ambiguous situations and enjoy helping others generate new ideas and create visions for the future.
- **Reflect:** When using the reflect style, you can be patient and reserved and be the center of attention for others. They listen with an open mind and gather information from a variety of sources. You can look at the problem from different perspectives and identify the underlying problem or issue.
- **Analysis:** Be structured, methodical and precise when analyzing. Plan ahead to minimize errors, consolidate information to see the big picture, and use critical thinking to understand the situation. Be methodical when analyzing details and data.
- **Thinking:** Your thinking style is skeptical, structured, linear and controlled. Use quantitative tools to analyze problems and formulate arguments with logic. Knows how to effectively communicate ideas and exercise independent judgment.
- **Decide:** Be realistic, accountable, and candid when using a decision-making style. Find practical solutions to problems and set performance goals. Focus can be selected.
- **Acting:** When it comes to acting, you are assertive, performance-oriented, and brave over time. Commit to your goals and objectives and find a way to reach them on time. Plans can be executed with limited resources.
- **Initiate:** The initiate style allows you to be self-motivated, shake off losses and "failures", and try again. They actively seize opportunities and participate without hesitation.
- **Balancing:** Balancing styles recognize blind spots in situations and bridge differences between people. You are imaginative and able to adapt to changing priorities.

Stages of the Experiential Learning Cycle

- **Tangible experiences:** Tangible experiences represent the actual experiences we learn. This is where we try new things, run into problems, and leave our comfort zones. These experiences can be anything in your personal or professional life. Through experience, we learn from our successes and failures.
- **Reflective observation:** Next, we need to reflect to learn from our experiences. The "reflective observation"

phase of the experiential learning cycle is reflecting on experiences that involve both behavior and emotion. At this stage, reflect on the experience. You can look back at what went well and what could be improved. It is also an opportunity to observe how things are done differently and learn from each other.
- **Abstract conceptualization:** Identifying and understanding the characteristics of an experience will help you determine what you can change next time. This is the time to plan and brainstorm steps for success.
- **Active experimentation:** The active experimentation phase of the learning cycle allows you to test your ideas. It is time to test our action plan in the real world.

Reflective Learning

Reflective learning is a form of education in which students reflect on their learning experiences. One theory of reflective learning calls it a deliberate and complex process of recognizing the role of social context and experience. The goal of this process is to clarify and understand oneself, which leads to a change in conceptual perspective.

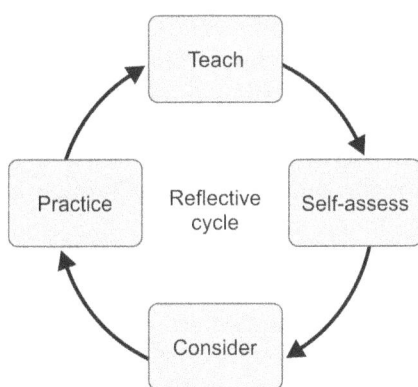

Fig. 4.12: Reflective cycle phases.

Examples of Reflective Learning

Doing something new whether there are gaps in knowledge, learn information that accompanies your hobbies, including which learning strategies you prefer to use.

Examples:
- Students taking a difficult course ask themselves what parts of the material they are having problems with and why, what they should focus on and how they can modify their learning to be more effective. you can find a way to do it.
- Interns who are learning to perform a variety of tasks in their new job can assess their ability to perform those tasks to know which tasks to seek help with.
- Athletes preparing for competition should reflect on which learning strategies are not working for them and why, and whether they can improve their use of those strategies or use them more effectively. You can replace it with a good one.

The Importance of Reflective Learning

Reflective teaching is the process by which teachers reflect on their teaching practices and find ways they can improve or change teaching methods to help students learn better. You can see this by looking at student reactions in class and test results. Teachers reflect on their teaching process and learn more about their practice to see if it helps their students' learning process. Through reflection and self-evaluation, teachers can improve their teaching.
- By reflecting on their teaching style, teachers practice doing their job well, providing students with effective learning experiences, and identifying strengths and weaknesses.
- Focus self-improvement for better educational practice and professional growth.
- Based on teachers' self-observations and self-evaluations of teaching methods.
- Openness to one's teaching practice and desire to maximize oneself.

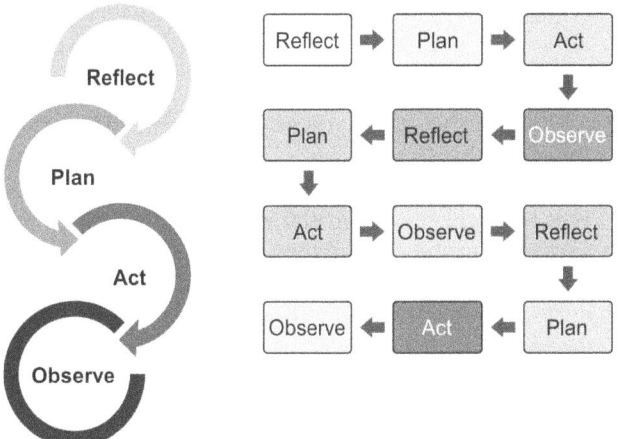

Fig. 4.13: Reflective teaching process.

The Importance of Reflective Coaching

The importance of reflective coaching is as follows:
- Reflective teaching leads to innovative methods and techniques of teaching by educators. This allows teachers to find innovative ways to make class activities interesting and fun for their students. In this way, students can receive satisfactory instruction.

- Reflective teaching also helps teachers develop problem-solving skills.
- Reflective teaching allows teachers to take responsibility for their duties and take seriously the future of their students.
- Seek feedback from students and colleagues.
- Use innovative teaching methods and techniques.
- Develop new teaching methods and strategies.
- Build good relationships with students.

Benefits of Reflective Learning

Reflective learning has many potential benefits.
- Help assess the situation by asking you to identify knowledge gaps or areas that need improvement.
- Helps you find ways to improve your learning process. For example, you can improve the learning process by asking them to identify which learning techniques worked for them and which did not.
- Helps you understand yourself better. For example, you can ask them to think about what kind of tasks or information they struggle with the most.
- Helps develop general metacognitive skills by training you to think critically about how you learn.
- By actively making the learning process feel responsible, you can increase your sense of autonomy and control.
- Gaining more control over the learning process, making it more conscious and effective, and increasing motivation to learn.

Theories of Reflective Learning

There are four theories that examine this type of learning.
1. **Dewey:** John Dewey's reflective theory is empirical. And about the difficulties that arise at certain times. This is a process of self-reflection that identifies and addresses problems and presents possible solutions to address situations. Furthermore, this theory argues that introspection is a continuous developmental process, as new events can redefine current knowledge and skills, which clearly shows a model in which the reflection occurs during or after the event. The first instance involves assessment and taking immediate action during an incident, and the second expresses the process of reflection as a post-event.
2. **Kolb:** Kolb and Fry proposed a comprehensive learning cycle framework in which all stages are equally important to becoming proficient.
3. **Pedler** has simplified this model to the next level.
4. **Finally,** there is the **Boud Keogh and Walker model**. It recognizes emotions as elements of the learning experience. Emphasizes the importance of emotions evoked when remembered.

Strategies to Support the Practice of Reflection

Reflection is not productive by itself. As a professional practice activity, this is what you need to deal with. Below are some strategies that can help you reflect your practice more effectively.
- Make time for yourself.
- **Tools:** Use tools such as: B. Model Diaries and Records. This helps formalize your work. You can also browse. You can experiment with different approaches to see what works best for you, and use different activities on a regular basis depending on your location.
- **Repetition:** Reflection is not a one-off activity, it is cyclical. As a result of reflection, confirm what you have done and reflect on it. This helps embed learning.
- **Share what you learn:** Find new ways (discussion group blogs) to share what you learn and get feedback from others.

Implications

There are several implications regarding individual preferences for reflective learning. Educators need to recognize that when students are actively learning, they may not approach new information in the same way. Similarly, reflective learners stand out from active learners in the classroom. No single teaching approach can appeal to both active and reflective learners. As such, educators need to design multimodal learning experiences with reinforcement activities that encompass different learning styles.

Pros and Cons of Reflective Teaching for Teachers and Students

Teachers can use this method to improve their teaching process. This includes providing direction, conducting self-assessment sessions, and better ways to focus on improvement and problem solving. We also need to focus on developing the analytical skills of our students. Over time, this technique helps teachers develop a critical eye for each issue.

Benefits of Reflective Teaching

- **Professional development:** Teaching promotes personal growth and allows you to know your strengths and weaknesses. The practice of reflection promotes professional development.
- **Lesson preparation and analysis:** Write down your goals and evaluate the results. Start with a reflective journal and write down your thoughts after each session.
- **Gives room to innovate:** It is not a complicated exercise, but it helps organized teachers grasp lessons and how to prepare. Evaluate the teaching after conducting the

session. Notice the positive experiences and challenges from the session. Take your time and work through the problem using different teaching methods. This leads to innovation and the two complement each other.
- **Facilitate teaching:** Practice should ensure that the learning experience is good for each student. Teachers should strive to create an interactive learning environment and motivation is the key to success. Reflection methods help you understand what your students are interested in and how you can change your message delivery to make it easier for them.
- **Strengthen student-teacher relationships:** Teachers value the bond with students and help students understand things better. Practice helps maintain relationships. This technique focuses on understanding and helping individual learners. Use strategies to analyze your performance and needs. Being in a comfortable classroom environment can improve student performance. Solve problems and implement new reflex strategies to activate each lesson.

This will encourage all students to actively participate in class. Start the lesson with a review session and repeat the last session. Try to do this in a fun and engaging way so that all students can participate. Ask questions and provide feedback to understand and improve problem areas.
- **Facilitate problem solving:** Experienced teachers develop ways to solve problems and overcome challenges effectively. Practical help teachers develop state-of-the-art strategies and provide individualized help to troubled students. This helps students deal with problems and master skills, and helps both teachers and students improve their intellectual stability.

Scenario-based Learning

Scenario-based learning (SBL) supports active learning strategies such as problm-based or case-based learning using interactive scenarios. Students typically progress through storylines based on unstructured or complex problems that need to be solved. Students are required to apply subject knowledge and critical thinking and problem-solving skills in safe, real-world situations. Often non-linear, her SBL can provide numerous opportunities to provide feedback to students based on the choices they make at each stage of the process.

Definition

Scenario-based learning (SBL) is an educational strategy in which learners choose their own path based on their choices. Learners are often placed in interactive scenarios based on real-life situations. This is an example of the increasing gamification of learning, a highly effective form of online training.

Principles of Scenario-Based Learning

Instructional designers agree that effective scenarios consist of five key elements tailored to the specific learning environment and skill training required.
- **Context:** Processing time to create a scene that gives the learner the opportunity to "read" the situation and environment.
- **Choices:** Choices presented at branching points in branching scenarios. They lead to consequences.
- **Consequences:** Consequences that can be positive or negative depending on your choice. There is not always a right or wrong answer.

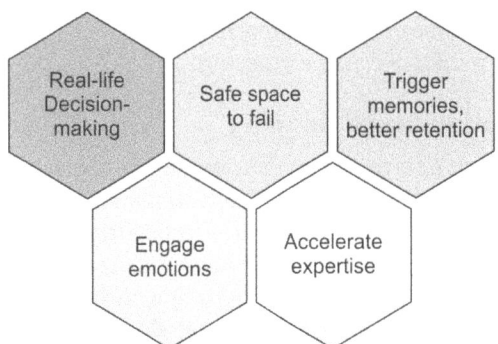

Fig. 4.14: Scenario-based learning (SBL).

Scenario Learning Example
- **Real world security scenarios:** Scenario-based learning is a good technique for teaching employees basic security practices. As such, scenario-based security training helps employees learn security measures in a contextual and easy way through real-world situations.
- **Skills training:** Skills training scenarios can be effectively used to provide customized skills training to professionals. Interesting scenarios make training content more engaging, memorable, immersive, and applicable, making the experience more fun and engaging for learners.

In addition to context, the course structure of skills training typically includes numerous exercises and gamification aspects. Certain courses have scenarios created using animated graphics and photographs of real people to simulate a real business environment and help learners make the right decisions.
- **Audio-driven scenarios with game elements:** Scenario-based learning is more effective when combined with

gamification components. This is especially useful when companies want to improve the performance and productivity of their sales teams. By adding gamification to sales simulation scenarios, sales people can practice and hone their skills in a safe and collaborative environment. These benefits can also be extended to other areas of life.

Benefits of scenario-based learning strategies are:
- Scenariobased learning is applicable to most corporate training needs. This strategy can be used to improve the learning effectiveness of both formal and informal training.
- Create a sticky learning experience.
- Make it easier for learners to solve problems.
- Provides guided learner exploration.
- Provides a safe practice zone for increasing proficiency.
- Allow learners to make mistakes and provide feedback to reinforce correct approaches.
- Can reinforce the main message.

Simulation-based Learning

Use simulation to assess the impact of process changes, new procedures, and capital investments. Engineers can use simulation to evaluate the performance of existing systems or to predict the performance of proposed systems by comparing alternative solutions and designs.

Simulation-based teaching is an educational approach that gives students the opportunity to practice the skills they learn in reallife situations. Educational simulations are teaching methods that test the knowledge and skills of participants by placing them in scenarios in which they must actively solve problems.

Meaning

Simulated teaching is a technique or feedback to elicit specific desired behaviors in students and teachers by playing the role of the teacher in their own group as an artificial classroom teaching situation her mechanism. In addition to enumerating strategies for modifying teacher behavior, modification can be made through participation in seminars, workshops, refresher courses, orientation programs, team teaching, conducting action research, etc. increase.

Simulation for Learning Purposes

Definitions of the two parts of this term "Learning" and "Simulation" are provided below. A broad definition has been adopted in the current entry, where learning is defined as the process of acquiring or improving knowledge and skills, whether cognitive, physical, social, etc. The various definitions that influence or consider a particular field reflect the field. For example, some researchers suggest that simulation is necessarily computer related.

Simulation Type
- **Identity simulation:** Identity simulation uses the real system as a model.
- **Replication simulation:** Replication simulation uses a behavioral model of the system under normal circumstances.
- **Laboratory simulations:** Laboratory simulations use laboratory replicas to characterize real-world systems.
- **Computer simulation:** A computer simulation is an abstract representation of a real system using a computer.
- **Analytical simulation:** Analytical simulation uses a mathematical model and tries to find a solution using analytical means.

Features of Simulated Teaching
- **Planning:** Simulated teaching requires systematic preplanning so that students can demonstrate the desired behaviors (skills) after completing the training. The plan should take into account the educational needs, interests, attitudes and conditions of the target group.
- **Participation:** Students are expected to actively participate in all activities. Simulated teaching requires strong student commitment and supportive behavior.
- **Feedback:** The quality and frequency of feedback plays an important role in simulation teaching. It brings about desirable changes in human behavior. Simulated lessons allow students to experience the results of their activities earlier than in real situations. The immediate feedback they receive has a huge impact on their learning.
- **Control:** Simulated teaching is based on a system approach to achieving specific goals set in front of the student. Simulated teaching allows teachers/trainees to decide what students should learn, in what order and under what conditions. You can set up simulated teaching so that you have full control over your learning. Students solve or encounter relatively minor problems before tackling more serious problems that require more advanced skills and experience.
- **Time:** Simulation education is a goal-oriented and flexible teaching method. Time can be shortened or extended, or both, depending on the goals to be achieved. A simulated lesson can be extended over multiple sessions if the goals to be achieved are complex or the skills to be mastered are difficult.
- **Safety:** Simulated instruction minimizes the risk of performing activities in artificial, simulated or laboratory

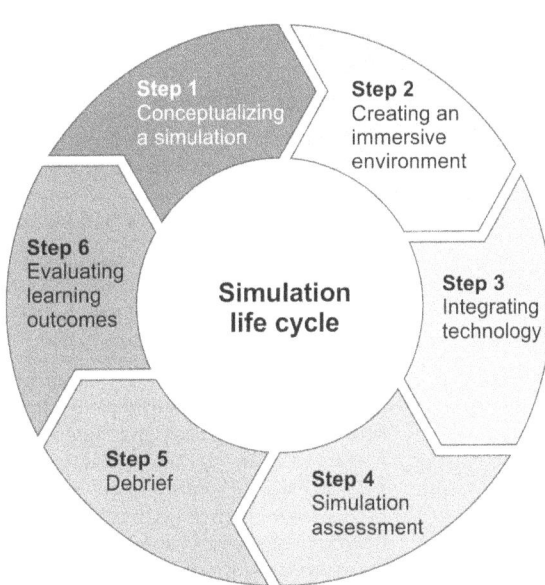

Fig. 4.15: Simulation life cycle steps.

conditions. By providing artificial situations and simulated experiments, can experience dangerous and dangerous situations such as operating a patient in flight or driving an airplane fighting in a war. Construction of a mock lesson: Five to seven student-teachers who were to practice social skills were involved in the construction of a mock lesson. The teacher is an actor, the two students who act as spectators, and the trainees who act as students are called foils, and there are 2 to 4 of them.

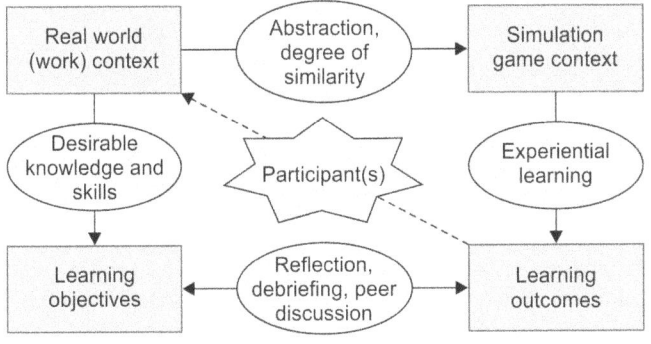

Fig. 4.16: Mock teaching process.

Procedure for Mock Teaching

Flanders recommends the following procedure:
- **Selection of teachers:** A small group of teachers is selected. Each person in the group is assigned a letter, such as A, B, C, D. Role assignments rotate for each character, giving each individual the option to be an actor or an observer.
- **Skill selection and discussion:** Select and discuss skills to practice. It also suggests topics for conversation based on your skill. Choose a topic for the first session and decide on subsequent topics so that each individual can choose a topic they are comfortable with in their role.
- **Decision-making considerations:** Decide who starts the conversation, who steps in, who ends the conversation, and when. A set of activities is thus defined.
- **Determining the evaluation method:** Determine the evaluation method, type of data to be recorded, recording method, etc.
- **Conducting practice sessions:** An initial practice session is conducted and the actors receive feedback on their performance. If necessary, the course of the second session will be changed to improve the training process.
- **Be willing to change procedures:** If necessary, change procedures and subjects to move on to the next skill in order to present each actor with a meaningful challenge and keep their interest as high as possible.

Applying Simulation-Based Learning

Simulation-based learning has been shown to provide the best learning outcomes in a variety of educational and work settings. This technique provides learners with a realistic immersive experience, enabling them to gain practical insights related to the subject matter or workrelated concepts. Regardless of the type of work, simulation-based learning is a powerful training tool that doctors, pilots, surgeons, and other professionals use to quickly gain experience in dealing with challenging situations.

Simulation Ideas for Nursing Education

Course	Topic(s) or concept(s)	Simulation suggestion
Pediatrics	• Immunizations • Culture • Assessment • Patient history	• Create a simulation for students to practice infant assessment in a clinic setting. • Create a challenge when parents state they do not want their child to receive vaccinations. • Add a cultural dilemma or language barrier.
School health	• Asthma • Patient handoff/transitions of care • Nurse role(s)	Create an unfolding set of simulations where a school age child has an acute exacerbation of asthma at school. The school nurse follows her asthma action plan, calls EMS and the child goes to the ED. There is a handoff to the inpatient unit or an observation unit where the child receives care.
Maternal health	• Laboring mom • Bathing • Post-partum care • Newborn assessment	Students need to understand the care of the laboring mom, so it would be important to learn to care for a mom in labor. For simulation centers that do have access to a birthing simulator there are options such as: • Mama Natalie® by Laerdal (less than $1000) • Parto Pants™ (Pronto) another low cost solution; worn by a student or SP. Both allow for normal or complicated deliveries. Newborn assessment can be done using a newborn simulator or even a doll that is appropriately sized.
Obstetrical emergencies	• Managing obstetrical emergencies • Postpartum hemorrhage • Teamwork • Communication • Situational awareness	Conducting a simulation on postpartum hemorrhage is essential in the maternal health curriculum. This simulation can be found in most vendor-offered packaged curriculums or other free resources. This teaches students to recognize and manage an area with a high rate of mortality as well as many other important skills.
Medical-surgical	• Cardiac • Respiratory • Sepsis • Stroke • Acute MI • Patient handoff • Medication management • Multiple patient management • Communication • Critical thinking	The importance of simulation at the medical-surgical level is focussed on: • Developing student clinical judgment and skills • Determining how to prioritize assessments • Gathering data • Making decisions • Implementing interventions correctly • Reflecting about what they are doing The content is less important. This is not the time to load content that does not seem to fit elsewhere. This is an opportunity to think about key patients for whom it would be great if every student had an opportunity to provide care.
Medical-surgical or advanced medical-surgical	• Stroke	Focus on a case to assist students to recognize signs of a stroke in a patient who is in the hospital for another problem, such as an elderly man who had a hip replacement and has a history of atrial fibrillation and sleep apnea. • This will teach students to recognize a stroke and learn how to react in a crisis. • This type of simulation generally requires a high-fidelity mannequin.
Leadership	• Impaired nurse • Nurse-to-nurse bullying • Root cause analysis for a sentinel event or medication error	In leadership courses, simulation can be used to address topics nurses face on the unit. There are articles and resources available to assist in developing simulation on these topics. Students find it beneficial to learn how to deal with nurse-to-nurse bullying and they need opportunities to role-play these types of strategies.

Benefits
- Motivating teaching is a means of motivating students.
- Provide students' teachers with opportunities to research and analyze important educational issues.
- Simulation establishes the link between theory and practice.
- Participants recognize their progress through various feedback methods. You can use social skills you have learned.

Cons
- Time consuming.
- Very expensive.
- Not all subjects in the curriculum are available for simulation.
- Simulation is not useful for young children because the mechanics are too difficult to understand.

- It requires a lot of preparation on the teacher's part. Few teachers are willing to do the extra work necessary to successfully apply a technique.
- In developed countries, advanced audiovisual equipment and computers are used for simulation. Currently, schools cannot afford to purchase these expensive audiovisual media.
- A final caveat that learning is a highly individualized and serious activity requires concentration on the part of the learner. Simulation is a game that reduces the seriousness of learning. Critics doubt that meaningful learning can be done through simulation.

Blended Learning

Blended learning refers to educational solutions that combine several different delivery methods, such as: The term blended learning is used to describe a learning process that blends various event-based activities. Inperson classes, live e-learning, or self-paced learning.

Definition

Blended learning can be defined as a delivery method that combines a variety of traditional and nontraditional teaching techniques, tools and approaches for designing, developing, managing and evaluating learning processes. A blended program is one where 30–79% of the program content is delivered online.

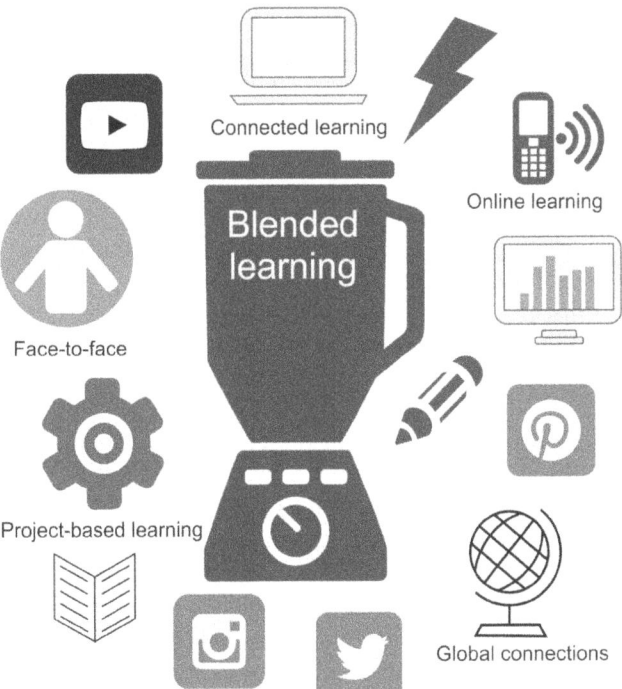

Fig. 4.17: Blended learning features.

Features

- Student involvement in learning
- Improved interaction between teachers and students
- Responsibility for learning
- Time management and flexibility
- Improving student learning outcomes
- Improving the reputation of the institution
- More flexible teaching and learning environment
- More open to autonomy and continuous learning
- Better opportunities for experiential learning.

Blended Learning Models

Here are the few most common types of blended learning frameworks. This model emphasizes online learning, rather than having learners attend classroom training and then self-paced online learning. Learners consume predetermined content at home or during free time before class, and class time is devoted to active learning and application of newly learned skills. This can take the form of discussions, case studies, or group projects.

- **Face-to-face driver model:** The face-to-face driver mixed learning model is the closest to traditional classroom training, as most of the training takes place in the classroom under the guidance of an instructor. This approach provides one-on-one, personalized support to learners who are struggling to grasp new concepts or who are falling behind in their training curriculum.
- **Rotation model:** In a mixed learning rotation model, learners are expected to follow a fixed schedule and rotate through both online self-paced learning and face-to-face interactions. The schedule is fixed but flexible. Incorporating a variety of training methods helps learners practice what they learn and close learning gaps. This makes it easier to track training progress as learners follow a fixed schedule.
- **Flex model:** The flex mixed learning model provides learners with a flexible and personalized learning experience specifically tailored to their needs. In this model, online learning can take the lead as the central vehicle for material throughout the learning experience, while instructors provide the necessary smallgroup support. Flex models allow students to customize the path and timeline they follow throughout the learning process.
- **Enhanced virtual models:** Enhanced virtual mixed learning models are very similar to flex models with online training as the main component. It is a model that is gaining popularity in the era of remote work. However, unlike the Flex model, learners must complete scheduled, instructor-led lessons in a physical or virtual classroom.

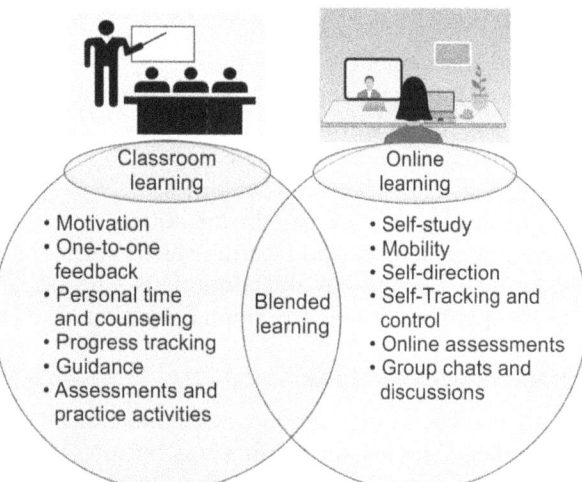

Fig. 4.18: Difference between classroom and online learning.

Benefits of Blended Learning

Benefits of blended learning for students include enhanced learning skills, increased access to information, increased satisfaction and learning outcomes, and opportunities to learn and teach with others will be recent research has revealed the following key benefits of blended learning:

- **Greater flexibility:** Technology-enhanced learning enables anywhere, anytime learning, allowing students to learn without barriers of time and space, but also supporting personal engagement.
- **More interaction:** Blended learning provides a platform that enables greater interaction between students and between students and teachers.
- **Expanding learning:** Additional types of learning activities increase learning motivation and help students achieve higher and more meaningful levels of learning.
- **Learn to be a virtual citizen:** Learners practice their ability to present themselves socially and academically in online research communities. Digital learning skills are becoming increasingly important for lifelong learning, and blended courses help learners develop the skills to use a variety of technologies.

Benefits

- **Facilitate collaboration:** Students and educators can connect outside the classroom with collaboration tools such as online discussion blogs.
- **Facilitate instant communication:** Online communication tools such as grading tools, discussion forums, interactive apps, and dropbox help teachers communicate effectively with students.
- **Greater flexibility and accessibility:** Teachers and students can access her learning materials 24/7 via LMS and more.
- **Individualized support:** Blended learning environments can be individualized to accommodate learners with varying coping skills.
- **Interactive learning experiences:** Technology enhanced learning aids such as interactive learning games, padlets and Pear Decks keep student sessions engaging and learning fun.
- **Track learner skills and outcomes:** Teachers can see how much time each individual has spent on assignments, glean meaningful insights from student data generated by online apps, and track effective activity and can determine which activities require improvisation.
- **Efficient student assessment:** Detailed reports and automatic grading with built-in rubrics enable comprehensive student assessment. These are useful for teachers as they are less effort and students are more aware of their progress as they get immediate feedback.
- **Improving computer literacy:** Students acquire computer literacy and real-world skills through blended learning so that they are better prepared for the future and make the most of the digital opportunities offered.

Disadvantages

- **Heavy reliance on technology:** Heavy reliance on the Internet for technology resources and tools that are key components of the combined lesson plan.
- **High cost:** Adopting advanced technology for blended learning in schools requires investment in infrastructure and equipment.
- **IT skills:** A lack of basic understanding of online tools and technologies can be a major obstacle for teachers. Technical training and support are essential for them.
- **Teacher overload:** To realize this paradigm shift in education, teachers must broaden their horizons, choose appropriate tools and apps, and strive to implement balanced and effective lesson plans must be unfortunately, conservative teachers may find this very difficult at first and not be prepared to adapt to this new culture.
- **Increased cognitive load for students:** Blended learning can be a new world of learning for students and it can take time to embrace and become accustomed to these new teaching methods.
- **Digital resources authentic and age appropriate:** As students access and use the Internet on a regular basis, they may be attracted to irrelevant and inappropriate things. Therefore, educating children about Internet

safety and how to behave responsibly online is a must for teachers.
- **Lack of supervision:** Teachers are concerned about student motivation when transitioning to blended learning, as there is less supervision compared to face-to-face classes and many students' performance may be slackened due to self-management.
- Learn flexibility that allows students to set their own pace leading to falling behind in the curriculum. These issues and principles can be examined with particular reference to the General Conditions. An educational environment and cultural context that will allow you to design your own system for evaluating educational practice, which will be of great help in promoting education at all levels of international significance.

CONCLUSION

Finally, it must be noted that maxims are our servants and masters. Also, as a whole, everything is connected. It should also be noted that children have different talents, interests, mental and physical requirements. Different sayings are suitable for different situations and different children. Therefore, it is important to use each maxim with caution.

REVIEW QUESTIONS

Long Essays
1. Define teaching and learning, explain teaching-learning process in detail.
2. Describe nature and components of teaching and learning processes.
3. Discuss teaching-learning strategies.
4. Define classical conditioning, explain the concepts and principles of classical conditioning.
5. Explain trial and error learning experiment and stages.
6. Enumerate modern learning approaches.
7. Define reflective learning, explain the importance of reflective learning.
8. Define scenario-based learning, explain principles of scenario-based learning.
9. Define simulation-based learning, explain the types, features and principles.

Short Essays
1. Importance of teaching in the learning process.
2. 6E's in teaching and learning.
3. Principles of teaching and learning.
4. Teaching and learning barriers.
5. John Watson's conditioning theory.
6. Operant conditioning.
7. Experiment by Pavlov.
8. Difference between classical and operant conditioning.
9. Trial and error learning.
10. Learning by insight.
11. Kohler's insight learning experiments.
12. Principles of experiential learning.
13. Forms of experiential learning.
14. Stages of the experiential learning cycle.
15. Importance of reflective coaching.
16. Theories of reflective learning.
17. Pros and cons of reflective teaching for teachers and students.
18. Benefits of scenario-based learning strategies.
19. Procedure for mock teaching.
20. Simulation ideas for nursing education.
21. Blended learning models.
22. Benefits of blended learning.

Short Answers
1. Desire.
2. Beliefs.
3. Interactive process.
4. Organized system.
5. Principles of learning.
6. Teaching principles.
7. Barriers to motivation.
8. Fixed internal schedule.
9. Skinner's operant experiments.
10. Thorndike's law.
11. Internships.
12. Field work.
13. Tangible experiences.
14. Reflective observation.
15. Abstract conceptualization.
16. Benefits of reflective learning.
17. Blended learning.
18. Enhanced virtual models.

Unit 2

Assessment of Teacher and Learner

Chapters

5. Assessment of Teacher and Learner
6. Curriculum Planning

KEYWORDS

Assessment: The systematic collection, review, and use of information about educational programs undertaken for the purpose of improving student learning and development.

Benchmark: A description or example of candidate or institutional performance that serves as a standard of comparison for evaluation or judging quality.

Knowledge: Recalling or remembering information without necessarily understanding it. Includes behaviors such as describing, listing, identifying, and labeling.

Comprehension: Understanding learned material and includes behaviors such as explaining, discussing, and interpreting.

Application: The ability to put ideas and concepts to work in solving problems. It includes behaviors such as demonstrating, showing, and making use of information.

Analysis: Breaking down information into its component parts to see interrelationships and ideas. Related behaviors include differentiating, comparing, and categorizing.

Synthesis: The ability to put parts together to form something original. It involves using creativity to compose or design something new.

Evaluation: Judging the value of evidence based on definite criteria. Behaviors related to evaluation include: Concluding, criticizing, prioritizing, and recommending.

Course embedded assessment: Reviewing materials generated in the classroom. In addition to providing a basis for grading students, such materials allow faculty to evaluate approaches to instruction and course design.

Direct measures of learning: Students (learners) display knowledge and skills as they respond directly to the instrument itself.

Goals for learning: Goals are used to express intended results in general terms. The term goals are used to describe broad learning concepts. For example: Clear communication, problem solving, and ethical awareness.

Indirect measures of learning: Students (learners) are asked to reflect on their learning rather than to demonstrate it. Examples include: exit surveys, student interviews (e.g., graduating seniors), and alumni surveys.

Learning outcomes (outcome behaviors): Observable behaviors or actions on the part of students that demonstrate that the intended learning objective has occurred.

Measurements: Design of strategies, techniques and instruments for collecting feedback data that evidence the extent to which students demonstrate the desired behaviors.

Portfolio: An accumulation of evidence about individual proficiencies, especially in relation to learning standards.

Quantitative methods of assessment: Methods that rely on numerical scores or ratings. Examples: Surveys, inventories, institutional/departmental data, departmental/course-level exams (locally constructed, standardized, etc.).

Qualitative methods of assessment: Methods that rely on descriptions rather than numbers. Examples: Ethnographic field studies, logs, journals, participant observation, and open-ended questions on interviews and surveys.

Reliability: Reliable measures are measures that produce consistent responses over time.

Student outcomes assessment: The act of assembling, analyzing and using both quantitative and qualitative evidence of teaching and learning outcomes, in order to examine their congruence with stated purposes and educational objectives and to provide meaningful feedback that will stimulate self-renewal.

Validity: As applied to a test refers to a judgment concerning how well a test does in fact measure what it purports to measure.

Chapter 5

Assessment of Teacher and Learner

Learning Objectives
- Teacher Evaluation
- Essential Characteristics of Teachers
- Teaching Styles—Formal Authority Demonstrator Facilitator Delegator
- Learner Assessment
- Learning Types
- Determinants of Learning
- Today's Generation of Learners and their Skills and Characteristics
- Motivational Factors—Personal Factors, Environmental Factors and Support Systems

TERMINOLOGY

- **Active learning:** Learning that engages students through a variety of activities and challenges their thinking.
- **Assessing for learning:** Key teaching strategies during learning to help teachers and students assess their progress in understanding and mastering skills and provide guidance and feedback for subsequent teaching and learning.
- **Closed question:** A question that can be answered with a single word (usually "yes" or "no") or a short sentence, with limited answer choices.
- **Critical thinking:** The ability to analytically judge and evaluate a particular claim or concept in the light of the evidence or larger context that underlies all rational discourse and investigation.
- **Feedback:** Information about how learners are progressing in their efforts to reach their goals. Feedback can also come from learners to teachers about how they feel they can help them learn better.
- **Formative assessment:** Activities that provide developmental feedback to students on their progress in a program of study and influence the design of next learning steps.
- **Open-ended questions:** Questions that cannot be answered in one sentence. "What do you think about global warming?"
- **Reflective exercise:** A process of continuous learning from experience in which teachers plan assessment and evaluation of practice, improving the quality of teaching and learning over time.
- **Reinforce:** Reinforcement or support (understanding or learning skills).
- **Self efficacy:** A learner's confidence in their ability to achieve goals through hard work and determination.
- **Subject curriculum:** The content and skills contained in the curriculum that apply to successive stages of student learning. These levels usually refer to grade levels and thus to specific ages of learners.
- **Summative assessment:** A final exam assignment, typically an exam or test, that measures and records the level of learning achieved for promotion to the next level or for certification.
- **Syllabus:** Complete description of qualification content assessment rules and performance requirements. Courses leading to awards or certificates are based on the subject curriculum.

INTRODUCTION

Assessment is integrated into the learning process. It is closely related to curriculum and education. As teachers and students work to achieve curricular outcomes, assessment plays an ongoing role in informing instruction, guiding students' next steps, and checking progress and performance. Assessment of Learning (AFL) is a teaching and learning approach that generates feedback used to improve student performance. Students become more involved in the learning process, gaining confidence in what they are expected to learn and at what level.

TEACHER EVALUATION

Teachers play an important role in shaping the thinking of children and shaping the quality of education. Teachers are expected to demonstrate an understanding of the subject matter. Build good relationships with students. Create an effective learning environment to ensure a fulfilling experience. Conduct student assessments. Work closely with your colleagues and community. Demonstrate professional commitment and accountability. Teacher assessment is a well-defined and systematic process used to access teacher performance in the classroom. Teacher assessment assesses a teacher's educational behavior against a set of standardized criteria determined by an assessment team.

Definition

- Assessment is the systematic basis for inferring student learning and development. It is the process of defining, selecting, designing, collecting, analyzing, interpreting, and using information to enhance student learning and development.
- Teacher evaluation is an integral part of maintaining a standardized education system. It helps educators track teacher performance and assess the overall quality of knowledge delivery.

Teacher Evaluation Techniques/Methods

Teacher Evaluation by Students

This is a common method of evaluating a teacher's teaching performance. By soliciting feedback from students on teacher teaching behavior and methods, you can gather decision-making information and meaningful insights. A student is the end-user (consumer) of the services provided by a teacher. This means that students can provide extensive data and feedback on how they perceive their teachers' teaching performance.

Benefits

- You can collect information directly from your primary end users (students).
- Student teacher evaluation is one of the most effective ways to determine if a teaching method is adequate.

Cons

- This type of rating can be very subjective. A student's personal preferences can cloud judgment.
- Students may find it difficult to assess teacher performance using the grading criteria provided.

Teacher Evaluation by Teachers

This is a type of peer evaluation that allows teachers to rate peers and provide feedback. this teacher evaluation method helps gather information about teachers' work ethics and behavior outside the classroom. Asking teachers to rate each other's performance is a great way to build team spirit and is widely recognized as one of the most objective ways to evaluate teachers. Teachers work closely with their peers and can provide effective feedback on their attitudes, behavior, skills, and abilities in the workplace.

Bonus/Benefits

- Teacher evaluations by teachers help improve team spirit in schools.
- This is a means of collecting meaningful data that provides insight into workplace performance.

Con

Workplace toxicity can lead to biased feedback during teacher assessment.

Teacher Evaluation by Management

This type of teacher evaluation is done by the school's Education Council. This council usually consists of the principal and faculty members. It is also the evaluation that determines the career of a teacher. One of the most common ways of conducting this type of assessment is to schedule one-on-one interviews with her members of staff (teachers) and the assessment team. During this conversational meeting, the assessment team can review the teacher's performance on the assessment parameters.

Bonus

- This gives you an objective view of employee performance.
- Management's evaluation of teachers helps the team to create realistic career development projections for each member of the workforce.

Cons

- In a toxic work environment, some members of the assessment team may use the assessment to resolve scorecards they perceive as hostile.
- Can lead to biased feedback and reviews.

Teacher Evaluation Criteria and Strategies

Teacher Evaluation Criteria and Strategies are dynamic and have evolved over time according to the needs of the institution. Some of the important criteria and their descriptors are listed below. Evaluators should check to see if teachers meet the same standards.

Place Effective Planning

- Follows the prescribed curriculum and lesson-plan
- Uses appropriate teaching aids materials and resources
- Plans assignments activities and resources appropriate to the abilities of the students including those with special needs
- Displays time-management and flexibility in planning
- Is able to plan student grouping based on instructional requirements.

Implementation of the Lesson

- Makes the lesson objectives clear to the students
- Is able to retain student attention
- Connects the lesson to previous and future lessons
- Provides appropriate and real-life examples
- Presents concepts clearly and logically and reinforces them
- Continuously monitors students' learning and provides feedback
- Smoothly transitions from one activity to another.

Student Interaction and Motivation

- Displays concern for students
- Uses students' interests and backgrounds along with intrinsic/extrinsic rewards
- Uses appropriate and encouraging tone/feeling
- Is capable of establishing a level of difficulty which promotes success
- Creates an engaging learning environment for each student to display initiative and be participative.

Subject/Curriculum Knowledge

- Exhibits accurate and up-to-date subject and curriculum knowledge
- Gives effective examples and illustrations
- Connects the learning content with instructional objectives
- Logically presents subject content.

Effective Communication

- Speaks clearly with proper pronunciation intonation and voice modulation
- Displays excellent presentation skills
- Interacts well with students by praising eliciting and responding to their questions
- Displays enthusiasm and involvement while delivering lessons
- Expresses ideas clearly and logically.

Student Achievement

- Clearly communicates performance expectations to students
- Ensures participation from all students
- Uses effective evaluative techniques to monitor student progress
- Gives evaluative feedback on time to determine level of learning
- Promotes 21st century skills by using higher order questioning techniques
- Creates opportunities for one-to-one discussion on student progress
- Has problem-solving skills to help students overcome their challenges.

Effective Time-Management and Class Management

- Schedules learning time and is punctual
- Keeps the management time and transition time to a minimum
- Manages discipline as per school policy and promotes self-discipline
- Constructively manages disruptive behavior demonstrating fairness and consistency
- Sets and communicates clear parameters for classroom behavior.

Interaction with Parents and Community

- Creates opportunities for community involvement with the school
- Communicates effectively with the parents in the best interests of the child
- Encourages and supports parent-teacher collaborative activities.

Interaction with Management and Peers

- Follows all policies protocols and procedures set by the school management
- Displays team spirit and cooperates well with peers sharing ideas and views with them
- Submits all reports and documentation on time
- Displays initiative for special events and activities.

Inclination towards Professional Growth

- Actively participates in professional workshops meetings training programs peer-reviews and self-appraisal
- Is engaged with continuing education
- Is associated with professional committees and associations
- Is upto-date with the developments in subject area as well as the education sector in general.

Ways to Conduct a Teacher Evaluation

- Decide on the type of teacher evaluation you want to carry out. You need to decide on who would conduct the assessment; that is whether it would be done by the students co-teachers or the management team.
- Define the parameters for the evaluation. This means that you should spell out the different criteria you would use for the assessment.
- Meet teacher assessment criteria and get everyone involved. If possible, convene a meeting and notify relevant parties to ensure transparency.
- Communicate the results of the assessment to the teacher, highlighting good achievements and other areas for improvement.

Benefits of Teacher Assessment

- Teacher assessment improves knowledge transfer by enhancing teacher quality. It identifies and addresses key educational challenges on an individual basis by helping teachers hone their skills.
- Helps stakeholders identify and reward the talent of outstanding teachers who deliver outstanding service.
- Regular teacher evaluations can identify gaps in teaching and learning practices that can contribute to poor student performance.
- Plays an important role in identifying curriculum loopholes.
- A well-founded teacher assessment exercise is a great opportunity for self-evaluation. Teachers can reflect on their strengths and weaknesses and work to improve.
- Provide useful and productive feedback that helps teachers grow and develop
- Provides insights for data-driven decision-making in the education sector.

Assessment Functions

Performs many functions listed below.

- **Detector:** Detects all activities under investigation. All activities are closely monitored, from planning to evaluating results. It also helps improve performance and achieve desired results.
- **Make a decision:** You need to decide what you need to do to improve. All decisions regarding assessment must be made by the teacher. It helps you focus on improving.
- **Screening:** Teachers should assess the potential for problems. They should do this using a simple yes or no. Assessment defines the problem, screening identifies and treats it.
- **Remedial course student evaluation:** It means that a student is below average. In this case, a remedial course should be offered. Additionally, these courses will help you improve your performance.
- **Lesson planning:** Lesson planning is the teacher's process. Helps teachers create plans for courses of study. In addition, it helps us meet the different needs of our students.
- **Feedback/answers:** This process helps validate how student performance is derived. It also identifies and acknowledges the characteristics of the student's work. Moreover, it helps students to improve their work.
- **Inspiration:** Inspiration and motivation are very important tools. This tool provides information about the environment and the type of task to help motivate you.

ESSENTIAL CHARACTERISTICS OF TEACHERS

- **Adaptability:** Adaptability is essential for teachers who need to continually evaluate what works and what does not work for their students.
- **Empathy:** Empathy is the ability to understand what another person is feeling or experiencing. Simply put, it is about putting yourself in someone else's shoes. As a teacher, it is important to practice empathy, not assumptions.
- **Perseverance:** Perseverance is key to being a role model and a role model for your students, as explained in our Learning Theory post.
- **Commitment:** Students are perceptive from a very early age and can quickly tell when teachers become bored or indifferent to their material.
- **Communication:** Communication skills should not be left out when talking about the good qualities of a teacher. A lot can go wrong in communication.
- **Social skills:** Social and communication skills are closely related. How well you communicate with your students and their parents determines the nature of your relationship with them. Interpersonal communication is important for building strong relationships.
- **Positivism:** Students often feel depressed and depressed. If teachers have the quality of always being positive, teachers can help students in many ways.

- **Fairmind:** Teachers must treat all students equally. Fairness is one of the most important characteristics of a successful teacher.
- **Consistency:** Consistency benefits both teachers and students. It helps teachers feel more organized. Being organized and well-planned relieves tension and stress.
- **Reward:** A pat on the back can make a big difference. Teachers should reward and recognize the efforts of their students.
- **Reliable:** A reliable teacher is someone who is dedicated to their work and can be trusted. Reliability is her one of the best qualities of a teacher. A reliable teacher knows how to make the right decisions and assessments.
- **Passion:** Passion is what every teacher should have. Teaching is not an easy task. There are many problems teachers face in their daily lives. There are many problems, from low student engagement to low interactivity. Today, online and live classes pose an even bigger challenge for teachers.
- **Motivation:** Low motivation for learning is one of the main concerns of all parents, teachers and students around the world. Teachers can make a huge contribution to motivating students. As mentioned above, even a little pat on the back can help.
- **Active listening:** Students often want someone to listen to them. You can be a good teacher only if you understand what your students need and that you need to listen to understand what your students want. Active listening is one of the most important qualities of an ideal teacher.
- **Caring:** Caring teachers foster healthy classrooms. Plenty of space for opinions, feedback, and errors. Students often need someone to talk to them about their problems and mistakes.
- **Honesty:** Students respect their teachers. Honesty is her one of the most important qualities that students need. It is very important to be honest with your students and colleagues. Honesty is often a package. It brings qualities such as responsibility, courage, and confidence.
- **Punctuality:** Being punctual and sticking to schedules and class schedules is one of the most sought after qualities of an ideal teacher.
- **Willingness to learn:** Teaching and learning go hand in hand. A good teacher never stops learning. The education sector changes daily, so teachers need to learn and improve.
- **Organization:** This quality helps teachers to be punctual and disciplined. Organization and planning are very important qualities of a good teacher. Imagine putting all your keys in a box without labels.
- **Ethics:** Ethics are a standard set of values and beliefs that teachers should follow. It is important that teachers have good ethics. Ethics tells us what is right and what is wrong and keeps us from doing wrong.
- **Dignity:** Respect for humanity is paramount. Learning starts with teachers, so it is very important that teachers respect everyone regardless of gender, caste or creed.

TEACHING STYLES—FORMAL AUTHORITY DEMONSTRATOR FACILITATOR DELEGATOR

Every teacher has their own teaching style. And as traditional teaching styles evolve with the emergence of differentiated teaching, more and more teachers are adapting their approach to the learning needs of their students. Everyone has different learning styles, so it is important to take into account different teaching styles. If you want to motivate your students and increase their participation and retention, it is important to consider different approaches that resonate with them. These different approaches can also help you achieve them.

Authoritative or Lecture Style

The authoritative model is teachercentric and often involves lengthy lecture sessions or one page presentations. Students are expected to take notes and absorb information.
- **Pros:** This style is acceptable for certain majors and classrooms with large student groups. The pure teaching style is perfect for subjects like history where you need to memorize key facts, dates, names, and more.
- **Cons:** Questionable model for teaching children as there is little or no interaction with the teacher. Also, you can sleep a little. Therefore, it is a better approach for older and mature students.

Demonstrator

In the demonstrator style, teachers still retain a lot of authority, but are more open to trying studentcentered teaching approaches, goes beyond lectures to include presentations, photographs, films, and experiments. As a result, it is applicable to more learning styles.
- **Pros:** This style allows teachers to incorporate a variety of formats such as lectures and multimedia presentations.
- **Cons:** Good for teaching math, music, PE, arts and crafts, but in large classrooms it is difficult to meet the needs of individual students.

Facilitator

Moving further towards a studentcentered approach is the teaching style of the facilitator. Facilitators encourage inquiry-based learning rather than oneway lectures.

Students learn by asking questions and discussing real-life case studies.
- **Pros:** Several other activities help improve problem-solving skills and help students understand the subject matter better through practical challenges. Help develop skills in finding answers and solutions through Great for science classes and similar subjects.
- **Cons:** Encourages teachers to interact with students and encourage discovery, rather than presenting facts and testing knowledge by memorization. Success is therefore somewhat difficult to measure concretely.

Delegator

The most studentcentered teaching style is called the delegator style (also called group style). Here the teacher exists only as an observer and it is the group of students who do all the work. Most delegatorstyle learning takes place peer-to-peer through frequent collaboration and discussion. The instructor is effectively removed from a position of authority and instead only facilitates discussion. Delegator style is ideal for lab experiments, group classes, creative discussions, and other peer-his-hers peer activities.
- **Benefits:** Guided discovery and inquiry-based learning puts teachers in the role of observers and inspires students to work together toward a common goal.
- **Cons:** Considered a modern way of teaching and sometimes criticized for undermining the authority of teachers. As delegators, teachers act more as advisors than as traditional authority figures.

Hybrid or Blended Styles

Hybrid or Blended Styles follow an integrative teaching approach that combines the personality and interests of the teacher with the needs of the students and a curriculum-based method.
- **Bonus:** Included! Teachers can also adapt their style to the needs of their students and the corresponding subject matter.
- **Disadvantages:** Hybrid styles run the risk of trying to say too much to every student, and teachers end up spreading minimal learning.

LEARNER ASSESSMENT

Learning assessment is an ongoing assessment that allows teachers to monitor students on a daily basis and modify teaching based on what students need to succeed. This assessment provides students with the timely and specific feedback they need to adjust their learning. Frequent monitoring of progress is an example of a learning test. The test regularly assesses student academic performance across benchmarks to determine if current teaching and interventions are having a positive impact on student performance or if adjustments are needed.

Assessment

- Teachers provide feedback to each student on how to improve their learning.
- Students will understand what successful work looks like for each completed task.
- Students become more independent in their learning by participating in peer and self-assessment.
- Overall assessments (e.g., exams and portfolio submissions) are also used formatively for improvement.

Exam Type

- **Diagnostic or preliminary screening:** A diagnostic or preliminary screening is conducted prior to the start of any educational unit or academic program. It helps you gather information about your learner's strengths, weaknesses, skills, and knowledge. Instructions are then developed according to the learner's needs.
- **Formative assessments:** These are ongoing assessments that support learning. Teachers conduct formative assessments several times during a unit lesson or course. They are specially designed for practice. Furthermore, the most important function of formative assessment is to monitor learning and provide feedback to modify instructions. It acts as a form of continuous learning, covering small areas of content while monitoring the learning process. However, such assessments do not award ranks or grades.
- **Summative assessment:** This type of assessment is intended to assess the level of learning at the end of the lesson. It seeks to measure learning effectiveness, student competence, and success. To do this, the method uses test tasks and projects to specifically assess and position students.
- **Confirmation evaluation:** Confirmation Evaluation, as the name suggests, is a method of checking the effectiveness of instruction one year after the end of the instruction period. The ultimate goal here is to see if the education strategy used is still successful and if the education is correct. They are therefore primarily a comprehensive form of comprehensive assessment.
- **Norms-based evaluation:** In this evaluation, teachers compare student performance against certain national average standards. For example, state average English grades.
- **Criteria-based assessment:** Criteria-based Tests assess a specific skill or knowledge against predetermined

learning standards. It tests a student's learning requirements and abilities at specific stages of learning. These tests assess students against specific goals, objectives, or criteria. In other words, it evaluates the entire curriculum.
- **Ipsative assessment:** Ipsative assessment test tracks learner progress relative to previous performance. Learners compare their previous results and try to improve. This type of assessment takes into account the fact that comparing yourself to peers is not always a good idea, as it can affect your self-confidence. However, comparison with an individual's past results can help improve the learner's overall knowledge and personality.

Assessment Cycle

- Basic building blocks of the assessment cycle.
- **Here four phases include:** Plan - Do - Check - Act: Plan - What do you want your students to learn? Do - How do you teach effectively? This phase includes the second and third basic components. Create experiences that lead to results.
- **Check:** Are my results met? This phase involves evaluating evaluation data (part of the 4th component).
- **Trading:** How will you use what you have learned? This phase involves enhancing and revising best practices to improve student learning (part of the 4th component).

LEARNING TYPES

Every student has a unique learning style that describes how they best process information and retain it in their memory for the long term. Everyone has a different set of learning styles, but most people have their own preferences.
- **Visual learners:** As the name suggests, they are people who learn best when they can visualize or imagine what they are thinking. In short, graphs, diagrams, and mind maps help you visualize and notice.
- **Auditory learner:** A person who learns by listening to and discussing topics. This is because conversations are easier to remember than letters and diagrams. The current classroom format is perfect for them as they can listen to explanations and ask questions in the classroom.
- **Kinesthetic learner:** Also known as a tactile learner, you learn by doing and can obtain information by recalling experiences and emotions while performing a task.
- **Writing learners:** Reading and writing learners are very familiar with the written language. They prefer to consume information by reading texts, and can absorb even more information by condensing and reconstructing it. The traditional college textbook and annotation process lends itself well to the literate style of learning.
- **Natural learners:** People who can learn naturally are called natural learners. In all other ways, their minds may be sitting in a classroom listening to a lecture, watching an educational film, going on an excursion, studying alone in another room, or doing group study. Holds information. These learners are best at gathering data through experimentation and experimentation practical.
- **Language learners:** These learners learn best through a variety of language skills such as reading, writing, speaking and listening. Her best learning methods include reading textbooks, listening to audiovideo recordings and lectures in the classroom, taking notes, and studying. She also likes other learning materials. Besides these, these learners can also talk (read aloud) about the topic.
- **Interpersonal learners:** These learners learn by relating information. I enjoy working in teams and groups that share information. Compare ideas. These people are often great leaders and team players because they learn best when accompanied by others from a member. These people are most likely to be found in the fields of social sciences and psychology, where things are done in groups. These people were setting difficult personal goals that were unattainable. Aside from external sources, these people are nurtured by internal forces and can be found in a wide variety of fields, including small business owners, entrepreneurs, and sometimes in creative fields. They usually dislike working in teams or groups, so they prefer to enter fields and industries where they can work alone without supervision.
- **Logic/mathematics learners:** These learners need to classify or classify things in order to understand the topic. These people understand patterns, numbers, equations, and relationships better than others. These types of learners are commonly encountered in various fields such as science, technical professions, and engineering mathematics.
- **Musical or rhythmic learner:** This is the type of learner who learns something using the rhythm or beat of a musical melody. I think there are some people who think that. It picks up information better with background noise. For example, this is like a musician learning to play music using different musical sounds, rhythms and sounds. Music is not a distraction, it is a learning tool for these types of learners.

DETERMINANTS OF LEARNING

Nurses have always taught patients and their families to learn about various aspects of healthcare. It is difficult to grasp the "moment of being taught" as much as the stay time is shortened.

- Learning needs (what)
- Willingness to learn (when)
- Learning styles (how)

Nurse Role as Teacher

- Provide meaningful information
- Recognize progress
- Provide feedback and follow-up
- Reinforce learning
- Client skills assessment

Learner Assessment

Principles that nursing effectiveness depends on the extent, accuracy, and extent of assessment.
- Prioritize behavioral goals
- Minimize client anxiety
- Prevent unnecessary repetition.

Learning Needs

Assess learning needs first to determine what needs to be taught and how much instruction is needed. must be determined. Learning needs are defined as knowledge gaps that exist between desired and actual levels of achievement.

Procedures for Determining Learning Needs

- Identifying learners
- Choosing the right attitudes
- About learners gathering important information
- Include health team members
- Prioritize needs
- Consider time management issues.

- **Identify learners**
  - Who is your audience? Individual patient groups for significant other patients.
  - Are their needs the same or different?
- **Please select your environment**
  - Create an environment in which learners feel comfortable sharing (disclosing) information and believe that their concerns are respected and taken seriously.
  - To build trust, protect privacy and confidentiality.
- **Collect key information about the learner**
  - The patient or family is the primary source of information for needs assessment.
  - Be sure to ask if any kind of social support system is available and how their social support system can help.
- **Involving members of the healthcare team**
  - Consulting with other professionals to understand the needs of patients and their families
  - Often provides insight into the learning needs of people with specific health problems or concerns.
- **Prioritize needs**
  - As Maslow's hierarchy of needs suggests, if basic needs are not met in the first place, learning of other information may be delayed or unfulfilled.
  - Prioritization helps nurses work with patients to set realistic and achievable learning goals.
  - Not all learners need to know everything, in order to give you a good assessment, here are some tips that will save you time in the long run.
- Learners should be given time to present their thoughts (actively involve customers).
- Conduct assessments at any time. Wherever possible.
- Provide lead time for clients.
- Minimize interruptions and distractions.
- **Lighthearted conservation:** Caregivers should rely on active listening using open-ended questions while conducting pt. use.
- **Questionnaire:** use checklist.
- **Observation:** Watching learners perform tasks is a great way to assess skills.

Readiness to Learn

Defined as the point at which a learner expresses an interest in learning or indicates what is needed to maintain optimal health. You can assess readiness for learning using the same methods used to assess learning. The timing of when classes should be held is very important. A learner who fails to accept information at one point may be more likely to accept the same information at another point.

Types of Readiness to Study

Four types of readiness to study:

Physical preparation

- Performance measures—sensory skills
- Task complexity—topic difficulty
- Environmental influences—environment conducive to learning
- Health status—energy available for learning

Accept medical care and pose fewer health risks than men

- Mental preparation
- Anxiety level
- Mild or severe anxiety can lead to learning disabilities
- Moderate anxiety drives someone to action
- Moderate anxiety is optimal for successful learning.

Support systems: A strong support system can reduce anxiety, but it can increase anxiety when it is absent. The

Teachable Moment is when the client is most receptive to learning.

Risk taking behavior: Health promotion nurses can help patients develop strategies to reduce risk in decision-making.

Developmental levels: Each level related to human development is taught.

Willingness to experience
- Understand how learners have dealt with past problems.
- Cultural context—assessing what the disease means to the patient's cultural perspective is important in determining willingness to learn.
- Control points—orientation of internal and external control points.

Knowledge readiness

Shows the learner's current knowledge base, level of learning ability, and preferred learning style.
- **Current knowledge base:** The amount of knowledge someone already knows to develop a willingness to learn based on this knowledge.
- **Cognitive skills:** Failure to match behavioral goals with learning potential.
- **Learning disabilities:** People with learning disabilities have special needs to teach.

Learning Style

Refers to the way an individual processes information. Each learner is unique, complex, and has different learning style preferences that distinguish one learner from another.

Six Principles of Learning Styles
- Client preferences
- Nurses do not have to use only their preferred style
- Help patients identify their preferred style
- Encourage clients to distinguish between different learning styles
- Become aware of the different methods and materials available
- Client will have chances to learn through their preferred style of learning

Mechanism Available
- Observation
- Interview
- Observation learning style tools
    Certain characteristics of learning styles are biological in origin, but others develop as a result of sociological and environmental influences.

Dunn and Dunn Learning Styles

The stimuli identified by Dunn and Dunn relate to the role of nurses as teachers. Nurses should consider the aforementioned characteristics when assessing a patient's or family's learning style.

Four Basic Stimuli Identified

1. Natural and biological environmental elements (sound, light, temperature and design) occur in home schooling and the like.
2. Sociological factors (the desire to learn alone or in groups).
3. Physical factors that are biological in nature and related to the learner's bodily functions (perception, time of day, mobility).
4. Psychological factors (indicating how learners process and respond to information).

Learning style interpretation must follow:
- Identify key elements of an individual's learning style through observation
- Ask questions to validate observations
- Tailor teaching methods and materials to those unique qualities
- Learning style assessment focus on and develop understanding from both caregiver and learner perspectives

TODAY'S GENERATION OF LEARNERS AND THEIR SKILLS AND CHARACTERISTICS

The world of work and communication is changing rapidly. As teachers, we must equip our secondary school student with the 21st century skills she needs to succeed in today's digitalized and globalized society.

Critical Thinking

- One of the most important 21st century skills we teach our learners is critical thinking. With so much information available online, it is important that young people analyze questions and challenge what is being said.
- You need to think outside the box.
- Encourage students to anticipate what will happen in reading and listening activities, give them challenging problems to solve in a variety of games and puzzles, and ask multiple answer questions to encourage critical thinking in the classroom and encourage thinking.

Communication

- Communication is a difficult skill for many students to master, especially in a second language, so it is important to practice it well.

- A good communicator not only speaks English more clearly and confidently, but also excels outside the classroom, whether in study, work or travel.
- Learners should be able to express their opinions on a variety of subjects, communicate with others, and work well in groups.

Collaboration

- This skill combines well with communication because good people work effectively with others to achieve common goals. Respecting the opinions of others and learning how to be a good team player are important to the success of your education also helps.
- Many students will need to work with people from different backgrounds and cultures.
- Incorporate frequent pair work in workgroups or collaborative projects into your lessons, and try to vary the students you work with so that you can work with different types of people.

Creativity

- Everyone has a creative side—may be they just do not know it.
- Similar to critical thinking, students should be encouraged to think of new and innovative ways to solve problems. Not only will it help you in other subjects in school, but it will also help you when entering higher education and the workplace.
- Traditional crafts are a good place to start, but there are many other things the class can do to spark creativity.

Cultural Awareness

- Learners should be able to understand the differences between themselves and people from other countries with different cultures and traditions.
- You can find common ground with everyone you meet, whether it is in your studies, work, or travel.

Digital Literacy

- Teenagers understand the digital world better than we do. That's why it is important to use technology in the classroom to motivate students and keep them motivated to learn.
- It should be remembered that many of the younger generation do not know life without Google social media and smartphones. It is therefore important that our teaching methods reflect this.
- Integrate your smartphone into your lessons to explore projects, review word definitions, and play interactive quizzes like Kahoot. Show real videos using interactive whiteboards or projectors, or let students create their own.

Skill categories: Each 21st century skill falls into one of three categories:
- **Learning skills:** Teaches students about the mental processes required to adapt and improve upon a modern work environment.
- **Literacy skills (IMT):** Focus on how students perceive facts, publishing channels, and the technology behind them. The focus is on identifying reliable sources and factual information to distinguish it from the misinformation flooding the Internet.
- **Life skills (FLIPS):** They are the intangible elements of student life. These intangibles focus on both personal and professional qualities.

Category 1: Learning skills (4 Cs). The 4 Cs of 21st century skills are:
- **Critical thinking:** Finding solutions to problems
- **Creativity:** Thinking outside the box
- **Collaboration:** Working with others
- **Communication:** Talking to others

Category 2: Literacy competencies (IMT) 21st century literacy skills:
- **Information literacy:** Understanding facts, numbers, statistics and data.
- **Media literacy:** Understanding how and through which channels information is published.
- **Technology literacy:** Understanding the machines that enable the information age.

Category 3: Life skills (FLIPS) is the last category. These skills, also known as FLIPS, are all relevant to your personal life, but they also affect your professional environment.

The four 21st century life skills are:
1. Initiative
2. Launching own projects, strategies and plans
3. Productivity: Staying productive when distracted
4. Social skills: Meeting and meeting others for mutual benefit networking

Learners Emotional Intelligence

Emotional intelligence helps students analyze situations better. It not only helps students to interact better with others, but also helps them to be more active solve academic problems EQ is defined as the ability to perceive, understand and manage emotions in a healthy and effective way. This skill helps students empathize with others and themselves and deal with difficult situations without tiring. It influences academic performance in interpersonal relationships and also influences the way students deal with pressure.

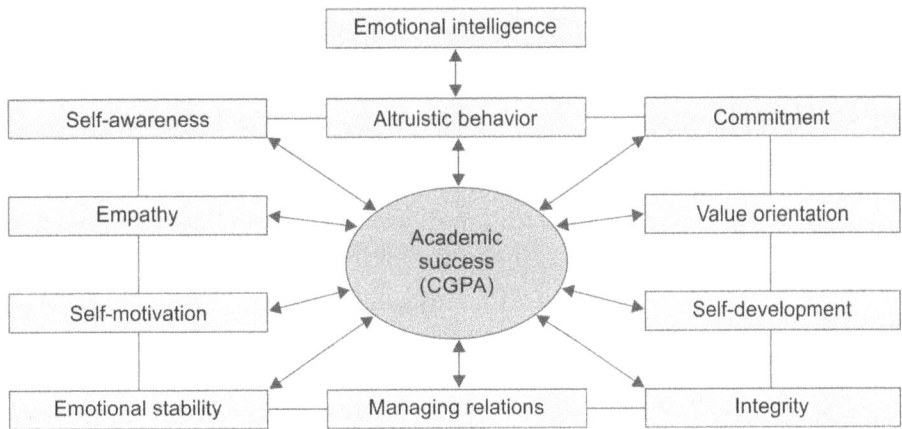

Fig. 5.1: Emotional intelligence in academic success.

Key Attributes

Five key attributes constituting emotional intelligence:
- Self-awareness
- Self-regulation
- Motivation
- Empathy for others
- Social skills/relationship building

Characteristics of emotionally intelligent:
Students have the following characteristics:
- They are positive
- Forgive quickly
- Recognize and improve your weaknesses faster
- Don't compare yourself to others
- Good listener
- Knows how to deal with toxic people.

Emotional Intelligence Symptoms

Here are the main symptoms and examples of emotional intelligence.
- Self-confidence
- Self-acceptance
- Ability to let go of mistakes
- Ability to embrace change
- Strong curiosity, especially about others
- Feelings of empathy and concern other
- Being sensitive to the emotions of others
- Taking responsibility for mistakes
- Ability to deal with emotions in difficult situations.

Components of Emotional Intelligence

Ability to reason with emotions, understanding emotions, ability to manage emotions.
- **Perceive emotions:** The first step in understanding emotions is to perceive them accurately. This often involves understanding nonverbal cues such as body language and facial expressions.
- **Emotions help us prioritize:** What we pay attention to and respond to. We react emotionally to things that attract our attention.

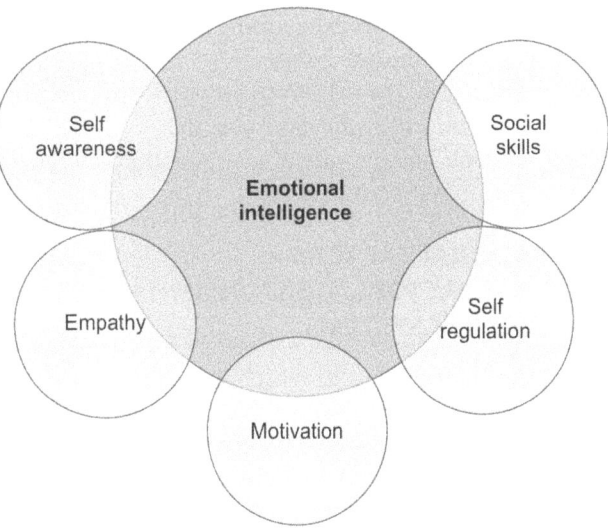

Fig. 5.2: Components of emotional intelligence.

- **Understanding emotions:** The emotions we perceive have very different meanings. When someone expresses anger, the observer must interpret the cause of that person's anger and what it means. For example, if your boss is angry, it could mean that he's unhappy with your job, got a speeding ticket on the way to work that morning, or had a fight with your partner.
- **Managing emotions:** The ability to effectively manage emotions is an important part and highest level of emotional intelligence. Properly regulating and respond-

ing to emotions and responding to the emotions of others are important aspects of emotion management.

Effective-use Emotional Intelligence

Emotional Intelligence can be used in many ways in your daily life. Here are some different ways to practice emotional intelligence.
- Can accept criticism and responsibility
- Can move forward after making mistakes
- Learn to say no when needed
- You can share your feelings with others
- You can solve problems in a way that works for everyone
- You can empathize with others
- You have excellent listening skills
- Do not judge others.

Benefits

EQ has many benefits for students. Key benefits of having good emotional intelligence include improved skills:
- **Leadership:** Emotional intelligence allows you to be a more effective leader.
- **Communication:** Understanding the feelings of others helps us communicate better.
- **Self-awareness:** The more aware you are of your feelings, the better you will understand yourself.
- **Self-control:** Being aware of your emotions also helps you develop self-control skills.

MOTIVATIONAL FACTORS—PERSONAL FACTORS, ENVIRONMENTAL FACTORS AND SUPPORT SYSTEMS

Motivation is the state in which a student maintains attention and behavior and provides more energy to complete a task. Therefore, it helps you stay active over a period of time. In education, motivation can have various effects on student behavioral preferences and outcomes.
- Allows you to complete those tasks in less time and maintains your attention for longer
- Minimizes distractions and helps you resist them better
- Information we keep and store
- Influences perceptions of how easy or difficult a task may appear.

Class and Curriculum Structure

- Children thrive with structure and struggle with confusion. Students feel more at ease when they feel and see that lessons follow a structure and curriculum and materials are prepared in advance.
- Feeling safe is fundamental to us is one of the most important needs. When this is provided in the learning environment, students are free to focus on their learning.
- Educators should plan their classes and curriculum to make students feel more at ease.
- All materials used in class should be prepared in advance.
- Teachers can also indicate course or class objectives at the beginning of the term or class.

Teacher Behavior and Personality

- If the student has negative feelings towards the teacher, such as fear or disgust.
- Teachers who favor certain students or use derogatory and degrading language can affect student motivation in class.
- On the other hand, friendliness, optimism, positive feedback and encouragement can have a positive impact on students' motivation to learn.

Teaching Methods

- Students are more likely to stay motivated in class when educators use different teaching methods. This creates diversity and avoids student boredom.
- Students in your class may have different learning styles. Teachers are therefore more likely to use different teaching methods to meet these needs.
- In some cases, enrollment in extracurricular activities and tutor support can help address unmet student needs at school.

Parenting Habits and Commitments

A significant number of parenting habits can indirectly affect a child's motivation, especially intrinsic motivation.
- Show interest in child's theme
- Ask about the day
- Active listening
- Helps with specific tasks and skills taught in school
- Attends parent meetings
- Encourages children to do homework and study for exams.

Family Problems and Instability

Lack of safety in the home, like in the classroom, can have a negative impact on motivation to study. On average, children who live with their parents do better than those who do not. Family conflicts and turmoil can lead to poor school performance. Here are some examples:
- Divorced
- Single or widowed parent
- Her not living with biological father or mother

- Not having contact with the biological father or mother
- Frequently moving from one home to another
- Being or having been involved with Child Protective Services.

As a result in certain instances additional support may be needed from schools to help students with their issues.

Peer Relationships

As children grow older the influence peers have upon them increases as well. Thus, problems and conflicts with peers can make students feel more insecure about their social status among peers, increase stress levels, and reduce educational motivation. and other peer problems can prevent serious problems.

Learning Environment

- The school environment or school climate is another factor that influences educational motivation. School environment refers to the various norms and rules that determine the overall atmosphere of a school.
- A positive school environment makes students feel safe, meets their basic needs such as daily meals, and provides the perfect environment for forming healthy social relationships.

- Too many classes and too demanding learning environment can reduce motivation in teaching. Adding a fun element to your class will lighten the mood, improve motivation and results.
- Providing plenty of play and rest time can also have positive effects.

Assessment

- Standardized assessment raises performance standards but can negatively affect student engagement.
- Students often lose motivation when tests are consistently too difficult. This does not give you a sense of accomplishment, and over time motivation to train wanes.

CONCLUSION

Effective teaching contributes to student learning regardless of the situation or condition. Effective education has the power to transform public education and ensure great public schools for all students, if schools also have strong leadership, adequate resources and meaningful stakeholder engagement. Teachers are responsible for making their practice as effective as possible. Teachers must also manage their own professions and share the responsibility of the school system to transform education.

REVIEW QUESTIONS

Long Essays
1. Define teacher evaluation, explain teacher evaluation techniques/methods.
2. Describe teacher evaluation criteria and strategies.
3. Enumerate teaching styles—formal authority demonstrator facilitator delegator.
4. Discuss in detail about determinants of learning.
5. Describe today's generation of learners and their skills and characteristics.
6. Enumerate the motivational factors—personal factors, environmental factors and support systems.

Short Essays
1. Teacher evaluation by teachers.
2. Teacher evaluation by students.
3. Effective time management and class management.
4. Benefits of teacher assessment.
5. Authoritative or lecture style.
6. Hybrid or blended styles.
7. Learner assessment.
8. Learning types.
9. Six principles of learning styles.
10. Learners emotional intelligence.
11. Components of emotional intelligence.
12. Effective-use emotional intelligence.
13. Learning environment.

Short Answers
1. Formative assessment.
2. Summative assessment.
3. Demonstrator.
4. Facilitator.
5. Delegator.
6. Diagnostic or preliminary screening.
7. Confirmation evaluation.
8. Norms-based evaluation.
9. Criteria-based assessment.
10. Ipsative assessment.
11. Interpersonal learners.
12. Kinesthetic learner.
13. Readiness to learn.
14. Critical thinking.
15. Digital literacy.
16. Emotional intelligence symptoms.
17. Class and curriculum structure.
18. Peer relationships.

Chapter 6

Curriculum Planning

Learning Objectives

- Curriculum Types
- Curriculum Objectives
- Factors Influences Curriculum Development
- Curriculum Features
- Principles of Curriculum
- Curriculum Types
- Core Curriculum
- Curriculum Design—Component Approach
- Curriculum Planning and Development
- Stages of Curriculum Planning
- Level of Curriculum Planning
- Curriculum Management
- Curriculum Process
- Writing Learning Outcomes/Behavioral Objectives
- Subject Classification
- Lesson Planning
- Course Planning
- Unit Planning

INTRODUCTION

Curriculum is the Latin word "currere" meaning a race, road, round, course, or slope spoken to achieve a goal that applies to study. If the teacher is the guide, the curriculum is the way. Curriculum is the overall structure of ideas and activities. Refers to the details of the specific training content, or course of study, that a student must complete in order to obtain various certificates or degrees from an institution.

DEFINITION

- A curriculum is an attempt to convey the essential principles and characteristics of an educational proposal in a form suitable for critical consideration and effective practice. **—Stenhouse (1975)**
- All learning activities planned and directed by the school, inside or outside the school, whether conducted in groups or individually. **—Kerr (1968)**
- Curriculum is the manifestation of the many components and factors that together enable the attainment of fully specified, selected and articulated goals of nursing education. **—Bevis (1982)**
- The systematic arrangement of a series of selected experiences planned by a school or defined group of students to achieve the goals of a specific educational program.
- Compilation of all ranges experienced by learners is done under the direction of the school. **—Lambertson**

CURRICULUM TYPES

Curriculum is the outward expression of the **community's ideas and aspirations**.

- Ongoing and continuous.
- Respond flexibly to changing social needs, national health scenarios, progress and trends in health science and technology patterns.
- Focus on social and health.
- Based on living conditions.
- Relates to the social, national and international needs of individuals.
- Ideal and practical approach.
- Depends on the philosophy and purpose of each course.
- It is intended to shift focus with respect to national health policy goals and consequent care demands.

- It is dualistic in the sense that it incorporates student ideas and course content.
- Contains two theories: Value theory and knowledge theory.
- Described in two ways (relative to children's themes and activities).
- Prepared by traditional authorities.
- It is based on children's interests, abilities, talents and needs.
- Curriculum is influenced by political, economic, philosophical and scientific factors.
- Curriculum is closely related to people's achievements and aspirations.
- A flexible curriculum designed to meet the evolving needs and skills of learners in the context of the needs of society availability of different knowledge and skills. The logical and psychological nature of learning.
- The syllabus represents the child's total living expenses. Schools should take responsibility for their development.

CURRICULUM OBJECTIVES

- Feed learners by bringing about desirable behavioral changes.
- To manage and handle life situations realistically and rationally without abandoning humanitarian principles.
- Help to:
  - Development of health workers at all levels.
  - Prepare each medical team member for the tasks they need to perform in their respective positions.
  - Student involvement in curriculum development.
  - A planned curriculum helps you achieve your educational goals.
- The curriculum is:
  - Designed to encourage, stimulate and inspire the full development of each student.
  - Create an atmosphere in which students learn to think. Be critical enough to be objectively constructively truthful for faculty and students to solve problems and develop thinking skills.
- Formation of values through intimate acquaintance with the humanities, arts, natural, social and religious sciences.
- Develop student personality such as sincerity, honesty, judgment, cooperation, kindness, goodwill.
- To create a community of scholars in which inquiry, curiosity, free inquiry and advances in knowledge take place.
- To give students citizenship in a democratic society where law, justice and responsibility exist.
- Meet the needs of students with wide range of abilities, aptitudes and interest.
- To discover milestones in human achievement.
- We will make appropriate decisions and judgments in a socially desirable direction.

FACTORS INFLUENCES CURRICULUM DEVELOPMENT

Loretta E Heidgerken (1965) identified six major factors that influence curriculum development in nursing education:

- **Philosophy of nursing education:** Philosophy of Curriculum Development or Educational Philosophy refers to the values that determine the goals, content, and pedagogy of an educational programme. The philosophy of nursing education is the determinant of the curriculum as it is the basis for the ultimate choice of curriculum objectives.
- **Educational psychology (knowledge about learning):** Educational psychology is the science of providing information about learning problems through experiments. It provides the data on which the principles of learning are developed. The principles of learning from the basis for developing teaching principles and methods.
- **Society (social change):** Society can be defined as a group of individuals who see themselves as a distinct group. They share common loyalty values, etc. that drive individuals to submit and even sacrifice for the common good of the group. These common elements comprise what humans have learned throughout history to do, believe, appreciate, and enjoy.
- **Students:** Students are learners of basic nursing education programs, most of whom are young female candidates in late adolescence, whose needs are consistent with those of this group. Although there are male candidates, enrollment in nursing schools and colleges is lower than female candidates. Nursing students, like all human beings, want to be accepted as different and unique, but they also want to share a common humanity with others. These young people are

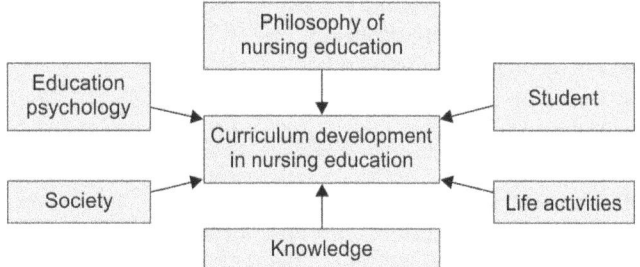

Fig. 6.1: Factors affecting curriculum.

characterized by their idealism, zest for life, generosity, and willingness to make sacrifices, all of which strongly motivate those who choose their profession to study nursing.
- **Living activities:** The term "activities" as used herein includes caregiving and personal activities in which the student is involved as a caregiver and as an individual. These are categorized into professional family, civic leisure, and spiritual service as sources of curriculum development goals.
- **Knowledge:** Knowledge can be broadly divided into descriptive knowledge and normative knowledge. Descriptive knowledge consists of statements about things that can be directly or in principle perceived. It includes facts, laws, rules, theories, principles, etc., that describe or state that things are or behave as they are.

CURRICULUM FEATURES

The university or school curriculum aims at the development of the learner:
- Language and communication skills necessary for social life and further study.
- Skills that facilitate mathematical operations and their application in everyday life and learning.
- Knowledge of the attitudes and habits necessary to maintain physical health and strength consistent with normal developmental patterns.
- Correctly understand the role and importance of sex in human life and maintain a healthy attitude towards sex and the opposite sex.
- Kindness, mutual help, compassion, self-discipline, self-criticism, self-control, humor, courage, love of social justice, and other qualities that make men socially effective and happy in a variety of social situations.
- Entrepreneurship and the dignity of manual labor necessary to increase productivity and job satisfaction.
- Ability to perceive and discover beauty in a variety of life situations and integrate it into one's personality.
- Understanding of the environment and its limited resources and the need to manage natural resources and energy.
- Evaluating the different consequences of large families and overpopulation, and the need to curb population growth.
- Understanding the diverse cultural and social systems of people living in different parts of the country and the cultural heritage of the country.
- Recognizing the need for a balanced integration between technology directed towards change and the continuity of the nation's cultural heritage.
- Knowledge of national symbols and desire and determination to uphold ideals of national identity and unity.
- Ability to appreciate and tolerate differences and different kinds of differences, and to choose between different value systems.
- Recognition of the need for equality and global brotherhood inherent in all people, with a strong commitment to human values and social justice.
- A scientific temper characterized by inquisitiveness, questioning and objectivity, eliminating ambiguity, superstition and fatalism.
- Knowledge of scientific research methods and their application to problem solving.
- Appreciation of sacrifices and contribution made by the freedom fighters and social workers in the country's freedom struggle and social regeneration and readiness to follow their ideals.
- Appreciation and readiness to practice in life the national goals of socialism secularism democracy and nonviolence.
- Divergent, independent thinking and the ability to discover new connections and combinations.
- Qualities and characteristics necessary for lifelong learning leading to self-study and the formation of a learning society.

PRINCIPLES OF CURRICULUM

Curriculum is a tool which considerably helps to inculcate those standards of moral action which are essential for successful living in society and for getting true satisfaction out of life.

Table 6.1: Principles of curriculum.

S. No.	Principle	Description
1.	The conservation principle	It has been stated that nations live in the present, on the past and for the future. This means the present, the past and the future needs of the community should be taken into consideration
2.	The forward looking principle	Children of today are the future citizens of tomorrow. Therefore, their education should be such as it enables them to progressive minded persons. Education should give them a foundation of knowledge, feeling and that will enable them to change the environment where change is needed
3.	Creative principle	The objective of education is to discover and to develop special interests, tastes, and aptitudes

Contd...

Contd...

S. No.	Principle	Description
4.	Activity principle	The curriculum should be thought in terms of activity and experiences, rather than of knowledge to be acquired and facts to be stored. Growth and learning take place only where there is activity. The curriculum must ensure the activity of body and mind. It should be the center of the curriculum
5.	Principle of preparation of life	This is the most important principle in the construction of the curriculum. We have to prepare him such a way as he is capable of facing the various challenges of the complex problems of the future
6.	Principle of maturity	Curriculum should be adapted to the grade of the pupils and to their stage of mental and physical development in the early childhood. The curriculum should harness the adventurous spirit of the growing child
7.	Principle of individual differences	Individuals differ in taste, temperament, skill, experience, aptitude, innate ability and in sex. Therefore, the curriculum should be adapted to individual differences. It should not be rigid
8.	Principle of vertical and horizontal articulation	Each year's course should be built on what has been done in previous years and at the same time should serve as basis for subsequent work. It is absolutely essential that the entire curriculum should be co-ordinated
9.	Principle of linking with life	The community needs and characteristics should be kept in view while framing the curriculum
10.	Principle of comprehensiveness and balance	The curriculum should be framed in such a way as every aspect of life, i.e. economic relationships, social activities, occupations and spiritual life, is given due emphasis
11.	Principle of loyalties	The curriculum should be planned in such a manner that it teaches a true sense of loyalty to the family, the school, the community, the town, the province, the country and the world at large. It should enable the child to understand that there is unity in diversity
12.	Principle of flexibility	Curriculum should take into consideration the special needs and circumstances of the pupils. Curriculum of the girls may not always be identical with that of boys. The special needs of both the sexes should be given their due consideration

Contd...

Contd...

S. No.	Principle	Description
13.	Principle of core or common subjects	There are certain broad areas of knowledge, skill and appreciation with which all the children must be made conversant and these should find a place in the curriculum. This is more important at higher secondary stage where there are diversified courses. These subjects are to be common to all groups
14.	Principle of leisure	The curriculum should prepare the child for the use of leisure time. According to Herbert Spencer. "Literature, music and art occupy the leisure part of life and should, therefore, occupy the leisure part of education. The capacity to enjoy leisure greatly determines a man's capacity to work. If leisure is spent in gambling, drinking and reading obscene literature, it will hamper progress not only of an individual but also the nation as a whole". The school curriculum should therefore, prepare the would-be-citizens to use effectively their leisure time
15.	Principle of all-round development	Principle of all-round development of body, mind and spirit. All kinds of experiences should be provided to the students so that they may develop their all powers
16.	Principle of democracy	Principle of democracy, secularism and socialism curriculum should be such as it trains the child to imbibe ideals and values of a democratic, secular and socialist state
17.	Principle of character building	Curriculum should provide those activities and experiences which promote human and social values. There should be provision for a number of co-curricular activities
18.	Principle of dignity of labor curriculum	Principle of dignity of labor curriculum should make provision for socially useful productive work. The students should be provided opportunities to learn from the use of hands

CURRICULUM TYPES

Along with the changes in the educational system in Japan and other countries, the concept and form of the curriculum have also changed. The modern concept differs from the traditional one. As new educational systems developed, new psychological, philosophical, and sociological principles modified the educational process. A new type of curriculum has emerged. Below, we describe key concepts and curriculum types that have evolved over time.

- Traditional or subject-based curriculum
- Action plan
- Experience curriculum
- Non-differentiated curriculum
- Basic education curriculum
- Life-centered or balanced curriculum.

Table 6.2: Curriculum types.

S. No.	Types	Description
1.	Traditional or subject-centered curriculum	The traditional curriculum which has been in vogue for sufficiently long time is conceived in terms of subjects. It is nothing but a statement of the subjects of study with indications of their extent and time limit. Each subject is separate entity and its nature and score is clearly defined. All stress is on the intellectual attainment of the child rather than on the values of studies for personal and social development
2.	Activity curriculum	It is a pity that even at present, educational system in India lays undue emphasis on verbal information, external examination and bookish knowledge and there is little attempt to see whether such knowledge and information produce the desired effect on the behavior of pupils. Thinkers like Rousseau, Montessori, Dewey and Gandhi realized that education which does not influence the child's conduct is not worth the time, money and energy, invested out it. The child is active by nature. He wants to know, handle and manipulate the things, around him, to satisfy his instincts of creativeness and curiosity. If constructive activities do not provide opportunities of expressing these tendencies. they may assume destructive form. So teaching through constructive and purposeful activities is quite in accordance with the nature and interest of children. Activity develops the constructive and creative urges of children and thus leads to full and all-round growth of their personality.
3.	Experience curriculum	A curriculum which gives rich and varied experiences of knowledge, skills, attitudes and appreciation is called the experience curriculum. Experience, in fact, is the product of the education process. No activity can be separate from experience. An educative and meaningful activity must end in a gainful experience. In words of John Dewey, experience is a matter of the interaction of organism with its environment, an environment that is human as well as physical that includes the materials of tradition and institution as well as local surrounding'. Such an interaction includes both "undergoing" and "trying" to do something with it. We also have trying situation and we meet the challenge. In both the cases, there is some gain either knowledge of skill or attitude.
4.	Undifferentiated curriculum	"Differentiation" means specialization and undifferentiation is the opposite of specialization. Undifferentiated curriculum, therefore, means a curriculum which does not aim at the specialized study of various subjects. Specialization should come at the higher secondary and the college levels. At the primary and junior secondary school stages, we should have undifferentiated or fused curriculum, which lays stress on the formation of worth-while habits, skills and virtues.
5.	Basic education curriculum	Basic curriculum should be interpreted in the light of the general principles of basic education which have been discussed separately—basic education, as conceived and explained by Mahatma Gandhi, is essentially an education for life and what is more, an education through life. It aims at creating a social order which is free from all exploitation and violence. This is the reason why productive, creative and socially useful work for pupils, without any distinction of class or creed, is placed as the very center of basic education. In this scheme of education, all knowledge, therefore, is related to activity, practical experience and observation. These aims and features of basic education must be kept in view while constructing its curriculum.
6.	Life-centered or balanced curriculum	After discussing the different types of curriculum we should not be in a position to decide as to what a balanced curriculum is. In fact, if we keep all the important principles of constructing curriculum in mind and then select activity and subjects for various grades of pupils, the result will be a "balanced curriculum". Such a curriculum will include all the aspects of human activity and human development and will, thus cater to the needs of both the individual and the society.

CORE CURRICULUM

In recent years, the term "core" has been used to deal with experience and develop the general competencies that everyone must have in order to live effectively in a democratic lifestyle. Applied to part of the experiential curriculum. These generic competencies are unlikely to be mastered in curriculum patterns based on collaborative learning. The term is general learning, meaning that the curriculum contains learning experiences that everyone, regardless of profession, must go through. The core curriculum also includes learning experiences to develop professional and diverse types of competencies, recognizing individual differences in interests, skills and abilities.

Core Curriculum Concepts

- Following John Dewey's "philosophy of experimentalism" was a core curriculum concept.
  - Focus on learning basic human activities.
  - Learning in the sense of continually reconstructing experience.
  - Troubleshooting.
- Dynamic changes in fundamental democratic values and political and social thought, cultural factors.
- Acceptance of cognitive learning theory. It is a dynamic and organic process.

Elements of the Core Concept

- General educational aspects of education as a whole, regardless of the student's social status or career choice.
- All students can benefit from it.
- Problem-focused.
- The learning process is important. To prepare for life in a democratic society, learners should experience first-hand the basic processes of democratic life.
- Collaborative preplanning by teachers. Teachers pool ideas to create resource units.
- Teachers and students plan each day in class.
- Emphasis is placed on the holistic development of the student (social, intellectual, physical, emotional and spiritual).

CURRICULUM DESIGN—COMPONENT APPROACH

That is, the way teachers plan their lessons. When teachers design a curriculum, they decide what needs to be done, who will do it, and what schedule to follow. The Core Curriculum consists of four main components that are cohesive and integrated. These components are purpose (objectives and goals), content (topic), learning experience, and assessment.

Definition

Curriculum design is the process of taking a subject and creating a plan for teaching that subject. This includes deciding which materials to use, how to organize those materials, and how to use them in the classroom to develop students' knowledge and skills.

Elements of Successful Curriculum Design

- **Clear goals:** Building a visionary core curriculum team is essential to providing momentum and energy to all efforts. This team should consider what the intended outcome of the curriculum is.
- **Strong beliefs:** Beliefs drive action. Therefore, a curriculum intended to ensure an experience for all students must demonstrate what the school district believes about the content of the curriculum and provide consistent behavior that aligns with those stated beliefs.

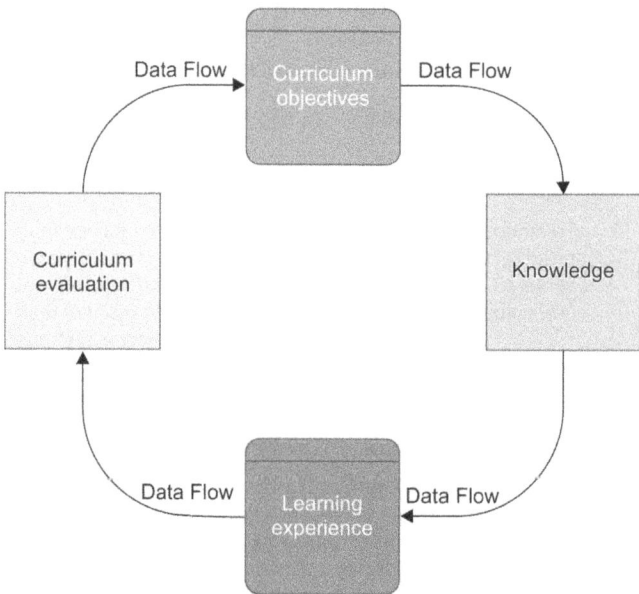

Fig. 6.2: Curriculum design.

- **Big ideas:** With clear purpose and shared beliefs, these long-term, transferable goals can be translated into big ideas for content areas specific to grade-level expectations and key learning focal points.
- **Sharing timely and targeted assessments:** Designing effective curricula that produce desired outcomes for your district is a daunting task, but the power of learning will help those whose children have the greatest impact. It is exciting because it is entrusted to your hands.
- **Common design review and annual revision time:** The curriculum design team is a key factor in the successful creation of a local his curriculum. Effective teams are made up of dedicated district educators who have grade-level expertise and are happy to review research and multiple resources.

Types of Curriculum Design

- **Subject-centered curriculum design:** Subject centered curriculum design revolves around a particular subject or subject area. For example, a subject-focused curriculum can focus on mathematics or biology. This type of curriculum design focuses on subjects rather than people.
- **Learner-centered curriculum design:** In contrast, learner-centered curriculum design considers each individuals needs, interests, and goals. In other words, we recognize that students are not uniform and adapt to their needs. Learner-centered curriculum design aims

to empower learners to shape their education through choice.
- **Problem-centered curriculum design:** A problem-centered curriculum focuses on teaching students how to see problems and find solutions to problems. In this way, students are exposed to real-world problems and help develop skills applicable to the real world.

Curriculum Design Principles

Curriculum Design Principles are broad guidelines that influence the structure of a curriculum. They are based on research and theory about learning and teaching and how people learn. These principles provide insight into what makes a curriculum effective for students to achieve desired learning outcomes.
- Create a curriculum-based on student needs, not teachers or schools.
- Decide which subjects and skills need to be taught and in what order.
- Create an assessment plan that matches what the student has learned and the skills they have learned.

How to Design a Curriculum

- **The curriculum design process involves various components, such as:** Reach the end of the course. These goals should relate to skills, knowledge, competencies, and attitudes.
- **Selecting assessment:** The next step in curriculum design is to select methods for assessing whether students have achieved the learning outcomes. Different assessments may be appropriate for different types of learning objectives. For example, an objective that requires a student to acquire a skill can be assessed by observing the student perform the skill, whereas an objective that requires the student to acquire factual knowledge can be assessed by written tests.
- **Developing lesson plans and learning activities:** The final step in curriculum design is to develop lesson plans to help students achieve their learning goals. A lesson plan may include materials such as handouts, reading materials, and videos, group discussions or lectures; and hands-on activities.
- **Establish a timeline for completion:** At this point, establish when each unit should be completed along with any other details such as holidays or special events that may affect your schedule.

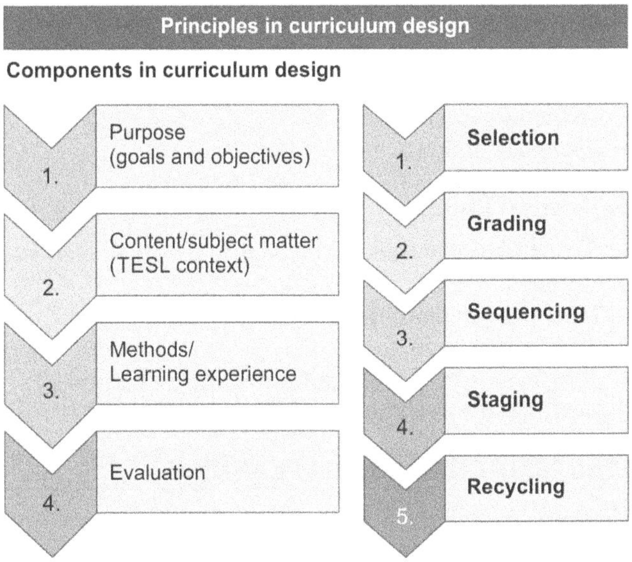

Curriculum Design Tips

Here are the most important curriculum design tips:
- Think about what you want to teach and how you want to teach it.
- Ensure that the curriculum can be taught large or small.
- Think about topics in different ways to help people understand the material. In this way, people are exposed to new information in different ways and see things from different perspectives.
- Always test your syllabus once it is complete to ensure that all information is clear, easy to understand, and covers all areas covered by the program.

CURRICULUM PLANNING AND DEVELOPMENT

Concept and Meaning

- The process by which participants at various levels make decisions about learning objectives in a teaching and learning context.
- The process of gathering, categorizing, selecting, reviewing, and synthesizing relevant information from many sources in order to design experiences that help learners achieve curricular goals.
- Methodical study and improvement of schooling in the light of established goals.

Features

- Continuous process
- Done on many levels
- This includes many group decisions on various plans and issues
- Ultimately, it is about the learner's experience.

Principles in curriculum design

Components in curriculum design
1. Purpose (goals and objectives)
2. Content/subject matter (TESL context)
3. Methods/Learning experience
4. Evaluation

1. Selection
2. Grading
3. Sequencing
4. Staging
5. Recycling

Fig. 6.3: Principles of curriculum design.

Syllabus Building Steps

- Syllabus topics and activities should be designed to build students' competencies in the areas of construction, observation, inquiry and problem-solving.
- Teachers should regularly evaluate the curriculum to reflect current trends and changes in the health field.
- Curriculum should be designed from a social perspective curriculum development is a continuous activity because society is not static.
- Nursing curriculum development is the school's responsibility. It is based on philosophical resource needs and other conditions.
- Core content is common to all state or national curricula as prescribed by statutory-bodies. Indian Nursing Council.
- The specific school curriculum and experience for students is developed by its own Curriculum Committee (Lead Administrator, Lead Teacher).

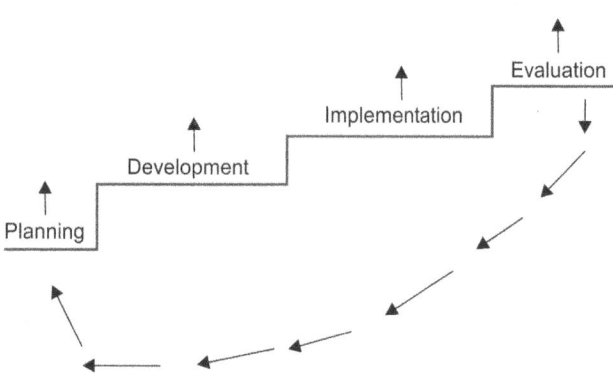

Fig. 6.4: Curriculum planning and development.

Plan

- State the philosophy of the nursing education program.
- Goals should be formulated based on community needs, resource availability, nursing roles, nursing philosophy requirements, and educational program goals.
- Involve influential figures in the preparation of curriculum development such as nursing instructor, nursing administrator, nursing administrator, nursing practitioner.
- Establishment of curriculum development committee.
- Establish organizational philosophy and policies.
- Student recruitment course type teaching methods groups involved duration human resource requirements examples: Instruction supervised clinical practice teaching/learning activities, selection of learning experiences theory and practice instruction hours.

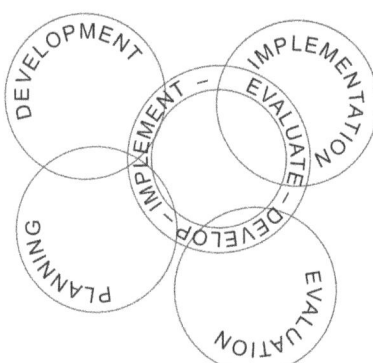

Fig. 6.5: Syllabus building steps.

Formation Stage

Organization and Procedures

- Theory
- Practical
- Supervised clinical practice
- Individual student rotation plan
- Preparation of materials and learning materials AV assistance.

The Curriculum Committee reviews progress, identifies bottlenecks, identifies the need for changes, and forms other standing committees to manage the curriculum.

Implementation Stage

- Practical implementation of teaching/learning activities (learner-centered and socialized methods)
- Conduct hands-on sessions in a laboratory or institutional setting
- Further development of teaching and learning methods.
- Assessment of academic performance
- Student counseling
- Health services
- Curriculum committee
- Necessary action.

Evaluation Phase

- Evaluate student learning through knowledge, skills and attitudes.
- Teaching and learning processes.
- Effective use of AV tools.
- Student activities in communities and institutions.
- How effective is the educational experience

STAGES OF CURRICULUM PLANNING

There are many ways in which curriculum planning may be approached. Torres and Stanton (1982) see the curriculum process as having four main stages as described in **Table 6.3**.

Table 6.3: Stages of curriculum planning.

S. No.	Stages	Description
1.	Directive stage	This initial stage lays the foundation for all other stages by identifying the beliefs. Knowledge and concepts that form the basis of the curriculum. This is done by the systematic gathering of information from the literature and also by the exploration of common beliefs about the nature of nursing. This leads to a statement of the philosophy of the curriculum, which in turn serves to influence each successive stage of the curriculum process.
2.	Formative stage	At this stage, the overall design of the curriculum takes shape and this design should reflect the philosophy described in stage one, as well as reflecting the nature of nursing. Objectives will be written for specific levels within the course as well as for overall course objectives and are derived from the broad characteristics identified in the previous stage. Content-mapping is used to select content elements for each aspect of the course and also gives staff and students and indication of the sequencing of topics.
3.	Functional stage	This is the stage in which the curriculum begins to assume a more practical form. Consideration is given to approaches by which the content can be organized and the notion of models of nursing is employed. The variety of teaching methods and learning experiences is also decided, to include both classroom and clinical methods. In addition, methods of validating learning are decided, using the behavioral objectives formulated in stage two. There are three types of evaluation to be considered: • Evaluation for continued learning. This is evaluation that provides feedback for students to improve their learning. • Evaluation for grading. Examinations designed for grading should not be viewed as a learning activity. • Evaluation for curriculum revision. This involves assessment of the total curriculum package and constitutes stage four.
4.	Evaluative stage	This can only occur when the curriculum is fully implemented and is thus a confirmative evaluation. There are three aspects to this: • Input evaluation. What the students bring to the course, such as mathematical abilities, problem-solving abilities and so on. • Throughout evaluation. All the tests and activities that students undergo as they progress through the course. • Output evaluation. Achievement of the characteristics identified in the directive stage. The Torres and Stanton process of curriculum seems to be finally based upon the behavioral-objectives model and is specifically tailored to the North American University system of nurse education.

LEVEL OF CURRICULUM PLANNING

The professional nursing curriculum includes all planned opportunities to study subjects that facilitate planning and implementation in all settings for a specific student group for a specific period of time increase. Here, three levels of curriculum planning related to levels of distance from the learning act itself are identified by Goodland (1961).

- **Social curriculum:** Social curriculum means a syllabus or part of a syllabus designed for a large group or class of students. Curriculum planned by an organization other than an educational institution. There are many such groups that put pressure on school and university curriculum development.
- **Institutional curriculum:** An institutional curriculum is a curriculum planned by faculty for a clearly defined group of students who spend a specific period of time at a particular institution, college, or nursing board.
- **Syllabus:** A syllabus consists of content, i.e., subjects and learning activities, planned day by day and week by a particular teacher for a particular group of students. Teacher planning instruction and clinical experience should be influenced by curriculum professionals.

CURRICULUM MANAGEMENT

There are three phases of curriculum management.

Curriculum Planning

It is the dynamic nature of human life, an essential feature of a managed curriculum program, and its attendant impact on the educational environment.

- Establish a new social order in India in accordance with the Constitution.
- Democratic way of life.
- Proposed national development.
- A scientific and national liberal approach to individual and national issues.
- Secular perspective and development of national integration.
- Improved economic living standards.
- International understanding, cooperation, world peace.

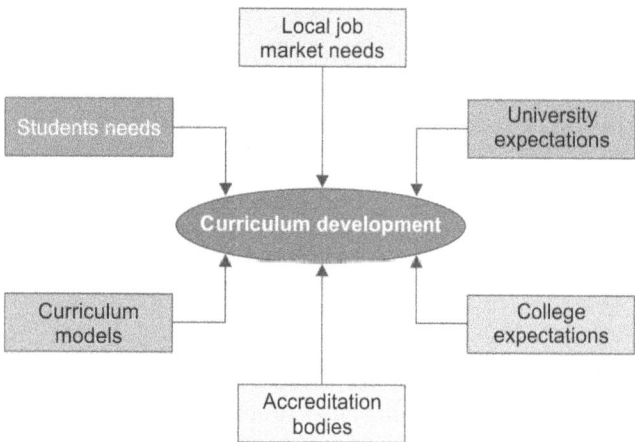

Fig. 6.6: Curriculum development.

Curriculum Organization

Requirements for all types of curriculum. Each course has a curriculum design for each subject. A detailed syllabus has been created as a basis for textbook development.

A highly centralized and decentralized system of curriculum construction, restructuring, and management is a functional aspect that must be met for effective implementation of a curriculum program.

State government education mechanisms have primary responsibility for curriculum design, for formulating education policies and their effective implementation, in order to provide adequate funding for the organization of educational programs in schools and colleges. Schools must be given the freedom to implement the curriculum.

The effectiveness of curriculum development depends on the quality of the:
- Prescribed curriculum.
- Types of manuals and textbooks available.
- Adequacy of instruction for teachers.
- Providing institutional support.

Curriculum Evaluation

The education administration shall be responsible for the evaluation of the curriculum. Provide feedback as needed for further revision and reform of curriculum implementation.

Curriculum assessment is done by:
- Face-to-face supervision program.
- Instruction and guidance under educational supervision.
- Planning methods for improving the effective implementation of the evaluated program.

CURRICULUM PROCESS

Curriculum is the summation of all the areas a learner experiences under the guidance of a school or university. It is the systematic arrangement of selected experience sums planned by a school or college or defined group of students to achieve the goals of a particular educational program.

Curriculum development is an ongoing activity. It should be designed according to the changing needs of society, namely, improvements in general education, changes in traditional practices, advances in medicine, research in nursing, and, from time to time, increased availability of resources. Whether the program is offered by a school, college or university, regular curriculum reviews and revisions are essential to keep up with all these developments.

Curriculum Process Stages

Curriculum is based on the philosophy and goals of the school, college or university and its construction requires an understanding of educational psychology and knowledge and skills in the principles and practices of nursing education. There are five steps in curriculum development.

The curriculum process has five phases, including:
- **Phase I:** Framing the statement of philosophy of the school or college or university.
- **Phase II:** Establish the purpose and goals of the school, college or university.
- **Phase III:** Selection of learning experiences to accomplish objectives and goals.
- **Phase IV:** Conduct selected learning experiences.
- **Phase V:** Overall program evaluation.

These phases can be described separately and considered sequential both in time and with respect to related operations. However, they are interrelated and interdependent, and are combined in a cyclical process such that the final stages influence the early stages over time. Each phase is mostly a logical progression of the previous phase. One cannot attempt work on a phase until work on the previous phase is complete.

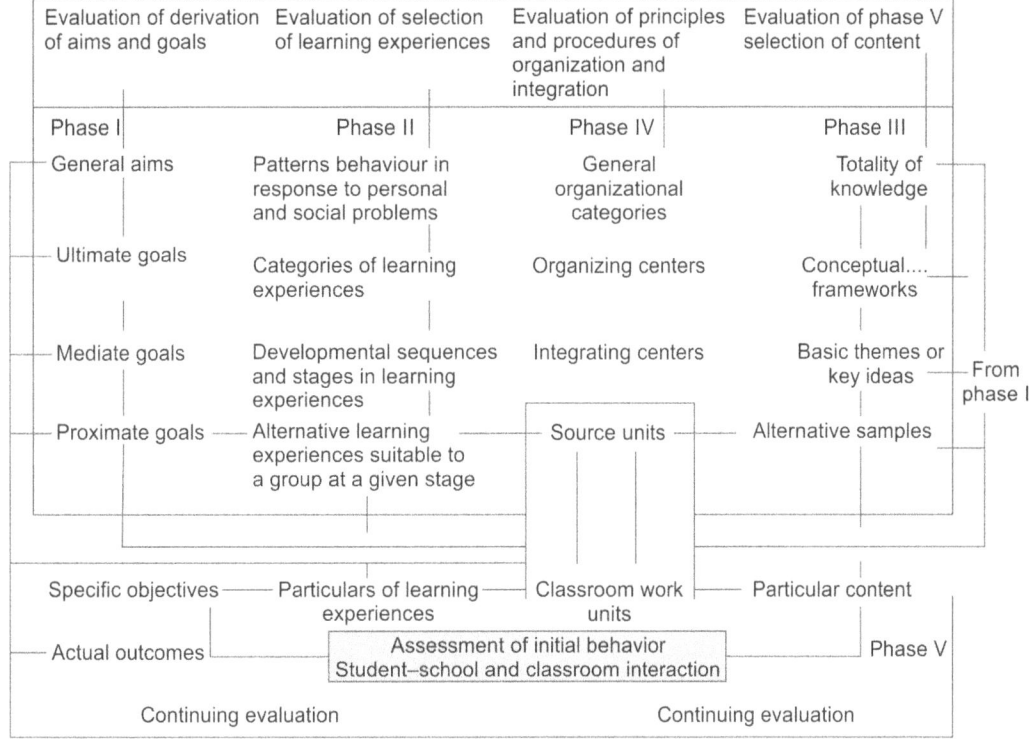

Fig. 6.7: Curriculum process stages.

WRITING LEARNING OUTCOMES/BEHAVIORAL OBJECTIVES

Learning outcomes and taxonomies of learning are central to teaching and learning in today's higher education. They provide an opportunity to achieve what is commonly referred to as 'curriculum alignment'. Curriculum alignment is a coherent structure in which objectives, learning outcomes, instructional strategies, content, and assessment are all aligned to enhance both curricular coherence and the learning that students do as a result of their learning to organize the curriculum. They are expressed in terms of the knowledge, skills, dimension and the application of knowledge and skills.

Formulate Goals

Educational goals describe the goals to which the educational process is directed, i.e., the learning to be gained from the lessons. Goals set by an educational institution or professional organization are usually called criteria. A taxonomy is a classification system based on an organizational scheme. In this case, a carefully defined set of terms, from simple to complex, concrete to abstract, provides a categorical framework for classifying educational goals.

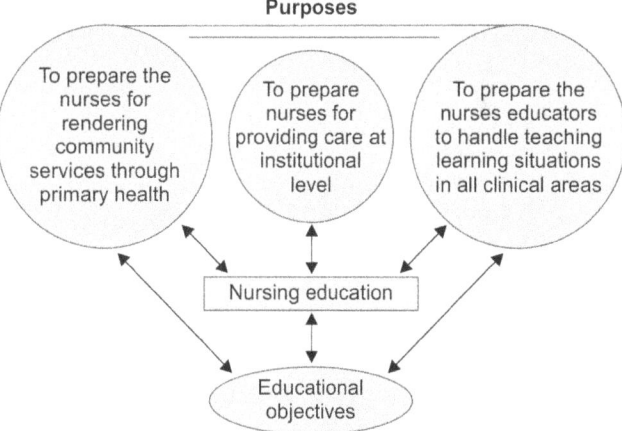

Fig. 6.8: Learning outcomes/behavioral objectives.

Definitions

- Outcomes desired by learners at the end of an educational program. At the end of the study period, the learner should be able to do what he could not do before.
  —**JJ Guilbert**
- A desired end result or goal is an expected or anticipated end result.
- "Objectives are behaviors that learners should exhibit". Objectives are for teachers and objectives are for learners

who are accomplished with the teacher's support and guidance.
- Representation of desired behavioral changes as a result of specific learner and teacher activities, a two-way process.

Meaning and Importance

Educational goals are expressions of what teachers expect from their students as a result of their education. In the educational process, learners must be able to demonstrate good possession of factual concepts, good ability to manipulate in more complex ways, and good ability to do things based on complex manipulation skills. Educational goals are political directions and form the basis of the entire educational structure. These are tangible and measurable expressions of cognitive or psychomotor attitudes that should be developed and statements that students can develop based on prescribed treatment or educational methods. or related to school. Relevance to the health needs of society is an essential quality of educational objectives.

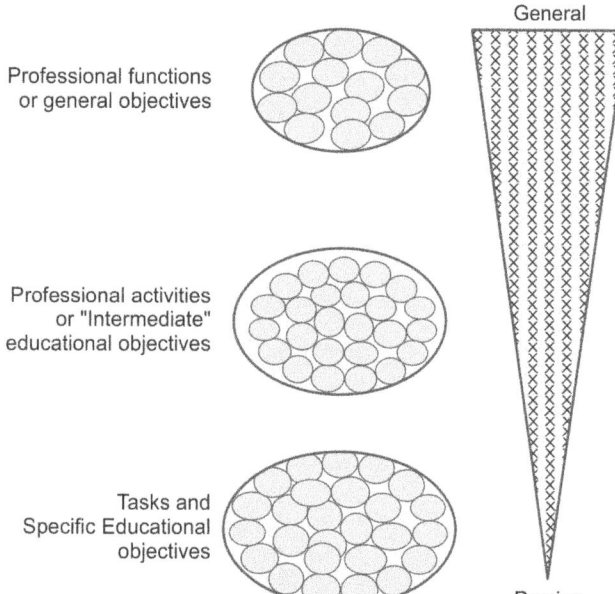

Fig. 6.9: Types of educational goals.

Type of Educational Goal

General Goals

- To provide individuals and communities with preventive and curative care in health and disease.
- Public health education depends on the general education level of the population. PhD students prepare or set goals.
- Obtain medical history and general health assessment.
- Safe and competent care in emergencies and acute illnesses.
- Provide supportive care to individuals with terminal chronic diseases.
- Provide health education guidance and counseling.
- Help people maintain optimal health.
- Take leadership responsibility for care planning and evaluation.
- Collaborate effectively with everyone involved in health issues.

Intermediate Goals

These components are professional activities that can be broken down into two more specific acts called professional tasks, as long as they can be measured against specific criteria. There may be several intermediate stages rather than a single stage.
- Place Intermediate goals reflect the health needs of populations living in specific situations.
- A goal is only a means or a working tool, not an end in itself.
- An object was created as a basis for selecting assessment instruments for measuring student performance.

Specific or Educational Purpose

Specific or educational purpose (professional task) definition: An educational purpose is a description of the outcome that education is intended to achieve. Defining goals helps identify the end result of instruction in terms of observable learner performance.

Characteristics of Specific Goals

- Must be written in terms of behavior (what students need to do).
- It should reflect the state (under what circumstances).
- Must reflect standards (what qualifications).
- If a reasonable number of behavioral changes are expected from a lesson, neither too much nor too little. Units are typically given 4–5 action objectives.
- Should be consistent with the theme of the unit and related to each other.

SUBJECT CLASSIFICATION

Description of Major Categories of Cognitive Domains

- **Knowledge:** Knowledge is defined as remembering what was previously learned. This involves searching for material ranging from specific facts to complete theories, but all it takes is memorizing the pertinent

information. Knowledge represents the lowest level of learning outcomes in a cognitive domain.
- **Comprehension:** Comprehension is defined as the ability to grasp the meaning of things. This includes translating material from one form to another (words or numbers), interpreting material (explaining or summarizing), and estimating future trends (predicting results or effects). These learning outcomes go far beyond simply memorizing material and represent the lowest level of comprehension.
- **Application:** Application refers to the ability to apply what is learned to new, concrete situations. This includes the application of rules, methods, concepts, principles, laws, theories, etc. Learning outcomes in this area require a higher level of understanding than what is not understood.
- **Analysis:** Analysis refers to the ability to break down materials into their constituent parts in order to understand their tissue structure. This may include identifying parts, analyzing relationships between parts, and recognizing relevant organizing principles. Learning outcomes here represent a higher intellectual level than comprehension and application, as they assume an understanding of both the content and the structural form of the material.
- **Synthesis:** Compositing refers to the ability to combine parts to create a new whole. This may involve creating your own communications (topics or speeches), work plans (research proposals), or a set of abstract relationships (schema for categorizing information).

Learning outcomes in this area emphasize creative behavior focused on formulating new patterns and structures.
- **Evaluation:** Valuation is the ability to judge the value of a material for a particular purpose (explanatory novel poetry research report). Judgments are based on certain criteria. These can be internal criteria (organizational) or external criteria (relevance to objectives), allowing students to determine or specify their own criteria. Learning outcomes in this area are highest in the cognitive hierarchy. This is because it includes elements from all other categories and value judgments based on well-defined criteria.

Description of the Major Categories of the Emotional Domain

- **Receive:** Receptivity refers to a student's willingness to pay attention to a particular phenomenon or stimulus (classroom activity, textbook music, etc.). From a pedagogical point of view, it is about attracting and keeping students' attention. Learning outcomes in this area range from mere awareness that something exists to selective attention on the part of the learner. Receiving represents the lowest level of learning outcomes in the emotional domain. Response refers to active participation on the part of the student. At this stage, he is not only interested in certain phenomena, but also reacts in certain ways. Learning outcomes in this domain are measured by tolerance in responding (reading assigned material), willingness to respond

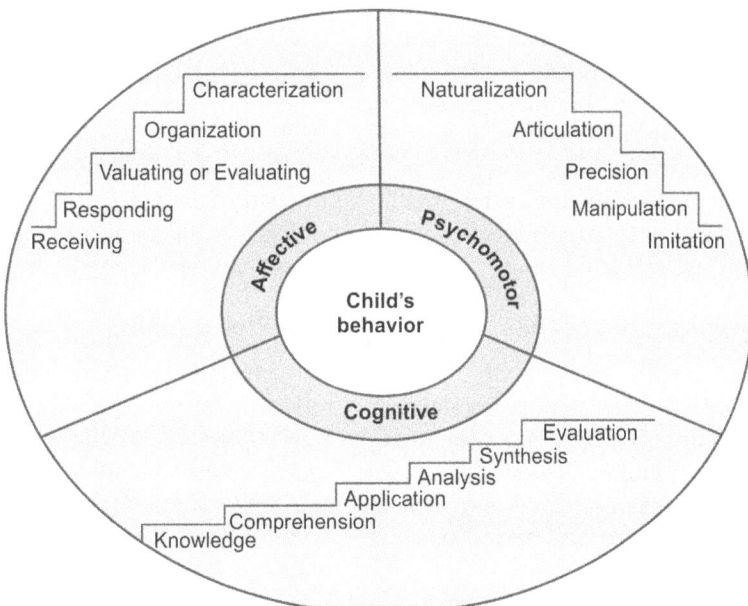

Fig. 6.10: Major categories of curriculum domains.

(reading beyond the task spontaneously), or satisfaction in responding (reading for pleasure or pleasure, etc). The higher levels of this category include educational goals generally classified as secondary interests. These emphasize seeking out and enjoying a particular activity.

- **Thanking:** Appreciation deals with the value or value that a student attaches to the phenomenon or action of a particular object. This ranges from simple value acceptance (the desire to improve the group's skills) to more complex levels of involvement (responsibility for the effective functioning of the group). Appreciation is based on the internalization of a set of specific values, but references to those values are reflected in students' apparent behavior. Learning outcomes in this area relate to behaviors that are consistent and stable enough to demonstrate value. Educational goals that are generally categorized as attitude and gratitude fall into this category.

- **Organization:** Organizations are interested in bringing together different values, resolving conflicts between them, and starting to build an internally consistent value system. Therefore, the emphasis is on comparing, linking, and integrating values learning outcomes may relate to conceptualizing values (acknowledging each individual's responsibility for improving relationships) or organizing a value system (creating a career plan that meets needs), both economic security and social services). Educational goals related to developing a philosophy of life fall into this category.

- **Characterized by a value or value complex:** At this level of the emotional realm, individuals have long had value systems that have controlled their behavior, and thus have developed a unique lifestyle. The behavior is therefore consistent and predictable. Learning outcomes at this level cover a wide range of activities, but the emphasis is on the fact that the behavior is typical or characteristic of the student. Teaching objectives that address students' common adaptive patterns (personal, social, and emotional) are appropriate here.

Description of the Main Categories of the Psychomotor Domain

- **Perception:** At the first level, we use sensory organs to obtain cues that control motor activity. This category ranges from sensory stimuli (stimulus perception) to cue selection (task relevant cue selection) to translation (the relationship between cue perception and performance actions).

- **Second set:** A set refers to the willingness to perform a certain kind of action. This category includes mental set (mental willingness to act), physical set (physical willingness to act), and emotional set (willingness to act). A key prerequisite for this stage is the recognition of cues.

- **Guided response:** Guided Response addresses the early stages of mastering complex skills. This includes imitation (repeating actions performed by the instructor) and trial and error (using multiple response approaches to find the right response). Performance adequacy is assessed by trainers or appropriate standards.

- **Mechanism:** This mechanism deals with performance acts in which learned responses become habitual and allow the behavior to be performed with some degree of confidence and skill. The learning outcomes at this level deal with different types of performance, but the patterns of behavior are less complex than at the next higher level.

- **Complex open reactions:** Complex manifest responses deal with the fine execution of motor behaviors involving complex motor patterns. Ability is demonstrated by fast, smooth and precise performance that requires minimal energy. This category includes uncertainty resolution (doing it without hesitation) and automatic performance (movements executed with ease and good muscle control). Learning outcomes at this level include highly coordinated motor activity.

- **Adjust:** Adaptation refers to skills that are sufficiently developed to allow an individual to adapt movement patterns to specific needs and problem situations.

- **Appearance:** Origination refers to the creation of new patterns of behavior that fit a particular situation or problem. Learning outcomes at this level emphasize creativity based on highly developed skills.

LESSON PLANNING

A lesson plan is a plan created by a teacher to organize a lesson. This is a plan of action and requires an understanding on the part of the teacher of the student's knowledge and experience of the subject being taught and the student's ability to use effective methods.

Lesson Plan Benefits

- Helps teachers to handle material in a systematic and orderly manner.
- It gives teachers confidence and self-confidence. She sets specific goals for student development through specific activities and other means.
- Promote continuity in the educational process and avoid unnecessary repetition.
- If well planned, student interest can be sustained throughout the lesson.

Lesson Plan Steps

To create a lesson plan you need to follow a few steps. These are:

- **Preparation/introduction:** In fact, this is a means of exploring the student's knowledge and helps guide the student through the lesson. Teachers must prepare their students to receive new knowledge. The teacher can start the lesson by asking questions to test the students' prior knowledge. This could expose their ignorance. The teacher arouses interest and curiosity for new things. You can also use charts, maps, charts and images.
- **Presentation:** Before presenting the subject, the objectives of the lesson plan should be clearly stated. This allows teachers and students to share common goals.
  - *During presentation*: This stage requires both teachers and students to actively participate in the teaching and learning process. Students need to acquire new ideas and knowledge.
  - *Discussion questions:* To keep your presentation interesting and motivate your students to learn, your presentation should include relevant examples from real-life situations.
  - *Supplemental materials:* Supplemental materials should be used to make lessons meaningful, clear, descriptive and comprehensive.
  - Blackboard outlines can be created in parallel.
- **Compare or relate:** This step is important when students are given examples and asked to observe them carefully and compare them with other examples and facts. These allow students to derive their own definitions and generalize.
- **Generalization:** This step involves reflective thinking. The knowledge imparted in the lessons should be thought provoking, innovative and stimulating to help students generalize untested formulas and more.
- **Application:** Students apply their knowledge to familiar and unfamiliar situations, testing the validity of the generalizations they have obtained. In particular, nursing students should develop the ability to apply the knowledge and skills acquired in class to their daily nursing practice in the ward clinic and at home. This makes learning more permanent and rewarding.
- **Summary:** This is the final step in lesson planning. Comprehension and comprehension of the material taught by the teacher can be tested by asking students appropriate stimulating and provocative questions on the topic. This also provides teachers with feedback on the effectiveness of the teaching methods they use. It also indicates if further explanation, clarification, etc. is required.

Recommended Performers for Lesson Plans

There are several performers that can be used as an overview for lesson plans. Whichever format you use, the key elements your lesson plan should include are:

- The relationship between the current lesson and the previous lesson
- Incorporating learning objectives (see student activities)
- Incorporate learning activities (see teacher activities)
- Teaching method used
- Use of audiovisual aids
- Lesson summary
- judgmental question
- Student tasks
- References on the subject of the lesson.

COURSE PLANNING

The course content and learning experience must be organized to achieve the educational objectives. Concepts of studentcentered learning, problem-based nurturing processes, and different learning methods may need to be considered to revitalize student teaching and learning activities. The key to successful education is good planning. Both teachers and students act as guides to create atmosphere.

Definition

A degree can be defined as a course of study leading to a degree or, in the case of a BSc (N) degree, a degree requiring the completion of several short courses.

Research Plan Objectives

- Ensure independence
- Stable
- Help solve the problem
- Support the curriculum process
- It guarantees future progress
- Bring improvements
- Facilitate the use of resources
- Contribute to the overall plan.

Course Planning Principles

- Identify behavioral goals to be achieved.
- Order: Sort content according to your learning experience, from simple to complex, known, unknown, or partial. It should be based on your time series learning requirements. Arrange content materials in some order.
  Example: A teaching bed plan teaches from a simple open bed, first to an inpatient bed, then to more complex beds

such as a postoperative bed, a fracture bed, a renal bed, and so on.
- Provide logical and psychological continuity:
  - Organize courses to focus on students rather than topics.
  - Must be adapted to the student's level.
  - Deviations from students (individual differences) must be tolerated.
  - Must promote logical memory and problem solving.
  - Helps consolidate logical and psychological demands, for example content.
  - Organize your content into smaller units.
  - Help students easily understand important concepts.
  - It avoids automized learning and repetitions.

  For example, teaching different types of diets be arranged from teaching about balanced diet fluid diet to different therapeutic diets prepared in various diseased conditions. The students may learn to prepare some of these diets.
- **Provide cumulative learning:** Provide reinforcement by continuing the use of these concepts and activities which have been acquired either through practice or through use in a new context such as reinforcement on communication skills problem solving approach community orientation and patient-centered teaching personalized care approach decision-making. For example, aspiring nurses learn to have the same bed bathing experience in their first year. This is enhanced in a variety of other clinical situations where patients with different conditions/illnesses need to undergo bed bathing with different techniques depending on tool availability, patient condition, etc. Concepts that require constant and continuous reinforcement are part of the core content of the curriculum.
- **Integration planning:** Integration or transfer of learning is not always voluntary.
  Note: Applying learning learned in one context to another context/area can lead to transfer of learning. Integration takes place within her one, but the teacher must plan the related courses horizontally so that knowledge can be transferred from one area to another. For example, we are teaching baby care in a midwifery clinic and bathing a baby at home in community nursing at the same time. "Reapplying the learning that anxiety causes stress and stress impairs the patient's response to recovery", actual patient care is the transmission of learning. The best way to preserve that is to use it.
- **Uniform curriculum:** Combine closely related subjects to reduce clutter in specializations and bring some unity to fragmented specialties increase. For example, gynecological nursing and obstetric care are an effective combination to reduce bulk. A focus center determines which ideas stand out from the ideas to build. It also reduces the unit to a manageable size and acts as an organizational center. The group title Behavioral Sciences combines psychology, educational psychology, sociology and economics.
- Choose an approach that is acceptable to all teachers. problem-solving.
- **Diversify learning methods:** Incorporate innovative ideas into learning methods. Group discussions, self-contained learning modules, and problem-solving approaches enable better learning. Planned tasks should be thought-provoking, not just copied from a book. Both teachers and students read nursing journals from India and encourage use of the library.

Study Plan Contents

In order to develop a study plan in an organized and systematic manner, there are several important things that should be included in the plan.
- Mention the goals or results that the course is trying to achieve-pediatric nursing, community nursing, midwives, etc.
- Indicates the learning level (Pt year 2nd year 3rd year).
- **For nutrition courses:** This is a brief description of the course (general purpose of the course). Example: This course is designed as a comprehensive wellness program.
- Refers to the placement of the course within the curriculum. The GNM program places courses in anatomy and physiology, physics, chemistry, and fundamentals of nursing in the year.
- Organize content by topic, unit, or lesson plan.
- Describe the materials and teaching methods of the resource. Clinical classroom teaching laboratory teaching including simulation and learner-centered teaching methods.
- Provide students with a plan of learning activities (such as assignments).
- Organization of ongoing and final evaluation procedures.
- Give references to both teachers and students.
- Schedule venue experience duration evidence of experience observation plan for rotation and clinical instruction for courses related to field experience, supervised and supervised practice.

Organizational Process Learning Experience

Specific Instructions for Organization

- Agreement on general organizational scheme a scheme should be discussed and agreed upon.

- We need to agree on general organizing principles: The structure and integration of the Church.
- Must include base units.
- You should create a flexible schedule that each teacher can put together.
- Plans should be used for specific activities in specific courses.

Course Plan Elements

Course plan contains:
- Purpose
- Learning level display
- Classification in curriculum
- Resource materials required for the course
- Unit plan
- Evaluation means
- References.

Course Planning Features

By Elliot and Mosier:
- Planning should be a continuous process.
- The plan should find a permanent place in the educational institution.
- The plan should consider resources and establish working conditions.
- Be realistic and practical.
- Active and ongoing participation of all interested individuals/groups is required.
- The content and scope of the plan should be determined by the needs of the individual or group being served.
- It requires engaging the services of professionals without allowing them to dominate.
- All individuals and groups should have the opportunity to understand and evaluate the plan.
- Curriculum must include continuous assessment.
- Subject to change for future promotions.
- Efficient and effective planning saves time, effort and money.
- Planning requires a redefinition of educational goals.
- Priorities need to be set.
- Educational opportunities need to be balanced.

Teacher's Role in Course Planning

- Teachers plan work units.
- Materials and learning activities should be selected according to the student's level.
- Careful planning is required.
- Gaps in thematic content and non-projective repetition should be avoided.
- Need to strengthen current level of learning.
- Need to set up a workgroup.
- The teaching and learning environment must be adjusted to advance student goals, but this is often not clear.
- Before you can plan, you need to set goals.
- She should have enough knowledge.
- You must have skills related to the subject you are teaching.
- The teacher's plan should focus on the overall goals of the course, unit and class plan.
- The course schedule should be prepared efficiently.
- Teachers carefully plan and incorporate conditions they know into the synthesis.
- She should be responsible for every step of the plan.
- She has to plan equally for all students.

UNIT PLANNING

Units range from small, covering just four hours of activity, to large, covering weeks or months of activity. For example, in normal labor, sessions may last 2 to 3 weeks as you learn about the stages of physiological change in the occupation and labor management including hands-on experience.

Multiple lessons may be required to complete the unit. A pure lesson is simply a collection of independent topics or lessons, but it should be well understood that they are integrated. Each lesson is part of the overall unit and leads to the development of subsequent lessons within the unit.

Features Unit Plan

- Takes place in terms of whole rather than fractions.
- Provides for verbal and horizontal organization of learning experiences.
- Take place effectively with understanding and acceptance of goals.
- Provide a solid basis for the evaluation.

Criteria for Good Unit Planning

- Students' needs, abilities and interests should be kept in mind.
- Diverse experience of excursions, experiments, demonstrations, projects, etc.
- The student's previous experience and background should be taken into account
- Lessons should be long enough to cover the student's interests.
- Students should have new experiences that they have never had before.
- You should include known related topics in your unit.
- It should relate to the student's social and physical environment.

Essential Activities for Unit Planning

There are specific activities for planning and developing all teaching and learning units.
- **Statement of choices and goals:** Educational goals are statements of outcomes in the form of desired behavioral changes that result from specific educational and learning activities.
- **Choice of content:** The knowledge or content building blocks of a unit plan refer to all knowledge in the form of facts, concepts, principles, etc., necessary to accomplish the objectives of the unit.
  Unit content and learning experience will vary depending on unit type, goals, and research areas.
- Time allocation and timing.
- Content structure of the unit.
- Selection of teaching and learning activities.
- Educational experience.
- Choice of evaluation method.
- Selection of references.

CONCLUSION

Curriculum can mean a learner's entire learning experience. It does not matter when the experience occurs. S does not imply the planning and organization of the experience by the school. Curriculum, on the other hand, means all the planned activities and experiences available to students under the direction of the school. The curriculum includes all the experiences students gain through a variety of activities in the school library, laboratory workshops, playgrounds, and informal contact between teachers and students. A well-planned and administered curriculum contributes to the development of a country and its people.

REVIEW QUESTIONS

Long Essays
1. Define curriculum, explain the objectives and types of curriculum.
2. Describe the principles of curriculum.
3. Explain core curriculum in nursing education.
4. Discuss curriculum design—component approach and principles of curriculum design.
5. Describe writing learning outcomes/behavioral objectives.
6. Describe the major categories of the emotional domain.
7. Describe of the main categories of the psychomotor domain.
8. Define lesson plan, explain the steps in lesson plan.

Short Essays
1. Factors influences curriculum development.
2. Curriculum features.
3. Types/classifications of curriculum.
4. Types of curriculum design.
5. Curriculum design principles.
6. Curriculum planning and development.
7. Stages of curriculum planning.
8. Level of curriculum planning.
9. Curriculum management phases.
10. Curriculum process stages.
11. Type of educational goal.
12. Describe the major categories of cognitive domains.
13. Course plan—principles.
14. Organizational process learning experience.
15. Features and criteria for good unit planning.
16. Essential activities for unit planning.

Short Answers
1. Philosophy of nursing education.
2. Elements of the core concept.
3. Elements of successful curriculum design.
4. Big ideas.
5. Subject-centered curriculum design.
6. Learner-centered curriculum design.
7. Problem-centered curriculum design.
8. Curriculum planning.
9. Curriculum organization.
10. Curriculum evaluation.
11. Intermediate goals.
12. Course plan elements.
13. Course planning features.

Unit 3

Teaching in Classroom and Skill Lab

Chapter

7. Teaching Methods in Education

KEYWORDS

Blended learning: It is an approach to education that combines online educational materials and opportunities for interaction online with traditional place-based classroom methods.

Demonstration: A session involving the demonstration of a practical technique or skill. Examples might include the demonstration of laboratory skills, clinical skills, and performance art or fieldwork techniques.

Didactic: While it is sometimes used informally to neutrally imply a method of teaching which is largely 'chalk and talk', its meaning is much more complex, often carrying moral or negative connotations.

Distance or remote learning: Distance learning and remote learning are terms that are used interchangeably by providers when describing teaching and learning activities.

External visits: A visit to a location outside of the usual learning spaces, to experience a particular environment, event, or exhibition relevant to the course of study.

Face-to-face delivery: Face-to-face delivery of education and training programs have been in common use for some time in the higher education sector.

Fieldwork: Practical work conducted at an external site. Examples of fieldwork might include survey work and other forms of data collection, excavations and explorations.

Learning lab: Refers to a location in a school, such as a classroom or dedicated section of the library, where students can go to receive academic support, or to the programs school create that deliver academic support.

Locus of control: It is a psychological concept that refers to how strongly people believe they have control over the situations and experiences that affect their lives.

Learning objectives: They are brief statements that describe what students will be expected to learn by the end of school year, course, unit, lesson, project, or class period.

Hidden curriculum: It refers to the unwritten, unofficial, and often unintended lessons, values, and perspectives that students learn in school.

Learning pathway: It refers to the specific courses, academic programs, and learning experiences that individual students complete as they progress in their education toward graduation.

Scaffolding: It refers to a variety of instructional techniques used to move students progressively toward stronger understanding and, ultimately, greater independence in the learning process.

Curriculum mapping: It is the process indexing or diagraming a curriculum to identify and address academic gaps, redundancies, and misalignments for purposes of improving the overall coherence of a course of study.

Brain-based learning: It refers to teaching methods, lesson designs, and school programs that are based on the latest scientific research about how the brain learns, including such factors as cognitive development—how students learn differently as they age, grow, and mature socially, emotionally, and cognitively.

Classroom management: It refers to the wide variety of skills and techniques that teachers use to keep students organized, orderly, focused, attentive, on task, and academically productive during a class.

Classroom observation: It is a formal or informal observation of teaching while it is taking place in a classroom or other learning environment.

Community-based learning: It refers to a wide variety of instructional methods and programs that educators use to connect what is being taught in schools to their surrounding communities, including local institutions, history, literature, cultural heritage, and natural environments.

Competency-based learning refers to systems of instruction, assessment, grading, and academic reporting that are based on students demonstrating that they have learned the knowledge and skills they are expected to learn as they progress through their education.

Criterion-referenced tests and assessments are designed to measure student performance against a fixed set of predetermined criteria or learning standards, i.e., concise, written descriptions of what students are expected to know and be able to do at a specific stage of their education.

Chapter 7

Teaching Methods in Education

Learning Objectives

- Importance of Educational Methods
- Teaching Objectives
- Types of Teaching Methods
- Classification of Teaching Methodology
- Factors that Determine the Choice of Teaching Method
- Characteristics of Teaching Methods
- Classroom Management
- Educational Management Strategies
- Communication in the Classroom
- Classroom Communication Facilitator
- Communication Barriers in the Classroom
- Information Communication Technology (ICT)—ICT Used in Education
- Classroom Teaching Method: Simulation, Peer Sharing, Case Study Analysis, Journaling, Debate, Gaming
- Interprofessional Education
- Programmed Lessons

TERMINOLOGY

- **Pedagogy:** Pedagogy is stimulation, instruction and encouragement to learn.
- **Demonstrations:** Demonstrations teach through exhibits and explanations. This is an explanatory process. It trains students in the art of careful observation.
- **Lecture format:** A lecture is a teaching method that consists of clarifying or explaining facts, principles, relationships that the teacher wants the class to understand.
- **Role play:** Role play is a discussion technique that maximizes group participation by acting out examples of the problem or idea being discussed.
- **Programmed instruction:** The process of assembling learning material in a series of small steps that allow learners to selflearn what they know, leading to new and more complex knowledge and principles unknown.
- **Discussion methods:** Discussions are cooperative when participants speak informally and conversationally, whereas debates are competitions between debaters and advocates. He opposes the proposal for an equal split of alternative hours.
- **Workshop:** A group of people working together to solve a problem in a specific area for a specific period of time.
- **Team teaching:** A form of classroom organization involving faculty members.
- **Case analysis methodology:** Addresses core situations that require several decisions. A group of students led by a teacher analyzes the case, discusses it and decides the problem.
- **Case incident method:** This is a case analysis remediation method focused on serious incidents for cases requiring immediate decision and action.
- **Bedside clinic:** A method of clinical education that requires the presence of the patient. Either the group visits the patient and continues the discussion, or the patient is taken to a conference room. It leads to mutual understanding and relationships.
- **Laboratory experience:** Students learn laboratory skills using dummies or manikins under the close supervision and guidance of clinical experts in their particular field. Experiences are selected according to student needs and curriculum requirements.
- **Supervised nursing internship:** After an internship, nursing students practice in an ideal setting.

- **Internships:** Teachers allow students to practice their skills here after acquiring knowledge and practice in any field according to the needs, requirements, and interests of the students. Instructors act as program coordinators.
- **Group meeting:** A meeting is a discussion in which two or more people meet in a formal meeting for the purpose of exchanging or disseminating ideas. This includes two-way conversation flow.
- **Cooperative practices:** Operate in partnerships between professional groups and/or between individuals, families, groups and organizations with communities.
- **Competency-based education:** defines course outcomes in terms of what students can do by the time they complete the course.
- **Continuing professional development (CPD):** It is the maintenance and development of practical competence through continuing postqualification learning.
- **E-learning:** E-learning uses web-based information simulation and communication technology.
- **Facilitation:** Allows students to learn from their own and others' experiences.
- **Formative assessment:** Contributes to student learning as students assess their progress and plan for improvement.
- **Interdisciplinary care:** It is sometimes used as an alternative to interprofessional care and can also refer to care between departments of the same specialty (usually medicine).
- **Interprofessional nursing:** Interprofessional nursing is the collaborative response to the needs of the community of individuals, families, groups, and dual or multiprofessional her members. Interprofessional education occurs when a student or two or more members of her profession learn from each other to improve the quality of cooperation and care.
- **Interprofessional learning:** It takes place between students or members of two or more professions to develop knowledge and competencies during interprofessional training or informally in an educational or practical setting. Interprofessionalism is the actual collaboration between members of two or more professions.
- **Interprofessional teamwork:** Brings members of two or more professions with complementary competencies into sustainable collaborative practice towards a common goal.
- **Interprofessional research:** It refers to either systematic and/or interprofessional research in interprofessional education and practice.

INTRODUCTION

Pedagogy is a systematic way for teachers to communicate, receive or share information. Jeffrey defines pedagogy as the process of imparting knowledge and skills that teachers apply in the classroom. It implies the use of guiding principles and theories. Teachers have to use a different number of methods to meet the needs of each student in the class. This is the hallmark of an effective and efficient teacher.

DEFINITION

- The method of teaching that most closely resembles the method of learning. —Burke
- Teaching methods include the principles and methods used by teachers to enable students to learn. These strategies are determined partly by the subject matter being taught and partly by the nature of the learner. Jeffrey defines pedagogy as the process of imparting knowledge and skills that teachers apply in the classroom.

IMPORTANCE OF EDUCATIONAL METHODS

The procedural aspects of the educational process refer to the methods and techniques that teachers or learners can use to achieve desired educational goals. Dimensions such as content, environment, relationships, and procedural dimensions are interrelated. The knowledge environment and human relationships all influence the procedural aspects of education. Education in nursing includes both cognitive and artistic aspects. Teaching competence and professional competence in teaching influence student learning. Art in the classroom is necessary and can be developed. Systematic investigation of teaching and learning methods and materials, and subject mastery are essential to the development of artistic education.

TEACHING OBJECTIVES

- Seek to develop a love of work
- Arouses the desire to work as efficiently as possible
- Develops clear thinking
- Offer reasonable opportunities to participate in projects and activities that are freely accepted and require cooperation and discipline at all times
- Expands students' interest
- Provides opportunities for students to apply their acquired knowledge and skills in practice
- Must be adapted to the age of 3A of student ability and aptitude
- *Regulatory enthusiasm:* Department of education officials are personally enthusiastic about conducting experiments within reason

- General support for the profession
- Teamwork and a sense of security
- Mastery of the subject-matter
- Provision for a good library and teaching-learning material
- Role of teacher training institutions
- Parental co-operation.

TYPES OF TEACHING METHODS

There are basically two types of teaching methods. The only key to classifying these two methods is the method of teacher–student interaction.

1. **Teacher centered method:** A method that assumes the teacher is central and the source of all material. There is no teacher-student interaction. Students are seen as emptyheaded or canned food that needs to be packed with knowledge.
2. **Student centered method:** In this method, the student becomes the source of the learning object. As Hudgins explains, students are given the opportunity to interact with the teacher's content and with themselves. From this well the trenches of knowledge are dug and great and wide paths of knowledge are created.

CLASSIFICATION OF TEACHING METHODOLOGY

- **Method of presentation:** High cognitive emphasis, low emphasis on student activities and experiences, e.g., lecture method.
- **Natural way of learning:** Learning happens in a natural way, e.g., trip.
- **Individualized methodology:** The emphasis is on each learner learning at their own pace, e.g., programmed instruction, case methods for self-study, and computer-oriented instruction.
- **Methods of encounter:** Mediation of experience through confrontation or encounter leading to changes in basic behavioral patterns and development of new perspectives, e.g., RPG simulation.
- **Detection method:** These methods have higher priority in all dimensions, e.g., problem-solving techniques.
- Group methods such as project methods, socialized classroom method.

FACTORS THAT DETERMINE THE CHOICE OF TEACHING METHOD

- **Teaching objectives:** Teaching objectives terms are used to describe procedures and expected results. This is the result of learning. Everything we learn in the classroom has subject goals, teacher goals, learner and school policy goals.
- **Availability of materials and learning materials:** Materials are directly related to educational goals and teaching methods. If the teacher does not have suitable materials to match his method, he should change the method to be relevant to his material.
- **Teacher competence and preference:** Teaching methods are determined by the competence and experience of the teacher using the method. There are also other methods that can distract your class if not used carefully. Teachers should therefore choose a method that suits their experience level and preferences.
- **Cultural aspects of society:** Address ethical issues related to gender. Some other ethics and religions prohibit mixing boys and girls. Therefore, the method used here prohibits students from sitting in groups.
- **Learner's age:** The method you choose depends on your age. Teenagers are very interested in experiments and demonstrations, but lectures can be boring. Children are also more likely to be influenced by concept caricatures than by experiments. In other words, learners' cognitive domains are influenced by the methods used. A learner's quick brain depends on the relevance method used and age.
- **Psychological needs of the student:** These will vary depending on what the student needs. Different students have different needs. Some struggle with stress, lack of love, and financial problems, while others need to escape humiliation. Bello said "A teacher's awareness of these psychological needs helps teachers choose ways to meet all needs".
- **National educational philosophy:** The National Educational Philosophy is what the nation sees as revolutionary ideas for the betterment of the nation. This goal is the economic, political and social content and purpose of the country.
- **Learning speed of learners:** Learners have different learning speeds, some are very talented (gifted students) and some are slow learners. The speed of learning has influenced the teaching methods and materials used.
- **Exam structure:** The curriculum determines the type and mode of examination structure. This has influenced the way teachers choose teaching methods. Many teachers preferred Q&A and lectures to essay questions. All of these methods were preferred due to the nature of the study.
- **Class size:** This number is fair enough to use all the methods. Large groups of learners are reached by lecture methods, but other methods are often applied to small groups.
- **Time limits:** Time is an important factor in determining how teachers present contacts. This depends on your

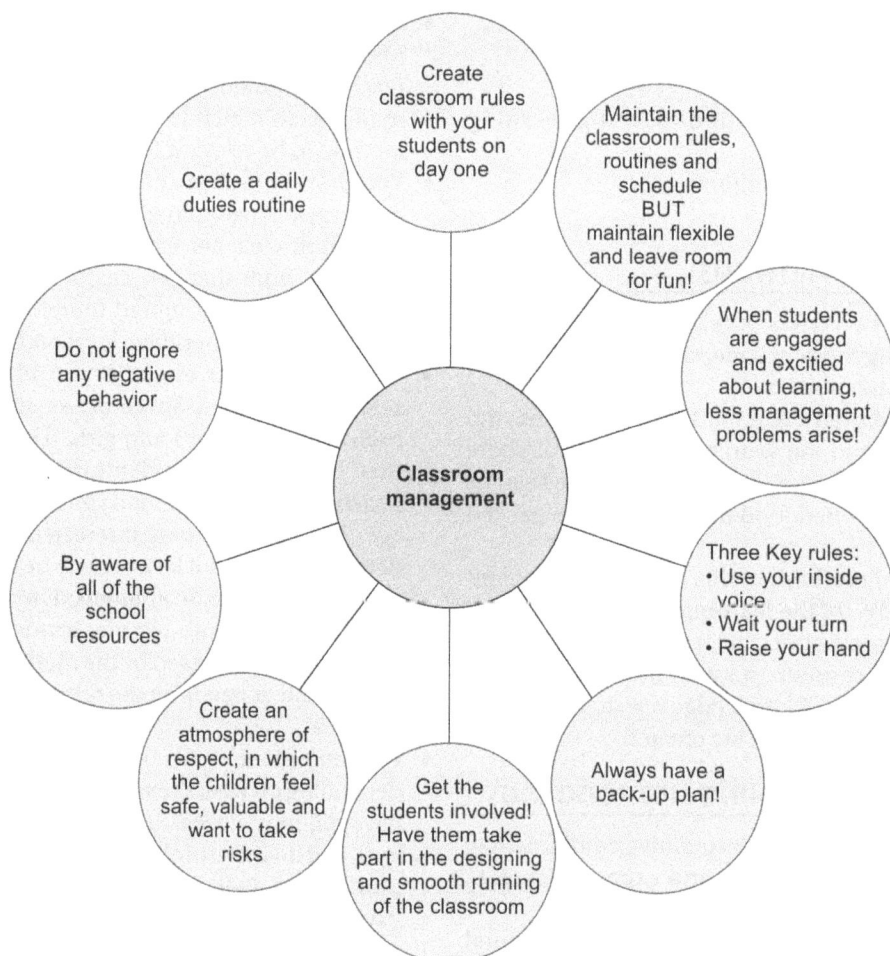

Fig. 7.1: Classroom management.

pros and cons. Some other methods are time consuming and others are time servers. The lecture method is a time saving method, but the experimentation is time consuming.
- **Type of content:** The type of subject determines the methodology used. Some of the themes are directly related to specific teaching methods.
  Example: A history theme can be presented through storytelling, but a chemistry theme requires experimentation and demonstration.
- **Student's learning style:** In this type of learning, some learn quickly by sight, others by hearing, and others by touch.

CHARACTERISTICS OF TEACHING METHODS

- Transfer of knowledge in an efficient manner.
- Instill in students desirable values and appropriate attitudes and work habits.
- Develop a true commitment to work and a desire to work as efficiently, honestly and thoroughly as possible.
- The principles of activity "verbalization and memorization" and "project method" should be incorporated into school practice.
- Provide opportunities for students to actively learn and apply what they learn in class.
- Clear thinking and clear expression must be practiced in speech and writing.
- Train learners in learning methods techniques to acquire knowledge through personal effort and initiative.
- A deliberate attempt should be made to adopt teaching methods in ways that benefit all categories of students.
- Students should be given opportunities to work in groups and to undertake group projects and activities in order to develop the necessary qualities for group living and working together.

THE BENEFITS OF CHOOSING THE RIGHT TEACHING METHOD

Teaching method is an important factor in students' understanding of the lesson. Bad results are obtained when teachers choose the wrong teaching method.
- **Manage class discipline:** Choosing the right teaching method will help the teacher to manage the class. Discipline will be good as students will participate effectively in class.
- **Eliminate boredom:** Lessons are interactive and engaging, giving teachers ample time to listen to students' needs. Therefore, learners feel healed of their psychological needs and emotional demands for learners.
- **Anger and stress relief:** Students develop strong friendships with their teachers and develop a habit of loving learning.

CLASSROOM MANAGEMENT

Classroom management refers to the various skills and techniques teachers use to keep students organized, attentive, and academically productive during class. When classroom management strategies are effectively implemented, teachers minimize behaviors that impede learning for both individual students and groups of students, and maximize behaviors that promote or enhance learning. In general, competent teachers tend to exhibit strong classroom management skills, but inexperienced or less competent teachers are characterized by clutter full of students who are not studying or paying attention.

Definition
- Richard (1990)—classroom management is defined as an organization and how teachers control student behavior so that teaching and learning processes are effective.
- Albert and Trautmann (1986)—classroom management is a skill that requires teachers to manage the spatiotemporal resources and behavior of their students in order to foster a learning environment.
- Classroom management is defined as the methods and strategies used by educators to maintain a classroom environment conducive to student success and learning. Many educational strategies are involved in classroom management, but the common denominator is making sure students feel in an environment where they can achieve something.

Meaning
- Class management is her one of the most important tasks of a teacher that determines the success of a lesson.
- Effective teachers appear to be effective with students of all ability levels, regardless of the degree of heterogeneity within the class.
- An effective class leader is someone who understands and uses specific techniques.
- Individual teachers can make great strides in student learning, even if the school they work for is not very effective.
- Select, develop and use the most effective educational strategies.
- Design educational curricula that facilitate student learning.
- Consider student needs collectively and individually on designing curricula.
- Enforce rules and regulations and impose disciplinary actions.

Classroom Operations Goals
- Encourage desirable student behavior
- Create a positive learning environment
- Build relationships between teachers and students
- Maximize the time allotted for learning
- Engage students in the teaching and learning process
- Reduce disciplinary problems
- Maintain an effective routine
- Students become more independent

Types
Comprehensive type of classroom management by identifying.
- Learning needs.
- Build good relationships with teachers, students, and peers.
- Use teaching methods that promote optimal learning by addressing the academic needs of individual students and class groups.
- Adopt organizational and group management practices that maximize task performance.
- Ability to use a variety of counseling and behavioral methods to assist students experiencing persistent or severe behavioral problems.
- Students in classes that use effective management techniques perform better than students in classes that do not use effective management techniques.
- Teachers will not be able to teach and students will be productive if there are no guidelines on how teachers should behave, when to move around the room, or if teachers and students are frequently in the way is not possible.

- Students in classes with rules and procedures in place may be inherently less confused than students in classes without rules and procedures in place.

Rules and Procedures

- Effective classroom management requires good rules and procedures.
- Rules and procedures vary from teacher to teacher and from classroom to classroom.
- The most effective classroom management includes the design and implementation of classroom policies and procedures.
- Rules and procedures should not simply be imposed on students. Good design of rules and procedures includes explanations and group input. Explanations are important to ensure that students understand the need for and accept the rules.

Classroom Preparation

- Have spare supplies in places in the classroom so that students who forget their supplies will not disturb other students.
- Be a role model for students by keeping the classroom clean and tidy.
- Make classroom attractive. Beautify your classroom with warm botanical corkboard banners and more.
- Organize the lesson to avoid confusion and encourage learning. For example, do not place a talkative student next to a sharpener. This creates many opportunities for destructive behavior.
- Teachers should be able to observe all students at all times and see the door from their desks.
- Students should be able to see the teacher/presentation area without moving or turning.
- Arrange the room for easy movement.
- **Key idea:** Make your classroom fun, engaging, and motivating and functional.

Building Good Student–Teacher Relationships

- Follow the golden rule—"treat all students with respect and kindness".
- Pick a few students for each lesson and find ways to reward them individually so that by the end of the week everyone in the class is rewarded.
- If students need help or just want to talk to you, be available before and after school.
- Praise students for doing well.
- Praise your students for their efforts.
- Establish the right level of dominance and collaboration.
- Create a one-on-one interaction with a student.
- Demonstrate student achievement in the classroom.
- Disclose appropriate personal information that the student may find helpful (e.g., tell a personal story to help illustrate a particular point in the lesson).

Instruction Hints

- Provide step-by-step instructions and avoid long, detailed instructions.
- Use visual aids to present and confirm concepts and instructions.
- Offer a variety of learning experiences, including peer teaching, collaborative learning, small group classes, and lectures.
- Provide homework and activities that are meaningful, relevant and educational.
- Teach students good study habits and offer different study suggestions.
- At the end of each class, ask them to summarize the lesson or activity.
- Give feedback to students (what went right and what went wrong).
- Help students set realistic goals.

Create a Positive Educational Environment

- Use humor.
- Greet students at the door and in the hallway.
- Show enthusiasm and energize.
- Provide each student with an opportunity for success.
- Demonstrate good listening skills by listening to students.
- Build anticipation for lessons and assignments.
- If a particular student is struggling, provide an adult and responsible classmate.
- Create rituals and traditions in your classroom that build a sense of community
- Encourage parental and community involvement.

Tips to Avoid Cheating

- Establish realistic and age-appropriate rules and procedures.
- Discuss with students the rationale and purpose of each rule. Incorporate students' opinions and ideas into educational policies and procedures as appropriate.
- Walk around the classroom, provide support, and monitor behavior during lectures and sedentary tasks.
- Separate lessons and assignments from behavioral problems.
- Plan your class time carefully and make extra plans in case you finish early.
- Offer extra activities when students get bored or finish all their work.

- Establish routines for transitions (such as leaving the room to the bathroom) and warn students in advance to prepare for transitions.
- Affirm and praise good behavior.
- When deciding whether to intervene in behavior, determine whether the problem is wholly "property of the teacher". Does the behavior only annoy you or harm other students.
- Establish a program that teaches students selfdiscipline and responsibility. If necessary, give students additional assignments that save time and help teach responsibility.

Dealing with Student Disciplinary Situations

- Act calmly
- Communicate in the most confidential, respectful, and positive way when correcting misconduct.
- All disciplinary action will be based on "the heat of the moment."
- Use appropriate humor to defuse conflict situations.
- If you or your student feel too emotional to handle a particular situation, suggest postponing the discussion until you are both ready to talk about it.
- Instead of blaming, use to explain why the behavior was destructive.
- Use positive selftalk to destress and stay in control. Mentally say things like "calm down" and "I am handling this situation well".
- Try to deescalate the situation by providing distractions. These distractions give people a chance to cool down.
- Exaggerate things to help students put the situation into perspective.
- Use stress management techniques such as deep breathing and tensing and relaxing muscles.
- Focus only on student behavior, not individual characteristics.

Classroom Climate

Classroom climate is the classroom environment, social climate and emotional and physical aspects of the classroom. The classroom environment is defined as the intellectual, social, emotional, and physical environment in which students learn. Student behavior affects how they interact with peers. Responsibility for influencing this behavior rests with the trainer. The way teachers structure lessons should lead to a positive environment rather than one that is disruptive and/or unconducive to learning

Manage Class Climate

- Incorporate diversity into your classes and use inclusive teaching methods.
- Use icebreakers and collaborative learning to provide opportunities for students to get to know each other.
- Include a discussion of diversity and disability in the curriculum.
- We apologize for the inconvenience.
- Establish ground rules.
- Regularly check the atmosphere in the classroom.
- Try to communicate with students

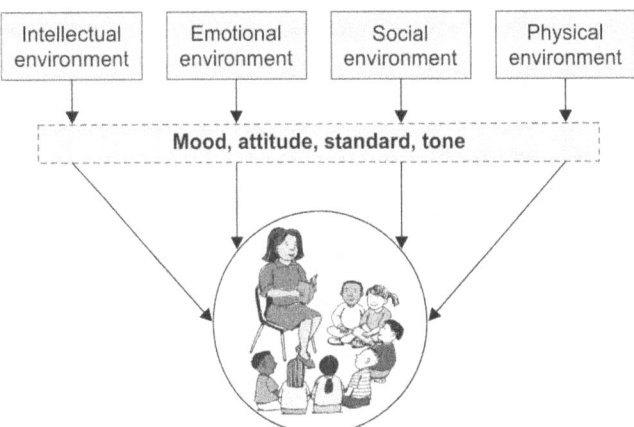

Fig. 7.2: Classroom climate.

Classroom Management: Principles and Strategies

Effective classroom management requires awareness, patience, good timing, boundaries, and instincts. Classroom management refers to the skills and techniques you use to make your classroom more engaging, organized and engaging. An effective teacher knows how to manage lessons and involve students in the learning process. Traditional interpretations of classroom management focus on the compliance aspect. It takes into account the rules and regulations that students should follow in order to bring more attention to their learning. The educational process is based on the personal commitment of teachers and the goals that teachers and students should achieve. The principles of education reflect the teacher's interest in his or her own educational task. A teacher proves to be a successful manager when he or she shows a strong interest in the lesson and the students.

- **Principles of clarity and content mastery:** The first principle of instructional instruction is that the teacher should be familiar with the subject matter. Must have a good knowledge of the school curriculum and subjects. Good knowledge means familiarity with a subject, which helps teachers to teach effectively in the classroom. Depth and understanding of the subject matter help teachers in two ways.

- **Principle of participation:** This principle enables teachers to make the teaching and learning process more participatory. Active student participation in class is a prerequisite for learning. The ability to ask questions, receive and give feedback can make teaching and learning a twoway process. Interactive teaching and learning is only possible if teachers carefully plan their educational activities.
- **Principles of democratic action:** Democracy is a way of life. How to work together to achieve common goals. Teachers provide all students with equal opportunities to participate in teaching and learning activities. Such behavior on the part of teachers fosters healthy positive attitudes towards student learning. Students learn how to find solutions to classroom problems by understanding each other's point-of-view.
- **Principles of teacher's behavior:** A teacher's behavior during a lesson should demonstrate a variety of positive qualities, such as selfconfidence and willpower. This indirectly creates a learning environment in the classroom and helps guide the classroom with desired learning behaviors. Positive traits in teacher behavior also help develop desirable behaviors in students. This is because the students constantly observe and analyze the teacher's behavior and compare it with the teacher's claims. With strong beliefs and a deep commitment to the tasks assigned to you, you can effectively manage your classroom. Teacher selfmanagement aims to give teachers control over their own behavior. This allows students to develop selfcontrol in their actions.
- **Principle of flexibility:** The principle of flexibility is not inconsistent with the principle of selfregulation. Teachers should demonstrate flexible behavior and be responsive to student ideas, plans, and observations. Teachers must be able to make necessary changes in their behavior and teaching/learning activities as the situation requires. This helps develop and use alternative strategies to achieve curriculum goals.
- **Principle of personal qualities:** A teacher's personal qualities (warmth, empathy, etc.) have a strong influence on student behavior in the classroom. Caring behavior of teachers demonstrate harmony and respect for each other dignity at work leads to peace and selfdiscipline, and indirectly controls undesirable behavior in students. Teachers play a key role in determining the psychosocial environment that prevails in the classroom.

Factors Affecting Classroom Management

- **Effective teaching:** Effective teaching supports teachers' efforts to promote both learning and discipline (order) in the classroom. Well-planned lessons with appropriate pacing, guided practice, individual student attention, effective and immediate feedback, etc., help teachers manage the classroom and thereby ensure desired learning.
- **Establishing and enforcing rules:** Teachers who set clear classroom goals and demonstrate some level of commitment to achieving those goals are better able to manage classroom activities. Therefore, teachers must demonstrate the will and ability to act when rules are broken. For example, ask them to raise their hand before speaking or asking a question. After raising their hand, students wait their turn to answer questions and participate in discussions. The process of establishing and implementing rules has both instructional and managerial value. Students will learn procedures to ensure their participation is effective and embracing their social environment.
- **Intervention management:** Clearly, the process of monitoring student behavior and intervening when necessary is one of the most challenging requirements for effective classroom management. When rules are categorized and classroom activities are properly conducted, the need for intervention is reduced. Typical misbehaviors such as inattentiveness, mild verbal and physical aggression, not bringing books, and not doing homework should be dealt with effectively.
- **Feedback on appropriate behavior:** Students expect ongoing feedback on the acceptability of their behavior in class. Learning success should be praised by teachers.
- **Educational environment:** The educational environment is also related to management. Many organizational factors create the right learning environment, including instruction, feedback, communication, and interpersonal relationships between teachers and students. Students do not want to study in a chaotic environment and teachers who have to teach problematic classes have to work under stress. Poorly run classes do not provide a comfortable and supportive environment for teaching and learning. A certain amount of calm and comfort is necessary for the mental health of both teachers and students. This includes the ability to plan lessons, organize and manage classrooms, and use teaching strategies to help students reach their end goals.

Techniques of Classroom Management

- **Behavior modification techniques:** The basic assumption behind this technique is that student behavior is a direct result of teacher behavior. It is the teacher's job to identify desirable and undesirable behaviors in

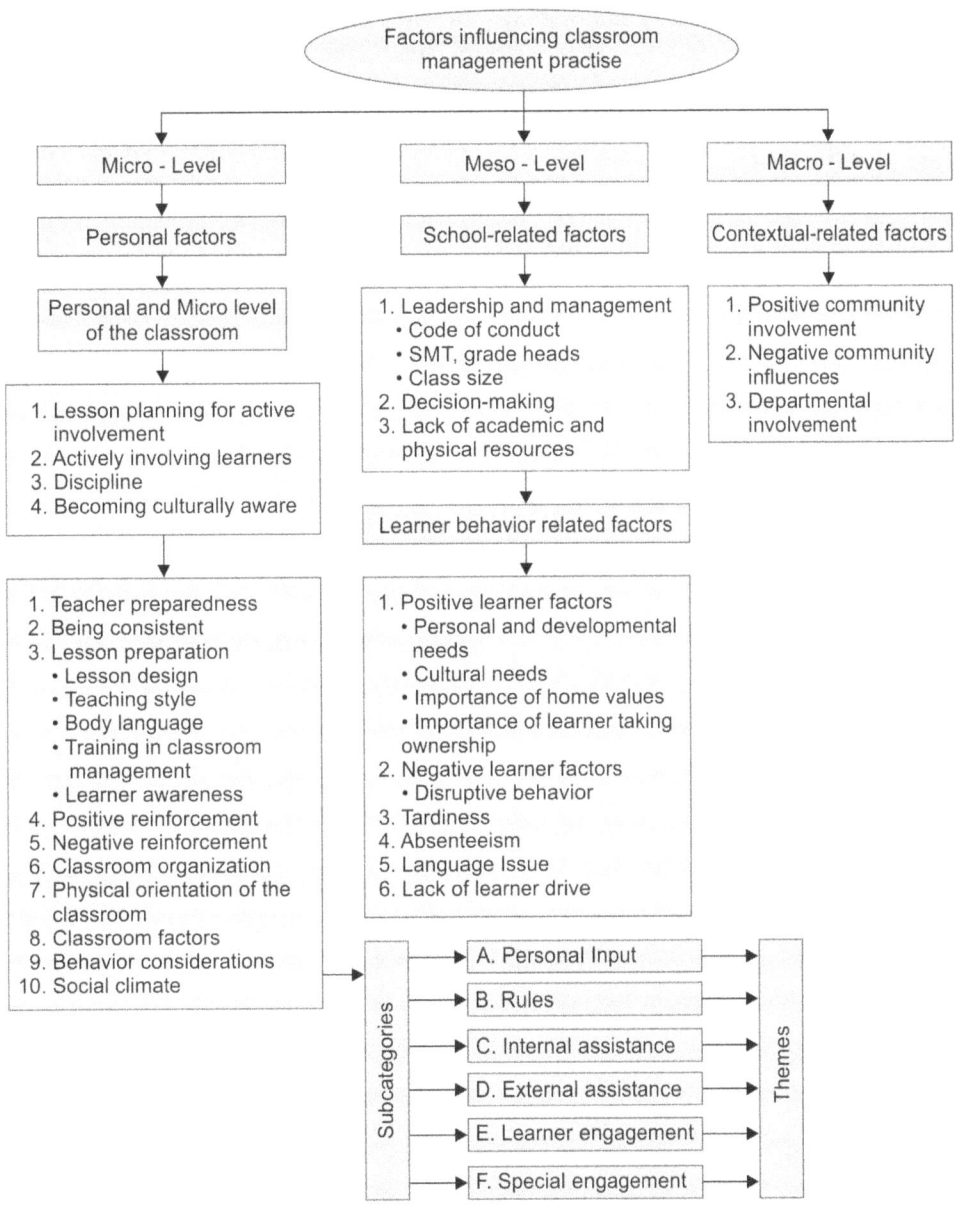

Fig. 7.3: Factors influencing classroom management.

the classroom. Teachers should ignore inappropriate/undesirable behaviors and reinforce acquired desired behaviors.

- **Student responsibility:** Some teachers believe that students should be responsible for their actions. The teacher's job is to make students aware of the expectations and consequences of their own desirable and undesirable behaviors. This method of classroom management promotes selfdiscipline in students. It is the teacher's responsibility to help students take more responsibility for their actions and develop plans to change unproductive behaviors.

- **Group activities:** Some teachers prefer working with groups of students to manage a class rather than individual students. They see their class as a peer influenced group. Students working together perform desired behaviors to earn a group reward. Students compete with each other. The seating arrangement should allow teachers to easily see all students. You can also use voice movements and tempo changes to refocus attention during class. We need to be aware of the tendency to create a monotonous environment in the classroom.

EDUCATIONAL MANAGEMENT STRATEGIES

Strategy 1: Create an Effective Learning Environment

This is especially true of teacher behavior during the first week of school. The effort and time you put into planning for the year and thinking about potential pitfalls will pay off in the long run.

- **Preparation:** Design the room so that students are close to each other and have easy movement.
- **Preferences:** Greet students at the classroom door and tell them what to do once they enter the classroom. For example, on the first day, introduce yourself, ask for your name, and assign seats.
- **Develop community:** Develop a set of written behavior expectations (rules and procedures) with the class that you can live with and consistently enforce.
- **Setting class rules:** Teachers are ultimately responsible for setting class rules. New teachers and teachers of new cultures should consult experienced teachers and follow their example to establish class rules.
- **Take back control of the classroom:** This happens to both inexperienced and experienced teachers. Identify problems and make plans to restore order.

Strategy 2: Establish Instructional Procedures

Instructional procedures communicate how daily activities are performed. Teach and model the procedure until it becomes routine.

- Write step-by-step instructions for the activity.
- Say the steps or read them aloud.
- Provide visual instructions in text or illustrations.
- Demonstrate or have students demonstrate each step.
- Practice with the whole class until each student masters the procedure and makes it routine.
- Relearn the procedure if necessary.

Strategy 3: Create a Motivating Environment

Following teaching conditions and strategies can help create a classroom environment that is conducive to learning.

- Create an inviting and enriching environment. Engage your students by asking them to decorate their own classrooms. Whenever possible, use student work as decoration to validate work and provide examples of good work.
- Develop the lesson at a level that challenges the student so that it is not too difficult or confusing.
- Give clear instructions. Ask students to repeat the instructions.
- Involve all students actively. For example, one student gives a presentation while another student takes notes or grades the presentation using a rubric.
- Structure the learning experience so that the student feels successful. She considers how she can participate in two or three of her levels, deploying activities at the appropriate level of difficulty and ensuring all students succeed.
- Set clear behavioral expectations and consistently reinforce expectations for different learning styles. For example, write keywords on the blackboard or use diagrams and pictures.
- Make learning really interesting by relating the lesson content to the student's life and the local environment. For example, associate lessons with local current affairs or share experiences of living in the area.

Strategy 4: Count Every Minute

- Start on time.
- Finish on time.
- By saving a few minutes of class time each day, you will have hours of additional academic instruction before the end of the school year.

To Maximize Your Learning and Teaching Time

- Plan each lesson in advance. A well-designed lesson plan has clear learning goals and provides meaningful activities that help students reach their goals.
- Before class, write learning goals, e.g., assignments, etc., on the chalkboard on flipchart paper or play cards. Tasks can be associated with the previous lesson or the current day's lesson.
- Save time by using the seating chart while students are working, or by delegating tasks to team teachers or student assistants.
- Assign this to distribute and collect papers and materials.
- Prepare emergency lessons and activities. If you run out of scheduled lessons for the day or need to fill time, make an organized plan. No time is wasted and students do not act out of boredom.
- Activities include books to read, fun worksheets, educational games, and art supplies for students who finish early. Use homework folders.
- Students place their completed homework in their portfolio and remove the checked work. When distributing worksheets, place a copy in the absent student's folder. The work is ready for student return.

Strategy 5: Get Everyone Involved

Challenging active thinking in students engages them in learning and develops critical skills. Expect both low and high performing students to participate in classroom discussions and answer questions.
- Ask a question. Wait 3–5 seconds (the wait time) before calling the student. Latency encourages more thoughtful responses and allows both slow and fast students to respond.
- Use the echo technique. One student answers and she has another student repeat it.
- Invite students to answer the questions.
- Praise correct answers. "Well thought!" "Great! Create aquestion box. Write each student's name on the box and draw their name to answer question
- Pose a question and move your gaze to several different students during the wait time before selecting a student to answer
- Correct students' wrong answers and encourage them to stay involved in the learning process.

Strategy 6: Instill Life Skills and Good Study Habits

Creating organized, learner-centered classrooms can teach students many important skills. Sometimes referred to as character skills or life skills, these skills enable students to become mature, self-confident, and successful adults who make positive contributions to their communities and society at large.

Here are some ideas for making extra effort to teach life skills:
- Use "teaching moments" to strengthen your life skills. For example, "If everyone helped clean up the classroom, we could go to lunch earlier".
- Emphasize different skills each week throughout the grade.
- Have the student write a story or role-playing game in which the character demonstrates one or more life skills.
- Create a life skills art exhibit by asking students to draw pictures or posters that illustrate life skills.
- Use the journal. Students write about people they observe demonstrating life skills and how they would like to apply the behavior in their own lives.
- Create a life skill ticket. When you see a student demonstrating a skill, circle the attribute and write the student's name on the ticket. At the end of the month, the student with the most tickets is selected as the "Student of the Month". Consider appropriate rewards.

Strategy 7: Be Creative

Teachers may think that your teaching methods are limited due to lack of resources:
- Search the Internet for resources such as photos, maps, activity ideas, craft instructions, and free downloadable materials.
- Find out which local or national professional associations or agencies have the material.
- The chalkboard can be written on, rolled up, taken to the classroom, hung on the wall, erased and reused. Search the internet for sources.
- Some faux leather fabrics are suitable as an alternative writing surface.

Strategy 8: Use Project Design and Management Techniques

Here are the steps you and your colleagues (and possibly your students) take to create and maintain projects that apply to class management.
- **Step 1:** Identify existing strengths and needs to facilitate teaching and learning.
- **Step 2:** Create a vision of what the ideal classroom would look like.
- **Step 3:** Collaborate with others to explore alternative ways to achieve your vision.
- **Step 4:** Prepare a classroom management plan.
- **Step 5:** Monitor consistent adherence to the classroom operations plan and adjust as necessary.
- **Step 6:** Evaluate to determine if the plan achieves the desired vision.
- **Step 7:** Celebrate achievements with students.

COMMUNICATION IN THE CLASSROOM

Communication is important in the classroom. Typically, only 50% knowledge and 50% communication skills are required to be successful in teaching. Therefore, the teacher should be proficient in all her four types of communication (listening, speaking, reading and writing) and know how to use these skills effectively in a school environment. The ability to do this has been shown to influence not only the academic success of students, but also the career success of teachers themselves.

Types of Communication in the Classroom

Classroom communication is important for effective student learning and should be introduced early in learning. Classroom communication falls into three categories: verbal, nonverbal, and written.

1. **Verbal communication** refers to sending and receiving messages through sounds and language. Teachers can address students or the entire classroom through verbal communication. For example, a teacher may ask a student to stand up, which is verbal communication.
2. **Nonverbal communication** refers to nonverbal communication through body language, gestures, facial expressions, tone and pitch of voice, and posture. For example, if a teacher nods their head when a student is speaking, this can be encouraging or indicate agreement with the student.
3. **Written communication** means sending and receiving information in writing. For example, teachers may provide written assignments for students to test their knowledge, or present lecture slides or notes for complex information.

Five Different Phases

According to Cole and Chan, a typical process of classroom communication (and communication in general) involves her five different phases:
1. Message
2. Message encoding
3. Message-transmission
4. Reading and interpreting messages
5. Feedback and evaluation

Types of Classroom Interactions

- Interactions in collaborative learning
- Interactions in discussions and debates
- Interactions in interactive sessions
- Conversation with learner interaction
- Interaction read aloud
- Interaction tell a story
- Interaction role play
- Interaction soliloquy.

Importance of Communicating in the Classroom

Increase, strengthen the connection between students and teachers, and create an overall positive experience.
- **Self-esteem:** People generally want their opinions to be heard. When a teacher shows interest in a student's opinion, the student feels that his or her thoughts and ideas are valued. This will boost your selfesteem and confidence. Confident students are less likely to guess their answers on tests, and confident students are more likely to speak up in class. Class participation leads to more learning throughout the class.

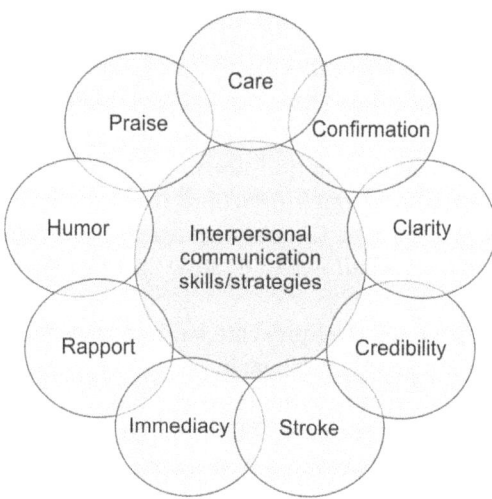

Fig. 7.4: Interpersonal communication skills.

- **Class performance:** Teachers who reward student communication and class participation will notice an improvement in overall class performance. A teacher can gauge the effectiveness of a lecture by student feedback. By asking questions a teacher can determine if students were able to retain the imparted information.
- **Professional growth:** A degree of communication is required in every profession and communication skills are necessary at even the most preliminary stages of career growth. For example an applicant must be able to communicate her skills and abilities during an interview in order to acquire a job.

Factors Affecting Communication

The factors influencing classroom communication can be listed in various heads such as factors related to the sender.
- How he perceives his world and himself
- Language competency
- Voice
- Facial expressions
- Emotions
- Energy level
- Age and experiences
- Attitude beliefs values

Factors Related to the Message

- Accuracy and precision of words
- Simplicity and clarity
- Appropriateness
- Imagination and originality
- Choice of medium length of communication

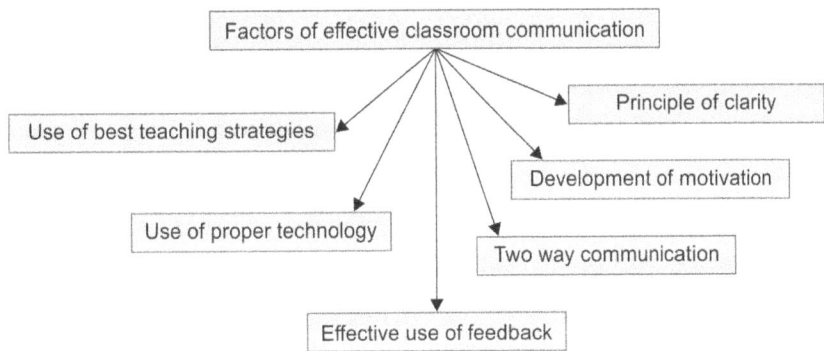

Fig. 7.5: Factors affecting effective classroom communication.

Factors Related to the Receiver

- Intelligence
- Attitude towards the subject or sender
- Age and experiences
- Self-esteem
- Motivational level
- Beliefs and values
- Previous experience
- Listening skills.

Barriers to Effective Communication

The process of communication can be affected by the following barriers:
- Linguistic incompetence
- Lack of clarity
- Lack of motivation
- Socioeconomic background
- Improper body language
- Distrust
- Low IQ levels

Along with the above listed barriers excessive verbalism verbosity confusion day-dreaming, limited perception and physical discomfort too act as barriers in communication.

Overcoming Communication Barriers

- Simplifying words
- Limiting emotions
- Actively listening
- Feedback.

CLASSROOM COMMUNICATION FACILITATOR

Teachers who foster the personal growth of their students are unique and dedicated. It takes confidence and a willingness to take care of yourself to begin the journey, then send students out on personal quests they may not be able to share. Perhaps sending students past their teachers without them realizing or appreciating what they have been given. It is that unconditionally undefinable difference between training and education, storytelling and education of bosses and leaders.

Facilitator Characteristics

Her six identifying teachers who are very helpful for personal growth features:
1. Effective listening
2. Honesty
3. Understanding
4. Respect
5. Intelligence
6. Interpersonal communication skills.

Communicator

- Make good eye contact
- Pay attention to what you say—specific words, body language and nonverbal expressions, pitch and timing
- The person try to get a sense of how
- Be concerned with how the speaker perceives the world
- Perceives people as being without critical overtones
- Confirms perceptions by asking people questions or reflecting back on what they have said
- As part of listening, seek to save real meaning and real needs.

Sincerity

- Face-to-face person-to-person encounters
- Minimal defensiveness or withdrawal, maximum true sharing
- Roles recognized as roles, not used to distance
- Feelings are admitted and recognized, those which are positive and those which are less comfortable but just as real—anger, sadness, weariness, joy, frustration, peace, need for solitude

- Human growth is a developmental stage, so there is peace in letting go, giving our children time to see things differently than we do.
- Your right to disagree will be respected and served peacefully.

Understanding

- Empathy represents true understanding—what can or should be felt being expressed in order to delve deeper into the student's emotions and eliminate self-protection and withdrawal.
- Engage students in learning to understand themselves and move toward understanding others.

Respectful

- Accepting the student's experience as important to the student
- Respecting others as part of the educational system and process
- This is often indicated by optimism, deep concern, and concern
- Positive appreciation, warmth, and respect gain the student's respect, but demanding or punishing respect leads to anger, and cheating leads to love and skill.

Main Duties and Responsibilities

- **Facilitate communication:** Facilitate communication between students and all members of the school in student communication mode. Reflect the content and spirit that is conveyed to the students. Vocalize student-to-person communication as appropriate.
- **Providing educational support services:** Reinforcing materials taught in class as needed.
- Maintain confidentiality between self-study students and all other persons involved in the education of students.
- **Promote intercultural understanding:** Educate hearing staff and students about deaf culture. Educate deaf students about hearing culture.
- **Monitor student comprehension:** Check student comprehension.
- **Provides access to the education system:** Interpretation at conferences and extracurricular activities.
- **Promote deaffriendly learning environments:** Maintain awareness of disruptive noise and lighting. Encourage the use of videos with subtitles.
- **Act as part of the education team:** Notify the education team of any concerns or issues that arise.

Areas of Responsibility

- **Supervision duties:** Communication Facilitators assist students individually or in small groups under the direct supervision of the class/program teacher.
- **Language skills:** Ability to read, write and understand simple instructions, short correspondence and notes. Ability to effectively present information to staff, parents, student's and administrators in individual and small group settings.
- **Reasoning ability:** Ability to use common sense to carry out detailed written or verbal instructions. Ability to deal with problems involving several concrete variables in standardized situations.
- **Other skills and abilities:** Ability to work with excellent students.
  - Ability to remain calm in stressful situations.
  - Ability to work effectively with student staff and the school community.
  - Ability to communicate clearly and concisely, both orally and in writing.
  - Ability to perform duties in accordance with all school district and intermediate unit requirements and department of education policy.

Essential Functions of Facilitators

- Assist students with the mastery of instructional equipment programs and materials assigned by the teacher.
- Reinforce lessons and instructs students individually or in small groups within a classroom setting assisting them in reaching classroom objectives.
- Helps develop communication and socialization skills. Teach students, and supervise student practice and assignments in various skills.
- Helps students complete homework and classroom projects in a variety of areas. Ensure students understand classroom rules and procedures. Help students answer questions by providing appropriate examples, emotional support, friendly demeanor, and general guidance.
- Support classroom activities by preparing, writing, duplicating, archiving, and grading lessons and school materials, student tests and assignments. Record student grades and attendance and files as assigned.
- Increase training and instruction in sign language.
- Observe and support student behavior in the classroom according to approved procedures and/or behavioral intervention plans. Supervise student outdoor activities as directed. Monitor and report student performance and behavioral progress. Create and publish citations as needed.

- Make sure the student explains and understands the lesson and homework instructions. Assist assigned teachers in implementing lesson plans, content standards, and classroom activities. Discuss lesson plans and materials with teachers to meet student needs.
- Use technology with communication devices and applications to support student staff and families.
- Communicate with employees and various external entities to share information and resolve issues and concerns.
- Enter and update student and various other data in assigned computer systems as required. Maintain automated records and files.
- Follow established practices and procedures to ensure student health and safety. Maintain a safe, orderly, and clean learning environment.
- Monitoring material inventory levels. Assist in ordering, receiving, and maintaining appropriate inventory levels of assigned consumables.
- Support the class teacher by setting up work areas, exhibits, and assignments.

COMMUNICATION BARRIERS IN THE CLASSROOM

Communication barriers in the classroom make it difficult for students to get the most out of their education. Some teachers are unable to create engaging lessons and have difficulty connecting with a student one-on-one with her. Students who do not deal with speech and language problems often have trouble communicating with teachers and classmates. Personality differences and peer pressure can make classroom interactions feel awkward and pushy.

- **Verbalization:** Excessive verbalization is no longer acceptable, especially in today's world of communication. It provides a much more efficient alternative to other representation formats. Such verbalization is undoubtedly an obstacle that limits effective communication in the classroom.
- **Fear:** One of the most important emotional causes of communication disorders is student fear. If a student is anxious and unsure, they are less likely to speak up in class. This is true even in situations where a student does not understand what the teacher is saying and needs clarification. Anxiety stops students from participating in group discussions because they do not want to be made the center of attention and they are afraid of other people's opinions of them.
- **Language:** Language is the primary way of communication thoughts and ideas. This can be a major obstacle to communication when teachers and students do not speak the same language. Communication problems arise when a teacher speaks *English* and a student speaks *primarily English* as a second language, as the student may not understand everything the teacher is saying.
- **Fourth expression:** Communication is never accurate. The caller tries to put his idea into words, and the recipient has to decipher the words to understand the idea. Communication barriers arise in the classroom when teachers and students cannot choose the right words to describe the ideas they are trying to convey. An example of this is a teacher who is a professional mathematician but is an ineffective math teacher because she can only communicate ideas using math jargon that students do not understand.
- **Listening barriers:** Effective and active listening is one of the most important factors in classroom communication, educational activities and classroom interactions. Take your time and listen to what the other person has to say. Do not think about your next reply when someone is speaking. Using certain words and body language can evoke negative emotions.
- **Perception barriers:** Perception can be a barrier to effective communication in the classroom. Different people receive or hear the same message, but interpret it differently. Attention to detail is also important. If you do not go deep into the topic, you may miss important aspects. Teachers also need to learn to focus on both positive and negative aspects of conversation. A distorted focus may cause the teacher to focus only on the negative aspects of the conversation.
- **Daydreaming:** A common (avoidable) obstacle to effective communication occurs when learners daydream, or engage in classroom activities. Students are not getting enough attention in the classroom when they think about the movie they saw the night before.
- **Apathy:** Student apathy arises due to the lack of available teaching materials, educational system, and effective teachers in the classroom. To eliminate the distance, teachers need to have movies, modems, filmstrips, charts, cassettes, TV recordings, and many other audiovisual materials. A variety of teaching methods and materials tend to increase students' interest and enthusiasm in their work. Because of this, you may lose interest in listening to your teacher's lectures. This type of barrier must also be considered in the classroom for proper communication between students and teachers.

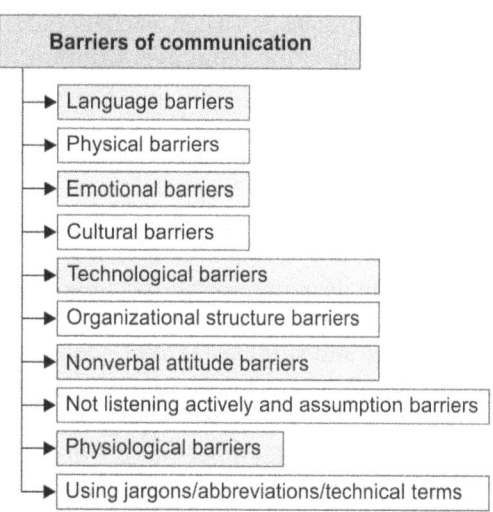

Fig. 7.6: Communication barriers in the classroom.

INFORMATION COMMUNICATION TECHNOLOGY

Information and communication technology (ICT) can simply be defined in its simplest form as an electronic medium for creating storing manipulating receiving and sending information from one place to another. It makes message delivery faster more convenient easy to access understand and interpret. It uses gadgets such as cell phones, the Internet wireless network, computer, radio television, satellites base stations, etc.

Definition

ICT is defined as a diverse set of technological tools and resources used to exchange information. These technological tools and resources include computers, the Internet (websites blogs and e-mails), live broadcasting technologies (radio television and webcasting), recorded broadcasting technologies (podcasting audio and video players and storage devices), and telephony (fixed or mobile satellite visio/video-conferencing, etc.).

ICT Stands

ICT is technology that supports activities with information. Such activities include the collection, processing, storage and presentation of data. Increasingly, these activities also include collaboration and communication. Thus, IT became ICT.

Information Technology Characteristics

- Real-time access to information
- Easy access to updated data
- Connecting geographically dispersed regions
- Broader communication media

The ICT system has six main components:
1. Information data transformed to be meaningful
2. Hardware: Physical component
3. Software: The name given to computer programmes
4. Information: Data that is converted to give it a meaning
5. Procedure: A series of actions that are performed in a specific order to keep the system running smoothly.
6. Human: Humans are the source of data.

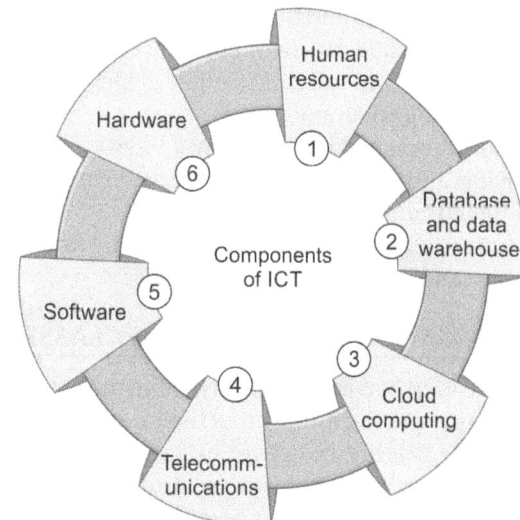

Fig. 7.7: Components information communication technology.

Teaching Technology Classification

Teaching materials can be classified in different ways. Edgar Dale's experience with cones provides one of his ways of classifying them. Educational technology is classified based on four key characteristics. That is, the stimuli provided to the learner's sensory control are categorized by the type and range of media they provide. The most common classification is based on the senses stimulated by teaching techniques. These are categorized as follows:

Visual (Oral) Print or Reproduction

- Textbook supplements
- Reference book, encyclopedias, etc.
- Magazine, newspapers, etc.
- Documents and newspaper clippings
- Programmed learning materials and self-study modules
- Case studies (reality simulations) and case reports.

Visual (Pictorial) Non-projected Two-dimensional

- Blackboard writing and drawing
- Charts
- Posters
- Maps
- Diagrams
- Graphs
- Photographs
- Cartoons
- Comic strips.

Audio

- Human voice
- Gramophone records
- Audio tapes/discs
- Stereo records
- Radio broadcast
- Telephonic conversation.

Visual Non-projected Three-dimensional

- Model
- Mock-up
- Diorama
- Globe
- Relief map
- Specimen
- Puppet
- Hologram.

Visual Projected (Still)

- Slide
- Filmstrip
- Transparency (OHP)
- Microfilm, microcard
- Motion picture film
- Television
- Close-circuit television
- Video cassette/disc.

Multi-media Packages (for More than one Sense)

- Slide + tape + workbook
- Radio + slide or posters (radio vision)
- Film + posters + workbook (print materials)
- Television + workbook (print materials)
- Any of the above + group discussion
- Any of the above + introductory and summarizing talk by teacher/leader of the group.

New Emerging Media (All of these are Multisensory)

- Teleconferencing (group discussion through telephones)
- Cable television
- Satellite television/communication satellites
- Computer networking
- Video discs
- Minicomputers/microcomputers/word processors.

Uses of ICT in Education

- **Planning tools:** Calendar and task manager very useful for scheduling exam deliveries, creating workflows, and more.
- **Data storage in the cloud:** Collaborate and access data from any device, anywhere. Tools that use this technology include office packs, storage, and more/or broadcast your screen by email.
- Interactive tables allow students to interact directly with the surface
- Enhance the learning experience and provide new skills
- Reach more students with massive open online courses (MOOCs)
- Facilitate undergraduate education
- Minimize costs and time savings associated with providing information and automating routine routine tasks
- Improving agency management to improve the quality and efficiency of service delivery.
- The importance of information and communication technology (ICT)
- To develop in students an analytical mind that helps them research problems and provide solutions from all related fields to use as learning tools.
- As an emerging discipline, it helps students innovate and develop new ways to solve problems scientifically.
- It makes information storage and retrieval easy.
- It enhances computer networking globally known today as internet and intranet.
- It accelerates economic development nationally as it is a virile source of national income for all nations that have fully embraced its usefulness.
- It creates gainful employment hence a viable source of livelihood.
- It makes comprehension of other subjects easy. Virtually all fields of learning are amenable to ICT such as the application of projector for teaching in the classroom.
- It creates an avenue for the exchange of ideas and inventions among information technology scholars locally and internationally.
- It is the basis for e-learning and online library. Hence information dissemination is easier than ever.

- Important to all forms of globalization and the achievement of the Millennium Development Goals.

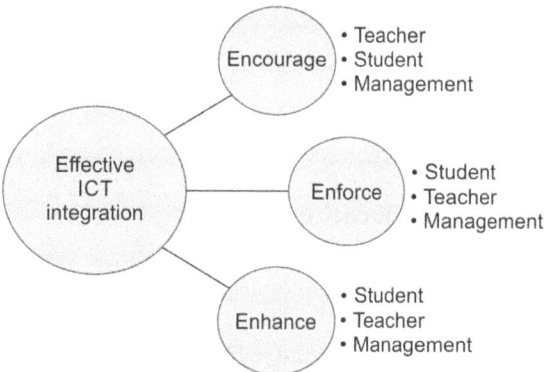

Fig. 7.8: Disadvantages of lecture method.

Benefits of Using ICT in Education

- Interest in learning is increasing. Traditional subjects become more interesting through the use of diverse resources such as videos, websites, graphics, and games. Multimedia content is a very useful tool for introducing students to various topics in a comprehensive and entertaining way.
- **Interactivity:** This allows students to explore fun physical and mental activities while learning. Educational games, interactive museum tours, and virtual labs.
- **Student collaboration:** Student collaboration is greatly improved by a variety of digital tools. They find it much easier to create team projects, collaborate, and learn from each other.
- **Promote creativity:** ICT tools stimulate the development of imagination and spontaneity in all class members.
- **Increased communication:** Close communication between students and teachers is facilitated in a more spontaneous and informal way through various channels.
- **Content personalization and timeliness:** In a digital environment, all information and resources can be updated in real time. Additionally, it is possible to adapt tools and content to local and nearby realities.

Information and Communication Technology Challenges

- **Expensive ICT materials:** Especially materials required for advanced level of practical ICT knowledge are expensive.
- **Universal acceptance as a required subject:** This subject has not yet been fully adopted by all cradle learning institutions worldwide.
- **Malicious takeover:** ICT is used by some people for malicious purposes, such as cybercrime and malicious programs that can cause serious damage to computers and similar devicesused.

CLASSROOM TEACHING METHOD

Classroom learning is a traditional mode of learning in which the learning environment is created within the physical walls of a classroom. As the name suggests, in-classroom learning, both the teacher and student need to be present physically inside the classroom. The main aim of classroom teaching should be to facilitate learning. Classroom: A classroom is a place where various activities are going on, where interactions take place, social situations are enhanced and norms are built-in instructional situations

LECTURE METHOD

The lecture method was the earliest known teaching method. Currently, this method is used on a large scale only in universities. Many young people cannot stand telling long stories because they have limited attention spans. The lecture method is a one-way communication system, only the teacher is active in the classroom and the students are passive.

Definition

- A lecture method is a lecture that provides specific information to a class, or a long, serious lecture
  —**Oxford dictionary**
- Lectures are a great way to inform a large number of people in a short amount of time —**A Adivi Reddy**

Purposes

- Lecture method is just a good way to make a large class more accessible.
- It draws students' attention to its essential elements and puts them at the forefront of research.
- It helps provide the students with a factual foundation upon which to build concepts using concrete examples.
- Students can actively participate in general information such as legislation.

Principles of Lecture Method

- **Principle of aim:** Lecture is based on aim; nobody likes aimless lecture. Even the best teacher will fail if his lecture is not based on some objectives.
- **Principles of activity:** If you want to learn a thing you have to actively participate.
- **Correlation principle:** A lecture is not an effective lecture, but a scientific plan. The subject to be conveyed should be well-planned.

- **Foresight principle:** A good lecture is always predicted based on the teacher's past experience. Certain predictors are created for the child's future.
- A good presentation requires effective preparation. In order to give a presentation, you need to prepare yourself physically, socially, emotionally, and mentally.

The main features of the teaching method are:
- Usually, an organizational presentation.
- It can be used for in-depth coverage of a topic.
- Suitable for large groups.
- It saves time.
- Results are easy to miss.
- Listeners may absorb information without thinking.

Benefits of Lecture Method

- Lectures help convey new information such as, concepts related to new political treatment protocols or professional practices. A lecture can convey information to a large number of people in a short time. The sequence is controlled by an educator who facilitates learning group comprehension. The material presented is typically not available from a single resource, but educators need to synthesize content from multiple resources in a logical format.
- The lecture method is excellent for presenting a lot of facts in a short time.
- Helps introduce new topics in summarizing the literature in a field that considers integrating various ideas and concepts into a coherent system of thought. It often useful for advanced students.
- Lack of personal relationships between instructors and students makes it difficult for lectures to meet individual needs.
- Lectures should be well-organized and ideas should be developed in sequence. Local experience should be used to explain the statement.
- Most thrifty intern in terms of space use and time with family.
- Increases passivity on the part of the student.

Advantages

- It can present topics of appropriate perspective and orientation and create a general overview of the topic's scope.
- You can present a lot of facts in an impressive amount of time.
- Lecture series can greatly increase interest in a topic.
- Interest breeds attention so you can secure and maintain greater attention.
- Speeches can be suitable for all listeners.
- The spoken word has a greater weight than the mute appeal by books.
- Lectures can be advantageously made use of for presenting a number of facts belonging to the different subjects and the impressions thus created would be of a longstanding value.
- Lectures facilitate interdisciplinary approach to topics.

Criticisms

- **Lectures are time consuming:** Lectures have no advantage.
- **Little student activity in lectures:** This may seem like a fundamental flaw, but it is not.
- **Presentation requires special skills:** This mistake is a testament to weak presentation, not method. A successful lecture requires familiarity with the material, but that is not the lecture's fault.
- **Students do not immediately analyze or summarize lectures:** If this is the case, it is generally not the method's fault, but the teacher's fault. If the teacher carefully plans the lecture, structures it with subheadings, and speaks slowly while emphasizing the main points, students will be better able to take good notes.
- **Lectures may not be well adapted to students' perceptual abilities:** It seems impossible for a teacher to lecture on a subject for an entire semester without gaining students' understanding, but this sometimes happens.
- **Lectures are likely to be sustained dictation exercises:** This is clearly not a weakness, but an abuse of the lecture methods, common in nursing schools.

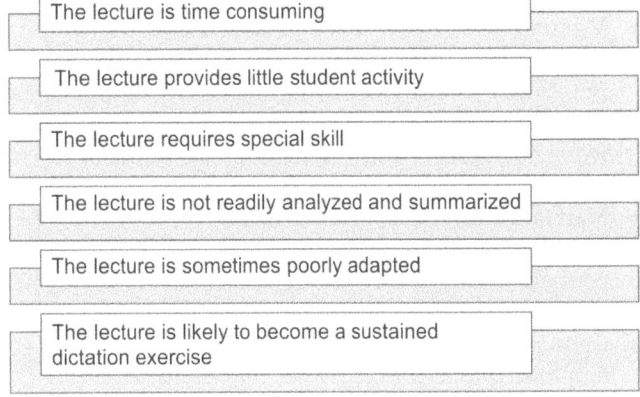

Fig. 7.9: Disadvantages of lecture method.

Tips for Successful Presentation

- Outline your lecture (using slides or handouts) and refer to it as you move from point-to-point.
- Repeat points in different ways.
- Use short sentences.

- Emphasize important points (with tone or explicit comments).
- Pause to give listener time to think and write.
- Use your speech as a compliment, do not just repeat the text.
- Do not rush the last part of the lecture. This is a common mistake made by teachers who want to give too much information in the allotted time.
- Being prepared reduces stress, frustration and uncertainty, but it is not consistently effective.

Cons

- It is a waste of time to repeat what has already been introduced in the book. This will break independent reads.
- To make the presentation effective, the teacher may be less concerned with the content and more concerned with manners.
- If the lecture is delivered too quickly, students will not be able to easily take notes and record important points.
- Lectures are designed to kill student imitation and weaken problem-solving attitudes.
- Lectures cause mental sluggishness in the classroom, i.e., failure to analyze the lecture will result in a loss of cooperation between the student's mind and the teacher.
- Lectures may lose track of materials and become information compilations.
- Dictation becomes more important as the lecture progresses.

Guidelines for Teachers

- Maintain good eye contact. Make the learners feel that what you have to say is addressed to them individually. Both your eyes and voice communicate with them. Their eyes, facial expressions and reactions communicate with you. Look for signs of misunderstanding, desire to participate, fatigue, or a lack of interest.
- Maintain a high level of enthusiasm.
- Speak in a natural conversational voice. Please clarify your words. Make sure the learner can hear every word spoken.
- Repeat gestures or change your tone of voice to emphasize your point.
- Carefully check the learner's understanding by observing their faces and asking questions throughout the presentation. Observing facial expressions for signs of suspicion or misunderstanding is not a surefire way to check a learner's understanding. The best time to clear the mental fog is when the fog is brewing. Mental fog tends to create mental blocks that prevent learners from concentrating on the material being presented.
- Teaching at the class level. Use verbal explanation questions and more that are tailored to the needs of the average learner in your class. Identify and prepare materials to illustrate your points.
- Encourage learners to think. Thinking as used here refers to creative thinking rather than mere memorization of previously learned facts. Stimulate learner thinking with a variety of educational tools. These tools include questions that make you think in the classroom.
- Provide examples that connect the topic to the learner's life.
- Arrange the content logically, systematically, and in order based on the previous content.
- Avoid regulation and try to be provocative.
- Maintain time designations.
- Various materials are available to support the content, such as transparencies, charts, posters, flannel, etc.

GROUP DISCUSSION

- A discussion is a focused conversation, such as a specific topic, question, concept, or problem with a genuine desire to reach a decision. This is essentially a collaborative problem-solving activity seeking consensus to solve a problem, rather than majority decision-making. In other words, working together to find solutions to problems of common interest, rather than just talking about problems, should be a clear goal that all parties can understand.
- You need a leader to direct and coordinate the process.
- Discussion points should be recorded during the discussion, on the board, or by a 'recorder' selected by the group.
- Anyone is welcome to participate.
- Shy people should be encouraged to contribute.
- All perspectives must be considered impartially.
- The discussion should be to the point.
- Discussions should properly end with a report, recommended decision, or a summary of the issues discussed.
- Group members should participate in discussions with a basic knowledge of the topic being discussed.

Discussion Techniques

A well-managed group discussions with the right resources are very effective in making decisions based on the ideas of all students. It is effective in changing the attitude and behavior of the students.

Group Discussion Rules

- The ideas and views expressed by group members should be clear and concise.

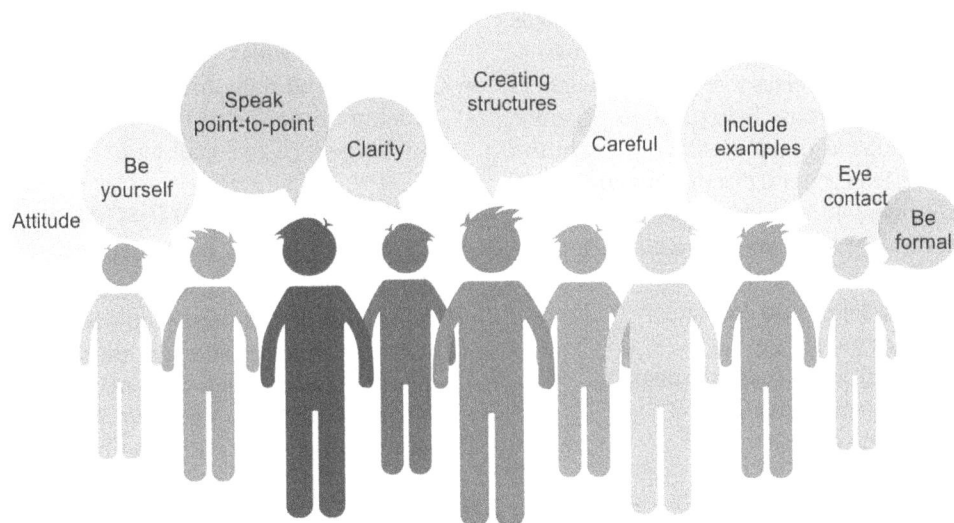

Fig. 7.10: Group discussion rules.

- The members have to listen to each other what is discussed among them.
- There should not be any interruption when the member of the group is discussing or speaking.
- Each member of group should accept the criticism gracefully, if by a member is done.
- The group discussion should reach a conclusion.
- The group discussions require members to make appropriate comments during the discussion.

Group discussion techniques include:
- Proper planning of topics including goals and guidelines. Proper planning of the environment in which the discussion takes place, i.e., the environment should not be a threat.
- In order for the group discussion to be successful, students should be well prepared for the topics they will discuss.
- The role of each member of the group leader and the role of the teacher should be clarified.
- The teacher starts the discussion with a short introduction of the topic.
- Students are asked to share their ideas and perspectives.
- The teacher acts as a moderator during the discussion.
- One of the students in the group records the steps.
- The teacher controls the group discussion by discouraging persuasive students and engaging passive students in the discussion.
- During discussion, the teacher clarifies difficult statements to avoid misunderstandings and confusion among group members.
- Teachers change the course of a discussion when it deviates from the set goals or wastes time.
- Teacher guides the students in relation to pros and cons of the view points and after analyzing the view points, a consensus is reached.
- After group discussion, a concluding note in the form of summary of the discussion, performance of students and a few words of appreciation to encourage the students to participate in forthcoming discussions.

Forms of Discussion
- **Class discussion:** Sometimes the teacher may select the discussion method for teaching a particular topic with the whole class participating as one group. This can be handled very efficiently if the class is not too large. The teacher, acting as leader, introduces the topic guide, leads the discussion, writes down the main points on the whiteboard, and helps the group to summarize. It is a convenient way to. It also serves as a learning experience for students on how to discuss.

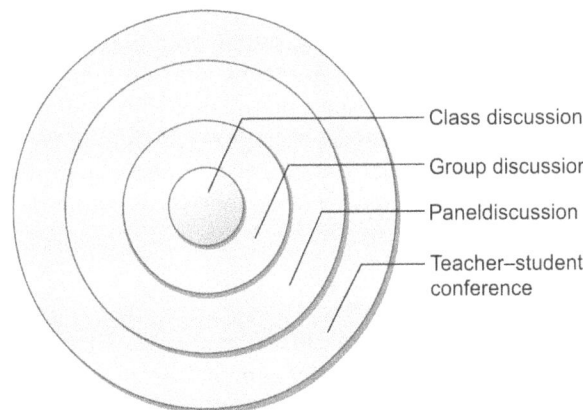

Fig. 7.11: Forms of discussion.

- **Group discussion (6–20 participants):** If the class is large, or if some aspect of the topic is to be discussed, it makes sense to divide the class into groups. Teachers introduce topics for discussion, help students organize groups, support groups as needed, take reports at the end of allotted time, lead general discussions, and make points. Each group should appoint its own leader and recorder. The following rules are followed during the discussion:
  - Express your ideas clearly and concisely.
  - Listen to what other people say.
  - Do not disturb others when they are speaking.
  - Make only relevant comments.
  - Take criticism seriously.
  - Helps draw conclusion.
- **Panel discussion:** A panel discussion is a small group discussion of four to eight speakers in front of a large audience. Panels retain the advantages of discussion groups when the audience is large and full participation is not possible. It is more formal than discussion and less formal than a lecture. Panels are composed of a small number of members who are willing to exchange ideas and opinions on a particular topic under the guidance of a chair. When used as a method of teaching, a panel can be a group of experts on the subjects. They prepared the topic in advance. The Chairman introduces the members/speakers, introduces the topic, allows the first person to speak, and initiates the discussion. This discussion takes place in conversation and the chairman keeps everyone on topic. If necessary, the moderator can clear up questions or misunderstandings, or offer alternative thoughts to ensure the topic is fully covered. Arguments may or may not be thrown openly on the floor. It is the chairman who takes the initiative and ultimately summarizes and concludes the discussion.
- **Teacher-student conference:** This is a private exchange of ideas and information to help the students function in a professional setting. It can be used to plan a more effective approach to coursework or to seek information about issues of a personal nature that affect a student's professional success. As a method of teaching, a conference is a meeting between a teacher and a small group of students to discuss a problem or selected situation, or before or after a visit.

Benefits

- Group discussion format that encourages active student participation and facilitates student learning.
- Help students develop problem-solving techniques.
- Empower group members.
- Provide opportunities for students to express their opinions and skills.
- Develop social skills and a sense of teamwork.
- Develop students' ability to compare and contrast knowledge on a given subject.

Disadvantages of Group Discussion

- The group discussion method takes time because it is difficult to finish the discussion within the time limit.
- Without proper student preparation, group discussion methods will not be effective and meaningful exchanges will not occur between students.
- The group discussion method is for larger groups, i.e., member exceeds 20 and is ineffective.

MICROTEACHING

A training process aimed at simplifying the complexities of the regular teaching process. It is difficult for teachers to simultaneously assess all student-teacher teaching abilities and make necessary corrections. By reducing teaching, teachers can easily identify deficiencies in performing a particular teaching skill, and help students master that skill by providing assistance in correcting identified deficiencies.

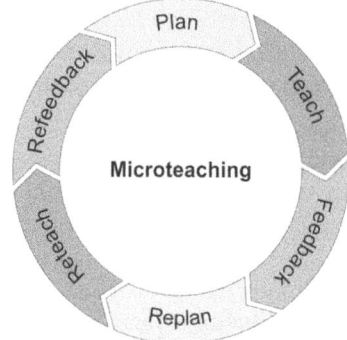

Fig. 7.12: Microteaching steps.

Definition

- Class size meets lesson time. We have 5–10 students and lessons are 5–20 minutes long.
- **DW Allen (1966):** Microteaching is an educational experience that reduces class size and time.
- **Allen and Eve (1968):** Microteaching is defined as a system of controlled practice that focuses on specific educational behaviors and allows teaching to be practiced under controlled conditions.
- **McAleese and Unwin (1970):** The term microteaching is most commonly applied to the use of closed-circuit TV to provide immediate feedback on future teacher performance in a simplified environment.

- **Clift et al. (1976):** Microteaching reduces teaching situations to simpler, more controlled encounters by limiting handson instruction to specific skills and reducing instruction time and class size. It is a shrinking instructional training method.
- **BK Passi and MS Lalita (1976):** Microteaching is a training technique in which a studentteacher must use specific teaching skills to teach a small number of students a single concept in a short period of time.

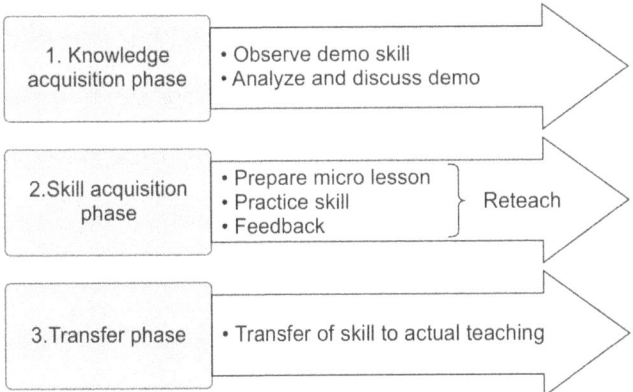

Fig. 7.13: Microteaching phases.

Microinstruction Features

- It is relatively a new experience or innovation in the field of teacher education, especially student education.
- This is a training technique, not a teaching technique. In other words, it is a technique or design used to train teachers (or teach teachers how to teach). It is not a method or method of teaching, such as inductive deduction or question-and-answer methods.
  - Practices one skill at a time.
  - Reduce class size to 5–10 people.
  - Reduced lesson time to 5–10 minutes.
  - Limit content to a single concept.
- Microteaching provides appropriate feedback to provide appropriate information on learner performance immediately after lesson completion.
- Lessons are said to consist of very specific skills. These skills cannot be acquired through traditional teacher education approaches. Microteaching provides an opportunity to pick one skill at a time, practice them through miniaturized encounters, and then learn other skills in a similar fashion.
- Microteaching is a highly personalized training device that allows you to impose a high degree of control over the practice of specific skills.

Considering the above characteristics and features, the term microteaching is used to train inexperienced or experienced teachers to learn the art of teaching by superimposing specific skills through "dumpy class encounters", in other words, it reduces the complexity of actual regular teaching in terms of size and content of teaching hours.

Phases

- **Orientation:** Initially, the teacher should be given the necessary theoretical background knowledge for microteaching through open and fair discussion of the following aspects:
  - Concept
  - Importance or justification for the use of microteaching
  - Procedure
  - Prerequisites and general conditions for adopting microteaching techniques
  - Analysis of teaching in partial teaching competence.

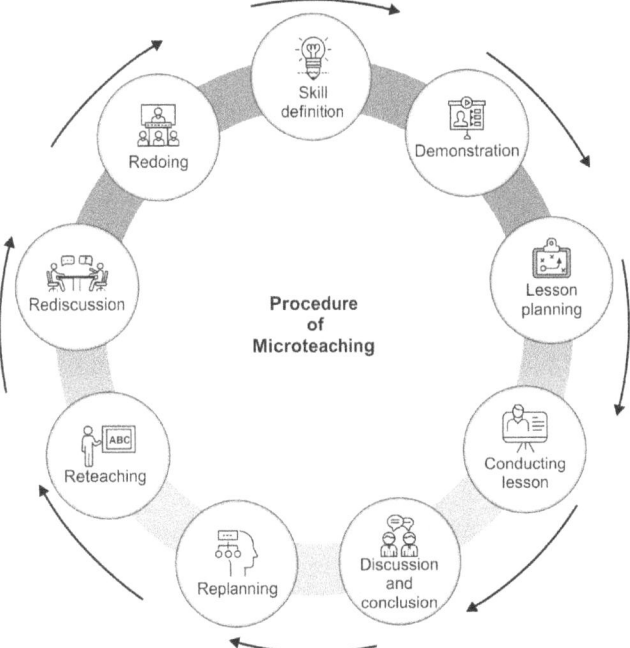

Fig. 7.14: Microteaching procedure.

- **Selection of specific teaching skills:** Teaching skills should be practiced separately. Teachers of students are thus persuaded to choose specific skills to practice. Additionally, they receive the necessary orientation and processing materials for practice. Most of these materials are described in the literature available at NCERT. The teacher can be given the background knowledge necessary to observe a model or demonstration lesson about the teaching ability of their choice.

- **Sample demonstration lesson presentation:** Here the student is provided with a demonstration or sample her lesson on how to use the selected Teaching Ability. This is also called "Modeling". Demonstration of desired behavior in relation to observer's ability to imitate. Depending on resource availability and the types of skills involved, demonstrations or model his lessons can be delivered in a variety of ways.
  - Provide materials such as manual illustrations and videotapes.
  - Film and videocassette displays.
  - Have the trainee listen to the tape.
  - Organizing live model demonstrations, i.e., teacher trainers or experts demonstrating the use of skills.
- **Observation and criticism of model lessons:** What you read, see, hear and observe here through the model source will be carefully analyzed by the trainee. In a demonstration by an expert or teacher trainer, the teacher is asked to write down their observations. Observation plans specifically designed to observe specific skills are distributed to trainees and trained in their use in advance. Observations of such model lessons and corresponding criticisms provide desirable feedback to model teachers.
- **Create microlesson plan:** In this step, the teacher must select concepts suitable for practicing the demonstrated skill and create a micro-lesson plan.
- **Create micro-class settings:** The default settings for micro-classes are:
  - *Number of students:* 5–10.
  - *Student type:* Real student, preferably classmate.
  - *Supervisor type:* Teacher educator and companion.
  - *Micro-lesson duration:* 6 minutes.
    Example micro-lesson cycle duration: 36 minutes.
- **Teaching session:** Here, the teacher presents her prepared micro-lesson for 6 minutes (specified schedule of teaching sessions) with 5–10 actual students or peers (teacher). Teach the composed micro-class). Monitored by both teacher trainers and peers with the help of an appropriate monitoring plan. If possible, the teacher can also record the lesson on video or tape.
- **Providing feedback:** The greatest benefit of microlesson is the ability to provide immediate feedback to the teacher on the teaching performance demonstrated in the microlesson. Feedback is provided on the use of component instructional movements that accentuate the actual skill so that he can modify the skill in the desired direction. This feedback in the Indian context is adequately provided by peers and teacher educators observing micro-lessons. Mechanical devices such as videotape, audiotape, and cable television.
- **Rescheduling (rescheduling sessions):** Considering feedback from varius sources, trainees attempt to reschedule microlessons in 12 minutes to do this.
- **Reteaching (Re-teach session):** In this 6 minutes' session, the student's teacher repeats a microlesson based on a prepared plan and reorganized framework.
- **Give ReFeedback (Re-feedback sessions):** Based on performance in repeated microlessons, the student's teacher receives refeedback in the manner previously described.

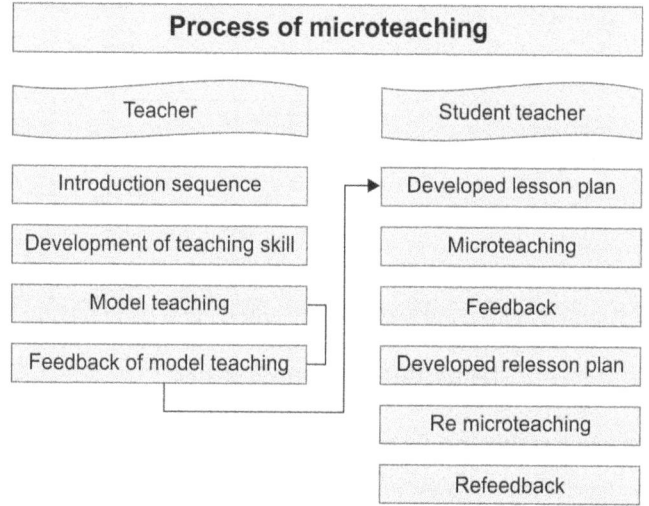

Fig. 7.15: Microteaching process.

- **Repeating microteaching cycles:** Microteaching cycles used to practice teaching skills consist of planning, feedback, replanning, and feedback operations. The cycle of microlessons repeats and the student's-teacher has to replan and teach the lessons until they have mastered the skill being taught.
- **Teaching skills integration:** The final step involves integrating the various teaching skills that the studentteacher has acquired individually. This helps bridge the gap between isolated teaching skills training and the real-life classroom situations that teachers face.

Advantages of Microteaching

Microteaching has the following advantages over traditional teaching methods in the Indian context:
- Cooperation between students and training institute staff. A microteaching approach that incorporates simulation technology can help educational institutions overcome the difficulties encountered in organizing student education.

- The microteaching approach replaces the holistic concept of education with an analytical concept. Here, a complex instructional task is viewed as a set of simple skills involving specific classroom behaviors. This will help you get the meaning and concept of the term education right.
- Microteaching helps reduce the complexity of regular classroom instruction. Classroom instruction will be curtailed or curtailed to reduce class size and teaching time.
- In microteaching, the student's teacher focuses on the practice of concrete, well-defined teaching skills, which are sets of observable, controllable, actionable teacher behaviors. As a result, it offers more appropriate techniques for learning the art of teaching than traditional programs (although you can master one teaching skill at a time).
- Microteaching helps systematic and objective observation by providing a specific observation plan.
- Microteaching serves as a practice focused on mastering teaching skills and teaching techniques. Here, trainees can try several options with limited time and limited resources. This is like learning the art of operating on a part of the human body from a student doctor in a medical lab before actually operating on a patient.
- Microteaching is economical in acquiring teaching skills. It saves time and energy for both the teacher and the student. Not only it is easier for teachers to handle small groups (5–10 students), it also poses less of a problem of class discipline and resulting mental strain than traditional practice classes. It also prevents students from being unnecessarily used as guinea pigs for teacher training.

SIMULATION

The word "simulate" means to imitate exactly. "Roleplay" during class stimulates students' interest. This skill is used in the classroom by teachers and students acting out roles without prior training, i.e., spontaneously or without rehearsal. From this, it is safe to conclude that simulation is a form of roleplay in which students and teachers spontaneously demonstrate this ability.

Simulated Teaching Definition

Simulated teaching is a learning and training technique that develops an individual's ability to engage in problem-solving behavior. It is defined as a roleplaying game in which the learner assumes a role in an artificially created environment.

Meaning

Recently, classroom simulations have entered pedagogy. Used at different levels of instruction. Teachers have practical training and also theoretical learning. Student-teachers must be trained in simulated situations before being sent to schools for teaching practice. He has to play the role of teacher in a manmade environment. After that he should be sent to school. In this way, teachers will be able to teach in a superior way.

Simulated play is the area of developing specific communication skills or carrying out educational processes in artificially created situations. In historical and literary subjects, the ability to simulate is used as a form of roleplay. With the help of different teachers, they imitate and act out roles.

Special Features of Simulated Teaching

- Simulated teaching creates a link between academic knowledge and practical application.
- A mock lesson allows you to identify and solve problems during the lesson.
- It helps to teach assistants to comprehend and cope with behavioral issues in school.
- Simulated teaching helps develop teaching strategy skills.
- It allows teaching assistants to assume the role of Student Instructor and Administrator.
- A mock lesson will boost the morale of the trainees.

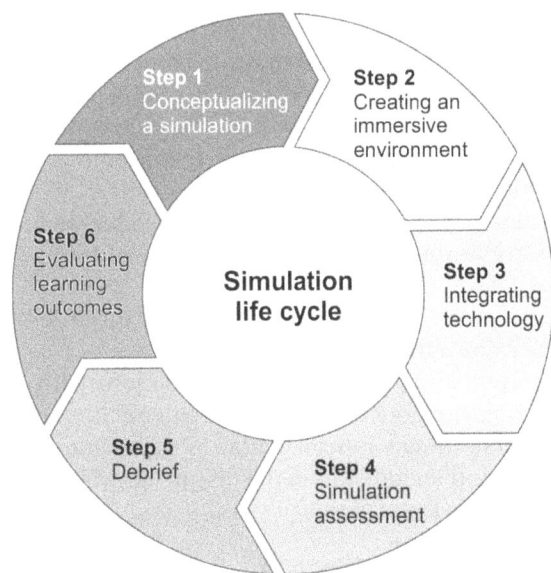

Fig. 7.16: Simulation cycle.

Simulated Training Steps

Below are the six steps typically performed in simulated training:

1. **Role assignment:** This creates the need to assign students to various roles, such as direct care providers and observers.
2. **Determining skills to practice:** In this phase, you decide which skills to practice and plan, and prepare for them. Each trainee selects topics based on their interests and intelligence.
3. **Preparing the work plan:** At this stage, decide who will teach first, who will watch first, and how each will teach/watch in turn.
4. **Observation technique decision:** At this stage, a decision is made about the type of observation technique. This also includes what kind of data we need to collect and how we intercept this data.
5. **Configure first practice session:** The first practice session begins and observations are recorded for evaluation of educational behavior.
6. **Procedure change:** The whole procedure is changed in this phase. There are teacher changes, observer changes, teaching ability changes, and subjects taught. Each student has the opportunity to play the role of teacher.

Implementation

Effective simulation requires three elements. Prepare students for active participation and report after the simulation.

Preparation

Classroom simulations are very effective in encouraging student participation, but many simulations require extensive preparation in the simulation classroom. Preparation depends on the type and complexity of the simulation.

- Facilitators read all the supporting material for the simulation.
- Facilitators do a trial run or participate in the simulation before assigning the simulation to students when possible.
- Facilitators ensure that university facilities support simulations when facilities are needed.
- Teachers integrate classroom simulations with other teaching methods such as collaborative learning.
- Teachers should anticipate how the simulation will go wrong and include this in the discussion with the class prior to the simulation.

Active Student Participation

Effective learning comes from simulations in which students actively participate.

- Students should predict and explain the expected results from the simulation.
- Every effort should be made to keep students from becoming passive during the simulation. Each student must assume a role they knew or did not know before the simulation.

Postsimulation Debriefing

Postsimulation discussions with students lead to deeper learning. Instructors must:

- Give students plenty of time to reflect and discuss what they learned from the simulation.
- Prepare questions to be asked during the debriefing to ensure students understand the consistency between the simulation and course objectives.

Simulation Methods in Teaching

- **Orientation:** The instructor will plan a comprehensive introductory event introducing the concepts of the model.
- **Demonstration:** After orientation, teachers present sample lessons for new teachers in the same class. All simulated educational processes are carried out there. Finally, the trainee analyzes the shown lesson to understand each element of the simulated lesson.
- **Group formation:** At this stage, the teacher forms groups according to the capacity of the classroom. This team consists of teacher-learners and monitors who ensure that the simulated lessons run smoothly.
- **Role assignment:** In this process, teachers assign tasks to team members. All trainees must take full responsibility. A trainee mainly fulfills her three roles: instructor, learner, and administrator.
- **Selection of skills for practice:** You can also explore skills and topics with your instructor to deepen your understanding. However, the theme should be such that it covers all skills at once.
- **Create work plan:** After selecting skills and subjects, the trainer creates a work plan for the simulated classroom exercise. The work plan determines who will start the mock class, who may interrupt the training session, and who will end the session. Ultimately, the schedule will determine when the session ends.
- The teacher should determine the observation technique. At this stage, observation strategies are determined. It specifies the type of data to collect and how to interpret it. This phase is therefore associated with the evaluation method.
- **Training session organization:** The first training session is planned with assigned responsibilities

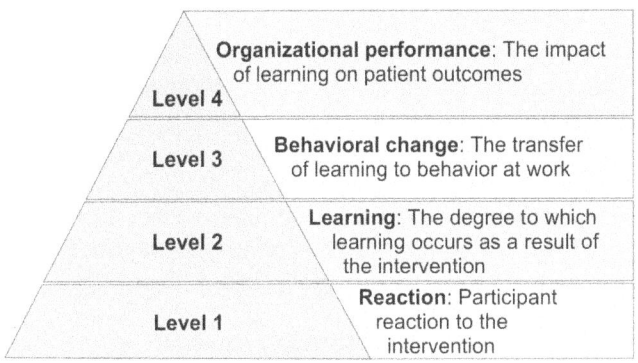

Fig. 7.17: Levels of learning in microteaching.

once all planning is complete. The teacher and other learners then provide brief comments on the teacher's performance.
- **Modifications of procedure:** After the lesson is over, there should be a discussion for the trainees to make corrections. The trainee then modifies the method based on the data obtained and organizes the next lesson.

Simulated Class Restrictions

- Not available for all subjects in the curriculum.
- This method requires a lot of preparation on the part of the teacher and may not be tolerated by the teacher.
- The observer playing the role may have misread it.
- Beginners may find it difficult to practice teaching techniques such as asking questions.
- There is no emphasis on delivering content.

DEMONSTRATION METHODS

Demonstration methods are of greater importance in nursing education than in any other discipline. This is a highly educational method and depends on the learning needs of the student's available time to teach. An experienced and competent teachers use different techniques depending on the subject.

Learning Objectives

- Provide a clear picture of relevant care.
- Make specific observations by the student.
- Thoroughly learn each procedure to provide trading status.
- Get a realistic picture of the process.
- Stimulate and encourage the development of student initiation.
- Encourage active student participation.

Definition

- A demonstration is an activity to illustrate or explain through an experiment or real application, during which a person shows, works and explains.
- Demonstration is a technique commonly used by all the teachers to teach various subjects.
- Demonstration method is self-learning by observation, using different senses.
- A demonstration is a visual representation of an idea, fact, or process.
- Demonstration measures are performances and actions to demonstrate the correct course of action.

Purpose

- A demonstration method is shown.
- Teach psychomotor skills.
- For new equipment/procedure orientation
- Provides gentle, loving care.
- Patient education.
- Facilitates learning by doing/imitation
- Use your sense of sight and touch.
- Presentation of processes and skills.

Type of Demonstration

- First personal demonstration, e.g., TPR.
- Second performance, e.g., lift and carry.
- Lecture with demonstration, e.g., television broadcast of CPR, rehabilitation procedures.
- Demonstration by practice, e.g., TPR in hospital wards and screening rooms.

Demonstration Features

- Before starting the actual work, he must tell the audience:
- Create an atmosphere that encourages questions and allows the audience to clarify their doubts.

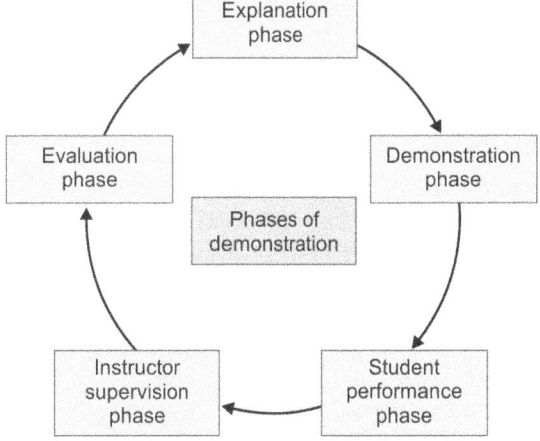

Fig. 7.18: Phases of demonstration.

- The demonstrator should be well prepared on the subject and take help from peers and teachers as needed.

Important Steps in Good Demonstration
- Initial assessment
- Prepare the patient unit and items.
- Procedure.
- Post-treatment of patients and items.
- Records and reports.
- Know the my students well. Who would you like to teach, What is the level of knowledge and literacy.
- Prepare your resources.
- Remember that changing people's practices is more delicate than surgery.
- Ensure that sufficient personnel, equipment, transportation, etc., are available before broadcasting the demonstration.
- By asking yourself questions, you are free to input knowledge as needed.
- Do not try to show too much. Usually one or two variables can be indicated at the same time.
- Observe and demonstrate interactions with variables.
- Demonstrate the effectiveness of the exercise by maintaining proper cheeks.
- Plan campaigns and communicate to ensure contact with targeted students.
- Choose your partners carefully. Make sure your employees are working with you.
- Keep them involved and informed.
- Consider location and accessibility for both non-professionals and VIPs.
- Include agency, individuals and others in all operations. The reliability of this lens has been proven.
- Arrange day trips and visits for potential users of the demonstration and its results.
- Keep records. Prepare a lecture.

Benefits
- **Multisensory activation:** the display tells you the description of each. This increases learning as more senses take advantage of learning opportunities.
  Teach students the skill of careful observation, a very important quality as a nurse. It is a method in itself, learning through observation and using multiple senses.
- It provide opportunities for observational learning. Students cannot only listen to explanations, but also see operations and processes. It projects mental images into the student's mind that reinforce oral knowledge.
- Clarify the underlying principles by giving the "why" of the process.
- Create interest with concrete illustrations.
- Combine theory and practice.
- Teachers are given an opportunity to assess the student's knowledge of the procedure and determine if retraining is required.
- The fact that students have knowledge and must be able to apply it immediately is a strong motivator.
- Student return demonstrations under teacher supervision provide an opportunity for intensive practice before students have to use the procedure on the ward.

Application of Demonstration Methods
- To demonstrate the use of experiments and laboratory equipment in scientific laboratories, medical nursing, etc.
- To educate patient/client on home treatment procedures.
- Demonstrating the procedure at the bedside or in the ward briefing room makes more sense.
- Establish more effective nurse-patient relationships to demonstrate different approaches to building support with clients.

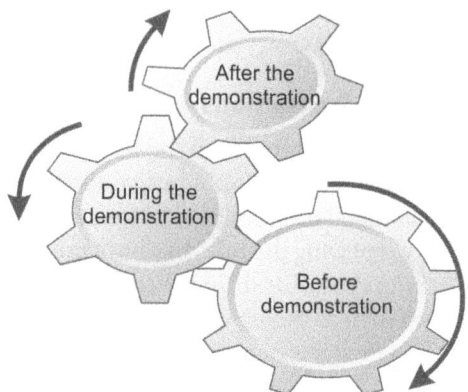

Fig. 7.19: Special care in demonstration.

Psychomotor Skill Demonstration Procedures
- Before demonstration:
  - Formulate action goals.
  - Conduct a competency analysis and determine the order.
  - Assess learner admission behavior and determine prerequisites.
  - Create a lesson plan with specific reference to:
    - Ensuring optimal visibility
    - Preparation of materials
- During demonstrations:
  - Communicate goals to learners.
  - Motivate by explaining why the skill is important.
  - Perform general skill at normal speed.
  - Write the series of subskills on the board as a checklist for step-by-step demonstrations.

- Slowly demonstrate each sub-skill in the correct order.
- Get feedback by asking questions and observing non-verbal behavior.
- Do not use negative examples or variations of techniques.
• After the show:
  - Provide immediate supervised practice with adequate time allowance.
  - Provide verbal rather than physical guidance.
  - Make the environment psychologically safe by providing a friendly atmosphere and constructive criticism.
  - Remember that your initial interest may wane. Offer motivation and encouragement.
  - Note that learners master this skill at different speeds. Therefore, individualize the plan for fast and slow learners.
  - Discuss.

Disadvantages of Demonstration
- Requires energy, time and skill.
- Poor demonstration yields poor learning.
- Demands the same condition where the skill is to be performed.
- Need interest, motivation and knowledge.
- Not all aspects of cognitive learning are covered.

RE-DEMONSTRATION

Return demonstration is an integral part of nursing practice that paves the way for future nurses to acquire knowledge of nursing procedures. This will give you an idea of what nurses in hospitals and communities do when caring for patients and how these procedures are performed.

Learning in almost every aspect of life is a process of trial and error, allowing individuals to gain insight from their mistakes. However, learning nursing skills, especially technical skills, directly from patients for the first time can pose significant risks to patient health.

Definition

A return demonstration (education) is an educational technique in which someone demonstrates what has been taught or shown.
- It helps reduce student anxiety when providing care, improve communication and relationship-building skills, increase dexterity when handling care equipment, and emphasize thinking and decision-making skills.
- Learners see rebuttals as tests to assess their performance, so validation may be required to reduce anxiety.

- Because the procedure is unfamiliar or new, learners need more time to practice the procedure thoroughly and reduce errors along the way.

SYMPOSIUM

A symposium is a type of socialized technology in which each participant is expected to present well-founded arguments or views on the issues under discussion. The perspectives can be presented by speakers or by reading papers. The facts and feel of each presentation will vary depending on the speaker and situation. This makes the format of the symposium constant, but flexible in method.

Meaning

Symposium is the Greek word for "drinking". Symposia were very common in Athens. Their joy was enhanced by pleasant conversations at the introduction of music and dance, and sometimes philosophical topics were discussed with them.

Derivation of word: Syn—together and posis—drinking.
- A drinking party with intelligent conversation.
- A conference or social gathering where ideas are freely exchanged.
- Conferences or meetings to discuss specific academic topics.

Definition

A symposium is a method of group discussion in which two or more people, led by a chairperson, give individual speeches addressing multiple aspects of an issue.

> **Characteristics of symposium technique**
> - It provides the broad understanding of a topic or a problem
> - The opportunity is provided to the listeners to take decision about the problem
> - It is used for higher classes to specific themes and problems
> - It develops the feeling of cooperation and adjustment
> - The objectives as synthesis and evaluation are achieved by employing the symposium technique
> - It provides the different views on the topic of the symposium.

Aim and Objectives
- Clarification of thoughts on controversial issues.
- Look at the problem from multiple angles.
- Acquire more knowledge, intellectual abilities and skills.
- Increase interest in the topic.
- Change attitudes and values toward common goals.
- For better personal and social adjustment.
- To get good cooperation.

Principles

- The Chairman should introduce the topic and lead the session.
- Discussions between symposium members are prohibited.
- The Chairman is responsible for the topics distributed to the speakers and allows sufficient time to present specific topics.
- The speaker presents the topic through a speech or presentation.
- The Chairman should start the symposium with a brief introduction of the topic and speakers.
- Finally, the Chairman is responsible for summarizing the topic.
- Clarify questions at the end of the discussion.

Members Who Attended the Symposium

- Chairman
- Chair speaker
- Audience.

Role of Chairman

- Topic selection
- Topic distribution.
- Guide the speaker towards goal.
- Group control.
- Summarize and draw conclusion.

CHAIRMAN QUALITIES

- Responsible for program planning and coordination
- A good guide
- Researcher
- Resource contact
- Representative of professional nursing organization.

Role of Speaker

- Topic preparation
- Topic presentation.

Role of Audience

- Listening the speach
- New question and final question clarification.

Uses

- Political rallies
- Professional conventions
- Association meetings
- Cooperative group
- Conference.

Technique

- Success is highly dependent on the personnel involved and the level of preparation.
- Experts with experience in different fields can provide more information.
- Good planning and organization.
- All members should know their goals.
- Teachers should confer with student representatives on the presentation of the topic before avoiding duplication.

Merits

- The symposium format generally provides a broader basis for discussion than the lecture format.
- More organized than other discussions.
- The advantages of professionally organizing political meetings are great.
- Stakeholders have different roles to avoid conflicts and misunderstandings between them.
- Audiences can gain a wide range of knowledge from different exposures.
- A disciplined method of teaching and learning.

Demerits

- No discussion among members of the symposium.
- The agenda is designated by the chair.
- Inadequate opportunities for active participation by all students.
- Speakers are limited to 15-20 minutes, so each one is severely handicapped in developing their topic.
- Defective program example.

PANEL DISCUSSION

A panel discussion is a discussion in which 4-8 qualified persons are seated to discuss a topic in front of a large group or audience. A panel discussion consists of a chairperson (moderator) and 4-8 speakers. The success or failure of a panel discussion depends on the moderator.

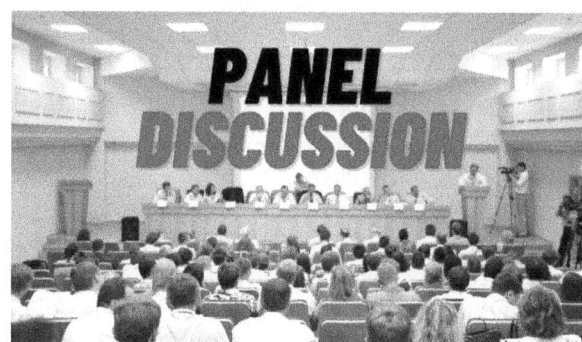

Fig. 7.20: Panel discussion members on stage.

Concept

- Panels are composed of a small number of members who are willing to exchange ideas and opinions on a particular topic under the guidance of a chairman. When used as a teaching method, a panel may be a group of "experts" in the field, or a select group of students who have requested and prepared objects in advance.
- The chairman initiates the discussion by introducing the members, announcing the topic, and mostly setting the boundaries of the discussion. After inviting the first speaker, the chairman remains seated.
- Discussions are conversational and moderators ensure everyone is on the same page. If necessary, the moderator can clear up questions or misunderstandings, or offer alternative thoughts to ensure the topic is fully covered.
- Panel discussions should provide a natural environment for the audience to ask questions, evaluate responses, and provide constructive input.
- The discussion may or may not be published. In this case, the chairman should continue to lead and summarize the discussion at the end by summarizing the main points.

Technique

- The chairman and 4-8 speakers are seated in front of a large audience.
- The chairman begins the session, welcomes the group, and introduces speakers.
- The chairman briefly introduces the topic, after which the panel invites the speakers to present their views.
- Panel discussions do not have a specific agenda, speaking order, or set of speeches. The chairman may interact with any of the speakers in the form of questions or brief statements on specific topics without the need for an order form, the chairman invites the audience to participate in the discussion and initiates the discussion.

Privilege

- If properly planned, it is a very effective method of parenting.
- Information reaches many people.
- Panel discussion spontaneity stimulates audience interest in participating in the discussion at the end of the panel discussion.
- The experts can have different opinions.
- It causes better discussion.
- Changing speakers frequently can help prevent distraction.
- It can produce better discussions than alone.
- Frequent speaker rotation prevents delayed attention.

Shortcomings

- Experts may not be good speakers.
- Personality may obscure content.
- Topics may not be in logical order.

SEMINAR

The word comes from the Latin seminarium, which means "seed." This teaching method is based on the teaching method of Socrates and the Greek work "paideia" which means the general knowledge or learning of values that every person needs. A seminary is a form of academic instruction generally offered either at a university or offered by a commercial or professional organization. It has the ability to bring small groups together for regular meetings focused on specific topics where all attendees are expected to actively participate. It is often achieved through ongoing Socratic dialogues, or through more formal presentations of research.

Definition

- A seminary is a group of members who come together to share current issues and to share their experiences, experiments, discoveries, etc., with others.
- Seminars are an advanced type of socialized technique. Each individual in the seminar group participates in conducting their own research or participates in larger projects.

Aims

- To give students the opportunity to deal with methods of scientific analysis and research processes.
- Promoting a greater understanding of desirable interpersonal attitudes, interests and development - desirable group processes.
- To help students develop the skills to read and understand oral scientific texts.
- Students can gain experience in self-evaluation and evaluation by others.
- Provide students with additional information, insights, and other approaches to solving problems.

Objectives

- To help participants learn the content.
- Background knowledge and skills in librarianship is required.
- Helps with problem solving skills.
- Help students engage in methods of scientific analysis and research processes.
- Promote student responsibility.
- Help students change attitudes and values.

Seminar Field

Seminar format makes sense in:
- Teaching professional development.
- Management skills.
- Ethical and legal issues.

General Instructions

- To develop an understanding of the ideas presented by the current work.
- Do not talk only to the teacher.
- Actively participate in your own learning.
- Think deeply about the issue in a clear and concise way.
- Speak more clearly.
- Listen to others.
- Listen carefully.
- Read carefully.
- Learn to justify/qualify opinions.
- Explore the extensive literature on this topic.

Seminar Elements

- Groups should be heterogeneous.
- Significant physical layout.
- We need a safe environment for free discussion.
- It must be surrounded by deep questions.
- Discussion of the profound works of human endeavor.
- Leaders are not active in discussions. He does not have his own opinion.
- The question level is high. More analysis, synthesis and evaluation. Less correct/incorrect answers.
- Arguments are always tied to argument work.
- Improves student motivation.
- Rarely used as a teaching tool.
- Seminar procedure/evaluation by participants.
- A solid learning experience for all involved.

Procedures for Conducting a Seminar

- Create a safe environment.
- Guide student expectations.
- Choose carefully. Assign it to a class.
- Carefully read and examine your selections and make notes if necessary.
- Prepare opening and closing questions.
- Prepare the room physically by arranging the chairs/tables in a circle.
- Start the seminar.
- Next, work on and evaluate the seminar as a class.
- Personally think about tweaking the experience for future use.

The seminar method		
Uses	Advantages	Dis-advantages
• To provide general guidance for a group working on an advanced study or research project • To exchange information on techniques and approaches being explored by members of a study or research group • To develop new and imaginative solutions to problems under study by the group	• Provides motivation and report. • Stimulates active participation. • Permits adaptive instruction.	• Requires highly competent instructor • Poses evaluation problems. • More costly than instruction, most other methods.

Fig. 7.21: Merits and de-merits of seminar method.

Seminar Paper Guide

- Seminar papers are short informal presentations on proposed topics and include an extensive literature review.
- Do not think of the presentation as a test. The act of investigating sources digesting information and summarizing other people's work will help to clarify these matters in your mind.
- Develop confidence in handling information making useful notes and presenting an argument.
- Topics can be chosen according to your interests or with the help of a tutor.
    - Read the set text from the course using critical theory.
    - Explanation of key theory and how to apply it to some fixed texts.
    - Response to one of the tutorial topics in the course materials.
    - Presentation of the history of the publication or critical reception of one of the texts set to music.
- A seminar presentation should not try to imitate an essay. Rather than asking general questions in your term paper, it is better to provide a smaller, more specific presentation.
- Do not write down the presentation verbatim. Create overview notes and use established texts of critical theory and your own extended notes as backup material to talk about those notes.
- If you have resources, provide copies of your outline notes to other members of the group.

- Overhead projection facilities are often available. Otherwise, a copy of the explanatory material is perfectly acceptable.

Seminar Benefits
- Seminars help students develop a sense of responsibility.
- Provide opportunities to participate in scientific analytical methods and research procedures.
- It helps to study the subject thoroughly.
- It helps to develop leadership skills.
- Effective problem solving.
- It helps to improve the curriculum through the profession.

Seminar Cons
- Only suitable for high school students as library work requires advanced skills.
- Advance planning is required.
- Members must bring presentation and discussion materials.
- Holding a seminar requires proper planning.

Member Roles in the Seminar
Students
- Expected to work in the library
- Collect relevant content
- Content should be clear and well-stated
- Use AV tools
- Should be well prepared before presentation.

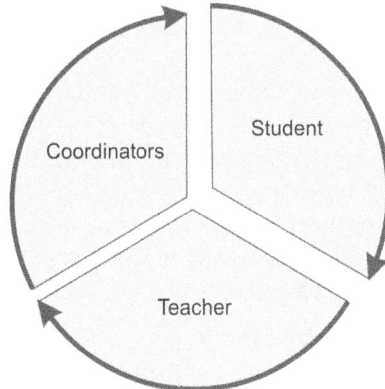

Fig. 7.22: Members involved in seminar.

Teachers
- Help the students to choose appropriate topics
- Guide the students to select content
- Suggest available sources of information.

Coordinator
- Selected issues are resolved, analyzed, critically evaluated and closed by the coordinator.
- The coordinator should hold the seminar.

WORKSHOP
A workshop is a meeting with a group of individuals in which various experts and consultants find solutions to problems that arise during a specific period of work. A key feature of the workshop is the full active participation of each participant. The overall focus of participation is working and learning from handson experience. One of the most common methods used in workshops is group discussion of selected issues. Group sizes are small enough to allow each member to participate fully and large enough for each member to benefit from each other's experiences.

Definition
- A workshop is a large group of people belonging to a particular or related field who meet to address a particular issue or problem and to develop recommendations for future action.
- The workshop is an initiation where people work together in small groups to find appropriate solutions to problems related to their field of activity.
- Workshop is the name of a noble educational experiment. Usually he consists of a series of four or more meetings, with the emphasis on individual work within the group, assisted by advisors and resource staff.
- A workshop is a meeting where experienced managers work together with experts and consultants to solve problems that arise during work or that are difficult to solve on their own.
- The workshop is an active participation of each participant. The cobblestone point of attendance is working and learning from hands-on experience.
- A workshop is a meeting where a group discusses and takes action on a specific topic or project.

Goals
- It helps to improve the knowledge.
- It improves the opportunities of learning.
- These techniques are used to encourage participation.
- Support those with prior knowledge of the subject, especially in departments, institutions and communities.
- This will help in the further development of policy programs and methods.
- More interaction and discussion among participants.

- It helps the participants to express themselves freely and exchange ideas.
- Problem solving is a collective thought process.
- Introduce participants to a systematic approach to educational issues.
- Stimulate specific suggestions from participants who want to achieve set goals, at least educationally.

Principles

- Workshops that allow participants to prepare and select goals to achieve are motivating.
- Workshops give participants an active role in making lessons more effective.
- Giving participants the opportunity to review their progress on a regular basis increases the speed of learning and improves the quality of knowledge and skills required.

How the Workshop Works?

- Free choice of personal goals: Choose the goals you want to achieve before the workshop ends, in order to ensure that the workshop fully meets your educational needs. You will be prompted to:
- Reading preparation tasks (based on practical exercises).
- Briefing.
- Hands-on exercises.
- Group presentation.
- Next business day preview.
- Individual Advice.
- Formative evaluation (prestudy evaluation, day evaluation, questionnaire, and long-term evaluation).

Benefits

- Training programs help to achieve educational goals.
- It improves learning activities.

Cons

- Time consuming.
- It must be monitored at all times.
- We need workers and enough materials.
- Mainly learning activities.

Evaluation and Workshops

As with all workshops, the evaluation process is very important. In addition, to evaluating how the objectives were achieved, decisions must also be made as to whether it makes sense to repeat various aspects with or without modifications.

EXHIBITION

Exhibitions are common place in our environment today. When walking through an exhibition, attention is often drawn to groups of objects or materials on display according to a conscious plan. Exhibitions held at schools usually convey something of value to the public and parents of students.

Property

- You should have a central theme with many sub-themes to focus on.
- Must be clean and clearly labeled.
- Color concept and size should be used for exhibition design.
- Please set-up the exhibition hall in a bright place.
- Exhibits must be displayed in a clearly visible location.
- To enable blended learning, we need to be able to relate different disciplines.

Purpose

- The purpose of the exhibition is to acquire the knowledge of students and make learning an adventure.
- Cultivate the imagination of students and train them to focus on facts and figures in a way that captures the attention of the audience.
- Articulate ideas clearly and effectively.
- Promote team spirit among students.
- Promote understanding.
- Outlined the actions taken and emphasized their importance.
- Influencing people to adopt better practices by inspiring them to think and act.
- Inform the public of a better standard by providing facts.
- Encouraging participation in and funding of public causes and activities.
- Give recognition to individuals or organizations by allowing them to display their products.
- Create a market for a particular product

The value of an exhibition is:

- Voluntary activities of exhibition participants are encouraged.
- Students are well aware of the results of various activities and processes.
- Team spirit is encouraged as running an exhibition is a community effort.
- Parents and visitors can get ideas for student work and facilitate contact between parents and the school.

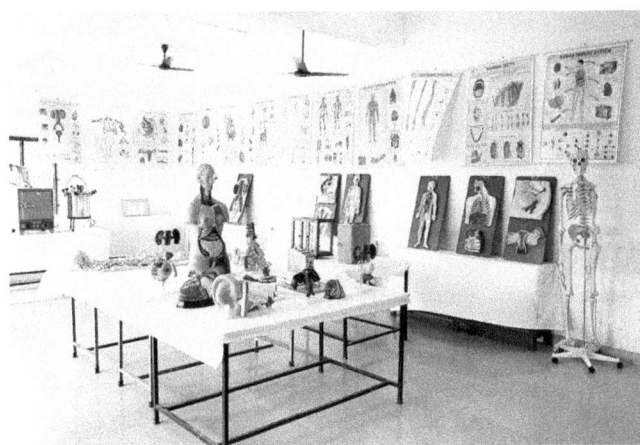

Fig. 7.23: Exibits in nursing.

Placement of Exhibits

- Popular difficult exhibits should be mixed with easy exhibits.
- Avoid packing too many exhibits into one room.
- Store the exhibits in a bright place.
- Dynamic and static exhibits should be mixed to avoid crowding.
- It is better to put one single idea in an exhibit.
- Colorful and moving exhibits will attract the attention of the people.
- Entire campus should be clean and should present a festive appearance.
- Student committees can be organized for various activities.
- There should be enough space for visitors to move around and for volunteers to stand and explain.

Exhibition Planning

Please note the following points when planning an exhibition.
- Use only one main idea for the exhibition.
- Place the exhibit where it can be seen.
- Look at the exhibits rather than read them.
- Keep labels short and simple.
- Labels should be consistent and legible.
- Movement attracts attention.

Benefits

- Creates a competitive spirit.
- Make learning activities more meaningful.
- Give concreteness to abstract ideas.
- Have a sensitive learning situation.
- Useful for international understanding.
- Reduced vocabulary.
- Great for teaching illiterate people.

Disadvantages

- Requires a lot of preparation and investment.
- Not suitable for all subjects and should not be used frequently or extensively
- The whole process is expensive.
- Many exhibits are routinely arranged without a specific educational purpose.

ROLE PLAY

Role play is a way for learners to participate in dramatizations without rehearsal. They are asked to play the character's assigned role because they think the character will actually act. This method is a technique that arouses the learner's emotions and evokes an emotional response. It is primarily used to achieve behavioral goals in the emotional realm.

Definition

- A role play is a spontaneous act out of a well-defined situation by two or more of her people, which is then discussed with the whole class. This is usually a teaching method that arouses the interest of the students and allows the teacher to assess the students' understanding, concepts are offered for discussion at the end and used to practice real-life situations.
- Role-playing is the technique of putting students in situations that the teacher wants to teach them.
- Role plays are based on specific themes and are performed in front of an audience to convey a message to the audience.
- Role-playing is a dramatization along with verbalization.
- Role-playing is relatively new educational techniques in which people spontaneously act out problems of human relations and analyze the enactment with the help of other role players and observes.

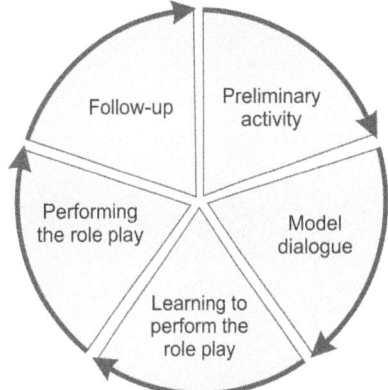

Fig. 7.24: Steps in role play.

Purposes of Role Play

- To develop communication skills for successful interpretation.
- Everyone working together towards a common goal.
- Try new behaviors in front of your peers.
- Experience the situation emotionally and develop insight into the problem.
- Develop new skills to deal with problems.
- Encourages thinking and creativity.
- Helps participants immerse themselves in the letters and understand their meaning.
- Creates the motivation and engagement necessary for learning.

Role-playing Game Features

- Role-playing should have clear goals.
- You need to analyze your needs in exciting real-life situations.
- Must promote independent thinking.
- An actor cannot project his life onto a character.
- Active audience participation should be encouraged.

Role-playing Steps

According to Richards (1985), the following are the role-playing steps:

- **Preliminary exercise:** The role play begins with a question. This is recognized by learners or teachers. Role play focuses on the needs and interests of the group. The group is somehow involved in the development of the background situation. The situation should increase the group's insight and deepen their ability to see the situation. Preparatory activities therefore include situation selection and participant selection. It is best to ask for volunteers unless you have a specific reason for being assigned a specific role. After the actors are selected, they are briefed on their roles and the group conducts a warmup session. This will prepare you for critical observation and analysis of the situation.

Role-play		
Uses	Advantages	Disadvantages
• Exploring and improving interviewing techniques and examining complexities and potential conflicts of groups • To consolidate different lessons in one setting	• Good energizers • Promotes empathy of trainees for other situation • Encourages creativity in learning	• Participants might be reluctant • May not work with trainees who do not know each other well

Fig. 7.25: Advantages and disadvantages of role-play.

- **Conversation examples:** It should be simple and clear so that the audience can understand the role play concept. Dialogue is also maintained so that no one in the audience is harmed.

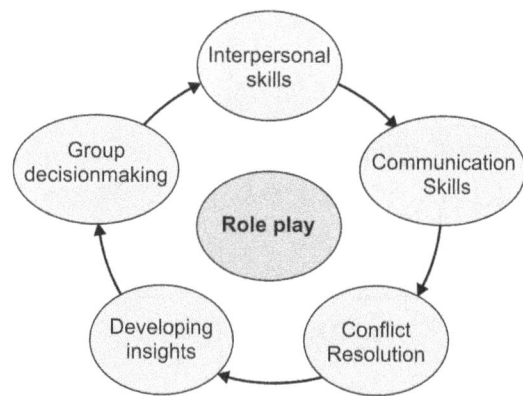

Fig. 7.26: Skills needed for role play.

- **Learning to perform the role play:** After the roles have been decided the participants are given written descriptions about their roles and setting. The scenes are described and discussed with them briefly. The actor should understand who he is and he should be given some time to think so that he can add some of his views.
- **Performing the role play:** The role play is performed under a director. The director introduces the scenes and the roles of the people involved. When introducing roleplay in groups, it's best to keep the problem and situation as simple as possible, involving familiar, nonthreatening situations. All members of the group should understand what is going on and be supported to actively participate. The members of the group play their respective roles and the audience actively participates in the drama. You have to pay attention to what is going on. Scenes should be brief. Elaborate dialogue and irrelevant material are avoided. Scenes are cut when they serve their purpose.
- **Follow-up:** After the role-play actions are completed, both the participants and the audience can discuss the actions. This gives them a chance to explore their own feelings and eliminates the possibility of feeling threatened if observed by the group. After the discussion, develop a plan to summarize and evaluate the lessons learned and provide a way to implement the implicit behavior.

Factors Affecting Role Play

- **Level:** Indicates the minimum level at which the activity can be performed.
- **Time:** Depends on whether students need to read articles, reports, etc.
- **Goals:** Goals show the broader goals of each activity.

- **Language:** Language indicates the language required by the student.
- **Organization:** Explain whether the activity is pair work or group work, and if group work, how many students are needed in each group.
- **Preparation:** View everything you need to do before class.
- **Warm-up:** Contains ideas to grab students' attention and intrigue them.
- **Procedure:** Activities are executed accordingly.
- **Follow-up:** Includes activities that are conducted after the roleplay is completed.

Benefits of Role-playing in Nursing
- Helps develop leadership skills and social interaction.
- Help solve the problem.
- Develops to perceive, observe and analyze situations.
- Practice your chosen behavior in a real situation.
- Helps identify critical issues.
- Promotes independent thinking and action.
- Helps nurses observe, understand, and resolve patient problems.

Roleplaying Cons
- It takes time.
- Requires careful planning, preparation and rehearsal.
- Learners may find it difficult to play their part.
- Group members may be too shy to participate.
- Role-playing games should not be used under time pressure.

Effective Role Play Guidelines
- Teachers should carefully plan roleplays. They must also be willing to monitor student behavior and reactions and make changes as needed.
- Including situations with conflicting emotions can create good scenarios.
- Her three levels of role play:
  1. *Briefing:* Set the stage and explain your goals. This is usually the shortest phase.
  2. *Run:* Complete the role play. It takes 5–20 minutes.
  3. *Debriefing:* Analysis of conversations and evaluation of roleplay experienceThis may take 30–40 minutes or more.
- The debriefing stage becomes more important when students are provided with a platform to clarify decisions.
- Video or audio recordings of role plays may supplement the debriefing phase. This method works best for small groups of students where every student participating in the role play can be an active observer.
- Students should be encouraged to react naturally to role plays and not to make mistakes.
- Criticism should be focused on the behavior demonstrated in the role play rather than directed at specific students.

The value of role plays for teachers:
Role plays help teachers in teaching and learning situations.
- Write down individual student needs in simulated real-world situations.
- Help students meet their needs by suggesting places. She can encourage a group of her peers to make her suggestions.
- Encourage spontaneous thought and action by staying behind the scenes and having students perform.

PROJECT LAW

Projects and project law apply to almost all teaching methods, old and new, and it is almost impossible to derive meanings for terms that are truly different. The term project in education was an application to objective forms of education developed by agricultural boys and girls clubs and vocational courses established in secondary schools. The essential elements of the project used here were personal activity and achievement of concrete results.

Definition
- **Stevenson (1922):** "A project is a problematic act carried out in its most natural setting."
- **Ballard HG:** "It is a part of real life that has been taken in."

Project Fundamentals
The learning activity should be:
- Inherently problematic.
- Focuses on specific achievability.
- You are intentional, natural and lively in your approach to achieving your goals.
- Directed and planned by students.
- Practical in nature with emphasis on a single complete unit of purposeful activity resulting in concrete achievement.

Criteria for Selecting a Project
Each potential project should be carefully considered considering the following questions.
- Is there a particular educational value? Is it worth it?
- Is it challenging and requires reasonable effort?
- Does it meet the student's needs and abilities?
- Will the cost and availability of materials and the time required for implementation related to educational value be derived?
- Is it feasible and practical?
- Did the students choose?

- Can you complete it by the end of the semester/year/semester?
- Are there targeted actions and clear goals?

Principles

The project method is based on certain principles.
- **Purpose principle:** Every activity has a purpose, and when doing a project, you should ask "why should I do it". "What is the purpose"? Then you can achieve your goal of creating projects that lead to learning.

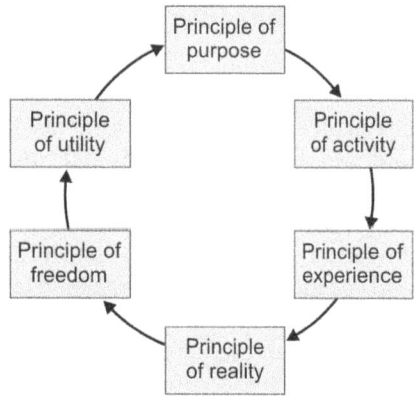

Fig. 7.27: Project law.

- **Activity principle:** "Learning by doing" ensures long-term learning. Children actively participate in physical and mental activities.

- **Experiential principle:** The project approach provides opportunities for learning through experiential group activities when systematically supporting the development of social skills such as: Communication among students, team spirit and good habits. By doing projects, children gain experiences that are also useful for self-study.
- **The reality principle:** The project methodology allows you to deal with real-life situations. This is like transferring classroom learning to a real-life situation.
- **Principle of freedom:** The project approach provides opportunities for children to be creative according to their interests, abilities and talents. Children can choose their favorite projects.
- **Utility principle:** Project law uses the utility principle to encourage children to work on a variety of projects that make a difference in their lives.

Project Method Features

The distinguishing features of this project method are:
- The purpose of this method is to teach children to enjoy life to the fullest by living in the here and now, not in the future or when they grow up, trust and supreme master, also one of the teachings we never aim for.
- The purpose of the project method is to bring out the children and give them opportunities to develop themselves.
- There are opportunities for self-expression.
- Project-based experimentation aims to reorganize the entire curriculum so that selected activities are core and knowledge acquired is incidental.
- The project method aims not only at the abstract solution of the problem, but at the whole set of activities belonging to the complete project. It's just a question. A situation that actually completes the associated activity, rather than just needing to be resolved. The underlying idea of this method was that children develop their knowledge by testing theories on practical solutions to problems, while learning to understand the principles involved. , should only be obtained based on the perceived needs of the student.
- Project or goal-oriented activities can be of any nature, annual and/or athletic. It can take the form of the preparation and performance of a play. The project methodology cannot be limited to "doing" type experiences. Because this goes against good pedagogy and sound psychology. "Projects can be excellent units of appreciation learning and attitude development as well as improving motor skills and technical knowledge.
- Making activities the only means of education inevitably permeates both the timetable and the regular classroom organization with which we are accustomed. For

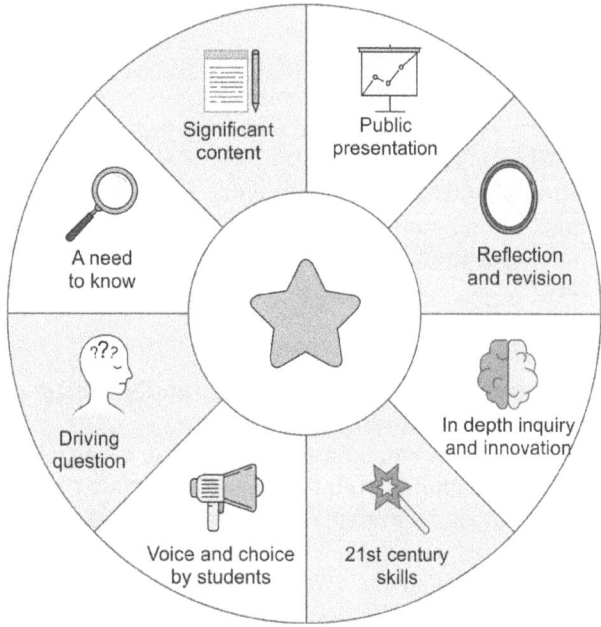

Fig. 7.28: Elements of project based learning.

example, in the preparation of a theatrical performance, the students have their roles, the actors learn and rehearse the roles, the young electrician and some painters prepare the effects, and the seamstresses make the costumes.
- Projects are play activities and the children involved in carrying out the projects can make many seemingly difficult and monotonous mistakes. There is a stark contrast between the boy building the bricks for the room and the workman doing exactly what he does. One plays and the other he works.
- The project method is a total dedication to the child's point-of-view. It seeks to provide students with complete freedom in choosing the problem to solve and the means to use to solve it. The basic principle is the educational use of the profession, designed according to general school requirements. As a result, student activity is centered on a series of impromptu projects rather than the more traditional nature of externally imposed assignments.
- In the project approach, the school's approach is determined by the workshop approach.
- Try to have a positive relationship with life. For Kilpatrick, a project is a heartfelt and purposeful act in a social setting.

Project Type

The project is classified as:
- **Individual projects:** Projects planned for each student.
- **Group project:** A class project.
- Projects are categorized by purpose and use.
- **Learning projects:** Projects such as lifting a fracture bed or CPR.
- **Projects that present solutions to patient problems:** These types of projects are aimed at intellectual development and emphasize the student's creative thinking.

Project Implementation Steps

Here are the steps in the project method:
- **Provide a situation:** Your school may have some situations that you can use as a project. Ask students to suggest a project they would like to work on. Have a general brainstorming session where the teacher can also come up with some ideas (although the teacher will never force the student to choose a project). It should be left to students to decide in which field they want to work.
- **Theme selection and goal development:** Specific topics should be selected from a wide range of work. After choosing a specific topic, you need to elaborate on the purpose of the project. Goals should be very specific.
- **Planning:** Teachers should motivate students to plan specific details of the project in terms of time, budget, acquisition and maintenance of items, etc. Ignoring planning details can lead to project failure. Plans should be discussed between teachers and students. A good plan with all necessary details is crucial to the success of your project.
- **Execution:** Project execution requires teamwork. For group projects, each participating student is assigned a specific task. If a student finds a problem while completing a project, the teacher should handle it and help the student solve it.
- **Evaluation:** When evaluating a project, both its purpose and plans should be considered. Evaluate whether the implementation went according to plan, whether there were any errors, and how to fix them. The exchange of experiences between students is very useful.
- **Records:** Students are required to keep records of all project-related activities. A project report should be prepared for future reference, detailing topic evaluation results, objectives, plan execution, and learning experiences.

Advantages

- Engage students.
- Allow students to think and act freely while working.
- Provide creative and constructive thinking.
- Helps the students think logically and be scientific before starting a project.
- Teaches the students to grade their completed work.
- Develops team spirit and collaboration among students.

Disadvantages

- It takes time.
- Sometimes students have the wrong idea about their semester projects.
- The cost of the project is too high due to material costs. Also, the materials to prepare the project may not be available.

EXCURSION/FIELDTRIP

According to Tagore's philosophy of education, a teacher is a person who is responsible for providing an environment in which students can engage in useful and constructive activities through their experiences and it is possible through excursions. Teachers cannot teach effectively in the classroom alone, but they can do so effectively if they do not ignore the experience of the outside world and its impact on students outside the classroom.

Definition

- A field trip is defined as an educational process in which students directly study objects and materials in their natural environment.
- Excursion is defined as the most specific and truly the best visual technique that puts students in direct contact with real life situations. **—Bhatia**
- An excursion constitutes a concrete learning experience in a real-life situation carried out with a specific purpose.
- An excursion can be defined as a combination of theory and practical experience.
- Excursions are basically visits to advanced model house demonstration plots for poultry farmers.

Objectives

- Put theory into practice.
- Evaluate the performance of new practices.
- Enrich your classes.
- Develop observation skills.
- Improve social interaction among the students.
- Assessment of students in domains such as cognition, psychomotor.
- Refresh students' knowledge.
- Get basic data.
- Develop student creativity.
- Get primary observations.
- Watch practice.
- Watch student performance.

Purpose

- To help provide initial, specific information to supplement and enrich face-to-face teaching.
- Direct contact with community conditions helps to relate and blend school life without subworlds.
- Helps better understand the economics of housing hygiene, etiology and disease factors.
- Develops keenness and observation.
- Excursions provide the most up-to-date source material for the course.
- Excursions provide active instruction that helps generate interest and motivation.
- Excursions provide an opportunity to solve problems that arise from individuals and groups in natural settings.
- Excursions help effectively connect educational content.
- Excursions help develop leadership skills.
- Excursions help develop the aesthetic sense of the students.

Types

- **Local school excursion:** This type includes a halfday visit to some of the school buildings and grounds to see procedures, equipment, and materials, e.g., measure distances, inspect trees, shrubs and flowers, and practice health and safety procedures.
- **Community excursions:** This type of excursion forms a fullday visit to nearby locations such as zoo museums, hospitals, etc.
- **Interschool or intercollegiate visits:** Medical students go to art colleges to exchange ideas and consult books for knowledge. A group of music or science students who meet with peer organizations from different schools to gain knowledge related to common interests.
- **Individual journeys:** This type of journey helps students take responsibility for tasks related to curriculum activities. For example, the trip is famous for collecting biological specimens and fossils for the study of natural sciences and anthropology.

Excursion Organization

Successful excursions depend on efficient planning.

- Determine the specific purpose of the field trip. Students and teachers should be clear about the goals and objectives of the excursion.
- Determine appropriate locations to visit and gather information about the locations to visit from various sources.
- Required travel authorization from relevant authorities.
- We need to ensure affordability.
- Organizing Committee Students should be formed to organize the trip.
- Teachers should act as guides and impart knowledge gained in school and on excursions.
- Evaluation of excursions after returning from trips.

Procedures for Organizing Field Trips

- **Knowledge:** Conduct research to obtain accurate information about visits that offer potential educational experiences to nursing students and analyze the educational value of field trips.
- **Relationship:** Develop and maintain amicable relations with the authorities in charge of the facility (or location) to be visited, and notify the relevant authorities in advance to avoid wasting time, energy, and materials.
- **Purpose:** Both students and teachers should be aware of the purpose of the field trip. It is the teacher's responsibility to ensure that students understand the purpose of the field trip in order to facilitate learning activities.
- **Time and transportation:** Necessary agreements will be made regarding meeting times, visit times, transportation, and costs.
- **Student preparation:** Student should be aware of the purpose of the trip and direct the student to write down specific point.

- **Supervision:** Excursions must be carefully supervised to protect students.
  - Do not get in or out of a moving vehicle.
  - Do not stick your hands or head out of a moving vehicle.
  - Cross the street at the green pedestrian crossing.
  - Be aware of potential hazards while traveling.
  - Always stay with group and never go alone. Please inform the group leader when going out in free time.
  - Students are responsible for their own health and safety during field trips.
- **Evaluation:** After the excursion, there will be a public discussion and students will be asked to submit their student papers. Student questions are clarified by the student's educational experience, and information gained through field trips is clearly related and integrated with subject activity.
  - Field trips will be documented for future reference. Any necessary changes for future excursions will be discussed through evaluation.
  - The excursion can only be evaluated through a group discussion, quiz program conducted by the teacher.
  - Knowledge gained from field trips can be drawn through flowcharts and photographs in the institution's magazine for future reference. After evaluation, the teacher concluded that the students had acquired accurate knowledge of what was observed through the meaningful excursion.

Responsibilities of Teacher

- Check attendance of all the students and ensure that no one is absent.
- Appropriate information for exiting the vehicle must be provided to the student.
- Review group member accounts and submit accounts.
- Guidance and supervision of students during travel.
- Safety rules that must be adhered to while traveling.
- Teachers should promote uniform discipline within the group.
- Carry a first aid kit and keep it in the vehicle while driving.
- Accuracy, clarity, and conciseness related to the learning experience on the excursion must be met by the teacher.

Responsibilities of Student

- Each student is responsible for knowing the location of the visitor vehicle used during travel time and where to drop off.
- Students must arrive on time and follow the teacher's orders and instructions.
- Students are required to wear appropriate attire for the location of their visit.
- A student should not cheat and be considerate to others and professional conduct is expected from all the students.
- Questions should be structured by the student in an appropriate manner and ready when the opportunity arises.
- All bags of the students should be labeled and should be ready for departure.
- Each student must record expenses and record the charges for the vehicle used for the trip.
- Each student should take notes whenever directed.

Benefits

- Observation of active participation in reality.
- Opportunities for collaborative group work and task sharing.
- Build self-confidence in students.
- Compare reality with theory.
- Develop qualities of observation and decision-making.
- Ensure close contacts with reality.
- It increases the variability.
- Evaluate the achievement of educational goals.
- A good way to motivate individuals.
- This is the most concrete and realistic visual technique that helps students give real meaning to their compact tendencies towards abstraction and simulate correct thinking.
- Free yourself from the monotony of daily classes.

Limitations

- Time and travel costs apply.
- Excursions are for a limited audience only.
- Effectiveness requires careful planning.
- Prior knowledge of the location should be made known to the teacher. Otherwise, they will not be able to answer the student's questions.
- A group discussion should follow the field trip, if full study is not possible.
- Finding the right location can be difficult.
- Scheduling is difficult.

Excursions and Nursing Education

- Facilitate the revitalization and enrichment of implementation of content areas in nursing education.
- As a nursing education field trip, students will visit clinics and visit various treatment units.
- Nursing students gain firsthand knowledge of the first aid activities of community agency health camps and

other functions associated with hospitals to assist these patients.
- It helps the nursing students to observe real thing and it helps them in active learning.

Following examples of field trip where nursing students can observe various situations:
- Rehabilitation centers.
- Water purification centers.
- Nursing home.
- Schools for children with disabilities such as deaf and blind.
- Industrial care field.
- Workshop with shelter.
- Trading companies such as milk centers.
- Specialized centers such as hospitals.
- Physical therapy in an outpatient program.

SELF-DIRECTED LEARNING

Self-directed learning (SDL) is a learning style in which the student is self-directed. This includes activities such as selecting, managing and evaluating your own learning activities. Teachers provide advice, direction, and resources to support students, while peers ensure collaboration.

Meaning

Self-directed learning is defined as the ability of individuals to proactively diagnose learning needs, develop learning goals, and pursue learning, with or without the help of others. It represents the process of identifying and selecting the appropriate human and physical resources for a company. Learning strategies, and implementation and evaluation of learning outcomes.

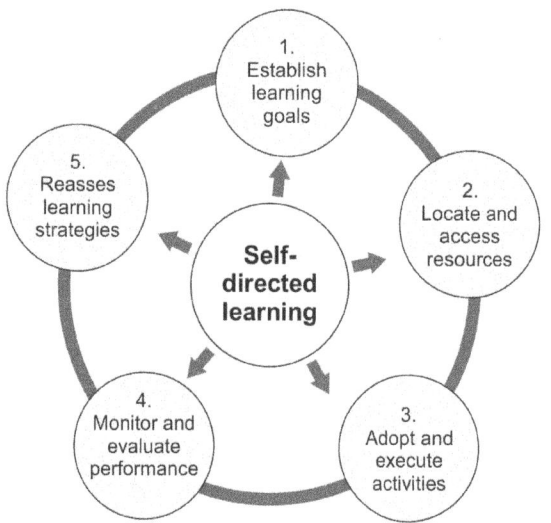

Fig. 7.29: Self-directed learning.

Goals

Merriam Caffarella and Baumgartner (2007) describe his three main goals for SDL:
1. Strengthen learners' ability to self-determine in their learning.
2. Encourage transformational learning.
3. Promote liberal learning and social activism as an integral part of SDL.

Features

Self-paced learning is an innovative departure from traditional classroom learning styles.
- **Flexibility:** SDL's most distinctive feature. Learners have the flexibility and freedom to design and build their learning. The constant development of information and communication technology has increased this flexibility.
- **Learner responsibility and autonomy:** SDL relies on learners to take responsibility for their own learning. Adult learners see learning as a tool that helps them solve real world problems and enable them to fulfill their personal and professional responsibilities and commitments. They are naturally motivated to learn and take responsibility for their learning efforts.
- **Learner empowerment:** SDL empowers learners to take responsibility for their own learning process and direct it in the direction they want. The training is developed with the learning style of adult learners in mind. That's why experiential learning and training that easily transitions from her desk to work is a key feature of her SDL.

Characteristics

According to Winne (2001), self-directed learners have the following characteristics.
- Regularly monitor progress towards goals
- Modify strategies to optimize progress towards goals
- Evaluate any obstacles and necessary adjustments.

Components

According to Zimmerman (2000), the components of self-directed (self-regulating) learning can be divided into three categories:
1. Prior thought processes and self-belief that exist before learning.
2. Achievement processes that exist at the time of the task.
3. Introspection processes that occur after task completion.

A Model of Self-directed Learning

According to Candy (1991), SDL is a comprehensive concept with the four dimensions, and also suggests that learners'

self-orientation may vary by content domain. The four proposed dimensions are:
1. Self-determination as a personal quality (personal autonomy)
2. Self-control as a willingness and ability to educate oneself (self management)
3. Self-directed instruction (learner management) as a form of educational organization in formal settings
4. Self-orientation as an individual, noninstitutional pursuit of learning opportunities in a natural social framework (autodidaxie).

Autonomous Learning Process
- SDL begins with a person taking the initiative with or without the help of others.
- SDL means a person diagnoses what they need to learn.
- SDL formulates learning goals.
- SDL identifies human and material learning resources.
- SDL selects and implements appropriate learning strategies.
- SDL assesses learning outcomes.

Student Roles
- Evaluate own learning motivation
- Define learning objectives and create a learning contract
- Monitor the learning process
- Evaluate and revise goals as needed throughout the session
- Consult with supervisor as needed.

The Role of the Supervisor
- An environment that builds collaborative learning
- Helps motivate and guide the student's learning experience
- Encourages student learning initiative

- Counseling is available as needed during the learning process
- Acts as an advisor rather than a formal instructor.

Benefits of SDL
- **Improved timing:** Cognitive flexibility theory is more effective when complex information is explained through analogies and examples from multiple perspectives.
- **Adapted to adult learning preferences:** SDL fits perfectly with the natural learning styles of adult learners who do not require supervision. This synchronicity removes resistance and motivates adult learners to seek learning.
- **Greater relevance to learner needs:** SDL enables self-paced learning according to individual needs and individual learning preferences. This makes SDL better suited to the needs of learners. Employees are also more relevant as they are motivated to learn from their experiences and apply their newly acquired knowledge to their jobs.
- **Facilitates knowledge updating:** Learners are at the forefront when they are motivated to learn and have tools and resources at their fingertips to set their own learning paths.
- **Improved professional skills learning:** Adult learners want to learn and master professional skills to keep up with the competition in the workplace. Being able to choose how they want to proceed is a great motivator. It also gives learners the opportunity to practice and master their skills by being able to schedule their learning freely without waiting for a trainer to organize a class.
- **Facilitates subject mastery:** It helps switching resources to analyze and summarize information, and building their own understanding. Mastery is better when you can learn the way you know it.

Disadvantages of Self-study
- Lack of self-discipline.
- Little personal commitment.
- Lack of variety and choice.
- No feedback from trainers
- Successful e-learning requires hard work.
- No peripheral benefits.

COMPUTER-ASSISTED LEARNING

Computer-assisted instruction (CAI), as the name suggests, describes the type of instruction that is assisted or delivered using computers as machines. This is one step further than using teaching machines, and perhaps two steps further

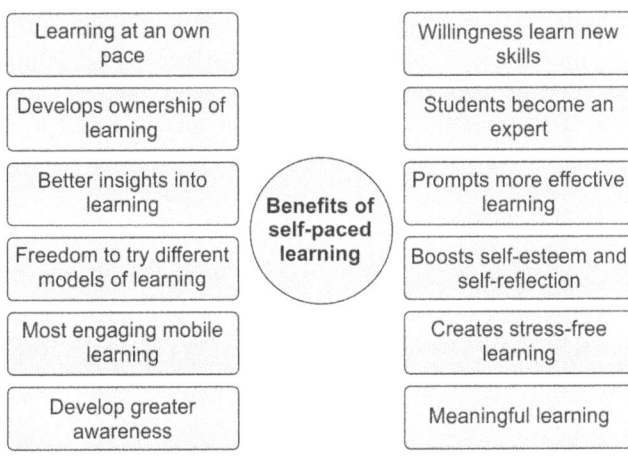

Fig. 7.30: Benefits of self-paced learning.

than using programmed textbooks to make the educational process as self-directed and individualized as possible. Computers will affect all areas of human activity, bringing about many changes in education, medicine, scientific research, social sciences, and more. Using computers in the healthcare system saves time and energy and helps nurses provide quality care.

Definition

- *Hilgard and Bower (1977)* "Computer-assisted education has now taken on so many facets that it can be seen as a simple off-shoot of the educational machine and the type of programmed learning introduced by Skinner." It is no longer possible".
- *Bhatt and Sharma (1992)* state that "CAI is the interaction between a student's computer-controlled display and responsive input devices to achieve educational outcomes."
- Individual students use and respond to the materials presented. These responses are tracked by a computer to determine the progression of future lessons presented to learners.
- The interaction between the individual learner and the computer device helps achieve set lesson goals.

Importance of Computers in Education

- The computer stores the progress cards and keeps them secret.
- Easy access to information files for reference and guidance.
- They engage students in tutor interaction and dialogue.

Types of Computer-aided Educational Programs

- **Logo:** Developed by Feurzeing and Papart, this system provides instructions that can be used to generate images with an oscilloscope or to build a small mechanical robot. Students often propose their own tasks and write corresponding programs.
- **Simulation and play:** This system allows the students to experiment in a symbolic way.
- **Controlled learning:** Controlled learning involves the use of interesting adaptive strategies. It includes both drills and practice. Drills and practice programs complement the regular curriculum followed by the classroom teachers.
    - *Basic assumptions:* The first assumption of CAI lies in its ability to provide qualitatively and quantitatively automated instruction to a sufficiently large number of individual learners simultaneously.

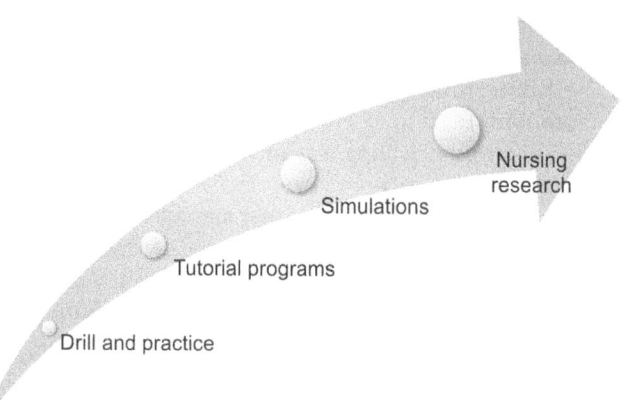

Fig. 7.31: Types of computer-aided educational programs.

- *Automatic learner performance recording:* How does an individual learner respond to presented material? What is its quarry and difficulty? What does that performance look like in terms of learning outcomes? All of these can be successfully and accurately recorded by computing devices. This greatly assists individual learners in further planning the instruction needed to make the right progress. This timely and accurate automatic recording is his second assumption underlying CAT.
- *Variety in the use of methods and techniques:* CAI does not mean that all learners will benefit from a single method, but that all subjects or subject topics can be addressed in a common method or strategy.

Using Computers in the Classroom

Computer-assisted education programs are very useful for self-paced learning. Below are some of the areas where computers have proven effective in the educational process.

- Drills and exercises:
    - The most common and easiest method
    - The learner is presented with a series of questions or problems on the material, for example, B calculation of drug dosage Calculation of infusion rate
    - Writing textbooks; collecting teaching materials
    - Building a library.
- Tutorials:
    - Show new material
    - Tutorial information
    - Feedback.
- Simulation:
    - Real life situations are presented to support learner problem-solving and decision-making in a safe environment.
    - Interactive video lessons provide learners with realistic simulations.

- Video image graphics can be incorporated into software design.
- Research:
  - Research the literature or search for related articles.
  - Data collection tools.
  - Dissemination of knowledge and results.
  - Table.
  - Preparation of research report project report.

Benefits of CAL

- Save time learning.
- Works wonders for processing performance data.
- Helps determine follow-up actions in learning situations.
- Large amounts of information stored on computers are made available to learners more quickly.
- Enables dynamic interaction between students and the curriculum.

Disadvantages of CAL

- Inadequate training of teachers and inadequacy of instructional material
- It is prohibitively expensive.
- Computers inject a non human quality into educational programmes.
- The computer does not recognize student emotions.
- The warm and emotional environment created by teacher-student interaction in the classroom is absent in CAL.
- CAT does not develop essential features of language ability CAT is a mechanical approach to teaching.

ONE-TO-ONE LESSONS

One-to-one lessons take place directly between one student and the teacher. Instead of being in groups with other students, one-on-one classes provide a distraction-free environment with more interaction.

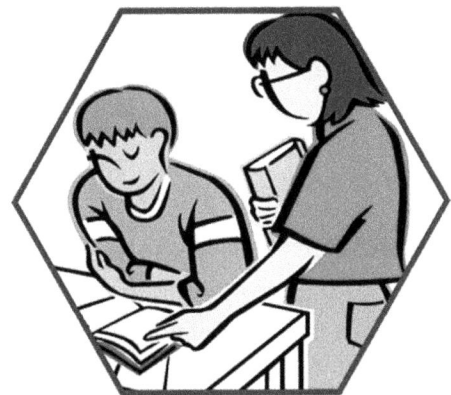

Fig. 7.32: One-to-one lessons.

Definition

A private lesson is defined as a placement with only one teacher and one student. It can also be defined as hiring a tutor to teach her one student only. This type of learning is contrary to traditional learning where a class of students is taught by one teacher.

Concept of One-on-One Instruction

- The teacher provides the student with their undivided attention.
- The student can ask an unlimited number of questions.
- Students and teachers get to know each other better (enhanced trust).
- Teachers show a genuine interest in their students, thereby improving classroom culture and class dynamics (in other words, creating a positive learning environment).
- By spending time with those who are struggling, teachers demonstrate high expectations of all student achievement (Ripple effect).
- The teacher provides advice on how to use metacognitive skills to overcome problems (e.g., a student may have no problem with mathematics, but may have problems applying mathematical processes) there might be).
- Teachers motivate students by helping them achieve small goals and publicly commenting on their achievement (and this awareness increases their self-esteem and confidence).
- Teachers provide explanations, modeling, and practical examples to meet the learning needs of students (e.g., students may have problems with only one aspect of a math problem).
- Teachers are involved in the 'one-to-one treatment loop' which is a continuous loop of diagnostic assessment treatment, formative assessment practices and feedback.

Advantages

- Students have the constant attention of the teacher so they can listen to and speak more English than they might in a group situation.
- Students can contribute to classes more and feel part of the learning process by bringing material like books songs or articles from local newspapers to class.
- Their strengths and weaknesses are addressed more consistently and fully without the competition of other students for the teacher's time.
- Become a better learner through learning training with your teacher.
- With less time pressure, you can go at your own pace and not feel pressured by other students' progress.

- Learners acquire language best through modified teacher input. This means that teachers can tailor the language to the student's level and maximize the amount and type of input from the teacher in one-on-one lessons to the student's benefit.

Disadvantages

- Many learners feel more comfortable practicing a new language and making mistakes in a dynamic group than in front of a teacher.
- Teaching can be physically and mentally demanding for both learners and teachers.
- Lessons can become boring if teachers do not come up with new approaches and learners do not respond to lessons.
- Connect with other learners to develop and support group dynamics.
- Possibly not giving the learner enough time for quiet study—important for handling the new language.
- The teacher may find it difficult to measure the learner's progress or level without the framework of a syllabus or other learners to compare with.
- The teacher may feel that they do not have the experience training or resources necessary for this kind of class and that they are only effective working with large groups.

ACTIVE LEARNING STRATEGIES

Active learning engages students in learning using activities such as reading, writing, discussion or problem-solving which promote analysis synthesis and evaluation of class content. Also provides students with informal opportunities for feedback on how well they understood the material.

Active learning creates the opportunity for deeper learning; however student resistance to this type of learning is often high. Active learning conflicts with students traditional views of teaching and learning.

Active learning refers to a broad range of teaching strategies that involve students in actively participating in learning during class time with the teacher. These strategies typically involve many students working together during a lesson, but may also involve individual work and reflection. These teaching approaches range from short, simple activities such as journal writing and pair discussions to longer activities and educational frameworks such as case studies, role plays and structured team-based learning.

Benefits of Active Learning

- The ability to process course material through reflection, writing, speaking, and problem-solving provides students with multiple learning opportunities.

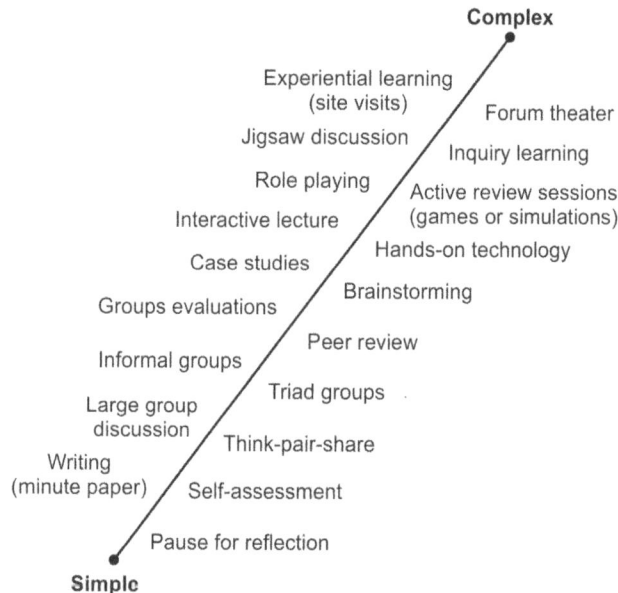

Fig. 7.33: Active learning strategies.

- Regular interaction with teachers and classmates around common activities and goals creates a sense of togetherness in the classroom. Materials help teachers focus their teaching in future lessons.

TEAM-BASED LEARNING

Team-based learning (TBL) is defined as "active learning that provides students with the opportunity to apply conceptual knowledge through a series of activities that include individual work, teamwork, immediate feedback, and small group teaching strategies".

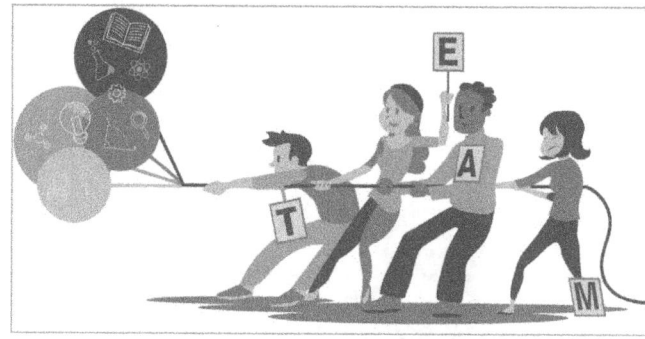

Fig. 7.34: Team-based learning (TBL).

Definition

TBL is an evidence-based collaborative learning strategy based on teaching units called "modules" taught in the three phase cycle of classroom preparation, proficiency testing, and applied exercises is classes usually contain modules.

Concept

TBL offers an innovative approach to student-centered learning and supports the flipped classroom approach to health education. TBL classroom activities offer interactive, expert-led lessons. This lesson allows many students to work in small teams and apply the content to a specific problem. This set of formats provides an opportunity to apply and build conceptual knowledge through a series of steps that include feedback on the anatomical readiness test and the application of knowledge through clinical problem-solving activities.

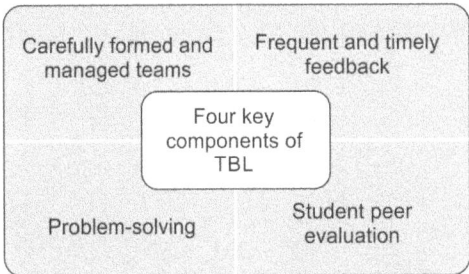

Fig. 7.35: Components of team-based learning.

- **Pillars of team-based learning:** Methodically formed and managed. Here it means that the trainer should consider her three factors:
  1. *Resources:* Each group must have adequate resources by being as diverse as possible. Indeed cultural and gender diversity can provide diverse input on how to solve problems improving both performance and learning.
  2. *Avoiding coalitions:* If two or more students are good friends in a romantic relationship or connected in some other way they might hinder the equilibrium of the group and the discussion making the others feeling at a disadvantage. Instructors should take into account these factors when creating groups to avoid tension and the forming of subgroups.
  3. *Time:* Students must remain in the same group for the entire course.
- **Responsibility:** Students must be responsible for the quality of their individual and group work. In total there are three types of accountability that an instructor should take into account when creating a TBL course.
  - *Individual preclass preparation:* Effective solutions to this problem involve clariying the class requirements assessing students' preparation (inclass quizzes, informal assessment or group activity) or including questions within the study materials
  - *Accountability towards the team:* Members must contribute to the team as equally as possible. Preparation for teamwork, class attendance and meeting attendance monitoring or positive contributions evaluation are effective ways in which students can contribute to teamwork.
  - *Accountability for quality team performance:* Accountability should be assessed. One way is to use a task that requires a team to create a product that can be compared to a product created by an expert. Another option is to use specific educational software to hold students accountable for team activities.
- **Feedback:** Getting immediate feedback makes TBL an effective practice. Especially since it not only improves learning and retention, but also has a positive impact on group development.
- **Assignment design:** Group assignments should foster both learning and team development.
  - Encourages students to have long and meaningful discussions about the product without a sense of urgency about the amount of work that needs to be done.
  - Allows the work to be divided evenly without students relying on the expertise of a single member or team who must undertake the bulk of the project.

Table 7.2: Phases or team-based learning.

Phase 1: Pre-class learning	Phase 2: Readiness assurance process	Phase 3: Application of course concepts	Phase 4: Peer evaluation
Independent student learning: Study materials provided, including instructor-set learning objectives	Individual and team multi-choice test: • Individual test answers submitted for grading • Teams take test and reach consensus by discussion • Team answers submitted and graded • Instructor feedback	Group assignment: • Cooperative problem solving • Instructor facilitated class discussion between teams	Formative and summative

Team-based Learning Steps

- **Individual preparation work:** Students are expected to use a variety of preparation materials in the form of readings, presentation slides, audio lectures, or video lectures. They should be set to a level appropriate for the students in your course.

- **Individual readiness assurance test (IRAT):** In class, students take an individual quiz called IRAT consisting of the 5–20 multiple choice questions based on preparatory material. Students form teams, take the same test, and submit responses as a team using scratchcards or the TBL-enabled software. Both IRAT and TRAT scores count towards a student's final grade.
- **Clarification session:** After the student has completed both the IRAT and TRAT, the student will have the opportunity to raise clarification points and ask questions about the quality of multiple choice questions on the test. Instructors can answer questions and facilitate discussion on the topics and concepts covered.
- **Advanced exercises:** Finally, students can work in teams on advanced exercises to apply and extend the knowledge they have just learned and tested. They need to arrive at a common answer to the application's question and display the answer choices in the classroom egallery walk. The trainer then facilitates a discussion or debate between teams to explore possible solutions to the application problem.
- **Peer review:** This final phase is an optional component of the team-based learning process. During or at the end of the course, some instructors conduct peer-reviews of the teams.

Benefits for students and facilitators include:
- Students receive multiple explanations of complex cases.
- Knowledge for educators and students
- Discussions and more lively discussion
- Role model for interprofessional collaboration
- Brings humorous into the classroom.

Benefits
- Students have the opportunity to receive immediate feedback on individual and team tests, thus enhancing their knowledge and preparation.
- A feedback-rich learning environment has a positive effect on content-related learning.
- Students in the TBL class are forced to make decisions and defend them logically with evidence-based counter-arguments.
- Highly adaptable to different space constraints
- Its properties make it suitable for training medical professionals.

Cons
- Fewer problems can be solved in one course because the whole team has to work on the same problem. This is because if each group in the course is solving a different problem at the same time, discussion between groups becomes less effective.
- Highly experienced and talented/and often advanced/teacher who thrives in a lecture format and believes it is the best way for students to learn.

PROBLEM-BASED LEARNING

Problem-based learning (PBL) is an education that encourages students to learn concepts and principles using complex realworld problems as a vehicle rather than the direct presentation of facts and concepts. Technique. In addition to course content, PBL promotes the development of critical thinking, problem-solving, and communication skills. It can also provide opportunities to work in groups, find and evaluate research material, and encourage lifelong learning.

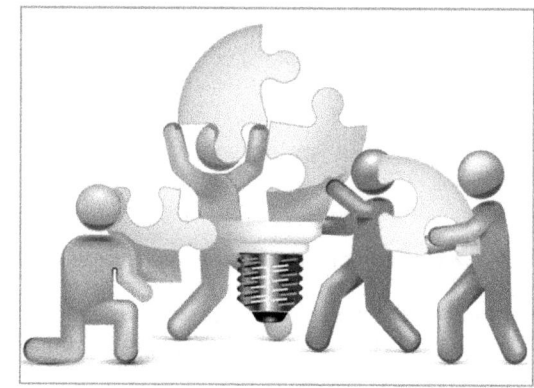

Fig. 7.36: Problem-based learning.

Definition
PBL is a student-centered approach in which students learn about a topic by working in groups and solving freeform problems. This problem promotes motivation and learning.

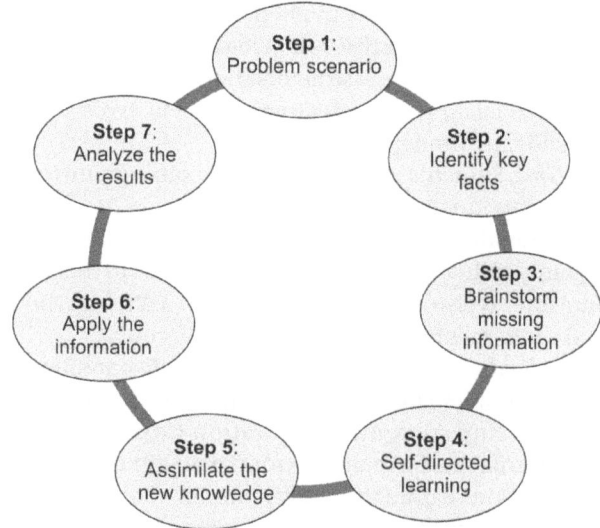

Fig. 7.37: Steps of problem-based learning.

Meaning

Wood (2003) defines PBL as the process of using identified problems in scenarios to increase knowledge and understanding. Here are the principles of this process:
- Learner-defined goals and outcomes.
- Students undertake independent, self-directed learning before returning to larger groups.
- Learning takes place in small groups of 8–10 people and is delivered at home, teacher facilitates discussion.
- Trigger materials such as paper-based clinical scenarios, laboratory data, photographs, articles, videos, or patients (real or simulated) can be used.
- Maastricht seven-jump process helps guide the PBL process.
- Based on the principles of adult education theory.
- Every member of the group has a role to play.
- Combining work and intelligence promotes knowledge acquisition.
- Teamwork in problem-solving learning that enhances communication with others and encourages independent responsibility for collaboration all skills essential for future practice.
- Anybody can do it, as long as it is the right one for a given cause and scenario.

Characteristics

Learning parallel to these goals:
- Learning is student-centered.
- Learning takes place in small groups.
- Teachers are facilitators or leaders.
- Problems create organizational focal points and incentives for learning.
- Problems are a vehicle for developing clinical problem-solving skills. New information is acquired through spontaneous learning.

Principles

Developed together as a team, these 12 principles form the basis on which this training was designed. The 12 principles are:
1. A prerequisite for learning is that learners take responsibility for their own learning
2. Be flexible in defining learning outcomes
3. Strive to be a role model
4. Learners will arrive at learning outcomes through variety of ways
5. Learn through reflection
6. Help students guide what they know and do not understand
7. Be a facilitator, not a teacher
8. Be moderate style from "follow me" to "collaborative experiment"
9. Learning through social processes
10. Creating physical learning environments for PBL
11. Students defining their own assessment
12. Learning skills for PBL develop

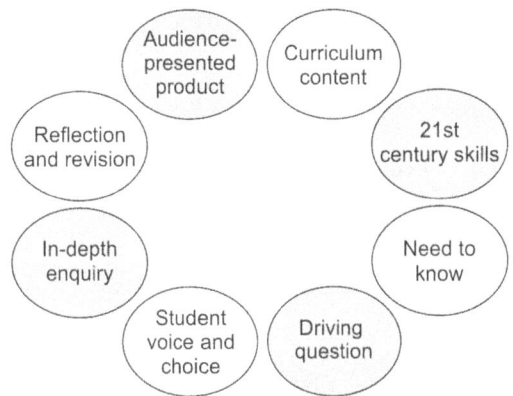

Fig. 7.38: Eight essential elements of problem-based learning.

Types

Three types of PBL are:
1. **Problem-stimulated PBL (PS PBL):** PS PBL uses relevant knowledge and information to solve problems. They are used to emphasize three basic objectives:
   a. Development of domain-specific skills.
   b. Developing problem-solving skills.
   c. Domain-specific knowledge interpretation.
2. **Student-centered PBL (SC PBL):** SC PBL has the same factors as PS PBL and adds one more factor, i.e., lifetime skill update. This factor benefits those who have long taught and practiced in a particular field. Keeping their skills up-to-date is important. This applies to doctors, engineers, managers, etc.
3. **Case-based PBL:** Case-based learning (CBL) is an established approach used across disciplines where students apply their knowledge to real-world scenarios, promoting higher levels of cognition. In CBL classrooms, students typically work in groups on case studies.

Steps to a PBL Approach

- **Step 1—examine the problem:** Collect the required information. Learn new concepts, principles and skills related to the proposed topic.
- **Step 2—show what you know:** Individual students and groups list what they already know about the scenario and list areas where they lack information.
- **Step 3—define the problem:** Contextualize the problem using what is already known and what information students expect to learn.

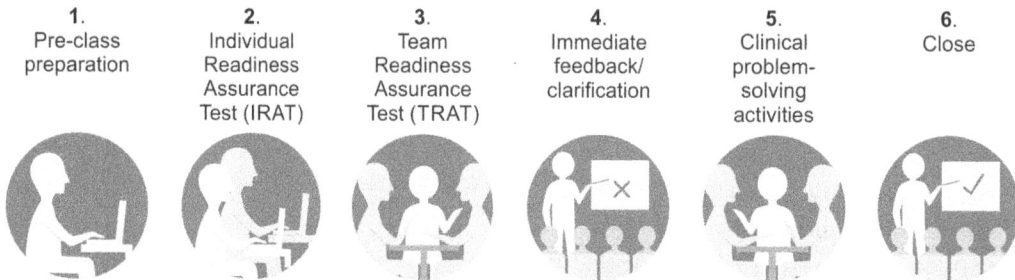

Fig. 7.39: Team-based learning steps.

- **Step 4—research Knowledge:** Find resources and information to help you craft compelling arguments.
- **Step 5—examine the solution:** List possible actions and solutions to the problem. Develop and test possible hypotheses.
- **Step 6—present and support the selected solution:** Clarify your conclusion and support them with relevant information and evidence.
- **Step 7—check performance:** It is easy to forget that this is an important step in improving your problem-solving skills. Students should evaluate their performance and plan improvements for the following issues:

Benefits of PBL

For Students

- A student-centered approach.
- Students generally find it more enjoyable and satisfying.
- Better understanding.
- Students with PBL experience value their abilities more.
- PBL develops lifelong learning skills.

Instructor

- Increased class attendance.
- This method offers a more substantial reward.
- Encourage students to spend more time studying.
- Provide interdisciplinary support.

For Education

- Prioritize student learning.
- Support student retention.
- Can be viewed as evidence of the institution's emphasis on education.

Risks of PBL

For Students

- Prior learning experience does not prepare the student for her PBL.
- PBL requires more time and takes away study time from other subjects.
- It creates some anxiety because it complicates learning.
- Group dynamic issues can undermine the effectiveness of PBL.
- Low knowledge of content available for study.

For Teachers

- Difficulty creating good problem scenarios.
- Preparation takes time.
- Students ask questions about the process.
- Group dynamic issues may require teacher intervention.
- New questions arise about what and how to measure.

For Educational Institutions

- Need to change the educational philosophy of the department, which is based on lectures.
- Faculty need training and support.
- Needs more instructors in general.
- Works best in a flexible classroom.
- Produces opposition from faculty who question its effectiveness.

Advantages

- PBL replaces traditional lectures with assisted learning, optional tutoring, on-site discussion and experience. This facilitates deep learning in detail.
- Direct lessons can be reduced. This encourages learner initiative. This will increase student motivation.
- Problem-based learning requires prior knowledge of problem solving. Therefore, the basic knowledge is constantly updated and revised.
- Problem-based thinking often stimulates critical thinking. Students try to think about different aspects of the project rather than following what the lecture teaches. Students will consider how, where and why the aspect of the problem introduced was introduced.
- Problem-based learners tend to have better information gathering skills and abilities than traditional learners.

This is because traditional learners tend to stick to only the books mandated by the curriculum and avoid exploring various sources of information. Problem-based learners, on the other hand, tend to be more hands-on, and PBL encourages them to think outside the box.
- Since PBL refers to life-based skills and practices, these skills can also be transferred to individuals through appropriate training and practice.
- All issues introduced in the PBL curriculum are open issues. This leaves more room for discussion and understanding of concepts, and you get more data.
- Another important element of PBL is the need for good communication skills. PBL enhances an individual's social skills as it includes peer skill comparisons and insightful discussions.

Drawbacks of PBL

- Good PBL design takes a lot of time and effort. Continuous monitoring and recording of students is required throughout the process.
- Not every teacher can be a good PBL adviser to her. They need dedicated, hardworking and trained facilitators.
- PBL requires more staff and more contact hours for preparation, discussion, and comparison of answers. Students and the advisors supposed to do timely and seasonable meetings once in a while.
- It is a known fact that PBL does not provide that many facts when compared with the traditional method so many of the teachers hesitant to take up this form of teaching.
- For a PBL curriculum to be effective, it must integrate multiple disciplines so that students can grasp different aspects of the situation.
- It is always difficult for coordinators to evaluate specific students within a team.
- PBL is also difficult for educational institutions because it requires different courses depending on the instructor.

Because the entire PBL curriculum reflects the ideals of students and how they should be educated.
- More and more coordinators need to evaluate and guide students' career paths, and coordinators also need people who create as many difficult situations as possible.

PEER SHARING

In peer teaching, the instructor asks the student a challenging question, the student answers the question individually, the student discusses the answer with their class partner, and finally the student answers the question again. A large body of evidence shows that peer instruction is beneficial to student learning.

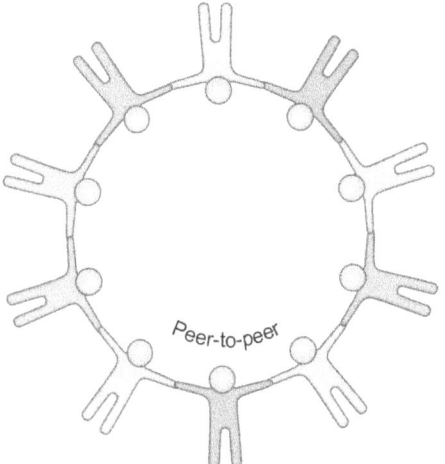

Fig. 7.41: Peer sharing and teaching.

Definition

- Peer learning is the process of learning from each other.

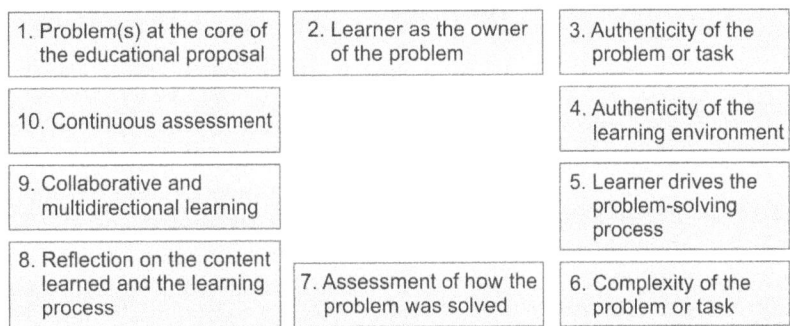

Fig. 7.40: Principles of problem-based learning.

- Peer relationships can also negatively affect social-emotional development through bullying, exclusion, and deviant peer processes.
- Universal school-based social-emotional learning programs promote healthy social-emotional development and provide a strong foundation for creating a positive peer culture.
- Children with peer difficulties often require additional systematic and intensive social skills coaching.
- Peers can be a powerful force that can promote or undermine group programs.

Examples of Peer Learning

- The senior year at the university works with faculty to lead a freshman experience course for new students at the university.
- An ESL student helps an english-speaking classmate learn to speak their mother tongue. A high school student who learned to code in a summer class helps his classmates learn to code in a group.

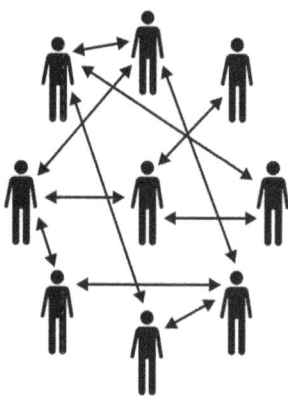

Fig. 7.42: Peer-to-peer model.

- A student who reads better than his peers is leading a discussion group on the assigned readings in english class.
- A fourth year medical student runs a clinical skills lab for other medical students.

Features of Peer-to-peer Learning

- It is about empowering students so that they can become more independent and responsible.
- Participants need to lead the meeting and make sure things go according to plan, so they become responsible and accountable for some of their work

Peer Teaching

- **One-way peer teaching:** In this type of peer teaching, only trained tutors can teach, and children with disabilities remain passive. This method is useful for teaching students with severe disabilities, such as visual impairment due to autism or cerebral palsy.
- **Whole class peer tutoring:** In this teaching methodology, the whole class is grouped into pairs or peers and taught by helping each other by prompting them to correct mistakes. This method is unique in that each student is given a cue card with assignments that focus on the goals of the chapter, and the tutor receives the cue card to mark the skills each student has acquired. The main advantage of this approach is that students are not singled out and all students must participate regardless of disability
- **Criss-cross or cross-age peer tutoring:** Cross-age peer tutoring is a tutoring method where children of different ages and ability levels work together on a task. An older or higher IQ student is assigned as a tutor and the other is assigned as a teacher. This method also helps improve interpersonal skills.

Importance of Peer Learning

There are benefits to breaking up large teams into smaller groups. Peer learning helps keep everyone on the same page for the next step. Each person is informed of what needs to be done as their performance affects everyone else's performance. When you are in charge of part of the job, others rely on you to do a good job.

All of this underscores the importance of peer learning in skill development:

- **Building interpersonal skills:** When they have to rely on each other for work, they tend to build trust and harmony. This is an important workplace skill that encourages building lasting relationships.
- **Improving communication skills:** Effective communication cannot be overlooked in a professional environment. From giving presentations to attending meetings to writing notes and emails, communication is a big part of our professional lives. Peer learning helps build skills to communicate effectively, clearly, and concisely.
- **Leads to effective teamwork:** Teamwork helps organizations achieve results. Building trust among teammates by learning and sharing knowledge with peers. Learn to rely on others for tasks you cannot handle yourself. They learn to ask for help and offer it when they need it.
- **Building a healthy work environment:** A healthy, harmonious and supportive work environment means optimal results and employee well-being. When employees have the autonomy to chair meetings, chair sessions, and take ownership of their work, they are more likely to stay to see results.

- **Promote growth and development:** Personal growth and development is a direct result of peer learning. Because there is a lot of room for improvement.

Benefits of Peer Tutoring

- Students are more creative in expressing ideas and grasping new concepts because they do not hesitate to ask questions.
- Peer teaching involves direct interaction between learner and student and teacher and student. This, along with interpersonal skills that actually allow them to say goodbye to so-called boring lectures and classes, helps promote positive learning.
- The burden of responsibility on teachers is reduced as they share duties that are beneficial to the children. But on the other hand, it strengthens the role of teachers in supervising and managing students.

Disadvantages of Peer Teaching

- **Amateur students:** Teachers share their tips and guidelines with students, but do not become experienced teachers (students).
- **Student reluctance:** The toughest responsibility that falls on a teacher's shoulders is the student's unwillingness to carry out their assigned duties.
- **Angry parents:** When parents learn about peer teaching, they may misunderstand the concept of peer teaching.

CASE STUDY ANALYSIS

The case method is a participatory, discussion-based learning method that develops students' skills in critical thinking, communication and group dynamics. It is a kind of problem-based learning. Teachers learn just like students. Due to the interactive nature of this method, teachers are constantly "encountering new perspectives on old problems or testing classic solutions to new problems.

Definition

A case study is an indepth study of a group of people or an event. Case studies analyze nearly every aspect of a subject's life and history to find patterns and causes of behavior. Case studies can be used in many fields, including psychology, medicine, education, anthropology, political science, and social work.

Objectives

General objectives of case studies are to:
- A description of each individual situation (case). Details of an individual, business organization, or institution.
- Identify the main problem of the case (the challenge question should indicate what the focus should be on).
- Analyze the case using relevant theoretical concepts of the unit or discipline.
- Recommend a course of action for this particular case (especially the problem-solving case study).

Benefits of Using Case Studies in Teaching

A major benefit of using case studies to teach is that students are actively involved in developing a foundation by abstracting from examples.
- Problem solving
- Quantitative and/or qualitative analytical tools depending on the case
- Decision-making in complex situations
- Dealing with ambiguity.

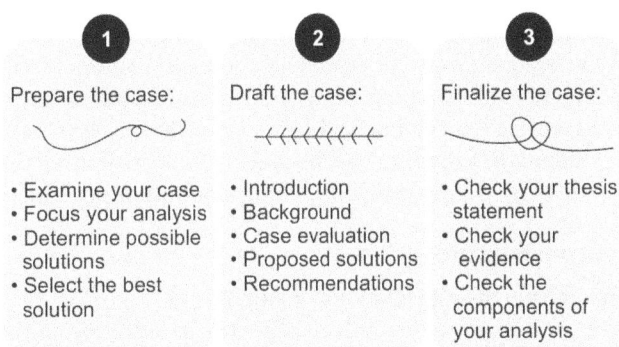

Fig. 7.43: Writing the case study analysis.

Cons

- Not always generalizable to larger populations
- Unproven cause and effect
- Science
- Can lead to distortion.

JOURNALING

The word "journal" comes from the French word "jour", meaning "a day". It is so named because the transactions are recorded daily in a journal. This is the original book of his entries for recording the trader's various transactions chronologically (in chronological order) and in detail. It is also called a diary because it contains a record of your daily transactions.

Definition

Journaling is the recording of thoughts, understandings, and descriptions of ideas and concepts on paper, usually in bound notebooks. Teachers ask students to keep journals with the understanding that students will share their journals with the teacher.

Meaning

Journaling is an effective learning and teaching strategy in teaching and nursing to achieve student learning outcomes. Research suggests that it enhances critical thinking and emotional expression, deepening the learning experience. It is most effective when used properly, and has benefits such as emotional exploration that addresses more learning and improved writing, and drawbacks such as being difficult to grade.

Purposes

- Some teachers allow students to write freely about the topic. Others provide writing prompts for students to respond to.
- Some teachers read every entry in a student's journal. Others read only excerpts selected by the student. Still others use journaling as an opportunity for free speech.
- Some teachers review and correct journal entries to help students improve her writing skills. Others use journals as one form of "uncorrected" writing that students produce.

Journal Features

The journal has the following features.
- A journal is the first successful step in a double-entry system. Transactions are first recorded in a journal. A diary is therefore called a book of original entries.
- Transactions are recorded on the day they occur. That is why diaries are called daybooks.
- Transactions are recorded in chronological order. So the journal is called Chronology.
- For each transaction, the names of his two associated accounts (indicating which is debit and which is credit) are clearly written on his two consecutive lines. This facilitates general ledger postings. For this reason, the journal is called the subsidiary ledger or subsidiary book
- There is a story under each entry.
- Amounts are written in two columns at the end—the debit amount in the debit column and the credit amount in the credit column.

Journaling Rules

Recording transactions in a journal is called journaling. The rule can be summarized as:
- Use two lines to write the names of the two accounts involved in each transaction.
- Write the name of the debtor or account to be debited on the first line and the name of the creditor or account to be debited on the next line.
- Next to the line starting in the Detail column, write the name of the account that will be debited and the name of the account that will be credited a short distance away from that line.
- Use "Dr" after each debit and "To" before each credit. The term "Cr." after credit is unnecessary because if one account is a debtor, the other account must be a creditor.

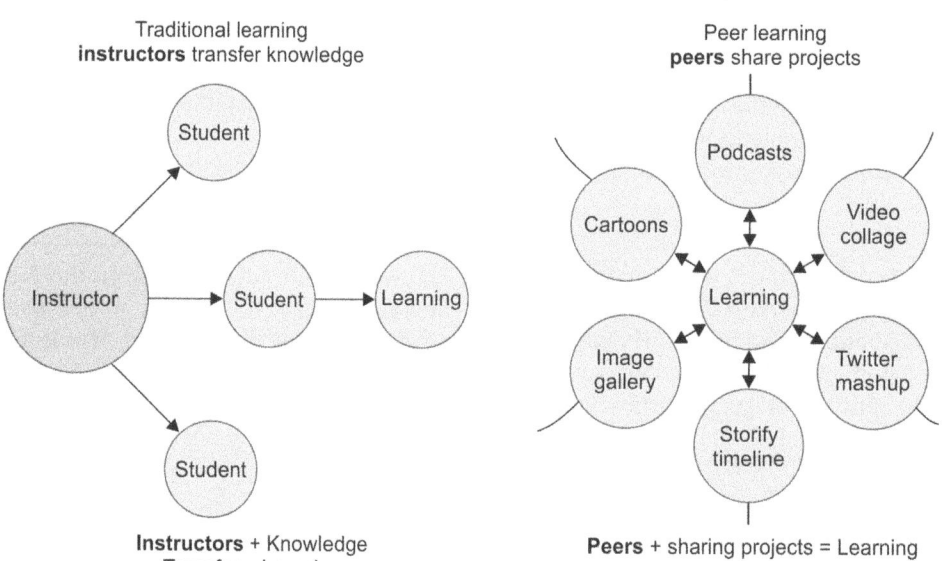

Fig. 7.44: Difference between traditional learning and peer learning.

- To separate an entry from another entry, draw a line under each entry that covers only the information column. The row does not reach the amount column.

Important for the Magazine

- The magazine encourages reflection on the one hand and active thinking on the other.
- The importance of the journal as a record of thoughts cannot be underestimated for teachers who value independent thought.
- Journals record a student's individual journey in the academic world. At the same time, it is also useful when a formal paper or project is being written.
  - *Title:* The title of your article is one of the first indicators your readers will understand about your research or concept. It should be concise, precise and informative.
  - *Keywords:* Keywords are an integral part of creating journal articles. When writing a magazine article, you need to choose the keywords you want your article to rank for. Keywords help potential readers find your article when they search on a search engine.

- *Abstract:* The purpose of the abstract is to present the main points of the research clearly and concisely. The abstract is the main element of the work that the reader will encounter, so it should always be well thought out. The abstract should be a short paragraph (approximately 300 words) summarizing the findings of the journal article.
- *Acknowledgments:* Acknowledgments may seem like a small aspect of journal articles, but they are important nonetheless. This is a place to thank people who do not qualify as coauthors but who have contributed intellectually, financially, or otherwise to articles.
- *Introduction:* The introduction is a central part of the article writing process. The introduction not only introduces the topic and its stance on that topic, but also (orients/contextualizes) the reasoning in the broader discipline.
- *Body:* The body contains the main arguments and proofs. Each paragraph contains different terms, with clear links between each paragraph.

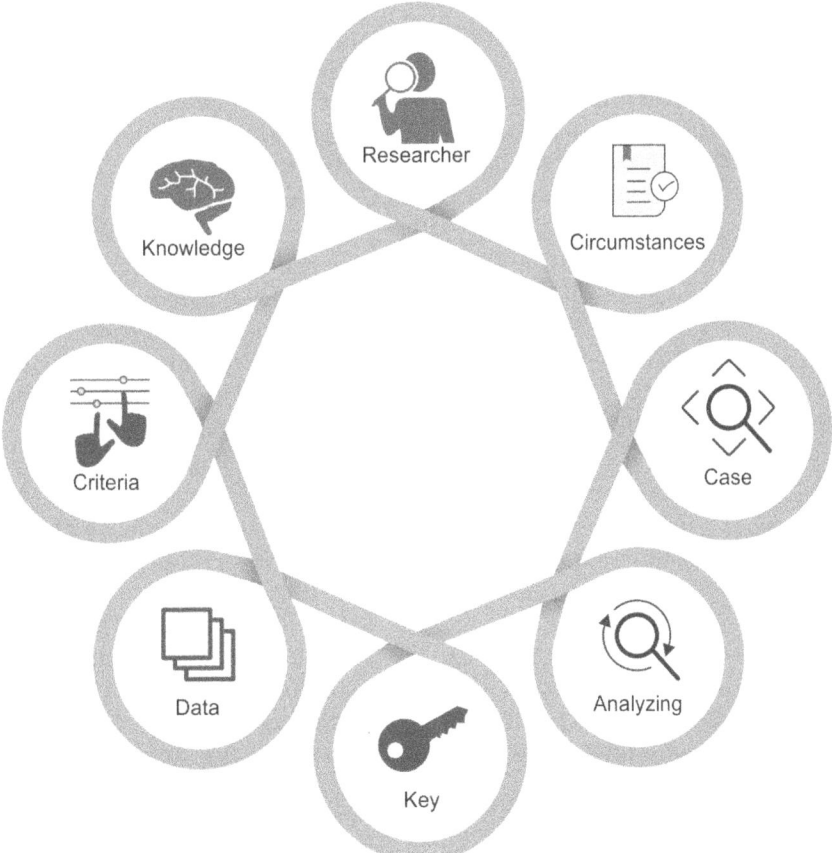

Fig. 7.45: Case study analysis model.

- *Conclusion:* The conclusion should be an interpretation of the findings, summarizing all the concepts introduced in the body of the text, from most important to least important. There are no new concepts introduced in this section.
- *References and citations:* References and citations should be balanced, current and relevant. Each field is different, but if possible, aim to cite references that are less than 10 years old. The research they cite should be strongly related to your research question.

Journal Organization

- Journals can be spiral bound notebooks or loose-leaf binders.
- Keep the journal in a designated place in the classroom or have students place the journal on their desks for easy access.
- Create lesson routines for magazine distribution and collection. For example, assign one student to be responsible for the magazine each week.
- If you want students to use their journals for multiple purposes, have them divide their notes into different sections. Sections can be labeled by subject. Or you can dedicate a section of your notebook to any kind of journal you ask your students to do throughout the year.
- Setup a system to identify each entry in the journal as follows. Write the date at the beginning of each entry. Students can use page numbers and clever titles. This is useful when students want to revise or reevaluate previous entries.
- Allow sufficient time for students to organize and write down their thoughts. Tell them how much time you give them to write and how much writing is generally expected. Apply the "do not speak" rule during journaling hours.
- Provide feedback in the form of written discussion questions, margin notes, or notes that allow students to read and think about their entries.

Types of journals students can use for development:

- **Bulleted lists:** Focusing on bulleted lists is a great way to personalize and track progress. Use this journal to create to-do lists, brainstorm projects, and record goals.
- **Transfer journal:** Write down the concepts and information you learned in class and think about how you can refer to them ("transfer") in the future.
- **Gratitude journal:** Being a student can be stressful at times. When you feel overwhelmed, it's good to remember to be grateful.
- **Duplicate your journal:** Write your concept or phrase on the left side of your notebook page, and your thoughts or reactions to the idea on the right side.
- **Question journal:** Write down questions about course material or internal questions you want to answer about yourself. Please come back to these pages to find out your answers.
- **Reading journal:** Write down what you read in class or what you read for fun. Write down ideas that come to your mind or information that you want to remember. Writing down your thoughts and perspectives helps you remember what you read so you can refer to that information later.
- **Idea journal:** Use the journal as a "brain dump" location. Write down everything you think or feel so that you can better process your thoughts and feelings. Letting the words flow in your stream of consciousness helps clear your mind.

Journaling in the Classroom

- **Be consistent:** Regular journaling will help your students become comfortable with the practice. You may want to set aside a special time for daily journaling or ask students to journal following a particular lesson. Try to allow journaling time at least once or twice a week (or every day if you can fit it in!). Be sure to give students at least 10-15 minutes to write so they do not feel rushed.
- **Give direction:** Make sure your students have a clear understanding of what and how you expect them to write. Set a minimum number of words sentences or paragraphs. Instruct students to write persuasive narrative and expository sentences so that they can practice these forms of writing. Mix and match these to keep your students interested and engaged. Just give clear instructions for each journaling task.
- **Use writing prompts:** Writing prompts give students a clear goal of what to write about. It also provides a way to evaluate what you will get out of a particular lesson.
- **Use free writing:** You may also want to ask students to freewrite on occasion. Leave the subject and content completely up to them; just give them some time to write about whatever they want.
- **Review student submissions:** Review student submissions regularly and respond as needed. Assessing student journaling can put students under pressure and make them less responsive.
- **Encourage self-evaluation:** Ask students to rate their own work. This can itself be a journaling task. Ask them to go through their journaling history and pick the parts they like and dislike. You can then write about why you chose those works and how you would modify future journaling tasks based on your evaluation.

Benefits

Keeping your journal online has many journaling benefits.
- Journaling is known to reduce stress levels.
- It gives you mental clarity.
- It helps you remember everything you learn daily
- It helps you visualize the life you desire.
- Good practice for self-reflection.
- Track your progress in a journal to help you set and reach your goals. For example, a weight loss diary.
- A convenient place to record ideas on the go and review them later.

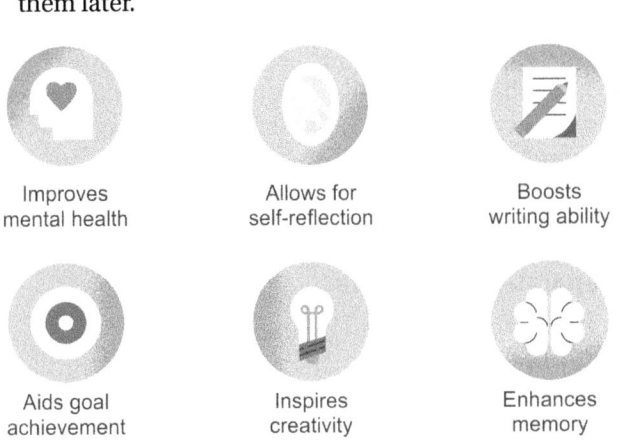

Fig. 7.47: Benefits of journaling.

Use of the Magazine

- Originally written book.
- Used to record daily transactions in chronological order.
- Full details of the transaction in the entry are displayed.
- Affects both sides of the transaction—debit and credit.
- It is the ledger that forms the basis for further processing of the recorded data.

Advantages

- All business related information is provided in chronological order.
- It gives complete information and explanation of a transaction.
- It facilitates error free recording of transactions.
- It also helps locating errors at the initial stage of recording.
- Facilitates correct posting and closing for financial reporting.

Limitations

- Journaling is not a straightforward process due to the prescribed accounting rules and concepts.
- Good for a small number of transactions, as it is inconvenient to record a large number of transactions.
- Account balances that require individual ledgers are not disclosed. Therefore, it cannot be used as a replacement for Ledger.

DEBATE

A debate is an argument in which two or more people take opposing positions on one or more issues in order to persuade an audience (or other supporters) to accept their position. Most people are used to participating in informal discussions such as: Trying to convince a friend why certain movie songbook artists, etc., are better than others. However, these often degenerate into things like circular reasoning and personal "attack" tangents, so formal debates often include rules to ensure the discussion stays on the original topic.

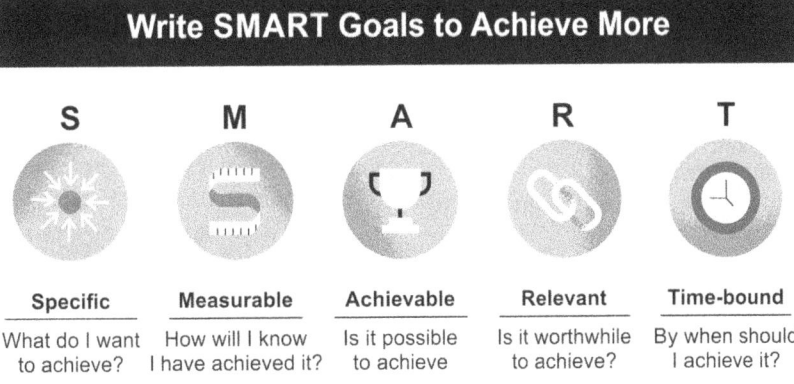

Fig. 7.46: Smart goals in journaling.

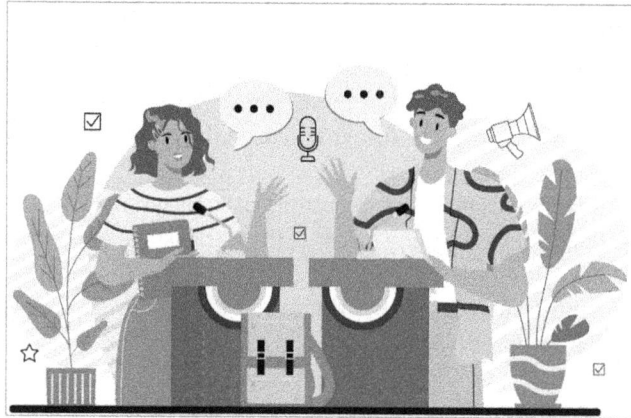

Fig. 7.48: Debate method of learning.

Class Discussions

Example: Class discussions are often best done in small teams.
- One team agrees and another disagrees. The rest of the students are non-debates.
- Before the discussion, allow time for the team to work together to identify arguments for or against a particular issue.
- Each member of the team is given the opportunity to present one argument on behalf of their team.
- Arguments should be timed approximately 3-5 minutes per person.
- Allow time for rebuttals and responses approximately 1 per person.
- Include the class in creating a clear set of rules timings and guidelines for the debate. Nondebating students should work together to create guidelines for how the debate will be judged evaluated and how feedback will be provided.

Student's Skill Development in Debate

Students who participate in debate programs will discover and develop the following skills:
- **Confidence:** Belief in themselves and their abilities and the desire to participate in all classes.
- **Curiosity:** Passion for discovery with effective tools for research organization and presentation.
- **Critical thinking:** How to explore the world through the lens of your inquisitive mind.
- Writing skills and strategies for discussing disagreements actively yet respectfully.
- **Control:** Eliminate the fears of public speaking.
- **Creativity:** The desire to explore create and invent.
- **Camaraderie:** Meet like minded peers at tournaments and build healthy bonds of competition.
- **Leadership:** Self-motivation and the ability to delegate assignments and manage peers.

Structure for Debate

- A formal debate usually involves three groups: one supporting a resolution (affirmative team) one opposing the resolution (opposing team) and those who are judging the quality of the evidence and arguments and the performance in the debate.
- The affirmative and opposing teams usually consist of three members each while the judging may be done by the teacher a small group of students or the class as a whole.
- In addition to the three specific groups there may an audience made up of class members not involved in the formal debate.
- Concrete resolutions are formulated and rules of debate are established.

Preparation for Debate

- Prepare resolutions for debate.
- Create a team.
- Establish rules for discussion, including scheduling.
- Research topics and discuss them logically.
- Gather evidence and examples of the position presented.
- Anticipate counterarguments and prepare counter-arguments.
- Team members plan the order and content of the discussion.
- Arrange for discussion.
- Establish expectations, if any, for evaluating debates. This pattern is repeated for the second speaker in each team. Finally each team gets an opportunity for rebutting the arguments of the opponent. Speakers should speak slowly and clearly. The judges and members of the audience should be taking notes as the debate proceeds.

A typical sequence for debate with suggested timelines is as follows:
- The first speaker on the affirmative team presents an argument in favor of the resolution. (5-10 minutes)
- The first speaker of the opposing team presents the objection to the decision. (5-10 minutes)
- The second speaker on the team presents additional arguments in support of the resolution, identifies areas of conflict, and discusses the possibilities raised by the other speaker (5-10 minutes)
- The second speaker from the opposing team presents further arguments for the decision, identifies another area of conflict.

- Rules may include short breaks for teams to prepare their counter-arguments (5 minutes)
- The opposing team initiates a rebuttal, attempting to defend the opposing side's claims and refute the claims it supports without adding new information (3–5 minutes)
- Affirmative team's first rebuttal (3–5 minutes)
- There should be no interruptions. Speakers must wait their turn. Teachers may need to enforce rules.

Post-debate Discussion and Evaluation

Allow time for debriefing and discussion after the formal debate. The audience should be given the opportunity to ask questions and express their own thoughts and opinions on the arguments presented. Members of the debate teams may also wish to reflect on their performance and seek feedback from the audience including the teacher.

Debating Tips and Techniques

- Preparing your debate topic
- Staying on topic
- Speaking slowly clearly and charismatically
- Confidence in a topic
- Consider your body language and what it tells your audience
- Listen carefully and take notes
- Anticipate questions before they are asked.

Advantages

- Acquire broad, multifaceted knowledge that spans multiple disciplines outside the learner's usual field of study.
- Enhancing learners' confidence and self-esteem.
- Provide engaging and active learner-centred activities.
- Enhanced higher rigorous skills and critical thinking.
- Improved ability to structure and organize thoughts.
- Analytical research of learners and improvement of note-taking skills.
- Developing effective speech synthesis and communication.
- Encourage teamwork.

Benefits

Debate benefits or maintenance include:
- Debating cultivates the habit of independent thinking in students.
- Debate fosters a healthy sense of competition.
- Debating is very useful in high school, but it is useful for everyone anyway, so it is used at all levels of education.
- Debates improve students' lecture skills as they eliminate hesitation.
- Debating develops students' intelligence and logic.
- Debating allows students to justify the question whether they agree or disagree.

Limitations

- Debate does not save time because it wastes time unnecessarily.
- Debate is not very useful for the lower classes.
- Real-life subjects are not the topic of middle school students.

GAMING

Game-based learning (GBL) is an umbrella term for the many ways games are used as educational tools. Learning and teaching with games is nothing new. Over the years, teachers have used physics, board, and card games in a variety of subjects to engage students and make learning more accessible. Digital technologies such as virtual and augmented reality are enabling teachers to bring more engaging learning experiences into the classroom.

Definition

GBL is learning using games, all within a game environment, with customized or thirdparty content. The goal is to encourage and motivate learners to acquire new skills, improve existing skills, and change behavior.

Meaning

GBL is also an active learning technique that uses games to enhance student learning. This is where learning comes from play, promoting critical thinking, and problem-solving skills. It can take place in digital or non-digital games and can include simulations that allow students to experience learning first-hand.

Examples

The most common examples of GBL are:
- **"War"** is a traditional card game that can have a mathematical twist. Check out our list of classroom math games to learn how to play.
- **Board games:** A game you play on a board that usually involves the movement of pieces. Chess and checkers are popular ones but there are hundreds if not thousands of board games for kids to explore.
- **Simulation games:** Games designed to accurately simulate real-world activities. Launched in 2000, The Sims is one of his series of most popular life. He simulation games about creating and exploring virtual worlds.

- **Word games:** Games typically designed to explore the peculiarities of language and the ability to use language on your own. Scrabble is an example of a traditional word game, but the Words With Friends app is a more modern one.
- **Puzzle games:** Games that focus on solving puzzles using spatial and pattern recognition, etc., solving sequences to complete logical words. For example, Sudoku and 2048 are popular math puzzles.
- **Role-playing game (RPG):** A game in which the player assumes the role of a fictional character and goes on an adventure. Dungeons and Dungeons is a popular fantasy tabletop role-playing game. Dragons, first introduced in 1974.

Purpose

According to students who participated in the study game, you can:
- Make complex ideas and topics more interesting and meaningful
- Help students become independent and engaged learners
- Provide opportunities to practice problem-solving and trial-and-error strategies
- Support different learners and different interests
- Encourage imaginative learning
- Enable students to work together toward common goals.

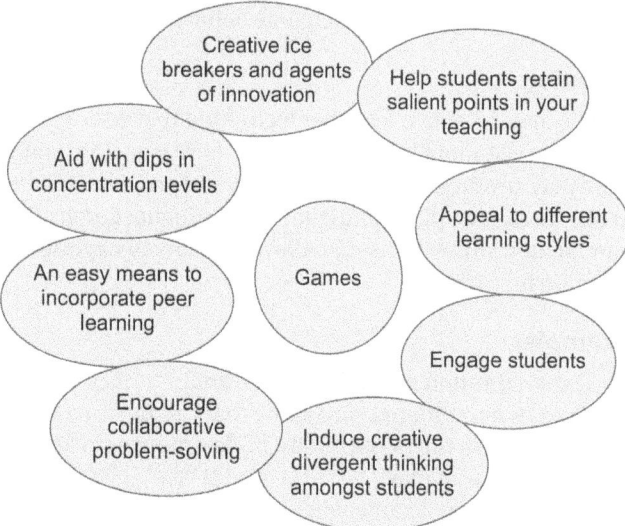

Fig. 7.49: Game-based learning (GBL).

Different Types of GBL

To better understand GBL, we can look at its different types given where the game takes place and the environment in which the students play. The three types of GBL are:

1. **Board games:** Monopoly can be considered an educational game. It has all the elements you need: story, characters, points, competition and many other aspects. There are many examples of Monopoly-like games for schools with modified rules for various subjects, such as History Monopoly and Math Monopoly.
2. **Real-life game:** The environment here is the real world. This is probably the most motivating, but also the most stressful type of play. This style requires students to move, act, and play with their bodies and minds. It is the most immersive and inspires students in almost every aspect of learning.
3. **Digital games:** The environment here is online. Digital games can be compared to board games. In fact, many of GBL's digital programs use online boards where teachers can edit or add learning content depending on the subject being played. This type of game also allows students to participate in the creation of the game, especially if the teacher cannot manage the online tools.

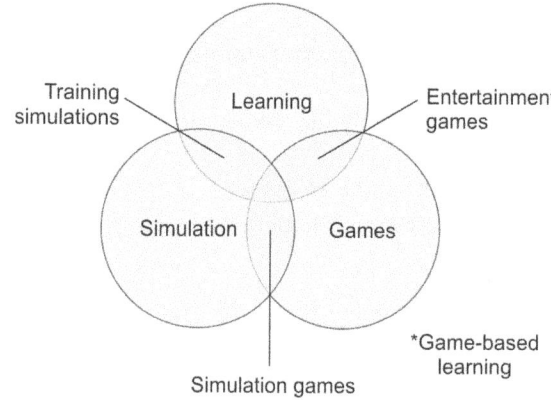

Fig. 7.50: Different types of GBL.

Theory

GBL theory involves new ways of training corporate employees. We are talking about using games to learn. The range of gamified content has grown and diversified with video games designed for nearly every audience and industry.

- **Constructivist learning:** Constructivism is premised on the need to provide students with the tools they need to develop their own ways of solving problems. This implies a participatory process in which students interact with their environment to solve the situations presented.
- **Practice and interaction:** Safe practice experiential learning and interaction are the underlying pillars of the theory of play-based learning. Learning through games allows students to experiment with non-threatening

scenarios and acquire knowledge through practice and social interaction with the environment and peers.
- **A motivating approach:** One of the strengths of GBL is its perceived ability to capture students' attention and ensure their full participation. The motivational approach of these games makes the learning process dynamic and interesting, and keeps students engaged as they progress toward their goals. In addition to its playful approach, GBL presents situations that require students to think and make decisions to solve problems. In this way, participants acquire knowledge and absorb concepts while developing cognitive skills derived from real-world critical thinking analysis and conflict resolution.
- **Feedback and self-control:** Unlike traditional teaching methods, GBL gives learners control over their own learning. With authentic games, students get instant, personalized feedback on their knowledge, allowing everyone to see what they are learning and what they need to work on more.

Benefits of Playing in the Classroom

- **Increased motivation:** Playing games in the classroom increases overall motivation. Playing games motivates students to study hard and participate in the challenges set. Games help students become part of a team and take responsibility for their own learning.
- **Regulated competition:** Students can be very competitive in the classroom, especially boys. Games are a great way to control peer competition.
- **Strategy simulators:** Most games require problem-solving strategy and planning. By applying different strategies in games, students can use their working memory to solve problems and increase their mental cognition.
- **Peer enthusiasm:** Using games in the classroom as part of teaching and learning creates a positive atmosphere around the classroom, motivates students through participation and creates a positive attitude towards learning. Games also create a positive memory and learning experience for students in the classroom.
- **Reduce stress:** Answering worksheet questions and creating pages of text can be very difficult and stressful for some students. It can also create a negative perception of the learning environment in students.
- **Stronger memory:** Playing a series of content-specific games will improve your memory. While playing the game, the student needs to memorize important details about the topic, but also needs to use her working memory to think and act quickly.

- **Class co-operation:** Students should work together as a team when playing against the teacher as a whole class, or in small team groups when playing together.
- **Warning note:** Playing the game requires students to pay close attention to detail. The game can change rapidly during play, so students need to pay close attention.
- **Friendly fun:** Play releases endorphins. Endorphins stimulate the brain and give students a sense of euphoria. This euphoria brings great happiness and excitement to the students in the classroom, creating a positive learning environment.
- **New knowledge:** Games are a great tool to reinforce new knowledge in the classroom. After introducing new content to your class, offer your students games that reinforce their understanding and connect them with what they already know.
- **Take it outside:** Games are not just for the classroom. Getting outside and enjoying nature can give your students a little head rest while reinforcing the topics they are learning.

Benefits of Game-Based Teaching Methods

- **Interesting:** Games offer a lot of variety in learning situations. Integrating games into the teaching and learning process makes them no longer monotonous, but interesting and engaging.
- **Motivation:** Games add variety to lessons and motivate students. Because games are fun. Students love playing games, so teachers can motivate them and get their attention.
- **Renewal:** Formal lessons can get boring and monotonous because they keep going at the same pace, but adding games can brighten up the classroom and renew the energy of the students.
- **Hidden exercises:** The game also has hidden exercises for specific speech patterns, vocabulary and pronunciation.
- **Improving various skills:** The game also improves the learner's attention span, memory, concentration, reading, and listening skills.

Disadvantages of Game-based Teaching Methods

- **Time consuming:** This method may take a little longer as the teacher needs to spend time preparing and organizing the game. Choosing the right game and planning its implementation can be difficult.
- **Distraction:** Games can distract learners from the actual educational goals and leave the outcome of the teaching and learning process unattained.
- **Resources:** Some games require a lot of resources and materials to give learners the best possible experience,

and some games may have insufficient resource availability.
- **Nonproductive:** The inclusion of games creates a relaxed environment and increases the amount of nonproductive interaction between teacher and learner, which some teachers may perceive as non-productive.
- **Loss of interest:** Complex games can make students more likely to learn the rules of the game and distract them from the topic at hand.

INTERPROFESSIONAL EDUCATION

Interprofessional education (IPE) is an important approach to preparing students for entry into the medical field where teamwork and collaboration are key skills. IPE is being promoted by many global health organizations as part of the redesign of health care systems, promoting interprofessional teamwork to improve the quality of patient care and improve health outcomes.

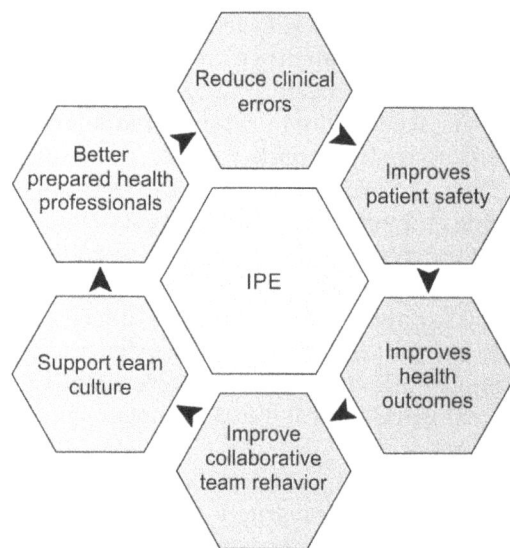

Fig. 7.51: Need of interpersonal education.

Definition

nterprofessional education occurs when students from two or more professions learn from each other, enable effective collaboration, and improve health.

Meaning

Interprofessional education is the study of students from two or more professions in the medical and social care professions together through all or part of their professional education. Refers to an opportunity to learn. Collaborative practice IPE is where two or more professionals learn together to improve collaborative care knowledge and skills and improve patient outcomes.
- The IPE is part of professional pre-registration programs (and some post-registration programs), especially nursing.
- IPEs come in many different formats, but most students find that the most effective format is a simulation.
- Most literature focuses on IPE and student assessment formats.
- Supports the effectiveness of IPE on patient and clinical outcomes hard evidence is inadequate.

Need for IPE

- Interprofessional practices provide collaborative, comprehensive care that is valued and expected by clients/patients.
- The goal of IPE is to train medical students with the knowledge, skills and attitudes necessary for interprofessional practice.

IPE Goals

The goal of the IPE is for students to learn how to function in interprofessional teams and to apply this knowledge and values to future practice. Ultimately, they provide interprofessional patient care as part of a collaborative team and improve patient focus outcomes. Interprofessional teams are made up of members from different health professions with specific knowledge, skills and competencies. The goal of the interprofessional team is to provide patient-centered care in a collaborative manner. The team sets common goals and uses individual expertise to achieve this patientcentered goal. Team members combine their observations and jobspecific expertise to collaborate and communicate as a team to achieve optimal patient care.

Key Challenges of IPE Facilitation

Although the role of facilitator is central to mediating group dynamics, team members are exposed to potential challenges that can arise in smaller teams. You will also have the opportunity to influence and solve critical issues. In student-centered learning, facilitators can find it difficult to support "teamwork" because not only do they need to support teams, but they also need to enable them to work independently. Often. Common barriers to effective teamwork include:
- Poor communication skills
- Different professional cultures
- Traditional hierarchies and assumed leadership.

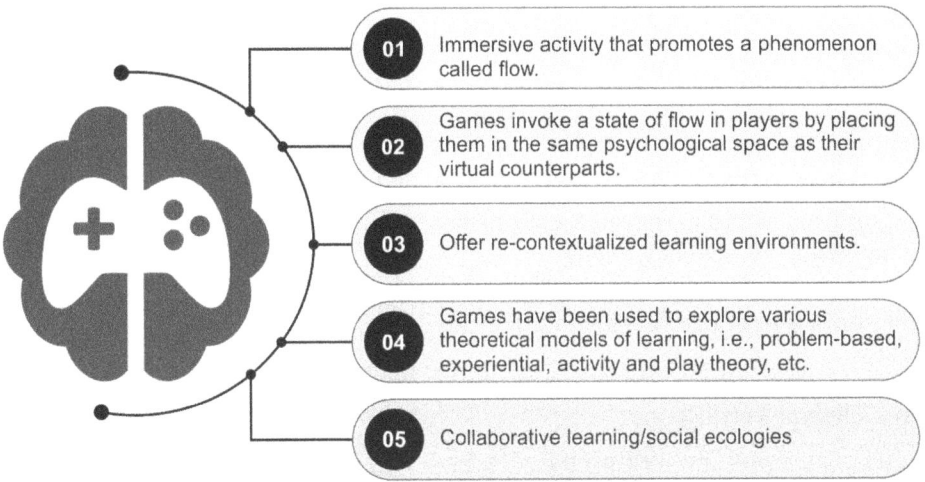

Fig. 7.52: Game-based learning theory.

Interprofessional education	Collaborative practice
Educator efforts 1. Staff training 2. Champions 3. Institutional support 4. Managerial commitment 5. Learning outcomes	*Institutional support* 1. Governance models 2. Structured protocols 3. Shared operating resources 4. Personnel policies 5. Supportive management
Curricular efforts 1. Logistics & Scheduling 2. Programme content 3. Compulsory attendance 4. Shared objectives 5. Adult learning principles 6. Learning methods 7. Contextual learning 8. Assessment	*Working culture and environment* 1. Communication strategies 2. Conflict resolution 3. Shared decision-making 4. Built environment 5. Facilities 6. Space design

Fig. 7.53: Difference between interprofessional education and collaborative practice.

Importance of IPE

Most health professional education is designed to develop the specialized knowledge needed to prepare newly qualified graduates for practice.

Achieving IPE learning goals can occur through planned shared learning experiences, but it can also occur through unscheduled encounters in which students are placed on clinical internships.

Agencies that support interprofessional collaboration work to develop and maintain effective interprofessional collaboration with learners, practitioners, patients/clients, families and communities.

Several options are available, including the Canadian Interprofessional Health Collaborative and the Interprofessional Education Collaborative (2016).

IPEs core competencies can be summarized in five topics:
1. Roles and responsibilities
2. Ethical practice
3. Conflict resolution
4. Communication
5. Collaboration and teamwork.

Preparation for Interprofessional Learning Activities

IPE offers opportunities for both formal and informal learning experiences. Informal experiences help students communicate and gain confidence in their field, while structured, formal experiences help beginners support their learning. When designing interprofessional activities, constructive coordination ensures that learning outcomes are directly related to activities and associated assessment tasks. This should be made clear to participating students at the start of the activity.

Moderation of interprofessional student groups is similar in theory and practice to moderation of interprofessional student groups, and the basics of planning and designing activities remain the same.

Promoting IPE

- Representatives, including students from various disciplines, are encouraged to participate in IPE programs and activities through collaborative planning, investment

of time, accountability, and commitment to promoting interprofessional learning.
- Facilitator's interprofessional leadership role modeling allows students to experience the collaborative nature of shared leadership that fosters trust and acceptance of interprofessional practice.
- It is important to promote scaffolding for student learning and support 'ownership' of student learning.
- Students should be encouraged to take responsibility for their own teaching and learning based on their current knowledge and skills.

Facilitating IPE in a Clinical Setting

Facilitators often feel competent and well-prepared to teach students in their field rather than students in other medical professions. Egan Lee et al. (2011) found that developing an interprofessional group of students in a clinical setting requires specific skills and attributes such as self-confidence, flexibility in managing professional conflicts, and commitment to IPE. Tips for fostering trust among medical professionals.
- Builds trust over time, be patient and work on building relationships
- A disagreement should not be interpreted as disrespect just differing opinion
- Offer your skills and knowledge with trust developing through your successes.

Common Barriers to Interprofessional Health Care

Organizational Barriers
- Lack of knowledge and appreciation of the roles of other health professionals.
- The need to make compelling arguments for team building to senior decision-makers.
- Lack of outcomes research on collaboration.
- Financial and regulatory constraints.
- Legal issues of scope of practice and liability.
- Reimbursement structures for different professions including which services receive reimbursement.
- Hierarchical administrative and educational structures that discourage interprofessional collaboration.

Barriers at the Team Level
- Lack of a clearly stated shared and measurable purpose
- Lack of training in interprofessional collaboration
- Role and leadership ambiguity
- Team too large or too small
- Team not composed of appropriate professionals
- Lack of appropriate mechanism for timely exchange of information
- Need for orientation for new members
- Lack of framework for problem discovery and resolution
- Difference in levels of authority power expertise income
- Difficulty in engaging the community
- Traditions/professional cultures particularly medicine's history of hierarchy
- Lack of commitment of team members
- Different goals of individual team members
- Apathy of team members
- Inadequate decision-making
- Conflict regarding individual relationships to the patient/client.

Advantages

Several advantages of IPE have been reported:
- Improved mutual respect and trust
- Improved understanding of job roles and responsibilities
- Effective communication
- Improved job satisfaction

PROGRAMMED LESSONS

Programmed lessons is a new innovation that is the result of experimental studies of the learning process in psychological laboratories. It is a self-study method for acquiring fact-based knowledge. An integrated teaching system that allows the use of programmed books that teach machine films on various forms of audio-visual equipment. Programmed instruction is self-directed instruction in which the learner reads the material in short steps at his/her own pace and immediately knows if the answer is correct.

Programmatic instruction is designed to monitor student response and provide feedback to students in patterns designed to maximize the transfer of learning. Attempts have been made since the time of Socrates. There have been attempts to systematically include the learner's own activities in the learning process.

Programmed statements are self-sufficient. It is so well planned and organized that, once programmed, it leads learners to successful learning without teacher intervention. Programmed education is a teaching technique that adapts to changing learning situations.

Definitions
- **Smith and Moore (1962):** Programmatic instruction is the process of placing the material to be learned into a series of sequential steps. It usually introduces students from familiar backgrounds to a complex and new set of concepts, principles, and understandings.

- **Jacobs et al. (1966):** Self-study programs are materials that students study. These programs can be used alone or in combination with other teaching techniques, with different types of students and learning content.
- **Espich and Williams (1967):** Programmed instruction is a planned series of experiences leading to stimulus response relational competencies that have been shown to be effective.
- **Leith (1966):** A program is a series of small steps in the material (called frames), most of which require responses by completing spaces within sentences. To ensure you get the expected answer, a hint system is applied and each answer is validated by knowing the outcome instantly. Such sequences should be treated as individual self-study at the learner's own pace.
- **Susan Markle (1969):** How to design a sequence of reproducible instrumental events to produce measurable and consistent effects on each acceptable student's behavior.
- **Gulati and Gulati (1976):** Programmed learning, as it is commonly understood, is a method of tutoring in which students are actively self-paced and see immediate results. Teachers do not physically exist. A programmer must follow the laws of conduct in developing programmed material and validate his strategy with respect to student learning.
- **NS Mavi (1984):** Programmed instruction teaches or selflearns live instrumental processes in the form of microsequences (topic segments) that the learner must read to get a correct or incorrect answer. It is a method for converting into materials that can be read by self-study. Answer or check the correct answer to fully master the concepts explained in the microsequence.

Program Statement Characteristics

- Programmed learning is a method or technique for giving and receiving individualized instruction, with or without teacher assistance, from a variety of sources, such as programmed textbooks or computers.
- In this method, the material is organized logically and divided into suitable small steps or segments of learning called frames.
- When sequencing a given unit of material, the programmer must consider the learner's initial start or start action and the end action or ability that the learner must achieve.
- In practice, the learner is presented with a framework, a small but meaningful section of the subject. Learners should read and listen and then actively respond.
- The learning system has reasonable provisions for immediate feedback based on reinforcement theory. For example, when responding to the first frame of programmed material, learners are informed of the correctness of their answers. If he is right, his answer is reinforced, and if he is wrong, he is able to correct himself by getting the correct answer and the learning material or program. Here students are motivated to actively learn and react.
- Provides self-clocking. Therefore, learning can be personal rather than general, depending on the learner's type of learning material and learning situation.
- Facilitates tangible learner responses that can be easily observed, measured and effectively controlled.
- It is intended for continuous evaluation to help improve student performance and the quality of the program material.

Program Teaching Principles

- **Small step principle:** This principle is based on the premise that people learn better when content is presented in appropriate small steps. Therefore, when preparing a program, programmers should strive to organize subjects into well-ordered and meaningful segments of information called frames. These segments must be presented to the learner for him to respond one at a time.
- **Active-response principle:** This principle is based on the assumption that learners learn better when they are active. Programmed learning allows learners to stay active by actively responding to each frame presented to them. Therefore, a good program should actively involve learners in the learning process. It should be designed so that the learner has little difficulty moving from one frame to another and remains meaningfully engaged and active by responding to the frames and acquiring knowledge incrementally.
- **Immediate reinforcement principle:** This principle is based on the psychological phenomenon of reinforcement. People learn better when they are motivated to learn by receiving information about the outcome immediately after answering. Therefore, good programs always take great care to provide immediate reinforcement by signaling the correctness of an answer.
- **Self-determined pace principle:** Programmed learning is a technique of tutoring. It is based on the basic premise that learning is better when individuals are allowed to learn at their own pace. A good program should always pay attention to the self-pacing principle. Materials should be programmed with the principle of individual differences in mind, and learners should be able to react and move from one frame to another at their own pace of learning.

- **Student examination principle:** For better learning, it is always good to strive for continuous evaluation of the learning process. The student examination principle meets this requirement. In program learning, learners must keep a record of their answers because they have to write their answers on the answer sheet for each frame. This detailed record will help you fix your program. It can also prove to be an excellent source of information for studying and improving the complex phenomena of human learning.

Program Teaching Benefits
- Students remain active and alert.
- Teachers are freed from their normal duties and can play an important role as mentors, motivators, and organizers.
- Social and emotional problems can be resolved.
- Domain problems were automatically resolved using self-study materials.
- Programmed lessons make learning interesting.
- Each student can work at their own workstation.
- Program instructions are useful in situations where human instructions are not available.
- Intellectual and some motor skills are taught more efficiently.
- More complex concepts may be known.

Types
There are two types of programmed instructions:
1. **Linear programming:** Linear programming is based strictly on the theory of conditioning learning. The main goal is to put the learner's behavior under control of different stimuli by using simple steps in sequence. Each step requires students to actively participate by providing answers.
2. **Branched programming:** Branched programming does not commit to learning theory. It is considered a technique for creating teaching materials covering a wide range of educational purposes. This is primarily for diagnostic purposes and is intended to allow students to provide the specific supporting material they need in selecting their answers.

Programmed Teaching
Programmed teaching is a new teaching method. This is a highly individualized behavior change education strategy. Used for educational purposes, but can also be used as a feedback mechanism to improve educational effectiveness. Theoretical knowledge of programmed instruction is essential for use as a feedback tool to modify teacher behavior in nursing education programs.

Program Instruction Assumptions
- Students learn better when they are motivated to learn by validating their answers
- Students learn better when content is taught in small steps.
- Students learn better when they minimize their mistakes while studying.
- Students learn better when a sequence of content is psychologically valid.
- Learning is effective when learners set prerequisites.

Program Education Characteristics
The main characteristics of the program education strategy are:
- Not an audiovisual device. It is part of educational technology, i.e., educational technology.
- Not a test. It is a new strategy for teaching and learning.
- It does not solve the education problem. A new educational problem. This is a new educational strategy to change learner behavior.
- You cannot replace teachers out of the classroom, but effective teachers can create great programs.
- Developing highly individualized instruction requires more creativity and ingenuity.

Steps for Developing Programmed Lessons
Developing programmed lessons is a very difficult task for teachers. Subject proficiency; for which knowledge and practice of programming education are essential. The following steps are important when preparing your programmed courseware.
- Select what to program.
- Target identification.
- Content analysis for developing course flow.
- Write the goals (appearance and end) in terms of behavior.
- Reference test structure.
- Determine appropriate program paradigms and strategies.
- Create a framework for your program and try it separately.
- As a group, try to revise and edit the program and develop a final proposal.
- Verification or evaluation of the master of the program on internal and external standards.
- Create a program manual.

Follow these steps to create effective program materials. This process is very time consuming and labor intensive. Program texts differ from traditional texts in that the practicality of the material is determined based on student responses.

Cons

- Requires an expert in programming instructions.
- Difficult and time consuming to prepare.
- No materials available.
- Requires special teaching ability.
- Requires a significant additional investment in teachers' time and money.
- No group dynamics.

CONCLUSION

From this chapter, all the nursing students will be able to understand different kinds of teaching methods in classroom and skill lab develop refined knowledge about information communication technology (ICT)—and its application in nursing education.

REVIEW QUESTIONS

Long Essays

1. Define teaching methods, explain the importance of educational methods.
2. Discuss the factors that determine the choice of teaching method.
3. Define classroom management, explain, goals, types, rules and procedures.
4. Describe educational management strategies.
5. Define information and communication technology (ICT), explain the characteristics and classifications.
6. Define lecture method, explain purposes, principles and benefits of lecture method.
7. Define microteaching, explain features, phases and advantages.
8. Define simulation, explain the steps involved in simulation method of teaching.
9. Define seminar method, explain the objectives, procedure and principles.
10. Define project, explain the features and principles of project method.
11. Define self-directed learning, explain goals, features and role of supervisors.
12. Define computer-assisted learning, explain the importance and types.
13. Define peer sharing, explain the principles, features and importance of peer learning.
14. Define interprofessional education (IPE), explain goals, challenges and importance.

Short Essays

1. Teaching objectives.
2. Types of teaching methods.
3. Classification of teaching methodology.
4. Characteristics of teaching methods.
5. The benefits of choosing the right teaching method.
6. Building good student–teacher relationships.
7. Dealing with student disciplinary situations.
8. Classroom management: Principles and strategies.
9. Factors affecting classroom management.
10. Techniques of classroom management.
11. Types of communication in the classroom.
12. Importance of communicating in the classroom.
13. Classroom communication facilitator.
14. Essential functions of facilitators.
15. Uses of ICT in education.
16. Communication barriers in the classroom.
17. Group discussion techniques.
18. Demonstration: Types and features.
19. Important steps in good demonstration.
20. Re-demonstration: Objectives and principles.
21. Panel discussion: Techniques.
22. Workshop: Principles, benefits and evaluation of workshop.

23. Role play: Purposes, steps and factors influences role play.
24. Field trip: Purposes, types and responsibilities of teacher in field visits.
25. Using computers in the classroom.
26. Concept of one-on-one instruction.
27. Active learning strategies.
28. Team-based learning steps.
29. Problem-based learning: Characteristics, principles and types.
30. Steps to PBL approach.
31. Benefits of using case studies in teaching.
32. Journaling: Features and rules.
33. Journal organization.
34. Journaling in the classroom.
35. Student's skill development in debate.
36. Game-based learning.
37. Benefits of game-based teaching methods.
38. Common barriers to interprofessional health care.
39. Facilitating IPE in a clinical setting.
40. Programmed lessons: Characteristics, principles and types.
41. Steps for developing programmed lessons.

Short Answers

1. Demonstrations.
2. Programmed instruction.
3. Discussion methods.
4. Case analysis methodology.
5. Case incident method.
6. Bedside clinic.
7. Competency-based education.
8. Interprofessional nursing.
9. Interprofessional learning.
10. Classroom climate.
11. Types of classroom interactions.
12. Factors affecting communication.
13. Barriers to effective communication.
14. Benefits of using ICT in education.
15. Define group discussion.
16. Panel discussion.
17. Teacher-student conference.
18. Disadvantages of demonstration.
19. Benefits of role-playing in nursing.
20. Criteria for selecting a project.
21. Benefits of CAL.
22. Benefits of active learning.
23. Team-based learning.
24. Benefits of PBL.
25. Important for the magazine.
26. Types of journals.
27. Debating tips and techniques.
28. Different types of GBL.
29. Disadvantages of game-based teaching methods.
30. Program education characteristics.

Unit 4

Clinical Teaching Methods

Chapter

8. Teaching in the Clinical Setting

KEYWORDS

Clinical Supervisor: Most responsible faculty member to whom the trainee directly reports during a training experience.
Clinical teaching unit (CTU): Teaching unit consisting of various levels of trainees who work with faculty members and interdisciplinary healthcare professionals to care for patients.
Clinical teaching unit director: A faculty member within the program responsible for the educational activities, supervision, and safety of trainees within a CTU.
Competence: Array of abilities across multiple domains or aspects of physician performance. Competence is both conditional on, and constrained by, each physician's practice context, is dynamic, and continually changes over time.
Competency-based medical education (CBME): Overarching term referring to a competency-based, outcomes-based model of medical training.
Indirect observation: Process of assessment where the assessor utilizes indirect methods to assess attainment of competencies (e.g., case presentation, chart documentation).
Authentic learning: Learning situations where students work on real-world experiences and challenges.
Benchmark: A standard for judging performance.
Blended course: A course that combines two modes of instruction, online and face-to-face.
Class period: A segment of time in the school day that is approximately one-sixth of the instructional day.
Core curriculum: The body of knowledge that all students are expected to learn in the subjects of English, Mathematics, History/Social Science and Science.
Counseling: Consists of professional advisement and interpretive services with children or adults for amelioration or prevention of problems that impact education.
Curriculum: A plan or document that a school or school division uses to define what will be taught and the methods that will be used to educate and assess students.
Curriculum alignment: Occurs when local curricula and classroom instruction include or exceed the content, knowledge and skills described by the standards of learning.

Deeper learning: Students demonstrate knowledge through six competencies: Mastering core academic content, thinking critically and solving complex problems, working collaboratively, communicating effectively, learning how to learn, and developing academic mindsets.

Digital learning: Any instructional practice that uses technology to support student learning, including digital learning content (which may include openly licensed content, software or simulations).

Electronic learning (eLearning): Education in which instruction and content are delivered primarily over the Internet; synonymous with online learning, cyber learning and virtual learning.

Full-time online program: A program that allows students to take a full load of online courses.

Mentor (online): A person working face-to-face with an online student to provide physical supervision and support. A mentor may or may not be a certified teacher but works in conjunction with the certified online teacher.

Non-academic competencies: Skills, habits, and attitudes students need to prosper both at school and in the wider world, such as persistence and creativity.

Norm-referenced tests: Standardized tests designed to measure how a student's performance compares with that of other students.

Online course: Any course offered over the internet; synonymous with e-course, virtual course and cyber course.

Online learning: Education in which instruction and content are delivered primarily over the internet; synonymous with e-learning, cyber learning and virtual learning.

Online learning program: An organized offering of courses delivered primarily over the internet; synonymous with eLearning program, cyber learning and virtual learning.

Pedagogy: Instructional methods, practices, techniques and strategies.

Planning period: One class period per day (or the equivalent) unencumbered of any teaching or supervisory duties.

Portfolio: A collection of student work chosen to exemplify and document a student's learning progress over time.

Professional/staff development: Training for teachers, principals, superintendents, administrative staff, local school board members and board of education members designed to enhance student achievement and is required by the standards of quality.

Project-based learning: An educational approach emphasizing creativity and critical thinking which uses broad, complex problems as a method for learning both content and skills.

Chapter 8: Teaching in the Clinical Setting

Learning Objectives

- Meaning of Clinical Teaching
- Clinical Learning Environment
- Factors Influences Clinical Learning Experience Selection
- Teaching Models in Clinical Use
- Clinical Learning Outcomes/Practical Skills
- Clinical Instructor
- Applying Clinical Teaching Methods in Education
- Clinical Education Issues
- Clinical Teaching Skills
- Clinical Teaching Challenges
- Clinical Teaching Strategies
- Patient Order/Assignment
- Clinical Meetings: Individual and Group
- Concept Mapping
- Problem-based Learning
- Process Recording Teaching

TERMINOLOGY

Preceptor: A physician who provides supervised, clinical-based training in which the learner is immersed in a physician's practice for a period of time.

Clinical supervisor: A clinician who oversees the clinical work of one or more trainees and is the attending physician.

Clinician teacher: A physician or senior resident who acts as a supervisor, imparts knowledge, provides feedback, and is an exemplary part-time teacher, emphasizing competence, professionalism, and enthusiasm for medicine.

Clinician educator: A physician with formal expertise in medical education (such as a graduate degree or other program) who consults and advises on educational issues and faculty efforts in the medical profession.

School of medicine: One or more individuals, usually in charge of teaching, research, administration, and clinical care, while attending the medical school of a university.

Role model: Someone who inspires learners and teaches by example as part of their professional work. It could be the teacher's supervisor or peer.

Mentor: A trusted individual or group of people who provide wisdom or advice on personal or professional matters.

INTRODUCTION

Clinical education is defined as teaching and learning that focuses on, and usually directly engages, patients and their problems. The clinical setting comprises inpatient, outpatient, and community settings, each with its own set of challenges. In such an environment, students learn what it means to be a real doctor. Skills such as history taking physical examination patient communication and professionalism are best learned in the clinical setting

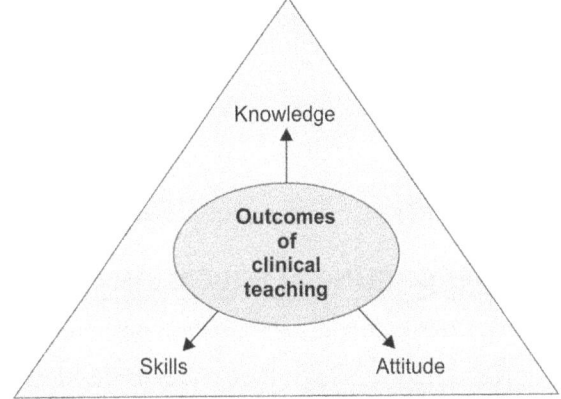

Fig. 8.1: Domains of clinical teaching.

medical knowledge is directly applied to patient care trainees begin to be motivated by relevance and self-directed learning takes on a new meaning.

Teaching in the clinical setting often takes place in the course of routine clinical care where discussion and decision-making take place in real time. Often the teaching will center on an analysis of actual patient care that the student has undertaken. This is the most common pattern for postgraduate trainees. Undergraduate students benefit from additional sessions specifically planned for teaching.

DEFINITION

The clinical teaching method in nursing is a type of group conference in which a patient or patients are observed studied discussed demonstrated and directed towards the improvement and further improvement of nursing care provided by the nursing student.

MEANING OF CLINICAL TEACHING

Clinical teaching is a teaching learning experience of the students in the clinical setting field such as hospitals clinics and community health centers, etc. Clinical instruction is planned by a nursing school/university tutor/lecturer and performed by a clinical trainer who accompanies the student in the clinical setting. Various other medical team members also participate in clinical education programs such as: examples—ward doctors, nurses, nutritionists, physiotherapists, etc.

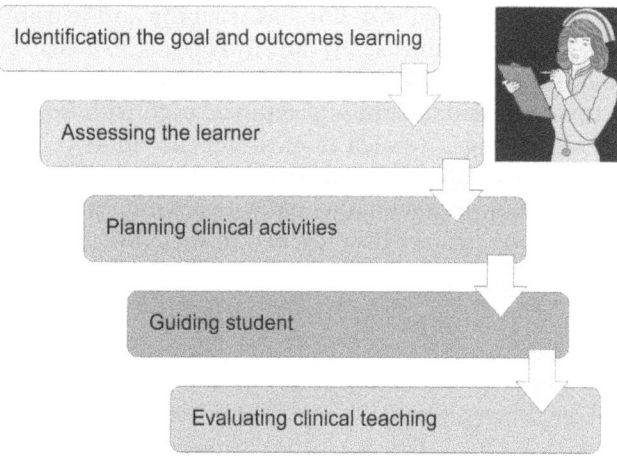

Fig. 8.2: Chart of process of clinical teaching.

OBJECTIVES OF CLINICAL EDUCATION

- Individualized care with a systematic, holistic approach.
- Acquire high technical skills.
- Practice different procedures.
- Collect and analyze data.
- Do research.
- Maintain high standards of nursing practice.
- Become self-employed and practice nursing.
- Development of cognitive, motivational, emotional and psychomotor skills.
- Students acquire skills such as surveillance.
- We will meet your needs.
- Improving standards in nursing practice.
- Development of different care delivery methods.
- To identify your problem.
- Learn various diagnostic procedures.
- Learn a variety of skills to teach clients, as well as other important health education techniques.
- Assistance in integrating theoretical knowledge into practice.
- Develop communication skills and develop interpersonal relationships.
- Maintain interorganizational relationships.
- Increase the ability and efficiency of performing various nursing procedures.
- Assisting physicians in assisting treatment.
- Learn management skills.
- Become a professional member.
- Face reality in the practice of the nursing learning exercises described in the course objectives.

USE OF CLINICAL EDUCATION

- Serves as a way to meet the individual needs of learners
- Creates optimal learning environments that facilitate learners' socialization as nurses.
- Promotes learner development by improving psychomotor skills and a positive attitude.
- Encourages students to face compassionate situations.
- Puts real-life experience and knowledge into practice.

CLINICAL LEARNING ENVIRONMENT

Nursing trainees are assessed in a clinical learning environment that applies their skills and knowledge to patient care. These environments influence the achievement of learning outcomes and influence student readiness for practice and satisfaction with the nursing profession. Articulating this concept into nursing education helps identify the antecedent attributes and consequences that influence students' transition to practice.

A good learning environment for students in clinical practice should include clear structures to provide students with an educational environment in which staff are interested in supervising students and easy to contact, as well as a strong relationship between educators and nursing teachers. It depends on the commitment and collaboration between them.

Definition

- A clinical learning environment (CLE) is essentially where students (and other learners) learn about patient care. From the bedside to her team's room, from the emergency room to the operating room, clinics and wards.
- A clinical learning environment (CLE) is defined as an interactive network of forces that influence clinical learning outcomes (CLO). The CLO is a statement of what students are expected to understand and demonstrate at the end of their clinical practice.

Attribute properties: The clinical learning environment contains four attribute traits that influence the student's learning experience.
1. Physical space
2. Psychosocial and interaction factors
3. Organizational culture
4. Components of teaching and learning.

Factors influencing the clinical learning environment:
- Stressors in the learning environment
- Inclusion
- Teacher-colleague relationships
- Professionalism
- Mental health/well-being curriculum
- Hours/shifts
- Feedback systems
- Pedagogy.

The importance of a good clinical learning environment:
- Effective learning puts the student at the center of the learning experience. Students are given the opportunity and space to take responsibility for their own learning, gain learning experience, and develop their own practice, all without compromising public safety.
- The level or format of supervision may be reduced or changed as the student gains competence and confidence.
- An effective learning environment provides opportunities for meaningful learning experiences that help students achieve learning outcomes. This means that it varies according to the student's learning outcomes, the stage of learning and the environment in which they are learning.
- A variety of settings enable effective learning experiences, allowing students to learn and enhance different skills in different environments and situations. The learning experience should cover the full range of nursing relevant to the student's field or area of practice.
- The culture of an effective learning environment should be learning-oriented and everyone in the learning environment should understand their role in enabling learning.
- An effective learning experience also takes into account equality and diversity considerations, or appropriate adjustments that need to be made in learning and student assessment.

FACTORS INFLUENCES CLINICAL LEARNING EXPERIENCE SELECTION

Learning experience selection deals with decisions regarding the theoretical and practical experiences that must be provided to students undergoing educational programs. This section will help you understand the conceptual basis and criteria for choosing learning experiences. Effective clinical teaching and learning are influenced by many factors. Clinical education is planned and delivered according to professional social, environmental, and educational expectations and needs, using the human intellectual, physical, and financial resources available in the context of the curriculum provided by faculty within the curriculum.

Principles for the Selection of Learning Experiences

- Selection of learning experiences should be made considering the philosophy, purposes and objectives of the program.
- Learning activities must relate to real life situations that students are expected to practice after earning the qualification.
- Selections should be made in such a way that theory and practice are effectively integrated, between what is taught in class and what is practiced in learning situations.
- Choose experiences that help students learn effectively and provide opportunities to perform the specific tasks of the expected job.
- Focus in choosing learning experiences. Learning situations and learning activities should focus on helping students learn.
  - Provides community-oriented services.
  - Meet national demand for medical needs.
  - Emphasis on primary prevention.
  - It provides care at all three levels of healthcare: primary, secondary and tertiary levels.
  - The values of case care; the arts of nursing and the science of nursing.
- Selected learning activities should be designed to promote logical and analytical thinking in students.

Criteria for Selecting Learning Experiences

- The learning experience chosen must be consistent with the school's philosophy and lead to the achievement of the program's ultimate goals.

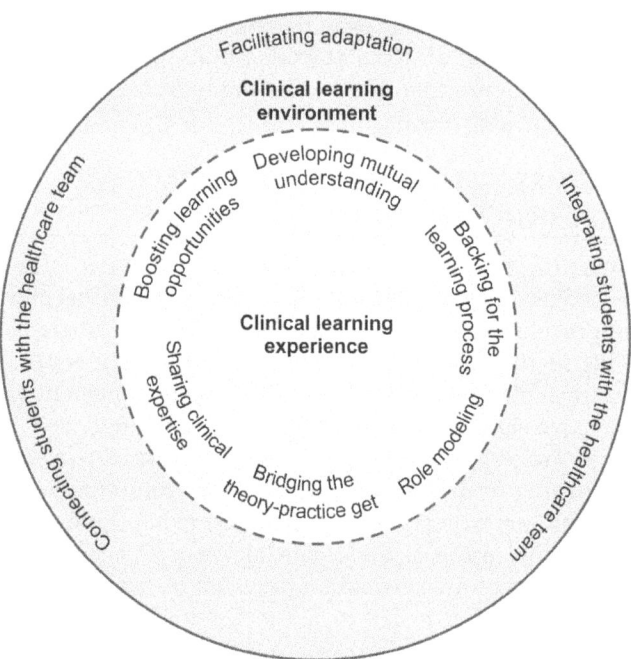

Fig. 8.3: Principles for the selection of learning experiences.

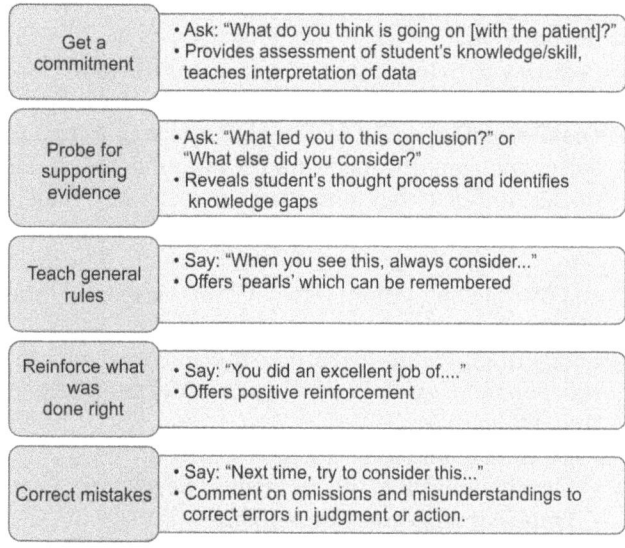

Fig. 8.4: Criteria for selecting learning experiences.

- The learning experience should be varied and flexible enough to take into account the learner's ability to change desired behaviors, not beyond individual developmental levels.
- You should choose learning experiences that provide students with opportunities to practice the behaviors included in the objectives. Adequate opportunities for self-reliance should be provided so that the transfer of acquired knowledge, skills, and desired attitudes becomes a habit.
- Learning experiences should provide opportunities to develop independent thinking and decision-making, sound judgment, intellectual resourcefulness, self-discipline, and firm resolve.
- The learning experience should be tailored to the student's needs so that the behaviors included in the goals are satisfying.
- The learning experience is arranged in a way that provides a continuous correlation and integration of theory and practice, and clinical learning experience.
- The learning experience is planned and assessed jointly by the teacher and the student. If teachers and students can plan assessments together, the variety of experiences offered can be effectively interesting and useful.
- Learning experiences are selected and arranged to give age appropriate emphasis and weight according to the relative importance of different learning experiences and content.

TEACHING MODELS IN CLINICAL USE

Two clinical teaching models have been used successfully for development by clinical teachers. Both models are behaviorbased and can be adapted by clinical teachers to any clinical situation. The first is the stanford faculty development model for clinical teaching and the second is the micro skills of teaching model, also known as the one minute preceptor.

Stanford Faculty Development Model

Categories are:
- **Foster a positive learning environment:** The learning environment is defined as the tone or atmosphere of the classroom environment. This includes whether it is stimulating and whether learners can easily identify and address their own limitations. It creates conditions for effective teaching and learning.
- **Session control:** This refers to how classroom interactions are focused and timed, influenced by the teacher's leadership style. It reflects the group dynamics that influence the efficiency and focus of all classroom interactions.
- **Targeted communication:** This includes defining and articulating what teachers and learners expect from learners. Goal setting provides structure for the educational process, guides teachers in planning lessons, and provides a basis for assessment.
- **Encourage comprehension and memorization:** Comprehension is the ability to analyze, synthesize,

and correctly apply; memorization is the process of memorizing facts or concepts. This category looks at the approaches teachers can use to describe the content being taught and interact with it in meaningful ways so that learners can understand and retain it.

- **Assessment:** This is the process by which teachers assess learners' knowledge, skills, and attitudes against pre-established educational goals. Teachers can see where learners are, which helps them plan future lessons and assess lesson effectiveness. Assessment can be formative to assess the learner's continued progress towards educational goals or summative for final assessment to measure the learner's achievement of the goals.
- **Feedback:** Feedback is the process by which teachers provide learners with information about their performance and potential improvements. It provides a teaching loop where teachers can guide learners to reassess their goal achievement using performance assessments.

The One-Minute-Teacher

Teaching "microskills", also known as the one-minute teacher due to the short amount of time available for teaching in a clinical setting provide a framework.

The original microskills model used a five-step approach.

- **Step 1—make a promise:** Teachers encourage learners to articulate their opinions regarding differential diagnosis and treatment, rather than stating their own conclusions or plans. Teachers need to create a safe learning environment so that learners feel safe enough to risk their commitments, even if it is wrong.
- **Step 2—seek supporting evidence:** Teachers should encourage learners to "think out loud" and give reasons to focus on the diagnosis, treatment, or other aspect of the patient's problem. Teachers should either validate the learner's commitment or gently reject it if it falls short.
- **Step 3—teach general rules:** Teachers can help learners understand how what one patient is learning can be applied to other situations. Learners are prepared for new information applicable to both specific patients and future patients. If the learner is doing well and the teacher has nothing to add, this microskill can be skipped.
- **Step 4—reinforce:** What you do well whenever a trainee does well in a patient care situation, it is appropriate to use this microskill. Effective reinforcement must be concrete and action-based, not vague. Positive feedback also boosts the trainee's self-esteem.
- **Step 5—right wrong:** Negative or constructive feedback is often avoided by clinical teachers, but is essential for good patient care. Encouraging self-assessment is a good way to get learners to identify their own mistakes, and once they do, they can receive positive feedback on their self-reflection skills. If any, it should be timely and fully action based.

DESCRIPTION OF CLINICAL LEARNING OUTCOMES/PRACTICAL SKILLS

Writing effective learning outcomes is essential for clinical practice skill. A learning objective is a specific, clearly formulated statement about a learner's observable behavior, which can be measured after completion of an educational activity. They form the basis of instructional orientation as

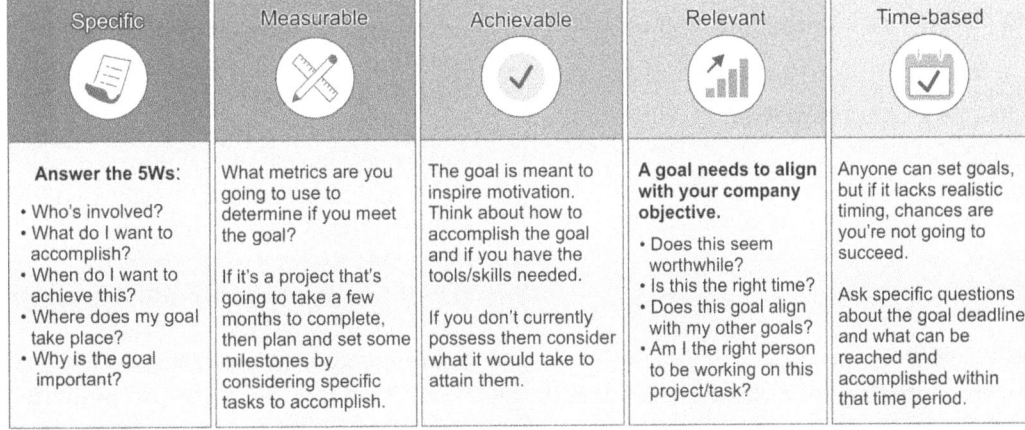

Fig. 8.5: Writing effective learning outcomes in clinical practice.

learning objective assessment instruments and teaching methods support each other for desired learning outcomes. A learning objective is a statement of what the learner should be able to do after completing the educational activity. A well-written learning objective outlines the knowledge skills and/or attitude the learners will gain from the educational activity and does so in a measurable way.

Well defined learning objectives describe what the learner must be able to achieve upon completion of the educational activity. Bloom's Taxonomy and SMART are two tools that educators may leverage towards writing learning objectives that effectively relate the intended outcomes to the learners simultaneously setting up the educators to successfully attain the learning outcomes within the time and resources provided. The successful academic anesthesiologist can align the instructional method assessment and intended learning outcome by using SMART learning objectives rather than learning goals.

CLINICAL INSTRUCTOR

The clinical instructor or primary nurse should select clinical areas where patients need appropriate care and provide students with opportunities to demonstrate high standards of nursing practice. Clinical instructors and lead nurses should consider the needs of students in developing individuals to higher levels of functioning. Select areas where instructors have the opportunity to teach and students have the opportunity to learn, according to the requirements set by the institution. Identify nursing staff (head nurses and nurse specialists) who are interested in participating in nursing discussions and participating in conferences, nursing rounds, and other meetings where clinical conditions are discussed. Competent teachers should be available. Primary nurses and trainers should work together to plan and deliver improved nursing practice.

Clinical Teacher Key Characteristics

- Clinical competence
- Non-judgmental
- Role model
- Enthusiasm
- Feedback skills
- Availability
- Respect learner autonomy

The most important attribute of a clinical teacher is to possess:
- Competence (clinical skills)
- Availability (physical availability at bedside at all times)
- Kindness (friendly gentle grace indicates warmth and kindness).

Clinical instructor functions:
- Set practice goals.
- Develop evaluation tools.
- Laboratory approval must be sought.
- Prepare a master rotation plan.
- Optimally set up the treatment area.
- Store equipment readily accessible for care.
- The clinical instructor has primary responsibility for planning the direction of the educational program within the clinical area of student's experience.
- Clinical trainers must adhere to standards of nursing practice.
- Clinical instructor has to direct and supervise the students in providing client's care.
- Assist in patient care and role model.
- Demonstrate nursing procedures on patients and ask the students to re-demonstrate procedures to develop skill and confidence.
- Improve research understanding for better patient care.
- Analyze difficulties and guide students accordingly.
- Maintain high standards of patient care.
- Encourage motivate and inspire students.
- Supervise and evaluate the performance of students.
- Maintain strict discipline.
- Maintain student files such as rota rolls, individual tasks, assessment tools, clinical teaching, and student performance.
- Conduct one-to-on-one interviews with students to resolve issues that arise and address their professional and personal needs.
- Attend scheduled lectures (by physicians) for students and arrange presentations on the subject. Bring in customers and have them ready overhead? projectors and more.
- Must attend faculty meetings.
- Draws the student's attention to the medical and nursing problems of the client to whom he or she is assigned.
- Help students develop the ability to tailor general care plans to individual patient needs.
- Help students develop lesson plans.
- Skillfully indicate which nursing procedures are of particular importance in each area.
- Help students learn new skills.
- Direct students to create and prepare their clinical assignments using library resources.
- Guide students in conducting nursing research activities.
- To develop the potential of each student.

Clinical instructor qualities
- Compassionate towards nursing.
- She should be a nursing professional.
- She must have good communication skills and build good relationships with the nursing staff.
- She must know how to provide care.
- Trust because the success of clinical nursing depends on the ability to engage physicians, primary nurses, nurses, other professionals, technicians and support staff, and to work well with others must be maintained.
- A reasonable theoretical background is required.
- Have advanced knowledge in advanced fields such as educational psychology and specialized fields.
- You should enjoy teaching students about hospital conditions.
- She should be appointed on the basis of her outstanding ability.
- Ability to put knowledge into practice.
- Ability to impart knowledge.
- Must have good teaching skills.
- Physically active.
- A very healthy healthy smile and a pleasant personality.
- Well-groomed (well-balanced).
- She is polite.
- Sensitive and caring.
- Must understand the overall care program.
- Must have detailed knowledge of the field in which she is employed.
- Should have a positive life philosophy.
- Must be familiar with teaching and assessment methods.
- Must maintain good working relationships.
- She should be responsible for all experiences in her clinical area.
- She must participate in professional activities.
- Maintain a favorable environment conducive to democracy.
- Freedom of expression must be protected.
- A clinical nursing instructor's primary responsibility is to teach nursing students in a clinical setting such as a hospital/clinic/community.
- Sufficient study time must be provided before grades are assessed.
- Teachers and learners share responsibility for maintaining this environment, but ultimately teachers are responsible.
- Build expectations that teachers and students will partner to achieve success.
- Educators should identify the knowledge skills and attitudes that are most important for students to learn. Learners should spend most of their time on this basic curriculum.

APPLYING CLINICAL TEACHING METHODS IN EDUCATION

Clinical teaching methods in teaching involve the use of models of the decision-making process used by physicians. Additionally, it utilizes the models used to train medical interns to enhance their clinical judgment and relevant knowledge. Several key features of the medical model help us understand classroom practice and teacher education.

How to Use the Clinical Teaching Method

- Teachers use evidence of what students have learned and want to learn to make instructional decisions.
- Current research is being used by teachers regarding effective practices in making decisions about how to work with students or groups of students.
- Integrate student information, characteristics and previous experience to make decisions about students and teaching methods.
- The impact of instruction on student learning is evaluated on a regular basis.
- Teachers must use professional judgment to understand students and determine what, when and how to teach.
- Through shared understanding and reasoning and commitment to practice, a strong link is established between the course and practical application.
- There must be a common community of practice.
- Requires professional discussion between novices and mentors, including clearly justified questions.

CLINICAL EDUCATION ISSUES

The following are examples of such issues, but are not exhaustive.
- Lack of clear goals and expectations.
- Teaching at the wrong level.
- Focuses on memorizing facts rather than solving problems.
- Lack of active participation by learners.
- Insufficient direct observation and feedback of learners.
- Not enough time for reflection and discussion.
- Lack of consistency with the rest of the curriculum.

Skills that Make Clinical Teachers

- Share a passion for teaching.
- Clearly organized, friendly, supportive, and caring.
- Empathize, give instructions and give feedback.
- Demonstrate honesty and respect for others.
- Demonstration of clinical competence.
- Use planning and orientation strategies.
- Has a broad repertoire of teaching methods and scripts.

- Work on self-evaluation and reflection.
- Uses multiple forms of knowledge. They adapt the lessons to the knowledge level of the learners.

CLINICAL TEACHING SKILLS

The clinical teacher utilizes a wide range of communication skills and behaviors and can be viewed as selecting specific techniques appropriate to the situation at hand. The repertoire of communication skills required ranges from a group that can be called "watchful silence" for passive teacher attitudes to what is called "cooperative negotiation" when teachers and learners have fairly similar attitudes. Groups, extending to groups with the term "persuasive". Conflict" is when the teacher takes an aggressive and dominant position in the relationship.

- **Aware silence:** Indicates that the teacher is paying attention and gives the learner time to think.
- **Chasing:** "nods and grunts" of understanding and general agreement.
- **Overt encouragement and advocacy:** Not completely fearless, but provides a supportive learning environment.
- **Surface paraphrasing and exploration:** To help the teacher gain additional general information from the learner.
- **Self-disclosure:** To strengthen the teacher's image and credibility by revealing personal experiences "war stories" difficult cases and mistakes.
- **Active listening:** To probe the learner's thinking for purposes of clarification expansion justification and correlation.
- **Intense paraphrasing:** This allows the teacher to more aggressively question the learner for specific information or for specific responses.
- **Open-ended questioning:** To expand the discussion and to stimulate the learner to consider several choices.
- **Giving positive and negative feedback:** This allows teachers to give negative information so that learners can improve their future performance.
- **Critical correction and closed question:** Provide learners with summative assessment (above) and learners' knowledge in a focused and convergent style.

CLINICAL TEACHING CHALLENGES

Challenge ancient knowledge and old attitudes to provide students with new knowledge and attitudes persuade to accept.

General

- Time constraints.
- **Work demands:** Teachers maintain other clinical research or administrative duties while called to teach.
- Often unpredictable and difficult to prepare.
- Multiple levels of involved learning (dormitory officers, etc.).
- **Patient-related challenges:** Short hospital stays. Patients very ill or unwilling to attend educational events.
- Lack of incentives and rewards for education.
- Physical clinical environment not comfortable for education.

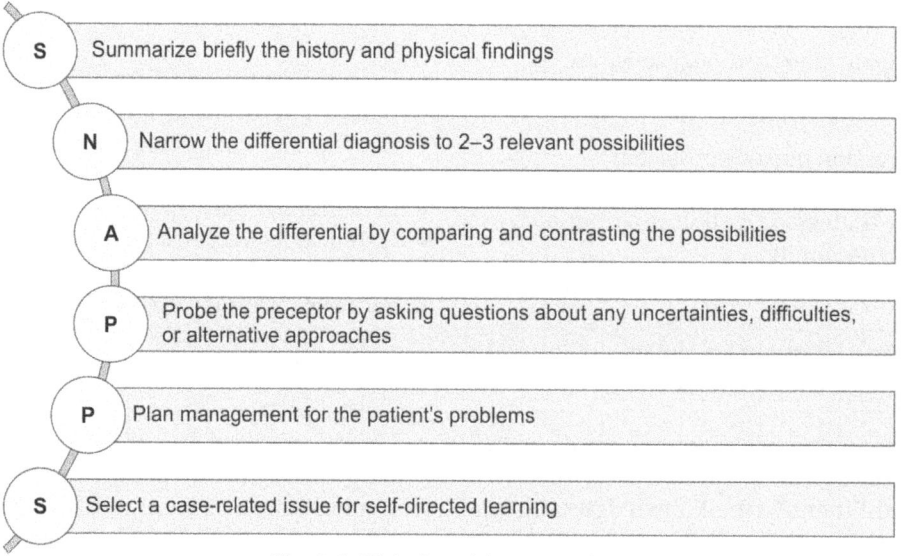

Fig. 8.6: Clinical teaching strategies.

Inpatient Education Challenges

- Difficult to set teaching goals, unanticipated events occur frequently.
- Station teams are usually made up of different levels of learners.
- Patients too sick or unwilling to participate in the teaching encounter.
- Patients are too short in hospital to follow the natural history of the disease.
- Teachers' dominance of face-to-face interactions can compromise student-patient relationships.
- Training Mistakes students and teachers make in front of patients and other members of the medical team who are anxious about hospitalization.
- Many clinical teachers tend to lecture rather than practice interactive teaching.
- Engaging all learners simultaneously can be difficult.
- Teachers need to pay close attention to learner fatigue boredom and workload.

Challenges of Outpatient Teaching

- Teaching time often short no time for elaborate teaching.
- No control over distribution and organization of time.
- Attending to several patients at the same time with multiple learners.
- Simple interaction between teacher and trainee.
- Patient care needs are usually a priority and need to be addressed.
- Multiple patient issues need to be addressed simultaneously.
- Learning and ministry occur simultaneously.
- Organic and psychosocial issues are intertwined.
- Diagnostic questions are often resolved with empiric treatment follow-up.

CLINICAL TEACHING STRATEGIES

Clinical teaching strategies involve interpersonal communication between teachers, students and study groups. This technique helps identify problems and teaches relevant skills to give you the knowledge to understand and solve them.

Clinical Skills in Clinical Teaching

- **Develop diagnostic thinking expertise:** Experience with a variety of analytical and nonanalytical strategies is required. Analytical techniques include the generation of formal hypotheses to keep diagnostic possibilities open and eliminate the possibility of premature conclusions during the inference process.
- **Current issue:** Helps improve pattern recognition by inducing memory. This will help you acquire relevant knowledge. Further research may be needed for semantic applications of clinical techniques if the performance is contextual.
- **Hypothesis generation:** This uses strategies such as contrasting approaches. The similarities and differences of competing diagnoses should be compared simultaneously. Using a contrasting approach, students can use ratios of key features of more common symptoms.
- **Evidence-based physical examination:** This has not been mainstreamed into educational practice due to the unwillingness to avoid the unreliable component of inquiry from clinical teaching and learning. Practicing and learning outdated operations leaves students with less time to acquire useful skills in clinical practice.
- **Psychomotor skills:** These are required to perform individual operations. These facilitate conscious piloting practice and recognition of abnormal signs.
- **Communication skills:** Building rapport with patients and ensuring teamwork with other healthcare professionals is critical to accurate and efficient data collection. Because communication skills are taught as a separate subject, students may be presented with advanced skills long before they apply them to clinical practice. This is a drawback in the medical field.

Principles for Improving Teacher

Learner relationships in clinical education:

- **Practical application of concepts:** Adults often want to apply what they have learned. This principle is less violated in clinical education than in other areas of medical education. Clinical teachers should aim to justify something that has not been shown to be directly or indirectly applicable in a particular clinical situation.
- **Interested in problem-solving, not just learning facts:** Clinical teachers focus on using theory, not just learning it.
- **Active participation in the learning process by setting learning goals:** Teachers have the appropriate knowledge and experience to negotiate goals, required resources, and overarching educational goals with learners. This is important to lead to better results through higher levels of motivation.
- **Feedback on progress:** Formative assessment is necessary to help students understand how they are doing. Clinical teachers make relevant comments, especially negative comments, to effect changes in student professional behavior. This will help you make better decisions and acquire skills. Such feedback bridges the gap between teachers and learners, leading to better learning outcomes.

PATIENT ORDER/ASSIGNMENT

Order means "a written assignment of duties to care for a group of patients by trained personnel assigned to the unit".

Purpose

- Delegate tasks to be done to nursing staff.
- Obtain cooperation from nurses by knowing and accepting the work to be done.
- To organize the work systematically.
- To prepare and motivate the nurses for delivery of care.
- To shoulder accountability.

Principles of Patient Assignment

- Prepared by the lead nurse for the individual nurse.
- Planned weekly and revised daily to ensure continuity of care.
- Must be balanced among nurses.
- Never assign the same task to multiple nurses rationale:
  - Each patient's need for care.
  - Skill experience capabilities of each staff.
  - Job description.

Factors Affecting Patient Assignment

- Patient characteristics.
- Nursing resource.
- Organization support.
- Type of nursing care delivery system.

Challenges In Patient Assignment

- Problem of personal management.
- Shortage of trained manpower.
- Lack of adequate training.
- No involvement in planning.
- No autonomy in nursing activities.
- Inadequate number of nursing staff.

Methods of Patient Assignment

- Case method nursing or total patient care.
- Functional nursing.
- Team nursing or modular nursing.
- Primary nursing.
- Case management or managed care.
- Progressive patient care.

Case Method

- The case method or total patient care method of nursing care delivery is the oldest method of providing care to a patient.

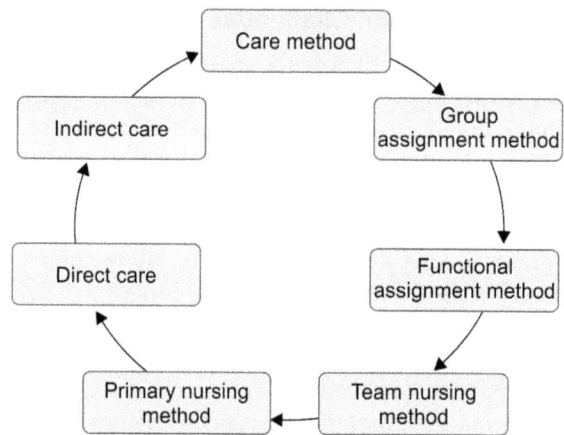

Fig. 8.7: Methods of patient assignment.

- In this method nurses assume total responsibility for meeting all the needs of assigned patient during their time on duty.
- The premise of the case method is that one nurse provides total care to one patient during her entire work period of one shift.
- This method was used in the time of Florence Nightingale and the patient was fully cared for at home.
- Nurses were 'employed' at the time, living with the patient's family and caring for the patient and family around the clock.
- A patient is continuously cared for by a nurse during her 8 to 12 hours shift. Nurses and patient families share mutual trust and work together toward specific goals.
- As a matter of principle, care is patient-centered, comprehensive, comprehensive and continuous.

Benefits

- Nurses can see better and respond to the holistic needs of the patient.
- Continuity of care is facilitated.
- Client-nurse interaction and relationships can be built.
- Clients feel more secure.
- Built-in accountability for the nurse's role.
- Family friends become known to caregivers and become more involved.
- You can evenly distribute the workload among staff.

Disadvantages

- Many clients do not require specific care.
- Needs modification if non-specialized medical staff is used.
- Major disadvantages if caregivers are untrained
- Cost effective when most of her assigned patients are sick.

Primary Nursing Care

- It was developed in the 1960s with the aim of placing RNs at the bedside and improving the professional relationships among staff members.
- This method is based on the concept of 'my patient – my nurse'. In this system of care, each registered nurse is assigned to a patient's care group to plan her full around-the-clock care and develop a care plan.
- He or she is responsible for coordinating and providing all necessary care that must be provided to the patient during the shift.
- In the absence of a nurse, the patient's inpatient care is taken over by an assistant nurse in charge of the nurse's absence, based on the original care plan created by the nurse.
- This type of care can also be used in hospice care and home care.
- Provides complete direct patient care.
- We need a nursing staff for all nurses.

Features

- The primary care nurse is responsible for her 24 hour period from admission or initiation of treatment to discharge or end of treatment.
- Primary caregivers provide all direct patient care during working hours.
- Other subordinate caregivers provide care when the primary caregiver is not at work.
- Establishing good communication is an important responsibility of primary caregivers.
- The primary caregiver is responsible for her 24-hour period from admission or initiation of treatment to discharge or end of treatment.
- During working hours primary nurse provides total direct care for that patient.
- When the primary nurse is not on duty care is provided by other junior nurses.
- An integral responsibility of the primary nurse is to establish a good communication.

Advantages

- Satisfaction for both patients and nurses.
- The relationship between nurses and patient is intimate.
- Autonomy for the nurses.
- Nurse is the person who is planning and providing complete care.
- She communicates with all other health team members involved in client care.
- Other health team members including physician tend to view her more knowledgeable and responsible.
- Patient receives quality and continuity of care.
- Reduces the number of errors than can result from a relay of orders.
- Increased satisfaction both to patients and nurses.
- Nurse can identify patient outcome as a result of their work.

Disadvantages

- More nurses are required for this method of care delivery and it is more expensive than other methods.
- Level of expertise and commitment may vary from nurse to nurse.

Functional Nursing

- It is task focused not patient-focused.
- In this model the tasks are divided with one nurse assuming responsibility for specific tasks. For example, one nurse may be responsible for hygiene and dressing, and another may be responsible for administering medication.
- Individuals can be very efficient at certain tasks and can get a lot of work done in less time (saving time).
- Helps organize unit and staff work.
- Make the most of people's abilities, experiences and desires.
- Organizations will benefit financially from this strategy. This is because patient care can be delivered to a large number of patients by mixing staff with large numbers of unlicensed assistants.
- Nurses acquire advanced skills by repeating assigned tasks over and over again.
- Less equipment is required and what is available is generally better maintained customer support can be personal and piecemeal.
- Continuity of care may not be possible.
- Employees can be bored and have little motivation to develop themselves or others.
- Employees are responsible for tasks.
- Clients may feel uneasy.
- Staff only know part of the care plan.
- Patients are confused because so many nurses are caring for them. Hospital director nurse, pharmacist nurse, union nurse, temperature nurse, etc.

Team Nursing

- Team nursing is based on the philosophy that groups of professional and non-professional staff work together to identify, execute, and assess comprehensive client-centered care.
- In team nursing, the RN leads a team of other her RNs, LPNs, or LVNs and nursing assistants or technicians.

- Team members coordinate and provide direct patient care to patient groups under the direction of her RN team leader.
- The nurse in charge delegates authority to her leader of the team who must be professional nurses. This nurse leads a team of typically 4 to 6 members who care for 15 to 25 patients.
- The team leader assigns tasks, plans care, and briefs team members on the details of care.
- Provides quality, comprehensive care to patients.
- Each member of the team can participate in decision making and problem solving.
- Each team members can bring specific expertise and skills to help in patient care.
- Improved patient satisfaction.
- Team members develop a sense of ownership and belonging.
- Workload can be balanced and shared.

Cons

- Establishing a team concept requires time and staff consistency.
- Unstable staffing patterns make team maintenance difficult.
- All employees must be customer focused.
- Low individual accountability and independence in nursing functions.
- Team leaders may not have the necessary leadership skills to effectively lead their teams and create 'team spirit'.
- Costs more because more people are needed.

Progressive Patient Care

- How patient care areas provide different levels of care. A central theme is better utilization of facilities, services and staff for better patient care.
- Here clients are evaluated for all care levels (intensities).
- As progress is made towards better selfcare (ethically less ill, more critical care and monitoring is required), staff will be deployed to provide the types of care needed.

The key elements of PPC

- Patients with acute myocardial infarction with life threatening arrhythmia.
- **Intermediate care:** Critically ill patients are transferred to intermediate care wards when their vital signs and general condition are stable.
- **Recovery and selfcare:** Patients are taught medication management, lifestyle modification exercise, walking, insulin sel- administration, pulse blood glucose monitoring, and dietary management.
- **Long-term care:** These wards care for chronically ill, disabled and incapacitated patients. Nurses and other therapists help patients and families manage walking, physical therapy, occupational therapy, and activities of daily living.
- **Home care:** Some hospitals/centers offer home care services. Hospital-based home care packages provide staff with equipment and supplies to care for patients at home. Paralytic patients postoperative mental retardation/spasticity patients and patients undergoing long-term chemotherapy.
- **Ambulatory care:** Outpatients visit hospitals for follow-up, diagnosis, treatment, rehabilitation, and preventive services. These areas are outpatient clinics, diagnostic centers, day care centers, etc.

Benefits

- Staff and equipment are used efficiently.
- Customers are best placed to receive the care they need.
- Maximize utilization of nursing skills and expertise.
- Clients are encouraged to engage in self-care and independence as needed.
- Efficient use and placement of equipment.
- Employees are more likely to reach their full potential.

Cons

- Frequent travelers may feel uncomfortable.
- Continuity is difficult to maintain.
- Difficulty building long-term caregiver-client relationships.
- Great emphasis is placed on comprehensive written care plans.
- There are often difficulties in meeting the administrative needs of staff evaluation and certification in an organization.

Case Management

Case Managers are responsible for tracking patient care and follow-up from the diagnostic stage through hospital rehabilitation to home care. For example, cardiac surgery patient case manager; assisting with diagnostic procedures; preoperative preparation for surgery; family counseling; postoperative care and rehabilitation.

Case Manager Responsibilities

- Evaluate clients and their homes and communities.
- Customer care coordination and planning.
- Collaborate with other health care professionals in providing care.
- Monitor client progress and results.

- Advocacy to clients passing through required services.
- Acts as a liaison with external payers when planning patient care.

Benefits
- Case management provides a coordinated caregiving experience that improves care outcomes, reduces length of stay, and efficiently leverages multiple areas and services.
- Provides comprehensive care for people with complex health problems.
- Seeks the active participation of the patient's family and various health care professionals.

Cons
- Nurse identifies major barriers to implementation of this service, financial barriers and lack of administrative support.
- Expensive.
- Nurses are client- and outcome-focused.
- Facilitate and encourage cost-effective coordination of care.
- Case management in nursing is a professionally autonomous role and requires clinical expertise and decision-making authority.

CLINICAL MEETINGS: INDIVIDUAL AND GROUP

Nursing meetings range from group discussions using problem-solving techniques and nursing processes to informal discussion of problems and sharing of knowledge and experience of common concerns. It is an educational method that provides opportunities for free exchange. Nursing conferences are so 'old fashioned' and equated with basic nursing education that their potential value in staff development and continuing education is often misunderstood. Within a facility, especially at the ward level, nursing conferences can provide a positive learning experience for all staff with common nursing issues in the care of a particular patient.

Individual Meetings
- Focus on the overall development of the individual student.
- Emphasis is placed on developing clinical skills.
- Addresses student nursing skill levels, performance and assignments primarily related to clinical experience.

Definition
- "A nursing conference is defined as the process in which students conduct group discussions using problem-solving techniques to determine options for the care of patients assigned as part of their clinical experience.
- Nursing conferences are designed around consultation visits by clinical nurses. More often, however, they are designed for the staff of a particular nursing unit and are designed around one aspect of nursing or to the scientific nursing problems presented by patients in that unit.
- Nursing conferences are "procedural conferences focused on evaluating nursing problems, finding possible solutions, and helping staff see their patients' problems from their perspective."

Purpose
- Emphasis on clinical skills.
- Recognize the skills and limitations of various team members.
- Assists in communicating student thoughts and views on issues related to the student's clinical posting.
- Provide opportunities for students to develop their clinical skills.
- Promote innovative and creative ideas among students.

Planning and Preparation
- Organizers should prepare well in advance of a particular meeting.
- Before presenting the student will have to collect all the data regarding the patient. She will have to work with that patient and collected information about the signs and symptoms since how long the patient is sick.
- Meetings should be planned and spontaneous in relation to the purpose of the meeting.
- Students should be given ample opportunity to work on the station for a reasonable amount of time before being assigned to speak at the conference.

Technology
- Nursing conferences serve as counseling tools for problem solving.
- Teachers need to be flexible and support students during discussions.
- At meetings, all students must participate in the discussion. Teachers engage all students by asking questions and providing guidance and referrals as needed.
- Teachers should maximize student potential during conversations. Give students enough time to think.

Phase
Nursing conferences serve as counseling tools for problem solving. There are 3 phases: (1) Initial phase, (2) work phase and (3) closing phase.

Initial Phase

The initiation phase can be defined as the first two minutes of the meeting. The task here is to address a specific patient-related issue. What happens in those few minutes often sets the tone for the entire session.

Work Phase

The task of the work phase is to reach agreement on problem identification and resolution. Once the patient was selected, we found that a lot of time was spent clarifying the issue during this phase. At some meetings there was disagreement among nurses and often the data were contradictory or incomplete. Asking direct questions that reiterate and summarize what the group has said helps keep the group focused on the discussion. If data about a patient are incomplete, the group may try to supplement it. If the consultant and group decide that the missing data is important to the solution, they would rather spend their time gathering facts than guessing. Meeting times can be used to determine what information is needed.

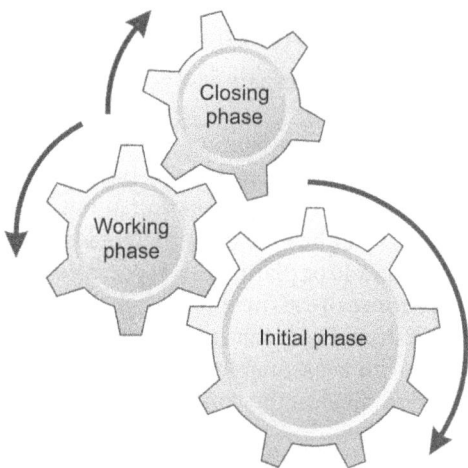

Fig. 8.8: Phases of clinical meeting.

Problems are recognized and groups are often able to come up with their own solutions. By offering concrete solutions to problem behaviors, employees feel like they are getting something from the group. Also, counselors who offer alternatives and support to disgruntled employees create trust and good service.

Closing Phase

After the group has come up with a solution to the problem and decided on a solution, the closing phase follows. The task here is to delegate responsibility for resolving the issue to one or more of her employees.

Benefits

- Helps students collect information in creative ways, students can validate data in relation to context and appropriateness.
- Provide students with a real, hands-on learning environment.
- Strengthen students' thinking ability, enhance their creativity and judgment.
- Offer free opportunity for reflection.
- Each member actively participates in the meeting.

Cons

- It is of little use if the student is unfamiliar with the situation.
- It is possible to use this office hour for face-to-face classes.

Conferences are an important method of clinical education. Nursing conferences are formed in formal or informal ways. Discussion uses problem-solving techniques and requires students to identify problems and solutions to those problems. Provide students with ample opportunities for reflection. Learning objectives are best achieved when used in a well-planned manner. These greatly improve student knowledge as many students contribute.

GROUP CONFERENCE

Although the concept of group/team as applied to the field of nursing is of relatively recent origin, our hospital wards have, almost from the beginning, had undefined relationships. There was a group of individuals with loose tissue patterns. Similar to nursing, the endless proliferation of advanced technologies aimed at the physical and psychological care of patients will eventually make it impossible for professional nurses to perform all the tasks of patient care.

Meaning of Meeting

A meeting is a joint deliberation. Conferences are at the core of the inservice care program. Many educational opportunities arise spontaneously at conferences and are invaluable in that they apply to specific patient issues. Group process techniques and interpersonal principles are an integral part of the process. Observations made during nursing team meetings provide a unique opportunity for nursing staff orientation.

Nursing Team Meeting Benefits

- Used for planning.
- As an educational tool, nursing team meetings provide valuable learning opportunities.

- Ability to observe, report, and analyze important findings, most tested when students face their daily responsibilities.

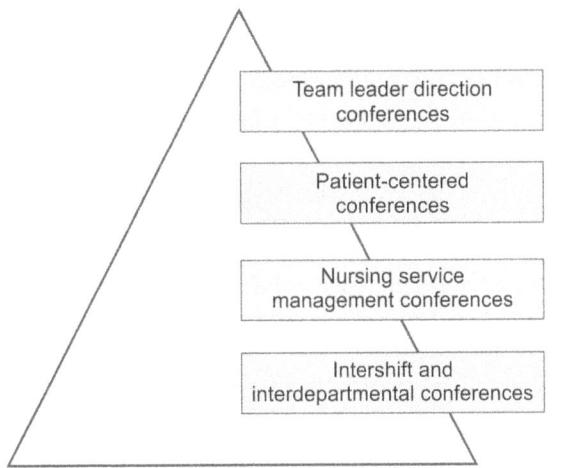

Fig. 8.9: Group conference.

Nursing Team Meeting Goals

Nursing Team Meeting

- Identify the patient's nursing problem.
- Recognize the skills and limitations of various team members.
- Helps communicate related care idea information.
- Using scientific information to influence causes of care
- Generalize specific information about facts.
- Assist with reporting, interpretation, channeling and enforcement of hospital and health issues.
- Teach team members what they need to do to fulfill their roles.
- Assist with joint care planning with other team members.
- It also maximizes team creativity.

Meeting Schedule

Time is set aside each day for Care Team members to meet as a group. During this time, patient issues are identified and investigated, and an approach is developed by the team. Care plans are revised or evolved as the patient's needs change.

Each member of the nursing team recorded patient responses to nursing questions and patient comments throughout her day and used individual notes to facilitate meetings.

Team leader uses her Kardex to read patient names and goals of care. The contracting member with that particular patient will discuss their response to treatment and any additional information from the patient or his/her family.

Problems are identified by groups. A plan is created to solve the problem. Kardex is revised and goals are changed by managers. The chief nurse acts as a resource, assisting the team leader and her team members in identifying issues of care and developing plans for her care.

The Nursing Team Meeting is the planning stage of the team and during and immediately after the meeting, the engagement of the nursing staff for the next day is developed.

Main Types of Meetings/Conference

- Team leader meetings are held at the start of the work shift and one hour before the end of the shift. The goal is to provide and receive relevant and accurate information about patient care and to create an environment that fosters collective and collaborative participation.
- Patient-centered meetings are meetings scheduled to identify problems and evaluate care. These meetings provide resources for all teams to contribute directly to patient group care and benefit from the experiences of others. Members as a group aim to formulate a nursing intervention for one or two patients and analyze the care provided. Clinical nurse coordinators and supervisors are important members of patient-centered meetings.
- Nursing leadership meetings should be part of each unit or section's scheduled meetings. Here, a supervisor supported by a clinical coordinator is in charge. Key topics discussed may include patient care standards and policy procedures, safety procedures, infection control, nursing audit and evaluation unit staffing actions, and description of new staffing policies.
- Intershift and interdepartmental meetings are required to communicate relevant information from one individual or group to another.

Professional Nurse Requirements

Nine requirements were identified by Chao and Wilkes nursing students at Columbia University.

1. **To identify patient care issues:** Team leaders are primarily listeners, and leaders can help the group develop an overall plan from various inputs. Gives the leader the opportunity to examine and evaluate the care provided to patients by her members of the team.
2. **Recognize the abilities and limitations of various team members:** Team leaders should use professional judgment in evaluating observational contributions and suggestions of other members when developing care assessments need to do it. Leaders should also help team members identify their own strengths and limitations in the areas of competence, knowledge, and judgment.

3. **Communication:** Professional caregivers should always pay attention not only to their own communication skills, but also to those of their team members. Communication requires two people, the speaker and the listener. Successful team communication depends on the extent to which the professional caregiver understands the abilities and limitations of her other team members. Leaders should be willing to apply approaches that facilitate communication.
4. **Use of scientific knowledge to influence the course of care:** This is an expression of the professional status of care. This ability makes it possible to plan comprehensive or individualized care. Professional knowledge and judgment are the skills of professional nurses who identify valuable cues in the work attitudes and thinking of nonprofessional members and identify and apply scientific principles that help them leverage their contributions. Reflected in directly protecting the ability.
5. **Generalizing from specific:** As leaders evaluate team members' contributions, they organize this information and present it in a way that will help team members in similar situations at a later date.
6. **Guidelines:** Guidelines are required guidelines and are therefore subject to interpretation. Team meetings are used to discuss hospital policy issues that apply to specific patients. An often-discussed policy is visiting hours.
7. **Encourage "maximum creativity":** The Team leader is responsible for creating a working environment in which her members of the Care Team can fully participate. You must know the needs of group members and help meet those needs. Through this process, team leaders help other members identify and solve problems and become more effective within their capabilities.
8. At the meeting, communicate what is needed to enable her members of the team to fulfill their roles: He has a broad scientific background and professional qualities that can be used in a variety of situations. Laymen rely on routines and techniques. It is important for professional caregivers to be aware of what instructions are given and whether the instructions are effective. A detailed briefing is not the responsibility of the meeting team leader.
9. **Plan care with other team members:** This is the main overall purpose of the care team his conference. Team leaders encourage all team members to participate in planning and guide the development of plans based on scientific principles.

Roles and Responsibilities

Faculty and students have a clear responsibility for ensuring meaningful clinical meetings.

Instructor's Role

- Make a plan.
- Be flexible in responding to situations such as emergencies and changing patient conditions.
- Set a positive tone for the clinical experience.
- Establish expectations for the conference.
- Create an environment conducive to openness trust sharing and discussion.
- Support and encourage students.
- Maintain focus of the group.
- Give yourself time to think.
- Provide constructive feedback.
- Encourage student learning in relation to course objectives and outcomes.
- Facilitate the transfer of knowledge.
- Model professional behavior.

Student Roll

- Arrive on time.
- Prepare.
- Be open minded.
- Participate in discussions.
- Accept constructive feedback.
- Demonstrate professionalism.

CLINICAL PRESENTATION/BEDSIDE CLINIC

Clinic means a group of clinical instructors and learners watching patients create or check physical. The process of discussing a preliminary diagnosis, diagnosis, or treatment options in the purpose of the bedside clinic is to improve the quality of care, enhance students' ability to solve care problems through detailed investigation and analysis of care situations, recognize the need to understand individual patients and their problems, It is about respect. Provides a learning experience for nursing students to gather information about their patients. Bedside clinics provide students with comprehensive preparation for effective participation in patient care. Helps develop student autonomy. Bedside clinics enable students to develop and maintain their professional skills.

Definitions

A bedside clinic is the process by which a group of clinical teachers and learners observes the generation or verification of physical symptoms in a patient and discusses preliminary diagnosis, diagnosis or treatment options in a clinical setting.

—Gaberson

Meaning

The bedside clinic is a method of clinical education. always presupposes the presence of the patient. A group visits the bedside or the patient is taken to a conference room. Nursing clinics are managed by a lead nurse or clinical trainer. At the nursing clinic, the patient's medical history and nursing history are briefly explained.

- A type of clinical teaching method in which a nursing administrator/tutor meets with her subordinates or nursing students and provides nursing instruction at the bedside in front of the patient.
- It is a teaching in the presence of the patient.

Purposes

- To portray nursing problem and to provide a complete picture of the related nursing care by associating with a specific individual.
- To improve the quality of nursing care.
- To improve students' ability to solve nursing problems through indepth research and analysis of nursing situations.
- Helps students develop their observation skills in a systematic and organized way.
- Understand each patient as an individual and recognize the need to respect their issues and perspectives.
- Provide a learning experience for nursing students to gather information about patients.
- Planning and implementing care plans according to patient needs and concerns.

Bedside Clinic Goals

- Discuss the benefits and challenges of bedside education.
- Research strategies for improving bedside education.
- Review bedside teaching techniques in the office.

Considerations when Conducting Bedside Clinics

- Select patients with typical medical conditions.
- Clinic groups should be large enough to gather informally around the bed for patient comfort.
- Consultation time is usually about 30 minutes, but it can be extended if necessary.
- Before starting the practice, the instructor should have a good knowledge of the patient's details, including personal characteristics, medical history, and medical conditions.
- Instruct the group on the necessary observations of the patient.

Practical Tips

It includes **12 practical tips** to ease teacher bedside discomfort and promote effective bedside instruction.

1. **Preparation:** Teachers should familiarize themselves with the clinical curriculum, diagnose different levels of learning, and strive to improve their own clinical skills.
2. **Planning:** Ende (1997) suggests that all clinical teachers ask themselves and attempt to answer the following questions prior to classroom discussion:
   - What do you want to achieve?
   - What is your perspective?
   - How are learners engaged?
   - How do you meet the needs of individual learners?
   - How are rounds organized?
3. **Orientation:** Teachers should understand learner goals, assign roles to each team member, ensure everyone is included, and set ground rules for the team.
4. **Introduction:** The medical team should refer the patient and the patient should be informed of the nature of the bedside examination. Example: The patient should be told that this encounter is primarily educational and that certain theoretical arguments may not apply to the patient's illness.
5. **Interaction:** Clinical teachers should act as role models in physician-patient interactions and instill a professionalism and humane bedside approach. Additionally, teachers should model teamwork and encourage positive team interactions, including professional interactions with nurses and other support staff.
6. **Observation:** Teachers do not need to host bedside shows and dominate bedside encounters. Observing trainee-patient interactions at the bedside is very informative and these observations can be used to plan future sessions.
7. **Guidance:** Clinical educators should avoid asking trainees impossible questions and actively prevent learners from overbidding by asking "read my mind" type questions. Acknowledging their own knowledge gaps allows trainees to acknowledge their limitations and ask questions. Teachers can demonstrate their willingness to learn by being willing to learn from their trainees.
8. **Summary:** The teacher's summary of what was taught in this encounter proves useful to the learner. Patients also need a summary discussion of what is and is not applicable to their disease and management.
9. **Debriefing:** Students should have time to ask questions, and teachers should be given clarifications and assigned additional reading.

10. **Feedback:** Teachers can learn from learners what worked and what didn't, and provide positive and constructive feedback to learners.
11. **Reflection:** Reflections about the bedside encounter coupled with learner feedback can help teachers plan the next encounter.
12. Preparation for the next encounter should begin with insights from the reflection phase.

Preparation for Bedside Clinic

- You need to prepare your device.
- Prior consent must be obtained from the patient and significant others.
- All appropriate treatments/medications administered during the interview must be completed prior to the interview.
- All patient reports can be prepared.
- The selected group must be small.
- It takes about 30 minutes.
- Patient selection should be appropriate to the student's knowledge.
- Patient and family consent is required.
- The clinical trainer should have a good understanding of the patient's problem and how to treat it.
- The environment should be conducive to teaching.
- Appropriate times should be chosen for classes to avoid unnecessary interference with the patient's daily life and the student's work.

Steps

- Students gather around the patient. All students must be able to see the patient and if procedures such as physical examinations are performed.
- The clinical trainer introduces the group to the patient and introduces the patient to the group.
- Describes treatment regimens and patient response to treatment based on history and patient data.
- In the meantime, you can engage the patient and ask them how they feel about their treatment and care.
- Discussion continues.

Method: Steps Required

- Place the student casually next to the bed.
- Necessary observations of the patient are instructed to the student.
- The clinical instructor first tells about the history the physical and mental condition of the patient.
- The nursing problems of the patient are presented to the students.
- Shows how to deal with such caregiving problems.
- Finally, summarize the patient's problem and treatment.
- The teacher asks for discussion.

Phases/Steps

- Introduction phase
- Discussion phase
- Evaluation phase.

Introduction Phase

- A prior permission is sought from the patient and the relatives for conducting bedside clinic.
- Information collected in this way is kept confidential.
- The facilitator provides an overview of the patient's site name and other details so that students can study the case sheet in advance before the discussion takes place.

Discussion Phase

- Discussions are initiated by teachers or students in charge of patient care.
- Do not criticize the patient's condition in order to humiliate him.
- Patients can participate in discussion groups as needed, depending on the patient's condition.
- Students are allowed to interact with the patient for further clarification.
- The discussion phase can last approximately 30-40 minutes.

Evaluation Phase

- The patient is released when the interaction ends.
- Further the students discuss on doubts and can clarify.
- The bedside clinic ends with a summary recapitulation of important aspects and feedback from the students.

Bedside Teaching Tips

- Preparation (What is the lesson goal?)
- Include all an Open-ended questions (What?)
- Speak out
- Admitting gaps in your knowledge correct mistakes complement achievements
- Observation is as important as education
- Best professional behavior
- Time management
- Reporting and follow-up

Benefits

- Participate in patient care.
- Foster student autonomy.
- Students can select patients with disease states of general interest.

- This helps students review and examine the quality of clinical practice.
- Bedside clinics allow students to develop and maintain their professional skills.
- Develop students' understanding of health, disease and the medical system.
- Bedside clinics develop clinical skills such as logical thinking, psychomotor and communication skills in students.
- Develop students' ability to critically evaluate and improve their own performance.

Cons

- Bedside clinics can be burdensome for patients.
- Its narrowness limits the use of the method.
- Bedside clinics are an expensive procedure.
- May compromise patient privacy.
- Leads to poor standardization.

BED SIDE CLINIC/BED SIDE TEACHING

Groups can visit clients or bring clients into the meeting room during discussions. This method is useful if some members of the group do not know the client, or if there are specific observations that need to be made to make the discussion more meaningful. The group knows the purpose of the visit and what needs to be considered.

Clients often participate in goal-oriented conversations. Teachers use this opportunity to demonstrate and help clients identify their own needs and address problems.

Clients should feel comfortable. We must avoid disturbing our customers.

Clients need to know the group and what is expected of them. A comfortable environment should be maintained and a minimum number of group members should be allowed.

Purpose

- Presentation of nursing problems typically associated with a particular disease or disorder.
- Delineate a caregiving situation and associate it with a specific person.

Benefits

- Stimulates student interest and ability to imitate.
- Encourage discussion among students about patient problems and their treatments.
- Gives teachers the opportunity to assess or assess the nursing knowledge and skills of students in the community.

- Each student will be given the opportunity to get to know the patient in general.

Cons

- Large numbers of medical team members can make patients uncomfortable.
- The patient may overhear the conversation and feel bad about their condition.
- Needs a well organized explanation. Otherwise, the essence of such gatherings is lost.

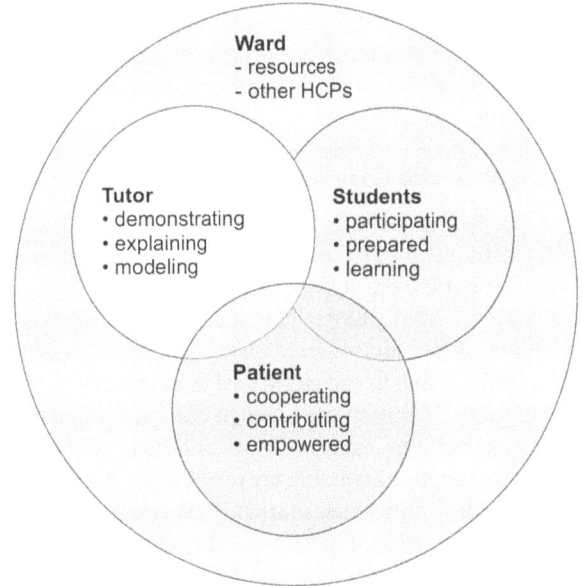

Fig. 8.10: Bed-side clinical teaching.

CASE STUDIES/CARE STUDIES

Students are given the opportunity to provide care to specific clients after 4–5 days of intense learning and general client discussion with attendees.

Definition

Case method is a clinical teaching method in which a student/teacher presents a case. This is an oral report of clinical cases compared to the literature.

Objectives

- To provide direct information about disease investigation treatment and care management.
- Thoroughly understand the specific patient landscape in the context of the disease and compare with the literature.
- Observe and interpret the patient's symptom response to assess prognosis.

- Compare cases with a specific diagnosis to another treatment with a similar diagnosis.

Case Analysis

Concrete cases for analysis and discussion by student groups under the guidance of an instructor. Students are presented with sufficient information to independently assess the problem or situation.

The case analysis method deals with core situations that require several decisions. Under the guidance of the teacher, a group of students analyzes the case, discusses the issue and decides. His main focus is decision-making. It focuses on learning concrete real-life problems and emphasizes problem-solving. About the different solutions used to solve the problem.

Objectives of the Case Analysis Method

- To develop the ability to move from known problems to new problems and to develop a spirit capable of wisely explaining the basis for decisions.
- Develop the ability to navigate a patchwork of evidence by selecting key factors from a set of facts and weighing their importance in the context of the evidence.
- Develop the ability to use ideas to compare them to the facts of a problem, examine ideas and facts, and discuss how to make them suitable for problem-solving.
- Extends the ability to use empirical data as a validity test for already generated ideas with the flexibility to modify goals and procedures as needed.
- Expand your ability to communicate thoughts to others in a thought provoking way.
- Develop the ability to frame general statements from problem-solving experience, using ideas in a theoretical form.

Critical Incident Technique

A critical incident technique requiring immediate decision and action is taken from the case and presented to the student for analysis and decision. At the time of presentation, they were given no background on the details of the incident. Facts about the case will be provided to the instructor. This can be requested by the student. The case incident teaching method is a modification of the case analysis method that focuses on serious incidents in cases that require immediate decision and action. No background information. It simply identifies the incidents that need resolution. Developed by Paul and Faith Pigose.

Medical history phase is:

- **Phase 1—events:** After discussing various factors that influence the behavior of adult patients in the hospital, events from living situations are presented to the class.
- **Phase 2—gather facts:** Students are asked what information they need before making effective decisions. The leader knows the facts of the incident and will pass them on to the group upon request. Group members summarize it.
- **Phase 3—determining causes and consequences of problems:** The group decides which areas of the problem require immediate decision and the consequences of not making a decision.
- **Phase 4—individual student decisions and reasons:** Each student was asked to write down what they would have done and justify their decision.
- **Phase 5—identify key decisions and issues raised:** By each student through group discussion. Identify and discuss key decisions made by individuals and categorize them. Next, we need to identify and summarize the process of thinking systematically about the incident.

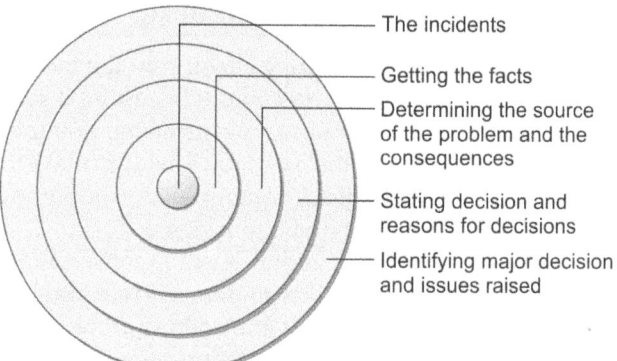

Fig. 8.11: Phases of clinical incident.

Benefits of the Drop Method

- It is useful to get knowledge directly from real situations.
- Recognize problems, discuss solutions, and develop insights.
- A sense of accomplishment increases as students present examples of others.
- Students will be given home schooling opportunities.
- Improves student confidence.
- Compare a patient's condition to the literature to enhance understanding.
- Develop presentation skills.

Restrictions

- Patients may feel uncomfortable and dislike losing their privacy.
- Inversions may be ineffective when presented in a disjointed manner.

- Large groups can be distracting, so groups should be small.

CASE PRESENTATION

Case Presentation is a learning method in which a student/teacher presents a case.

Meaning

- Detailed oral presentations of clinical cases for learning purposes are called case presentations.
- This is a form of teaching-learning activity conducted by teachers/students on the overall patient condition while comparing it to the pictures in the book.

Purpose

- To provide an ideal environment for learning disease research, treatment and care management.
- Know the actual situation first hand.
- Thoroughly understand the picture of a particular patient in the context of the disease and compare it to the picture in the book.
- Get a realistic picture of the patient's current condition and the care provided.
- Achieve active participation by stimulating and encouraging the development of intuition and skills in each member of the group.
- Signs Symptoms Observe and interpret patient response and treatment results.

Case Presentation Stage

Teacher Presentation

- Be aware of student goals and levels.
- Check case availability.
- Select the appropriate housing.
- Familiarize yourself with the theoretical aspects of the disease.
- Learn the case for yourself first.
- Please let your students know in advance.
- Select the appropriate cases (patients) based on the nursing student's level and their specific learning goals: knowledge attitudes and practices.
- The patient's condition must be recognizable.
- Receiving appropriate medical care suitable for education.
- Informed patient consent for case presentation is obtained and patient cooperation is encouraged.
- Please ask the staff at each station.
- Build a good relationship with the patient.
- Make a plan to look at the points and ask questions for discussion.
- Teachers should create an open and non-authoritarian atmosphere in which students can discuss cases freely.
- Treat students with respect and tolerance.

Audiovisual Aid Preparation

- It should be relevant to the content and condition of the patient.
- Must have an attractive design.
- Can be in the form of either flashcards or charts.
- Must be visible to everyone (everyone in the presentation). Therefore, good lighting is required.

Physical Set Up

- The presentation can be done near to the patient. So it should have adequate lighting.
- It should be free of noise.
- Cleanliness must be taken care of.
- Ensure patient comfort.
- Make sure there is enough space next to the bed.
- About 6 to 8 students can effectively learn from her presentation of the case in the station set up.

Procedure

- It should match the student's learning goals and the patient's condition.
- Correlation and integration must be done between the patient's condition and the book image.
- There must be unity, continuity and order in the presentation.
- Should be flexible to allow students to reflect on questions etc.
- Make it audible.
- Introduce each other to the patient and student group.
- Follow the order shown in the format.
- Talk to the patient and make relevant observations.
- Help students observe relevant signs and symptoms and clarify important medical history.
- State what medical care or care was provided and why.
- Link findings and care to the literature.
- Discuss care with ideal care.
- Encourage objective assessment of care.
- The presentation should interest students and encourage active participation.
- Use appropriate visual aids for the patient's condition.
- Case presentations are 30-40 minutes long.
- Involve the patient in the case presentation process.
- Lecturers should minimize their contribution to the discussion, but at the same time be ready to summarize the situation at any time.

- Graduate with nursing practice and future plans for nursing.
- Check the patient's health status and thank the patient for his participation.

Case Presentation Format

Medical History

- Identification data
- Socio-economic status.
- Family history.
- family medical history.
- Personal history.
- Menstrual history (female patient).
- Marital history.
- Obstetrical history.
- Previous medical history.
- Current medical history.
- Current surgical history.

Information content about this disease must be written in the format:
- Case definition
- Review of anatomy and physiology.
- Type (if available) (Book Image/Patient Image).
- Incidence (picture of book/picture of patient).
- Risk factors (picture of book / photo of patient)
- Photo of etiology (picture of book / photo of patient).
- Pathophysiology (pictures from book/pictures of patients).
- Clinical manifestations (picture from book/picture of patient).
- Diagnostic assessment (book photo/patient photo).
- Complications (picture from book/picture of patient
- Management (picture from book/picture of patient).
- Nutrition management.
- Drug management.
- Surgical management.
- Nursing management.
- Health education.
- Summary.
- References.

Advantages

- It is useful to get information directly from the actual situation.
- Recognize problems, discuss solutions, develop insights, and find connections.
- Students feel a sense of accomplishment when presenting cases to others.
- Helps students receive and care for patients without worrying about the future.
- Helps educate and rehabilitate families.
- Helps build good interpersonal relationships.
- Develop personal skills, knowledge and personality.
- It improves good speaking and organizing ability.
- It improves self-confidence.
- Gives an opportunity for teacher to check knowledge level of the student.
- It is helpful to correlate and integrate the patient picture and book picture. So that the student can understand well and the doubts will be clarified on the spot.
- Students can learn from each others.
- Student can take responsibility for their own learning.

Disadvantages

- An unorganized content can frustrate the listener.
- Patients can observe the discussion.
- The patient may feel uncomfortable.
- When the group is this large, students may not be able to speak or argue loudly, which can lead to loss of attention and distraction.
- If schedule in the morning the case presentation will not be effective it will be uncomfortable to both family and also hospital staff who will be busily doing procedures.

CASE STUDIES

Nursing case studies are one of the most common and useful teaching methods in the clinical field. It is a form of quantitative and qualitative analysis that involves a very careful and thorough observation of the patient and their situation.

Meaning

- A case study is a focused study of a phenomenon involving subjective and objective information.
- Case studies are analyzes of individual patient nursing problems arising from diagnosis, physical and emotional management, and affected by personality and socioeconomic development.
- Case studies are close cumulative clinical studies of patients.
- A case study is a fairly thorough study of an individual or group.

Criteria for Good Case Studies

- Continuity.
- Data integrity.
- Validity of data.
- Confidential records.
- Analysis and scientific synthesis.

Source of Case Data

- Personal record diary pre-existing condition.
- A member of the health team.
- Parties.
- Official record.
- Subject himself.

Principles

- Should include patient supportive and therapeutic care.
- The focus should be on the patient's individual needs and how they are met.

Steps for Nursing

- **Case selection:** When assigning patients, the student's knowledge level is considered. Case selection should be based on the level of care required. Example: Completely unrelated patients are not assigned to case studies.
- **Data collection:** Data collection is divided into two aspects:
  1. *Subjective data:* Information provided by the patient himself.
  2. *Objective data:* Data documented by observation, research, or intervention.
- **Tests:** Patient tests include anthropometric, biometric, clinical, and dietary tests. History related to current and past conditions is collected using appropriate formats.
- **Diagnosis and identification of random factors:** Laboratory tests and invasive procedures identify random factors.
- **Nursing process:** Nursing process involves patient assessment and the development of nursing diagnoses based on the assessment, planning, and delivery of care.
- **Evaluation and follow-up:** Here the effectiveness of the care provided is judged.

Type of Case Study

- Oral case study.
- Written case studies.

Forms and Presentations

- Written case studies are usually best documented in narrative format.
- Some form of outline should be used to guide the beginner. Older students can use the outline as a guide, but should be allowed to use their own initiative and creativity in writing their research.
- An oral case study is a case study that one or more students present to the clinical instructor in the form of an oral report.

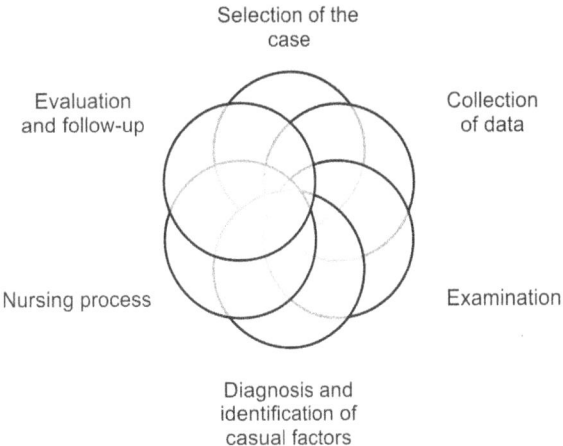

Fig. 8.12: Case study method in nursing.

Examples of Merits of Nursing Care Cases

- Case studies help students plan and provide comprehensive nursing care to their patients.
- The student will be able to supervise and follow-up on services for 3 to 5 consecutive days.
- It also helps develop self-expression in sentences related to patient care.
- Helps students develop clinical knowledge by comparing idealized book pictures with real patient conditions.
- Students' focused efforts to define and solve problems improve nursing outcomes.
- Students are better able to understand and appreciate human personality and the factors that influence it.
- Collecting and organizing information enhances students' understanding of disability-related nursing issues.
- Helps students learn and apply nursing problem-solving approaches.
- Considers individual research differences.
- Provide an opportunity to write a self-portrait.
- It provides a source of material for future references.

Disadvantages

- It is more time consuming and a costly method.
- It leaves no opportunity once the study is completed to branch out and incorporate new ideas.
- Rewriting to an acceptable form takes a lot of time.

CARE PLAN

The planning process leads to successful achievement of goals and objectives, gives meaning to work life, and directs the operational activities of the organization. Further planning leads to efficient and effective use of resources and helps formulate forwardlooking actions and the future direction of the agency. Therefore, the highest quality care can only be achieved when patient needs are individualized through appropriate and systematic care planning.

Meaning

Nursing is the diagnosis and treatment of human responses to actual or potential health problems. A care plan serves as an organizational framework for the delivery of care. A care plan is a systematic way for nurses to plan and implement patient care. It includes a problem-solving approach that enables nurses to identify patient problems and potentially at risk needs (problems) and plan and assess care in a science-based manner.

Definition

- A nursing plan is a systematic way of practicing nursing that provides a means for nursing professionals to demonstrate accountability and responsibility to clients and families.
- A care plan is a blueprint that supports a patient's adaptive response to illness (NANDA).
- A care plan is a document that reflects a patient's joint communication and informed consent.

Principles of Care Planning

- Diagnosis of physical and mental conditions and planning of medical care should be considered when nurses develop plans for use in patient care.
- The plan of care should embody the health concepts and values of both patients and caregivers.
- The patient's primary concern should be addressed.
- The plan of care should be based on the patient's resources and capabilities.
- A care plan should be the result of a shared decision-making process that allows the patient and community caregivers to respect the individuality of the patient.
- The treatment plan should reflect the patient's informed consent.
- Care plans should motivate the patient to carry out the plan.
- Care plans should take into account the patient's individual characteristics, nationality, age and disability.
- Statements should be short and concise.

Care Product Plan

- **Patients:** Developing an effective treatment plan requires the active participation of patients. Patients are the best source of information about needs and changes associated with changing health conditions. Similarly, the patient's values and beliefs should not be ignored. The values and beliefs that patients need strongly influence the issues addressed in collaborative patient care planning.
- **Expertise:** Nurses share professional recommendations with patients on issues they consider important. They discuss the level of happiness they think the patient can achieve. They share ideas for implementation in care and patient behavior to achieve that level of well-being.

Patient Care Planning Development

This stage of care planning seeks for nurses and patients to review nursing diagnoses and agree on a general method of implementing the outcomes and evaluation criteria to be included in the plan. The five dynamic and interrelated phases of assessment, diagnosis, planning, implementation, and evaluation should be considered when developing a care plan.

Evaluation

This is an initial care plan in which caregivers systematically collect, validate, and communicate data about clients to create a database of post-illness client wellness health practice levels and associated experiences and expectations.

The evaluation phase is divided into:
- Data collection.
- Data validation.
- Data clustering.
- Data document.

Data Collection

There are two types of data.
1. **Subjective data:** Subjective data are collected from interviews and medical histories.
2. **Objective data:** Data collection is via:
   - Physical examination.
   - Behavioral observation.
   - Diagnostic and laboratory data.
   - Medical records.

Other Members of the Health Team

Nursing diagnosis

This step allows nurses to customize patient care. During the diagnostic phase, nurses use their scientific and professional knowledge to analyze and interpret the data collected about their clients. Next, the nurse identifies the client's health problem and creates a nursing diagnosis that forms the basis of her plan of care.

Nursing diagnosis steps are:
- Recognize the client's problem.
- Formulate nursing diagnoses.
- Document diagnosis.

Planning

Planning is a category of nursing actions in which client-centered goals are set and strategies are developed to achieve those goals. Planning requires nurses to make conscious decisions and use their problem-solving skills to design care for each patient. During planning, priorities are set, goals are determined, expected outcomes are created, and a care plan is developed.

Planning procedure
- Identify customer goals.
- Determination of expected results.
- Consultation.
- Write a care plan.
- Set the priority.
- Choose a maintenance method.
- Select an action.

Implementation

The implementation shall execute the care plan created in the previous component of the care process. Implementation is a category of nursing actions that involve initiating and completing actions necessary to achieve expected nursing outcomes. Performing includes providing support or guidance in performing activities of daily living. Counseling and briefing family clients providing direct care to achieve client-centered goals, monitor and evaluate staff work, and record and share information related to the client's ongoing health.

Nursing practice types include:
- Perform nursing actions.
- Re-evaluate your customers.
- Review and change existing care plans.

Assessments

Assessments measure a client's response to nursing interventions and the client's progress in achieving goals. Ratings determine whether customers improve, remain stable, or deteriorate. Another aspect of evaluation is the measurement of quality of care in healthcare facilities.
- Examine the goal statement to identify exactly the desired behavior or client response.
- Assess the client for the presence of this behavior or response.
- Compare established outcome measures to actions or responses.
- Rate the agreement between the outcome criteria and actions or responses.

Evaluation Step
- Compare customer responses with expected results.
- Analyze reactions to findings and conclusions.
- Change the care plan.

Care Plan Benefits
- A summary structure that provides all patient information at a glance.
- Describes the patient as a person to her, describing her background, interests, known concerns and fears.
- In addition to describing the patient, the portrait provides suggestions for a personalized approach and identifies salient symptoms the patient is exhibiting. This allows new caregivers to have enough information to provide care and avoid interruptions to continuity.
- Collaborative team working with patients and their families.
- Students can schedule proctors based on their priority.
- Students will learn handson about the signs and symptoms associated with patient conditions and develop effective plans.
- Students will be able to assign and directly apply all steps of the nursing process they have read theoretically.
- Students can prioritize care plans according to scientific principles.
- Developing a patient care plan not only helps students absorb information, but also provides a means of communicating student knowledge to faculty.

Common Student Problems
- **Incomplete database:** Collecting insufficient data will cause many errors when creating care plans.
- **Categorize outcomes as nursing behavior rather than patient behavior:** Reporting nursing behavior rather than patient behavior is most common when students view nursing as task-oriented rather than problem-solving endeavors.
- **Selection of patient behaviors that are neither observable nor measurable:**
  - Consider the patient's resources and preferences.
  - The number of specialists is not enough to prepare the declaration of practice.

Cons Care Plan
- Time consuming.
- It cannot be formulated under emergency conditions. Cardiac arrest.
- Insufficient resources to execute all plan.

NURSING ROUNDS

There are several methods that can be used effectively in clinical teaching. Nurse rounds are conducted for staff/students by the lead nurse/nursing instructor. To be successful, all caregivers must be willing to participate in the care discussion.

Definition

Nurse rounds are conducted by the head nurse/nursing Instructor to help her staff/students clearly understand the disease process and the effects of each patient's care.

Importance of Nurse Visits

Familiarize nurses with all patients on the ward so they can better understand each patient and deliver more targeted care.

Purpose of the Nursing Visit

- Observation of the patient's physical and mental health and progress of daily living.
- Observe the work of the staff.
- Specifically monitor the patient and report to the physician, wound drainage bleeding, etc.
- Refer patient to staff and vice versa.
- Execute the plan developed for patient care.
- Assessment of treatment outcome and patient satisfaction with treatment.
- Ensuring patient and staff safety measures.
- Nurse/student orientation at handover/handover regarding patient treatment, care provided and patient status.
- Educate nursing students and hospital assistants about specific conditions.
- To check any preventable conditions present in the patient such as bedsore, foot drop, etc.
- Identify emergency equipment stored near the patient and verify its safety and functionality.
- Compare clinical manifestations of patients with disease to give students better understanding and insight.
- Prescribe changes in care procedures.

Visit Type

- Rounds with the doctors.
- Rounds to discuss psychological problem of patients.
- Social service rounds.
- Medical rounds for nurses.
- Rounds with the physical therapists.
- Nursing rounds.

Nursing Rounds

- In nursing visits, patient history and medical aspects of care are included only as background for understanding care.
- The nurse/teacher who cared for the patient during the week can provide background information and identify the points of care they consider most important.
- You are then responsible for answering class questions, including questions from the head nurse.
- Another way to conduct rounds is for the lead nurse/teacher to involve each nurse in the group to share what they know about the patient and their care. Other students make additions, suggestions, and help answer questions.
- This method is a means of testing a student's knowledge and proficiency for all patients on the floor.
- Learn and prepare for the efficacy and effects of medicines.
- Students will be notified prior to the round so they can be prepared.

Preparation by Chief Nurse/Nursing Educator

- In preparation for the visit, the nurse selects a patient to discuss, depending on the allotted time.
- Rounds must not exceed 20 minutes.
- The head nurse should read the patient's progress and anticipate care and its effectiveness.
- She will give at least a week's notice of the ward rounds and the kind of preparation the nurses will do. That is, do you need to know the complete or brief history of every patient on your ward and your own patient.
- Patients with similar diagnoses but different history, treatment, prognosis may be selected, or different conditions present on the same ward may be selected for educational purposes.
- Rounds for staff nurses should be held separately from those for students since the background of the 2 groups vary widely.
- Rounds for students in their first clinical term may need to be held separately.

Factors to be kept in Mind when Planning Nursing Rounds

- To consult student's previous clinical experience to avoid repetition and to add to earlier experience.
- Consider the value and availability of clinical materials.
- Demonstrations should not have teletelic effects on the patient.
- Explain the plan to the patient.
- Introduce the patient to the group.

- Make the patient feel important.
- Hold a post-event meeting for wrap-up and clarification.
- Record home visits in ward textbooks and summarize nursing points emphasized.

Ways of Conducting Rounds

- When true ward rounds are conducted the teacher with the group of nurses goes to the patient's room.
- Outside the door out of his hearing they discuss the objectives after which they go into see the patient and talk for a few moments with him.
- They then move on to the next patient.
- Discussions should be short and contain only the important points. When the purpose is to visit all the patients on the ward.
- Home visit nursing is done in the form of a report on the condition of the patient, the details of the treatment, the prognosis, etc.

Procedures for Conducting Nursing Visits

- Information about visits should be provided to students to assist them in preparing for the learning experience.
- Students follow the carewrap. A clinical trainer or ward manager will stop by each patient's bedside and briefly discuss the most important care issues.
- Trainers can ask each nurse in the group to share what they know about the client and their care.
- A student who has been caring for a patient for approximately one week should present the case to the entire group of students so that all students are aware of the case and its overall condition. If cardinal signs are identified with the client's permission, they are shown to the entire group. The background information is presented, followed by additions and suggestions from the group.
- The case presentation should be concise and address only issues and situations of immediate interest.
- Nursing rounds are carefully selected, well organized, clear, interesting, client specific, and only 3-4 minutes long.

Nursing Visit Benefits

- This method is a means of testing a student's knowledge and proficiency with the whole patient on the floor.
- Students who are notified prior to the round will benefit most from hands-on instruction.
- No other type of visit is a substitute for a nursing visit.
- It is always very beneficial for the lead nurse to participate in regular nursing rounds with the clinical educator.
- Intelligent nurses with creative skills can find many ways to successfully support nursing students in developing their nursing skills.

- Helps direct new nurses/students to patients.
- An interesting strategy involving student teachers and patients.
- Provide realistic learning situations.
- Assessment of nursing activities allows assessment of nursing staff failures and successes in nursing practice.

Nursing Round Disadvantages

- Patient confidentiality is compromised.
- Patients may overhear conversations and may be reluctant to be talked about as being deaf.
- If the group is large, the teacher may not be able to speak loud enough to be heard and may distract the person standing on the edge.
- There is a distraction at the station.
- An unprepared nursing visit has little teaching and learning value.
- Quality of nursing rounds on nursing educator/nursing administrator quality and presentation.

CONCEPT MAPPING

A concept map is a way of presenting information, knowledge, or facts in a graphical format. It consists of concepts and the relationships between them. Concepts in maps are all we want to talk about. Real objects, abstract concepts, events and even facts. Concepts are usually represented by text in rectangles and relationships as directed links between rectangles with arrows to indicate reading direction.

Concept maps have proven to be an effective teaching and learning tool for medical students. They can be used to reinforce students' meaningful learning, allowing students to practice more often to better understand concepts.

Definition

- Concept mapping is an educational strategy for individual and group learning that involves synthesizing knowledge and creating meaning by connecting concepts.
- A concept map is a visual organizer that helps students develop a better understanding of new concepts. Using the graphic organizer, students think about concepts in different ways.
- Concept maps are learning and teaching strategies that bridge the gap between people learning and meaningful learning topics. Concept maps in nursing are used as a way to combine theory with practice, case management, academic writing, and as a learning method for nursing students.

Concept Map Purpose

- **Dive deep into the topic:** When creating a concept map, start with the overall concept and identify subtopics.
- **Organize your thoughts:** When you and your team attend brainstorming sessions and workshops, you're bound to have a lot of ideas. This big mess can be hard to deal with, and concept maps can help make sense of them in a visual and easy-to-understand way.
- **Remember important information:** Studies show that visual learning produces better memory than auditory learning. So when you and your team work on a problem and need to understand a topic, concept maps improve both understanding and retention.
- **Understand relationships:** Emphasizing relationships is the biggest advantage of concept maps. Because it shows not just the ideas, but how they relate to each other. This helps you and your team uncover connections you might not have identified on your own.

Types of Content Maps

There are different structures and formats you can use to create concept maps. The four most common types are:

1. **Spider card:** This card is so named because it looks very much like a spider's web. Start with a central idea and branch radially into subtopics. Subtopics can branch into smaller subtopics.
2. **Flowcharts:** You may have seen flowcharts, but you may not have known that they are actually some kind of concept map. This concept map shows the steps in the process. Arrows usually represent different choices or actions to be taken, much like choosing your own adventure.
3. **Hierarchical map:** A hierarchical map is a type of conceptual map that shows the order of something. For example, think of your company's organizational chart. Here is an example of a hierarchical map showing people's roles and their dominance.

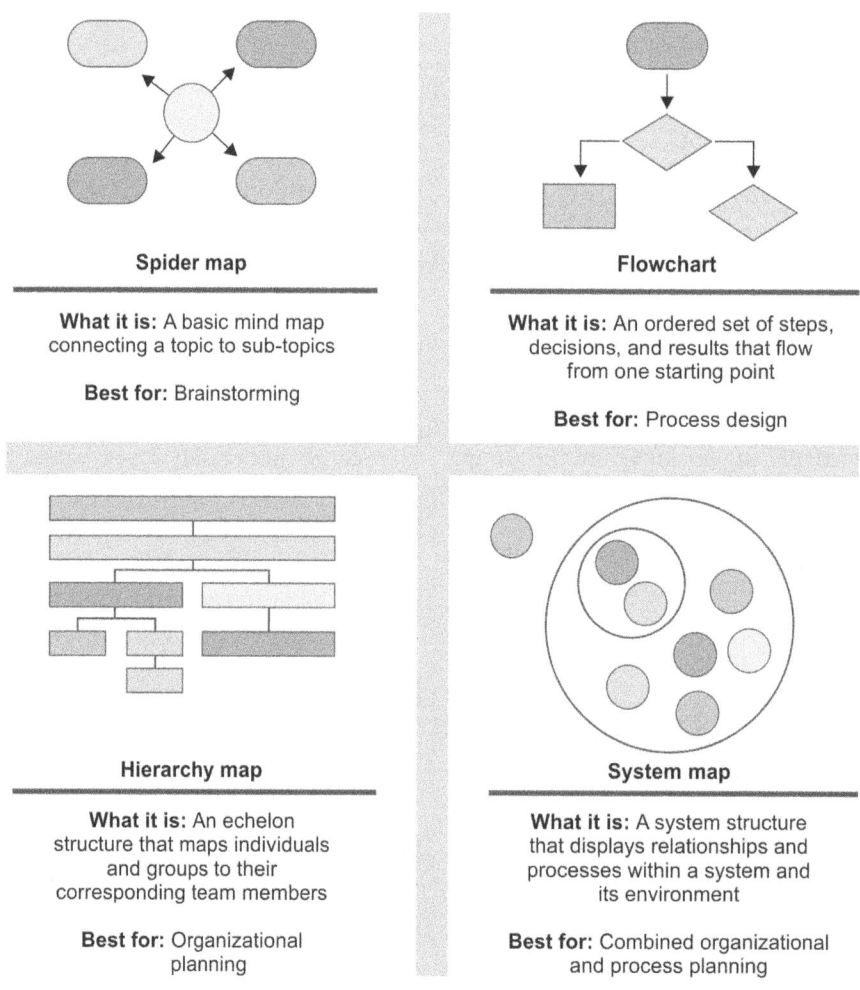

Fig. 8.13: Concept mapping.

4. **System maps:** System maps are arguably the most complex of all kinds of concept maps because they show all the different parts of a concept and how they relate to each other. Connection lines may contain to indicate positive or negative correlation. They often look like webs, but they don't necessarily have to move outward from the center like spider maps do.

Steps to Create a Concept Map

- **Selection:** Write down key terms, concepts, and keywords related to your topic.
- Identify general intermediate and specific concepts and rank them from most abstract to most concrete.
- Cluster: Circle to group terms.
  - Over the most common concepts.
  - Intermediate concepts
  - Specific concepts at the bottom.
- **Placement:** Place concepts on the schematic by drawing lines between related concepts.
- **Connect and name:** Use lines and prepositions to connect and name concept.
- **Self-assessment:** Modify the concept map based on your assessment.
- **Peer evaluation:** Get feedback from peer groups.
- **Finalize:** Finalize the concept map based on self and peer review and critical analysis.

Concept Mapping Tips

The following approaches are used to develop nodes and links:
- Top-down approach
- Working from general to specific
- Free association approach
- Develop links and relationships from brainstorming nodes.
- Different shapes of nodes to identify different types of information
- Different colored nodes to identify previous and new information
- Cloud nodes to identify questions.
- Question nodes that gather information.

Create a Concept Map

- Select a topic to investigate. The size of the topic does not matter as it is intended to be granular. It may be part of a lecture or material covered in multiple lectures.
- Write down the most important concepts from the text on a notepad or highlight them to identify particular emphasis from the script.
- Sort concepts (and facts) from most general to most specific.

- Place the concept map with the most common concept on top. Link it to a noninclusive concept and enclose the text in a circle or other shape. If necessary, label the lines with connective words that describe the relationship. Arrows can indicate direction, cause, effect, etc.
- Try to branch at each level of the hierarchy using multiple links.
- Identify and draw the interconnections between related concepts. This is a powerful step in developing integrative thinking.
- Alternative patterns: A "spider" or cluster pattern can be constructed from the center outward.
- Leave white space to grow your map for:
  - Further development
  - Remarks
  - Action points
- Extend the map over time (may be even a trial!)
- Compare the map to other maps. Gain insights from different groups or across your organization.

Using Concept Maps

It is important that teachers take the time to introduce charts and diagrams to young students before using this strategy. There are several ways to create concept maps.
- As you read, model how you identify the main ideas and concepts presented in the selected text.
- Organize your ideas into categories. Remind your students that as they continue to read and add information, the organization can change.
- Use lines or arrows on the map to indicate how the ideas relate to specific categories or main concepts. Limit the amount of information on the map to avoid frustration.
- After students have completed their maps, encourage them to share and reflect on how they created connections between concepts.
- Encourage students to summarize what they have read using concept her maps.

Benefits of Concept Mapping

- Breaking down and understanding complex ideas.
- Understanding relationships between ideas at a glance.
- Brainstorming or organizing ideas.
- From simple tasks to complex systems. Illustrate different processes.
- Understand how different parts of the system work together.

Benefits of Concept Mapping to Learning

- It is active learning. Decisions must be made to create a map.

- Organize information by grouping facts and concepts. Learning is at a higher level than simply memorizing facts
- Show the relationship between facts and concepts by interconnection.
- Simple visualization promotes long-term memory. Exam insights are faster and more effective. Guide reading to prevent linear focus. Reading is encouraged to answer the question, as it requires looking for groupings and comparisons.
- Promote independent life-long learning.

PROJECT

The project method is a teacher-supported, collaborative approach in which students acquire and apply knowledge and skills to define and solve real-world problems through extended learning. Through a process of inquiry. Projects are student-centered and follow standard parameters and milestones clearly established by the instructor. The main idea of project teaching is the opportunity for students to demonstrate their knowledge and scientific practice skills through self-study.

Definition

- "A project is a part of life that is handed down to school in a project way of life learning". —**Ballard**
- "Project law is a heartfelt and deliberate activity in a social setting." —**Williams Kilpatrick**
- "The project method is a questionable act completed in a natural environment." —**Stevenson**

Project Features

- This method aims to teach learners how to make the most of life.
- An attempt to use experience trust and the best master whose lessons are unforgettable.
- The method gives opportunity for self-expression.
- The experiments of the project aims at resetting the whole curriculum and has potentials to break all barriers.
- The project method proposes the whole sequence of activities and involves a complete understanding.
- A project can be a large unit of appreciation learning or of attitude development that increases motor skills and technical knowledge.

Types of Projects

- **Types of projectors:** Projects that give students the opportunity to build or create: Building a house or garden and running a model of the textile factor are project types called.
- **Consumer type:** Projects in which students are attuned and enjoy direct experience with prospective consumers. For example, projects related to home/home visits to assess older people in the community.
- **Problem type:** The project where or the solution to the problem was found.
- **Drill type:** Drill type projects include activities aimed at developing more advanced skills. Example: Students are given a project that develops their ability to perform an experiment or procedure.

Principles for Effective Use of the Project Methodology

Preparation is key: Students should participate in the discussion of project goals. Ensuring the group's involvement from the planning stage through the first stages of the project is essential. Students should participate in discussions about project goals. Ensuring group participation at the planning stage is essential. Students should be involved in planning what the project will look like, the time frame, the cost, the extent of the impact on others, and how it will be evaluated. Teachers are a constant source of encouragement and resource in carrying out projects. Remind students of deadlines. A project evaluation is a critical view of the work done. Students and teachers decide whether the project was successful, met the goals set, and what areas were lacking.

Fundamentals of Good Projects

- Projects should emphasize current and future values and experiences that complement and extend rather than replicate learning gained outside of school.
- Project should be related to a larger theme and the knowledge gained should be applicable in a variety of ways.
- Projects must be timely.
- Projects should be challenging.
- The project should be executable.

Teacher's Role in Projects

- Teachers skillfully guide project selection.
- Students need help when they need it.
- Teachers should be good prompters.
- Teacher-student relationships should be much more intimate and informal than in a typical classroom setting.
- Teachers act like friends with rich and mature experience.
- Teachers act like directors. That is, the teacher's knowledge must be complete and specific.
- Teachers must be keen observers.
- Teachers should be repositories of information and knowledge.

Project Law Issues

Project law has a lot of value. At the same time there are problems too. Some of the problems that are focused are that the project becomes an end in itself at times and one forgets that it is primarily a teaching technique. To overcome this the project must be determined by the objectives of the class; sometimes students lose interest as projects take a long time to complete.

Using Projects in Teaching Nursing

Utilizing the steps of the project method effectively several projects individual and group can be used as a teaching method. Information attitude habit and service project can also be used.

Values for Project

There are many values for projects. Some of these are student participation and interest. Give students room to think and act, and ensure individual differences. cooperative spirit, etc. The benefits relate to two aspects. The resulting learning process that is valuable to the class/others.

Benefits

- Follows the laws of psychological learning (law of preparation, law of practice, law of effectiveness).
- The project format gives students freedom.
- Adapts to psychological maturity methods.
- May improve social value.
- Facilitates learning through hands-on problem solving.
- Training for social adaptation.
- Protect learners from dishonesty and superficiality.
- She is training for a democratic way of life.
- Facilitates learning through hands-on problem solving.
- Establish internal benchmarks.
- I feel satisfied with getting all the work done.
- Great for science crafts, hands-on geography, and dramatic writing.
- This process is economical. Students show more interest and learn in less time.
- This method helps students and teachers grow. Learners who are stimulated and encouraged by exploring many sources will eventually approach other areas of learning in a similar fashion.
- Teachers gain a better understanding of children's creative development.

Disadvantages

- The role of communication in the teaching and learning process is subordinated to the glorification of active learning.
- Time consuming, limited by availability and material cost.
- In most institutions, the practical difficulty of covering the curriculum has eliminated the project approach as a basis for teaching.
- This method is only an opportunity for practitioners.
- May be too ambitious. beyond the capabilities of the student.
- Gaps in student knowledge.
- Very limited ability to link to academic subjects.
- The project method can disrupt the normal course flow.
- It is difficult to ensure systematic progress of guidance.
- Projects can be taken over or abandoned at will
- The project approach often fails to fully master the learning tools that are essential for subsequent teaching of students.
- A complete reorganization of the school is required for new teachers.

DEBATE

Involving students in discussions and debates helps students develop a deeper understanding of the content and connect it to their own experiences. Learning is enhanced when students are encouraged to form opinions and develop their own ideas about the content. Incorporating discussion and debate style activities into the classroom encourages students to think more deeply about connections and gain broader insight into shared ideas and the diverse perspectives of others.

- In today's complex healthcare environment, it is important to prepare students to be critical thinkers and effective communicators. In addition to strong psychomotor skills, future healthcare providers will be able to confidently and effectively communicate not only with patients, but also with a wide range of stakeholders, including policy makers, payers, and other health professionals. must have the ability to take.
- The teaching method of debate will prepare students with such skills. Debates have the ability to reinforce and enhance knowledge in a topic area to engage students in the learning process to verify that students have the ability to analyze incorporate and apply the literature to various situations to heighten organization and listening skills and to boost confidence when challenged on issues by others.

Benefits of Debate

- **Critical thinking:** Debating instead of arguing helps defuse an escalating situation. With debates students can develop essential critical thinking skills the ability

to make well arguments in addition to questioning behind a particular conclusion. Critical thinking also helps students develop an interest in new ideas and a questioning attitude. As critical thinkers, students can be more humble.
- **Clarify your thoughts:** Discussions help you better explain different topics. From planning your discussion to choosing the right words, a wise debate helps you identify your audience and set the right tone. Their ability to articulate their thoughts and produce well-planned and sharp arguments is an important element of discussion.
- **Understanding complex situations:** Debating also helps students understand complex issues. Taking the time to carefully research a topic and carefully framing your points will lead to better discussions. Debating teaches students to summarize complex information, be creative, and practice different kinds of comprehension.
- **Develop courage:** Most students like to develop courage when speaking and arguing with others. Debates require careful preparation and a little courage to stand in front of like-minded people and say the opposite.
- **Synthesize knowledge:** Topics of discussion are diverse across multiple disciplines. Thus, class discussion allows the debater to gain knowledge outside the normal subject of the student. Debates provide students with an opportunity to explore real-world issue.

GAME

Game based learning (GBL) is a type of game play that has defined learning outcomes. Generally game based learning is designed to balance subject matter with game play and the ability of the player to retain and apply said subject matter to the real world. These games also known as "serious games" are educational tools that employ gamethinking and mechanics where the principal intent is not amusement or pleasure and are designed for the express goal of improving medical education.
- Game-based learning in education is an approach to learning in which aspects of games are inherent in the learning activities that are used to teach students about a variety of topics.
- They are competitive and use entertainment as a learning tool to encourage students to interact with each other.
- This type of learning often involves placing students in separate teams, includes materials and activities that compete with each other to meet certain rules or expectations.
- For example, a teacher could divide the class into her two teams to hold and receive points each time someone from each team spells a vocabulary word correctly.
- Teams can score more points by using more difficult words and the team with the most points at the end of the class will be declared the winner.

Goal
- To provide educators with strategies for developing comprehensive and evaluative play-based learning methods in nursing and healthcare play-based settings.
- Demonstrates how to integrate game-based learning into existing curricula.
- Provides theoretical and practical examples of how game-based learning techniques can be used in nursing and clinical teaching.

Elements of Game-based Learning
There are several key elements involved in game-based learning activities, including:
- **Competition:** In situations like this, the winner is usually based on point accumulation or performance. Healthy competition in the classroom can motivate students to engage more in learning activities, leading to more learning. Competitions also help students focus on their learning goals and collaborate with their teammates.
- **Participation:** Game-based learning activities are also used to encourage participation or to help students bring their attention and effort to educational activities. Enhancing student engagement is one of her ways to make students more involved in learning and increase children's curiosity and imagination. For example, a teacher may design a game-based learning activity in which students compete to find the most creative way to explain the main points of a story read in class. These types of activities encourage students to think about concepts in ways they otherwise could not.
- **Immediate rewards:** Another aspect of play-based learning is often giving students immediate rewards. Rewarding students immediately keeps their interest in learning activities. Providing instant rewards is also a way to give students immediate feedback on their correct and incorrect answers to tests and quizzes. Research suggests that under some circumstances providing students with immediate feedback can promote long-term learning. Giving students immediate rewards can also reinforce positive behavior such as completing assignments on time or cooperating with other students.

ROLEPLAY

Roleplay contexts are intended to reflect interactions between caregivers and patients to achieve desired treat-

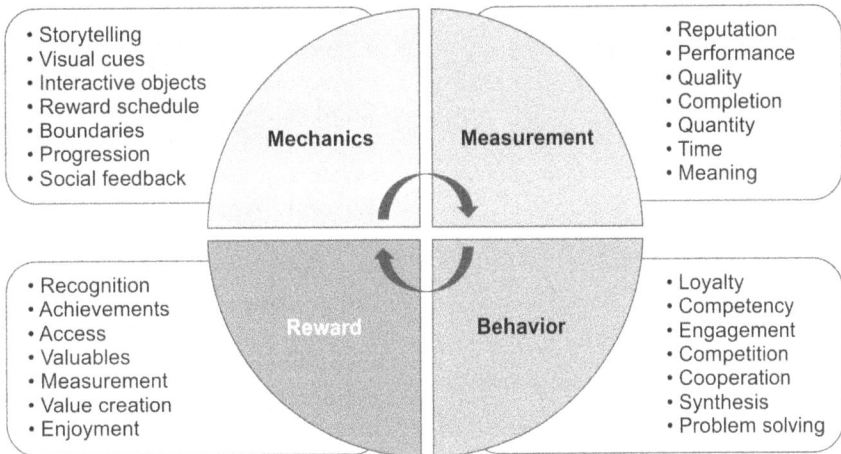

Fig. 8.14: Gamification model.

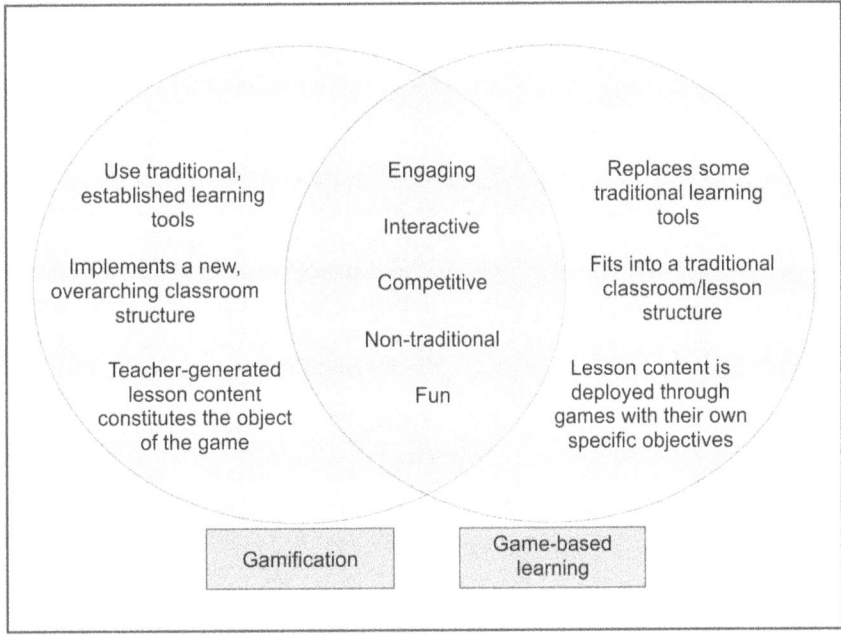

Fig. 8.15: Gamification and game-based learning.

ment outcomes. Enabling healthcare professionals to use effective communication skills while interacting with patients is critical.
- Roleplay situations are intended to reflect the interactions between caregivers and patients in order to achieve expected treatment outcomes.
- Key themes that emerge from the roleplay situations are self-disclosure and trust, respect, truthfinding and integrity, power and interpersonal conflict, empowerment and thought support.
- Self disclosure is an important theme in roleplay situations because it enables patients to trust their caregivers. Furthermore, roleplay situations require caregivers to respect the patient, but sincerity is closely related to trust, which affects caregiver credibility.
- Providers must be open to interacting with patients to avoid interpersonal conflict.
- The use of roleplay situations between nurses and patients is very important as it can contribute to the realization of desired treatment outcomes.

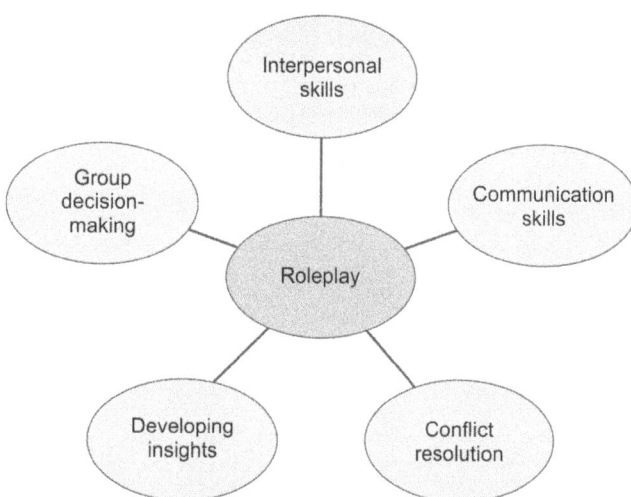

Fig. 8.16: Skills needed for roleplay.

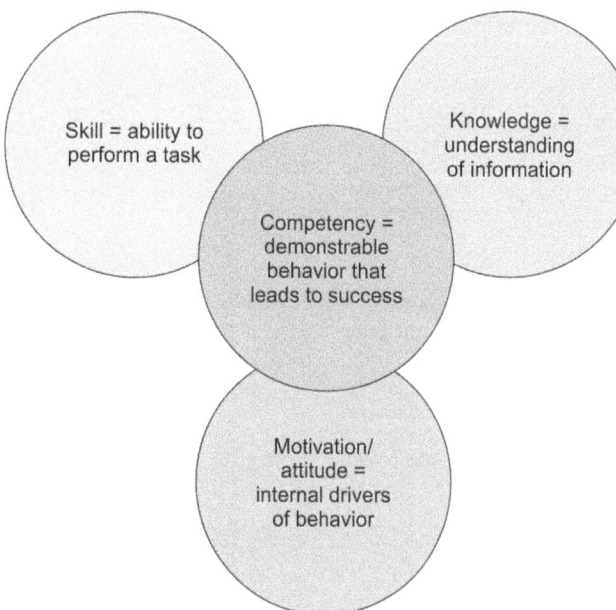

Fig. 8.17: Roleplay competencies.

Five reasons to add role-playing to your health simulation repertoire:
1. **Roleplaying provides an opportunity to take perspectives:** Roleplaying allows students to explore different "perceptual positions" and you can improve your awareness and understanding of yourself. Role-playing also builds empathy and appreciation for other perspectives.
2. **Roleplay simulations bring learning to life:** As students put into practice the skills they've learned in practice, they form a deeper cognitive connection with the material. Roleplay learning can be transformative by exposing participants to new insights beyond their own experience.
3. **Good roleplaying requires good listening skills:** It is important not only to understand the other person's words, but also to pay attention to his body language and nonverbal cues. Participants should be able to focus and pay attention to each response from other actors and respond appropriately in relation to it.
4. **Roleplaying is easy and safe:** Role-playing provides a safe and supportive environment to experience these situations for the first time and builds confidence in team members who can help them in the field. No matter how bizarre the situation in this controlled environment is, nothing strange has yet happened in real life. Roleplays help learners develop creative problem-solving skills while navigating challenging situations. Role-playing games are most useful for preparing for unfamiliar or difficult situations.
5. **Confidence through role-playing:** Preparing for situations through role-playing builds experience and confidence in dealing with real-world situations, allowing you to develop quick, instinctive and correct responses to situations.

Caregivers must be able to communicate effectively with patients to achieve desired treatment outcomes. To this end, the use of role-play situations between nurses and patients can contribute to the realization of expected treatment outcomes. However, a theoretical underpinning is essential for effective interactions between patients and caregivers.

PROBLEM-BASED LEARNING

Problem-based learning (PBL) has been identified as an approach to improve nurse education. It can be used clinically by teaching nurses how to apply theory to clinical practice and developing the problem-solving skills needed to overcome internal environmental constraints training.

Definition
Problem-based learning is a student-centered teaching learning strategy in which students solve problems together and this reflects their experience. In Problem-based learning, the starting point is the problem, question, or puzzle that the learner wishes to solve (DL Bound 1985).

Purpose
Problem-based learning is an approach that develops students' ability to critically apply accumulated knowledge to real clinical problems, motivates learning, develops clinical reasoning skills, and promotes self-reliance.

Components

PBL is the process of acquiring and understanding knowledge, skills and attitudes in unfamiliar situations and applying that learning to the situation.

PBL has four components:
1. Non-lecture format and teacher acting as a facilitator
2. A representation of a real-life situation or problem in everyday life.
3. Group work and group discussion.
4. Student solutions for selected pages problem.

PBL Functionality

PBL started due to a problem. The problem chosen is a real complex situation. Students are not given all the information they need to solve the problem. Students are encouraged to work in groups and identify resources on their own. The resulting learning of PBL is positively integrated, cumulative, and connected.

PBL Instructions
- Describe problem
- Organize ideas
- Ask questions
- Assigning responsibility for questions and discussing resources
- Survey questions summarizing and analyzing results
- Finding and reporting survey results
- Integrating new information and refining questions
- Solving problems.

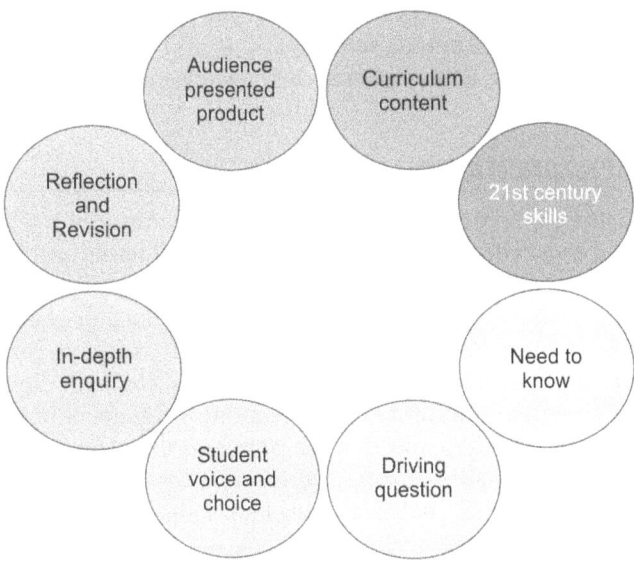

Fig. 8.19: Eight essential elements of problem-based learning.

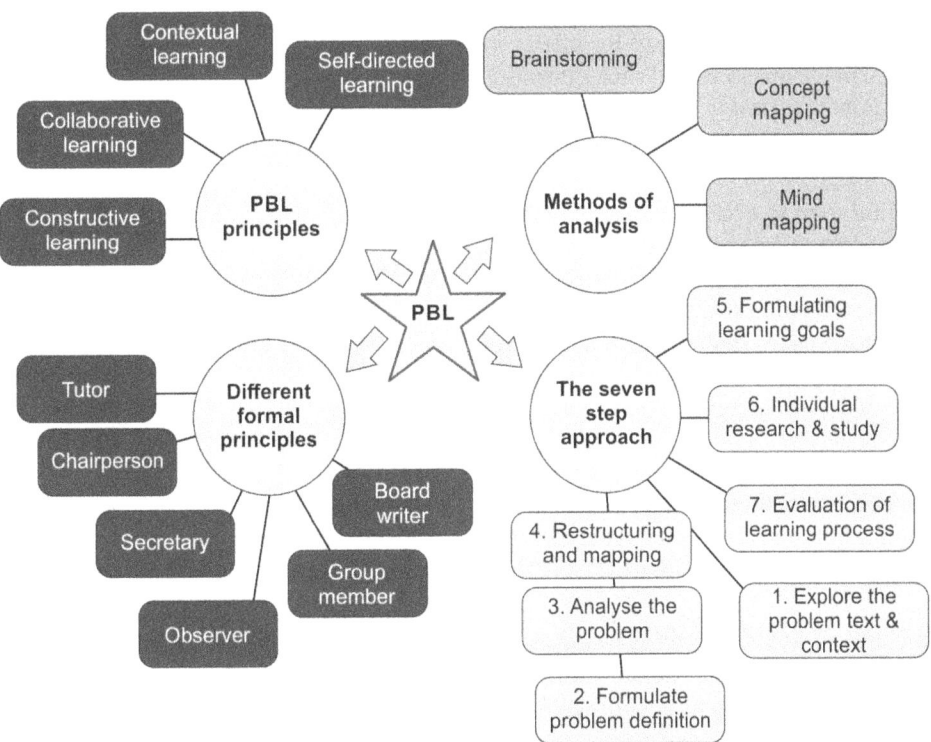

Fig. 8.18: Principles and steps of problem-based learning.

Advantages of PBL

- This helps students acquire subject knowledge.
- Students are continuously motivated to learn. The PBL method is relevant to the real world, so when students study using her PBL method, their memory improves.
- It promotes students' thinking and social skills.
- Promote student professionalism and promote trust and competence among students.
- Encourage the integration of knowledge from different subjects.

ASK/QUESTIONING

Asking questions is one of the most commonly used and most effective teaching strategies at all levels and in medical education. The concept of questioning may seem like a simple practice, but many medical educators have no training. When conducted effectively, surveys can produce positive results regarding learners' concentration and content comprehension. Nursing students should be encouraged to question the problems they encounter during clinical internships. Exploring different responses is the best way to analyze existing knowledge and integrate it into clinical practice.

Question Planning

An effective classroom voting session requires advance preparation. While some teachers may be adept at improvising questions, many teachers find such questions to be poorly worded, not organized in a logical order.

Levels and Types of Questions

- Questions should be used to achieve a clearly defined goal. Teachers should ask questions that require students to use the thinking skills they are trying to develop.
- Bloom's taxonomy is a hierarchical system for ordering thinking skills from lowest to highest, with each level requiring mastery of a lower skill.
- It is not essential that the instructor be able to tailor each question to a specific level.
- Taxonomy is introduced as a tool to help define the types of thinking skills a trainer expects from a student and to establish consistency between the trainer's goals and the questions he or she asks.

Strategies Used when Students Respond

- **Reinforcement:** Instructors should actively reinforce student responses and questions to encourage future participation. Trainers can reinforce with positive remarks and positive nonverbal communication. Appropriate nonverbal responses include smiling, nodding, and maintaining eye contact, while inappropriate nonverbal responses include looking at notes or looking at a board while the student is speaking or ruffled documents.
- **Probing:** A student's initial reaction may be superficial. Teachers should have students examine the first comment using a questioning strategy called probing. Probes help engage students more deeply in critical analysis of their own and other students' ideas.
- **Coordination/refocusing:** If a student provides an answer that appears to be out of context, the instructor should refocus and encourage the student to connect their answer to the content being discussed. This technique is also used to draw attention to new topics.

WRITTEN ASSIGNMENT

Clinical assignments are performed by program faculty with approved student-only affiliates on campus. Students who successfully complete the program on campus in the fall semester participate in a graduated clinical internship in the spring. In most nursing courses, students complete some type of written assignment. These assignments enable students to develop critical thinking skills, experience different styles of writing, and achieve other course-specific outcomes.

Writing assignments with teacher feedback help students develop their writing skills. This is an important achievement in any nursing program from entry level to graduate level. This chapter focuses on the development and evaluation of written assignments for nursing courses.

Purpose of Written Assignments

Written assignments are an important teaching and assessment method in nursing courses. They can be used to achieve many learning outcomes, but should be carefully selected and designed with the lesson goals in mind. For writing, students can call her on:

- Criticize and synthesize the literature and report your findings.
- Seeking criticism and synthesizing evidence in nursing practice.
- Analyze concepts and theories and apply them to clinical situations.
- Improved problem-solving and advanced thinking skills.
- Gain experience in organizing your thoughts and communicating them to others in a clear and coherent manner. and
- Develop your writing skills.

Types of Written Assignments

Many of the assignments written in the clinical course help students reflect on their care plan and identify areas that need further guidance. Some assignments, such as the Reflection Journal, also encourage students to examine their own feelings, beliefs and values, and reflect on their learning in the course. The assignment is suitable for assessment of nursing education. Some of these tasks provide information about how well the student has learned the content, but do not necessarily improve her writing skills. For example, structured tasks involving short sentences or phrases, such as care plans and recording assessments and physical examinations, do not facilitate writing skill development nor provide sufficient data for writing assessment.

- **Care plan:** A care plan is a written care plan for an individual family or community that reflects the care process. Components of the nursing process include evaluation of nursing diagnoses, planning with goals and measures, implementation and evaluation.
- **Case study answers:** Tasks that require case study answers must be written in complete sentence structure using correct grammar and spelling. A citation or reference list of resources may be required or included.

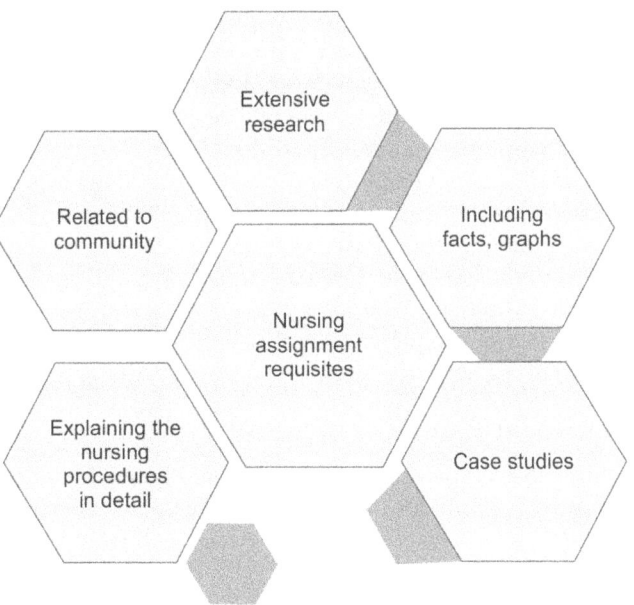

Fig. 8.20: Types of written assignments.

- **Discussion forums:** Discussion Forums provide an asynchronous online communication tool that allows students and faculty to initiate conversations in the form of posting messages and answering questions. Individual conversations in discussion forums are called threads. In a tiered discussion forum, comments are evaluated for content and reflective nature.
- **Electronic medical record documents:** Electronic medical records (EMRs) allow the entry, storage, and retrieval of health-related information during patient care. An EMR is a database with defined input fields for health information. Entries must be correct, especially for medical terms. EMR enables both portability and multiparty access. Students must comply with their institution's confidentiality standards and policies.
- **Multimedia presentations:** Students may be asked to give presentations in a variety of formats to demonstrate their integration of knowledge and communication skills. Multimedia presentations can include formats such as Power Point, Prezi Video, Wiki, and YouTube. As instructed by faculty. Text and images must be professionally clear and concise.
- **Reflective journal:** A form of writing that is detailed and often includes reflection on what the student has observed during the experience in a clinical setting. The journal contains personal experiences, observations from clinical practice, and theoretical approaches to the topic. In this style of writing, students connect thoughts and actions. Students are encouraged to post freely in their journals. Journaling is done in first person. The average length of a journal retrospective is 200-300 words.
- **Research papers:** The most formal of all papers written in nursing. One research paper uses the format of the American Psychological Association's Publishing Manual. Letters typically include a summary body of the title page and a bibliography. The paper has a goal or paper statement to guide the reader and reviews current evidence-based on peer-reviewed literature in the area of interest.
- **Research posters:** Visual presentations outlining scientific questions or issues. The poster will include the author's name and school affiliation in the title, research question, methods, results, conclusions, literature citations, and acknowledgments. A poster contains graphics, photographs, or other visual aids that represent the presentation of the material.
- **Curriculum booklet or curriculum:** A curriculum booklet or curriculum is a document, usually one or two pages long, that addresses the needs of the patient population. Topics are usually related to the disease course or treatment plan prescribed for the patient. The language of the material is visually appealing, the content is accurate, and it corresponds to the educational level of the population.

Writing Advice for Nursing Students

- Follow the instructions for the assignment. See syllabus and rubric.
- Review and search for resources. Internet Research Library APA. Read magazine articles, paying attention to both style and content.
- Define a specific focus or narrow aspect of the topic.
- Write for your audience. A fellow professional nurse.
- Writing should reflect the ability to introduce topics, balance ideas with concrete discussions relevant to nursing practice, support topics of interest, and draw clear conclusions.
- Letters should be logical and clearly and simply show the connections within and between paragraphs that flow from one point to the next.
- Writing should reflect critical thinking. Details should link to general concepts.
- Letters must have proper sentence structure. Grammar, spelling and punctuation must be checked carefully and accurately.
- The letter must represent the student's original work. You can use the ideas and words of others in support by summarizing or citing references. Students must cite original sources and follow academic rules for obtaining appropriate credits.
- Lettering follows APA style and format unless a different style and format is specified for a specific purpose.
- Take your tasks seriously. Do it on time and to the best of your ability.

PROCESS RECORDING TEACHING

The art of effective communication is a dynamic process. Some come naturally, while others can only be acquired through hard work. Student nurses often communicate with patients in a very superficial and stereotypical way rather than having a meaningful therapeutic quality. Therefore, student nurses need to be more perceptive in order to bring about constructive intervention through verbal exchange.

Definition

- Walker defines a process record as "the language between nurse and patient".
- Hudson defines a process record as "a record that accurately records the conversation between a nurse and a patient while they are together.
- Conen defines process recording as a "teaching and learning tool." Others used terms such as "interpersonal records." "Instead of process documentation, such as patient care interaction interviews. This process documentation is used in the artistic realm of nurse-patient relationships, but it is also widely used in the field of psychiatric nursing. Regardless of the field in which nurses work, nurses must be aware of the dynamics of human behavior and be able to apply their own behavior and communication.

Uses of Process Logs

There are three main uses:
1. As a teaching and learning tool.
2. As an evaluation tool.
3. As a therapeutic tool.

Different Phases of Process Mapping

- Prepare students for process mapping.
- Records of nurse-patient interactions.
- Evaluation of nursing-student interaction.

Student Guidelines

How to handle records (always use initials when referring to the patient's name):
- You should write down your goals.
- Note the key factors in shaping the patient's personality (obtained from the patient's history).
- Please mention the treatments the patient is receiving, both past and present.
- Must include the date of the process record.
- Time spent with the patient should be recorded.
- Prior to the interview, you will need to write a brief description of the setting and situation.
- Identify patient needs (expressed by patient behavior).
- Identify and give examples of mental mechanisms that the patient seems to use.
- When you have completed the process log, indicate how well you achieved the goals you set before starting work.
- As a learning experience, evaluate the process log at the end of the task.

Statement of Goals or Objectives

Since the therapeutic interaction should be goaldirected, objectives should be stated in relation to the outcome so that the process can be effectively assessed. Examples of goals are:
- Know the patient's anxiety level.
- Helps patients express their feelings about hospitalization.
- Evaluate your feelings and thoughts about specific events.

Nurse-Patient Interaction Record

A true record of what the nurse said and did, what the patient said and did.

Therapeutic Relationships

A therapeutic relationship is a relationship between two or more people for the purposes of behavior change, anxiety relief, support, encouragement, nurturing, and guidance. In a therapeutic relationship, helpers and helpers are involved.

The most important skills in interpersonal therapy are behavioral observation and understanding and communication are very important.

The goal is change towards the client's growth, but in the process the therapist may gain more understanding of himself, his interaction patterns, etc.

The therapeutic relationship, learn how to deal with problem situations, find new ways to deal with them, and move towards your own full development. The therapeutic relationship can be more burdensome for caregivers than other cares. Caregivers must offer a part of themselves, not medication or therapy. You need to be mature, have a fair self-image, and have certain skills and attitudes to be able to offer a piece of yourself.

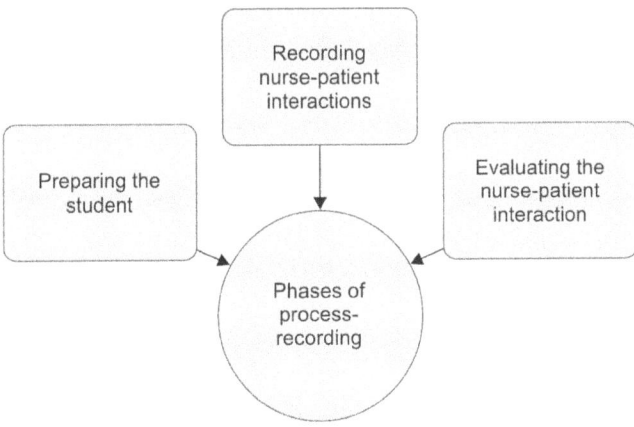

Fig. 8.21: Phases of process recording.

Stages of Process Recording

He has three main stages in process recording:
1. Student preparation for process records
2. Records of interactions between nurses and patients
3. Assessment of care-patient interactions.

Student Preparation

Teachers should help students define goals to be achieved in the nurse-patient interaction. Teachers should discuss process logs as a teaching and learning tool. Teachers should help students learn how to write process logs.

Recording Nurse-Patient Interactions

There are four key parts to recording nurse-patient interactions. We have the following records:

1. The exact verbatim report of nurse-patient conversation.
2. The student's conscious feelings and her interpretation of the patient's feeling.
3. Analysis for meanings and clues to patient's needs.
4. Instructor and student evaluation of the overall process recording experience.

Process record requirements

- At least two people.
- Reassurance of the patient regarding confidentiality of the interview.
- Recording of all verbal interaction.
- Notation of thoughts feeling and action's of student nurse.
- Representation of patient non-verbal communication.
- Record the interaction as soon as possible after the interaction (note the time between interaction and actual recording)

Evaluating the Nurse-Patient Interaction

After the interacting data have been collected by the student the teacher and the students should analyze the data during which the objectives should be kept in focus.

The teacher should correct the recording and help the student to advance to the stage of self-evaluation.

Merits

- Improves the skill of communication and technique of interaction.
- It reinforces more specific therapeutic conversations.
- Improves ability to handle stressful situations.
- Helps to understand the psychopathology of various illnesses.
- Understand how the mind works.
- The patient learns to listen to others.
- Provides links to theory and practice.

Cons

- Time consuming
- Possibility of transforming therapeutic relationships into social relationships
- Strict confidentiality is required.

CONCLUSION

Clinical teaching in nursing is a kind of group meeting that observes, examines, points out and guides one or more patients towards the improvement and further development of nursing by nursing students. Nursing's learning process is very unique. Nursing students, like general education, must be able to perform professional activities in reallife situations where it is all about understanding principles in the laboratory and on nonhuman objects. Nursing learning experiences should provide opportunities to apply theoretical principles to real-time bedside/community situations on a daily basis. This unit explores a variety of clinical teaching methods.

REVIEW QUESTIONS

Long Essays
1. Define clinical teaching methods, explain meaning, objectives and uses of clinical education.
2. Describe the factors influences clinical learning experience selection.
3. Explain the teaching models in clinical use.
4. Describe the clinical learning outcomes/practical skills.
5. Enlist the functions of clinical instructor.
6. Define patient's assignments, explain principles of patient assignment.
7. Describe the clinical meetings: Individual and group.
8. Define nursing rounds, explain the purposes and procedures for conducting nursing visits.

Short Essays
1. Clinical learning environment.
2. Importance of a good clinical learning environment.
3. Principles for the selection of learning experiences.
4. Criteria for selecting learning experiences.
5. Stanford faculty development model.
6. Clinical teacher key characteristics.
7. Clinical instructor qualities.
8. Applying clinical teaching methods in education.
9. Clinical teaching skills.
10. Clinical teaching challenges.
11. Clinical teaching strategies.
12. Principles for improving teachers skills.
13. Benefits and disadvantages of case study method.
14. Team nursing.
15. Progressive patient care.
16. Case management.
17. Group conferences: Role and responsibilities of the instructor.
18. Clinical presentation/bedside clinic.
19. Bedside clinic/bedside teaching.
20. Objectives of the case analysis method.
21. Case presentation stage.
22. Case presentation format.
23. Principles of care planning.
24. Concept mapping: Purposes and types.
25. Steps to create concept mapping.
26. Benefits of concept mapping to learning.
27. Principles for effective use of the project methodology.
28. Problem-based learning.
29. Elements of game-based learning.
30. Process recording teaching.

Short Answers
1. Preceptor.
2. Clinical supervisor.
3. Clinician educator.
4. Clinician teacher.
5. Mentor.
6. Clinical education issues.
7. Challenges in patient assignment.
8. Methods of patient assignment.
9. Factors affecting patient assignment.
10. Primary nursing: Features and advantages.
11. Functional nursing.
12. Case manager responsibilities.
13. Bedside clinic goals.
14. Preparation for bedside clinic.
15. Critical incident technique.
16. Benefits of the drop method.
17. Criteria for good case studies.
18. Patient care planning development.
19. Care plan benefits.
20. Benefits of concept mapping.
21. Teacher's role in projects.
22. Benefits of debate.
23. Advantages of PBL.
24. Ask/questioning.
25. Clinical assignments.
26. Purpose of written assignments.
27. Types of written assignments.
28. Stages of process recording.
29. Evaluating the nurse-patient interaction.

Unit 5

Educational/Teaching Media

Chapters

9. Eductional/Teaching Media
10. Still Visuals
11. Moving Visuals and Audio Aids
12. Electronic and Telecommunication

KEYWORDS

Educational media: Educational media refers to channels of communication that carry messages with an instructional purpose. They are usually utilized for the sole purpose of learning and teaching.

Desirable teacher behavior: There are some behaviors the teacher must follow while teaching in class.

Instructional media: Play a major role in the classroom communication process. This unit has focused on the nature and characteristics of media which you should be generally using in the class.

Electronic media: These include audio media, visual media and audiovisual media, projected media and nonprojected media.

Audio media: These are the teaching-learning devices that appeal to the auditory sense. In other way, these media can be heard alone, it carries sounds, for example audio tapes, record player, radio, etc.

Live classroom: The live classroom facility enables a learner to take class in real time. This online virtual classroom is a significant shift from traditional blackboard classroom.

Digital media: Digital media is a fast and efficient form of mass media. It encompasses all types of social media, blogs, forums, web portals, and others.

Multi-touch technology: This is a major transformation from blackboard, white board smart board to mobile devices. This multi-touch screens helps the learner to feed inputs which boost interaction of learner in classroom environment.

Digital daily: The learning process has transformed from textbooks to digital books. Electronic digital papers are thin and extremely light-built. They come with a lightweight, durable frame and are portable.

Social media: Digital awareness and social media understanding are much needed to assist students connect with others. Students can shoot queries in global communities with large, knowledgeable audience to answer and guide them.

Models: Unlike charts and posters, models are three-dimensional visual aids. Models provide representation of the real things in all respects except size and shape.

Computer-based instruction: Computers have great usefulness in the classroom. They can give instruction to students, call for responses, feedback the results, and modify students' further learning accordingly.

Digital media in education: Digital media in education is measured by a person's ability to access, analyze, evaluate, and produce media content and communication in a variety of forms. These media may involve incorporating multiple digital software's, devices, and platforms as a tool for learning.

Media education: Media education is the process through which individuals become media literate—able to critically understand the nature, techniques and impacts of media messages and productions.

Mass media: Mass media refers to the news and information that reaches a large number of people, while local media, e.g., newspapers, and regional television/radio stations, serves the needs of the communities or urban areas in which they are located.

Internet: The internet refers to the global communication system, including hardware and infrastructure, while the web is one of the services communicated over the internet. The internet allows the transfer of data, information, and communication worldwide, connecting organizations, devices, and people in a decentralized and distributed manner.

Chapter 9

Educational/Teaching Media

Learning Objectives
- Brief History of AV-Aids Use
- Importance of Audiovisual Aids
- Categories of Educational Media
- Important Values of AV Resources
- Teaching Aid/Materials
- Teaching Aid Issues
- Classifications of Teaching Aids
- Cone of Experience
- Importance of AV Aids in Educational Communication
- Role of Educational Media in Teaching
- Psychological Basis for AV-Aids

TERMINOLOGY

- Educational media is defined as any device, content material, method, or experience used for teaching or learning purposes.
- Materials are used to explain content, coordinate, activities, and provide new and exciting learning methods for review purposes. They help implement educational strategies and activities.
- **Print media:** This includes—books magazines, magazines newspapers, workbooks and texts. They are easy to use and inexpensive.
- **Nonprinted media:** This includes projected and nonprojected media.
- **Electronic media:** This includes audiovisual media, projected media, and nonprojected media.
- **Audio media:** These are auditory teaching and learning devices. Another way these media can be heard in isolation is sound transmission. From tapes, turntables and radio.
- **Visual media:** Media that appeals to the eye (eyes) or can be seen, e.g. TV computer whiteboard.
- **Audiovisual:** Means materials that provide learners with an audiovisual experience through simultaneous auditory and visual stimulation, television videotape and closed circuit television (CCTV).
- **Projected media:** Projected Media belongs to a group of educational resources and may only be accessed by projecting the content onto a screen or wall using a projector device specifically designed for that purpose.
- **Non-projection media:** These tools do not require projection to a screen. These do not require a light source. This includes 3D objects, 2D objects, prints, charts, models, etc.
- **Multimedia:** Multimedia combines five basic media types (text, video, sound, graphics, and animation) in learning environments to provide powerful new tools for teaching. Multimedia includes any combination of text, audio, still images, animated video, or interactive forms of content.
- **Motivation:** Motivates and engages students in learning.
- **Clarification:** Using materials to help teachers understand the material.
- **Direct experience:** Materials provide students with direct experience.
- **Hearing aid:** An educational device that only listens to messages.
- **Visual aids:** Materials that can be viewed while listening to the message.
- **Non-projected aids:** Visual aids that are simply presented without a projection device.
- **Projection aid:** A visual aid that is projected and magnified by focusing light.
- **Presentation aid:** A visual aid positioned for viewing by the audience. You understand the message by looking at it.

- **Presentation aid:** A visual aid presented or projected for viewing by a viewer that explains or presents a visual message in a way that the viewer can understand.
- **Chalkboard:** Probably the simplest, cheapest, most practical, and most widely used non-projected visual aid in extended education.
- **Whiteboards:** Modern classrooms are equipped with whiteboards, also known as marker boards or multipurpose boards.
- **Bulletin board:** A board for displaying messages.
- **Flannel board:** A visual aid in which a message is written or drawn on thick paper and presented to the audience in stages by an enhancement agent and synchronized with the lecture.
- **Flashcards:** A short visual message on a posterboard card that flashes (flips over in short intervals) in front of the audience to emphasize key points in a presentation.
- **Posters:** Printed messages placed in public places to raise people's awareness.
- **Charts:** Symbolic visual aids containing images of relationships and changes used to summarize or display the history of large amounts of information.
- **Multimedia:** A combination of multiple media, but can include multiple forms of media, including audio, text, still images, animation, graphics, video, and film.

INTRODUCTION

Materials are tools that teachers use in the classroom. Index cards, card cassettes, chalkboards. Educational materials, like many educational materials such as games, are designed to help learners improve their reading and other skills, explain or reinforce facts and ideas in skills, and relieve anxiety, fear, or boredom. It is a tool used by teachers. Audiovisual aids or equipment, or technical media or learning devices, help teachers clarify and create connections, establish accurate concepts, interpretations, and assessments, and make learning more concrete, effective, interesting, stimulating, meaningful and lively additional equipment. They help complete the learning process of the triangle of motivation, clarification, and stimulation. The purpose of teaching with technical media is to level the channel between what is learned and what is worth learning.

The basic assumption underlying audiovisual materials is that learning-clear understanding-arises from sensory experience. Teachers have to show and tell. Audiovisual materials offer great advantages in storing information learning and eliciting thinking an reasoning activities, interest, imagination, better assimilation, personal growth and development. Tools inspire you to learn the why, how, when and where. Hard-to-understand principles are usually revealed through the clever use of well-designed materials.

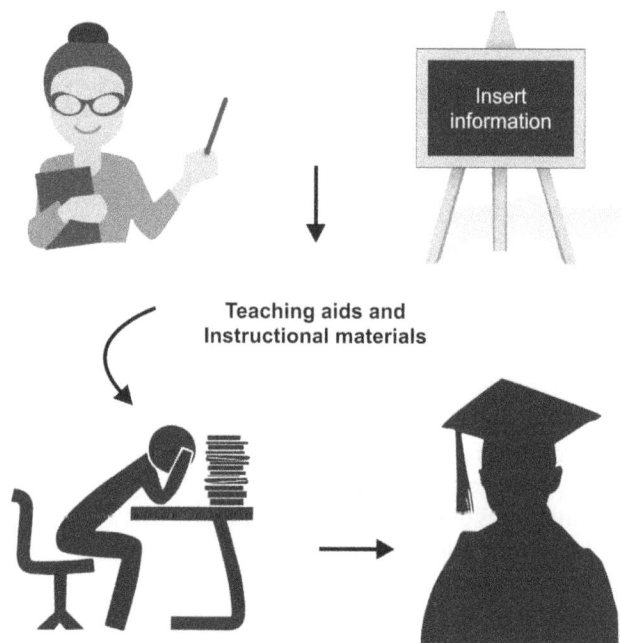

Fig. 9.1: Teaching aid and instructional media.

BRIEF HISTORY OF AV-AIDS USE

- The Dutch humanist theologian and writer Desiderius Erasmus (1466–1536) discouraged memorization as a learning technique, advocating that children should learn with the aid of pictures and other visual means.
- John Amos Comenius (1592–1670) authored a book titled his Orbit sensulium pictus (World of Sensory Objects) containing about 150 photographs relating to aspects of everyday life. This book is considered the first illustrated textbook for children's education. The book became widely known and was used in children's educational centers around the world.
- JeanJacques Rousseau (1712–1778) and other educators stressed the need for pictures and other playthings. Rousseau criticized the teacher's use of language and emphasized "things". He argued that the educational process must be tailored to the learners' natural curiosity.
- Pestalozzi (1756–1827) implemented Rousseau's theory in the "object method". He taught based on sensory perception.
- Eric Asliby (1967) identified his four revolutions in education. The fourth revolution in home to school education, the invention of the written word as a means of education, the use of print and books, and finally the use of electronic media. Radio, television, tape recorders, and computers in education.

DEFINITION

- Educational media refers to communication channels that convey messages for educational purposes. They usually serve the sole purpose of learning and teaching.
- Materials are tools that help teachers manage the learning environment and activities more productively. Props are physical objects commonly used in storytelling and demonstrations.
- An audiovisual aid is a sensory object or image that initiates, stimulates, and reinforces learning (Burton).
- Audiovisual aids are aids to help you complete the triangle learning process, motivational classification and stimulation. —**Carter V Good**
- Audiovisual media are tools that support the communication of ideas between individuals and groups in a variety of educational and training settings. These are also called multisensory materials. —**Edgar Dale**

IMPORTANCE OF AUDIOVISUAL AIDS

Audiovisual aids are aids that help you complete the learning process. This means motivational stimulation and clarification of completed learning.

The term "audiovisual communication" is used for materials used in educational settings to promote the understanding of spoken and written language. The fact that the term is used to cover the full range of descriptive materials such as visual materials, auditory materials, and combinations of the two.

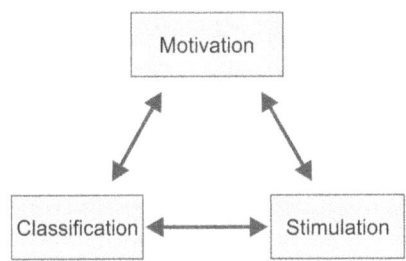

Fig. 9.2: Basic of audiovisual aids.

Audiovisual communication tutorial: We also refer to course information, ideas, and other content created for use with such programs as software, and audiovisual aids and devices as hardware. Audiovisual communication appeals to hearing and sight. Audiovisual materials are commonly used as learning materials to complement books and formal classroom instruction. Comenius was the first educator to create and use an erotic encyclopedia. He found that learning adapted to their experience. It is more effective to keep students' attention focused and make learning fun.

CATEGORIES OF EDUCATIONAL MEDIA

- Display materials such as black boards, that pictures, chalk boards, etc
- Printed materials such as textbooks, dictionaries, newspapers, magazines, official documents, and reference materials
- Graphic materials such as graphs, charts, diagrams, posters, maps, and cartoons
- Audiovisual materials Radio, telephone, television, cassette recorders, computers, etc.
- Filmstrip or slide projectors, microprojectors, opaque projectors, and overhead projectors.

IMPORTANT VALUES OF A-V RESOURCES

- **An antidote to verbal teaching diseases:** Helps reduce vocabulary. They help convey clear concepts and help achieve accuracy in learning.
- **Best motivator:** Students are more interested and enthusiastic, are more observant.
- **Clear image:** Find a clear image when you see, hear, touch, taste and smell. Learning through the senses is the most natural and, as a result, the fastest.
- **Surrogate experience:** Handson experience is arguably the best educational experience. However, it is neither practical nor desirable to give students such an experience.
- **Diversity:** Chalk and talk do not help. Audiovisual materials add variety and put different tools in the hands of the teacher.
- **Freedom:** Audiovisual aids allow children to move, talk, laugh and comment freely. In such an atmosphere, students work not because teachers want to work, but because they want to work.
- **Opportunities for handling and manipulation:** Many visual aids provide students with ways to handle and manipulate objects.
- **Memory:** Audiovisual aids stimulate the whole organism's response to learning situations and thus help improve memory.
- **Based on teaching principles:** The use of audiovisual materials enables teachers to follow teaching principles such as known knowledge, learning by doing, from concrete to abstract.
- **Helps to get attention:** Attention is a real factor in the teaching and learning process. Audiovisual materials help teachers create a caper-friendly environment and maintain students' attention and interest in the lesson.
- **Helps to modify new learning:** Should learning gains be anchored in students' minds? Audiovisual materials help

achieve this goal by providing learners with a variety of activities, experiences and stimuli.

- **Saves energy and time:** The use of audiovisual equipment makes it easy to explain, understand and process most concepts and phenomena, saving both teachers and students a lot of energy and time.
- **Realism:** The use of audiovisual materials makes the learning situation real. By watching a film about life in the tundra, students can learn more effectively in about two hours rather than weeks of reading.
- **Liveliness:** Audiovisual materials add liveliness to the learning situation. Movies about the Buddha provide a vivid depiction of the life and teachings of the Buddha.
- **Addressing individual differences:** Learners are highly individual. There are also ear ones. Some people find visual demonstrations helpful, others learn better by doing. A variety of audiovisual materials can be used to meet the needs of different types of students.
- **Encouraging healthy interaction in the classroom:** Audiovisual materials promote healthy classroom interaction to effectively achieve classroom learning goals through a variety of stimuli that provide active student participation and proxy experiences.
- **Access to education:** Audiovisual devices such as radio and television can help provide educational opportunities to people living in remote areas. It also helps promote adult education.
- **Cultivate a scientific disposition:** Students develop a scientific disposition by observing evidence and phenomena instead of hearing facts.
- **Advanced skill development:** Vocabulary facilitates memorization. The use of audiovisual materials stimulates students' imagination and thinking ability, challenges students' creativity and invention, and other advanced intellectual activities, and assists students in developing higher abilities.
- **Learner reinforcement:** Audiovisual aids have been shown to be effective reinforcement, increasing the likelihood of recurrence of relevant responses and providing valuable support to the teaching and learning process.
- **Active transitions in learning and training:** The use of audiovisual materials enables appropriate positive transitions in classroom learning and training so that other conceptual principles can be learned and practiced in life. Help solve the problem.
- **A positive environment for creative students:** Balanced, rational and scientific use of audiovisual materials motivates, engages students' attention and interest, and harnesses their tremendous energy provide a variety of creative opportunities for learning and stay engaged in educational activities. In this way, the entire classroom environment becomes conducive to creative discipline.

TEACHING AID/MATERIALS

Materials are an integral part of every classroom. The many benefits of educational tools include helping learners improve reading comprehension, explaining or reinforcing skills and concepts, differentiating instruction, and reducing anxiety and boredom by presenting information in new and exciting ways. including helping to reduce The teaching and learning process depends on the different types of equipment in the classroom. Currently, there are many assistive devices, such as audiovisual aids.

Teaching Material Functions

- Stimulate students' inspiration and curiosity about the subject.
- Provide opportunities for students to participate in a variety of activities.
- Keep topics simple and fun.
- It makes the difficult parts of the chapter easier to understand.
- Increase student interest in the subject.
- Makes an impact in the classroom and makes teaching and learning more impressive.

Need for Teaching Materials

- Everyone tends to forget. With proper use of the material, more concepts can be retained permanently.
- Students learn better when properly motivated by a variety of teaching tools.
- If the student sees, hears, tastes and smells correctly, the material forms the correct image.
- Materials provide complete examples of conceptual thinking.
- Materials create an interesting environment for students.
- Materials help students increase their vocabulary.
- Materials help teachers take their time and make learning lasting.
- Teaching aids provide direct experience to the students.

Characteristics of good teaching materials are:

- Materials should be large enough for the students using them to see.
- Materials are useful and always serve a useful purpose.
- The materials are up-to-date in every respect.
- Materials are simply cheap and can be improvised.
- The materials are accurate and realistic.
- Materials are based on the mental state of the learner.

- The purpose may be useful, but it is not mere entertainment.
- The materials will help you achieve the specified learning objectives.
- The materials are very useful and can be used in many classes and at different grade levels.
- Supplemental materials are useful to supplement the course, but do not replace the teacher.

Classification of Teaching Aids

Teaching aids can be classified as audio aids, visual aids, audiovisual aids, and activity aids.
- **Hearing aids:** like radio tape recorders. It is a useful tool for learners to acquire hearing knowledge.
- **Visual aids:** These are things like charts, photographs, models, epidiascopes, microprojectors, film strips, etc. Represents a tool that helps learners navigate through visual learning experiences.
- **Audiovisual aids:** These are all devices and aids, such as television movies, video films, creatures, etc., that give the learner the opportunity to accomplish an objective using both hearing and sight.
- **Activity tools:** Activity tools are tools that help students learn by participating in helpful activities. These tools facilitate learning through seeing, hearing, and doing.

The Importance of Materials

Materials play a very important role in the teaching and learning process. The importance of educational tools is:
- **Motivation:** Teaching tools motivate students to learn better.
- **Clarification:** Teaching materials allow teachers to clarify material more easily.
- **Discourage cramming:** The material promotes proper student understanding of discouraging cramming.
- **Increase vocabulary:** Learning materials help students increase their vocabulary more effectively.
- Save time and money
- **Classroom lively and active:** Materials make the lesson lively and active.
- Avoid dullness.
- **Direct experience:** Materials provide students with a direct experience.

Effective Materials

Effective materials have the following characteristics:
- They should be meaningful and purposeful
- Must be exact in all respects.
- They should be easy.
- Be inexpensive.
- Must be large enough to be clearly visible to the intended student.
- They must be up-to-date.
- Easy to carry.
- They should be appropriate to the intellectual level of the student.
- Learners should be motivated.

Principles for the Use of Materials

- **Principles of choice:** Materials are effective only if they match the educational goals and characteristics of a particular group of learners, the following points can be maintained.
  - Must be suitable for the learner's age level, grade level, and other characteristics.
  - Must be interesting and motivating as well as have a specific educational outlet.
  - They must be genuine and true representatives.
  - It should help you achieve your desired learning goals.
- **Principle of preparation:** This principle requires the following points to be adhered to:
  - When creating aids, locally available materials should be used whenever possible.
  - Teachers must be trained to create tools.
  - Some tools must be provided by the teacher.
  - Students can participate in creating resources.
- **Physical management readiness:** This principle relates to the placement of tools to keep them safe and facilitate learning for teachers to use.

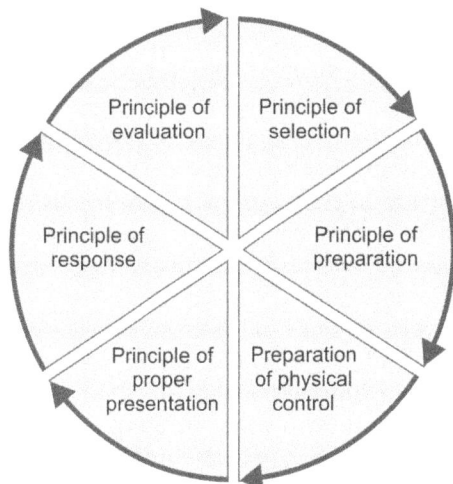

Fig. 9.3: Principles of using AV aid materials.

- **Fair presentation principle:** This principle includes:
  - Teachers should carefully visualize the use of the material before the actual presentation.

- Familiarize yourself with the use and handling of the resources demonstrated in the lessons.
- Handle the aids with care to avoid damage.
- Resources must be properly displayed so that all students can see, observe, and get maximum benefit from them.
- All kinds of distractions should be avoided as much as possible so that you can give your help enough attention.
- **The responsive principle:** This principle requires that teachers lead students to actively respond to audiovisual stimuli in order to obtain the maximum benefit from learning.
- **Principle of evaluation:** This principle states that both audiovisual materials and accompanying technology must be continually evaluated in order to achieve their intended goals.

Selection of Materials

Teachers need to know how to use the appropriate materials in a particular teaching-learning situation that best fits the lesson. As one issue or guidance, science teachers should keep the following principles in mind while carefully choosing appropriate materials to teach a particular subject.

- **Relevance:** The tools you use should be relevant to the topic at hand.
- **Suitability:** It should suit the topic as best as possible by making its study quite comprehensive interesting permanent and effective.
- **Educative:** The aid should have specific educational value besides being interesting and motivating. In no case it should be confined to mere entertainment
- **Best substitute for the first hand experience:** The aid should be so chosen as to prove a best possible substitute in terms of reality accuracy and truthful representation of object or the first hand experiences.
- **Learner-centered:** Supporting materials should be chosen that match the age level, baseline, core instincts, interests, and other unique characteristics of the students in the class.
- **Simplicity:** The tools you use should be fairly simple in structure and use. It should also be able to convey its meaning as simply as possible.
- **Environmental orientation:** Supporting materials should be appropriate to the needs of the student's physical, social and cultural environment.
- **Practicality:** Tools should be selected considering the specific situation, available resources, and purpose for which they are served. It should not be too expensive to buy and collect, use or demonstrate in the classroom. It should reflect the availability of weather conditions, climate requirements, teacher and student responses, and other resources available at the institution and in the classroom.
- **Achieving goals:** Supporting materials should be chosen in a manner that helps to successfully achieve the learning or teaching goals stated in each topic.

Advantages of the TA Benefits

TA are:
- Supplement to oral description.
- Materials make learning permanent.
- Materials offer variety.
- Supplemental materials help to hold the student's attention.
- Materials save time and energy.
- Materials promote healthy interaction in the classroom.
- Materials help teachers create situations for teaching beginners.
- Materials help create a positive environment for the discipline.
- Teaching materials help to counteract individual differences.
- Materials are useful for students' language training.
- Materials help children retain language content longer.
- Materials enliven the learning situation.
- Materials help to embody abstract ideas and make learning more effective.
- Materials are a great substitute for real objects because they make learning just as meaningful.
- Teaching aids help develop a variety of skills such as: How to chart topics among students.

Use of Materials

- Materials should be concise.
- Materials should be relevant to the lesson objectives.
- The material should be a large door that all students can see.
- Teachers must use appropriate teaching materials for the benefit of their students.
- Materials should be prepared and planned in advance.
- Materials should be selected according to the physical and intellectual level of the students.
- Materials should be colorful and have a direct impact on the lesson.
- Materials should be meaningful and interesting.

TEACHING AID ISSUES

Although these tools are becoming more popular by the day, there are still some issues that need to be resolved.

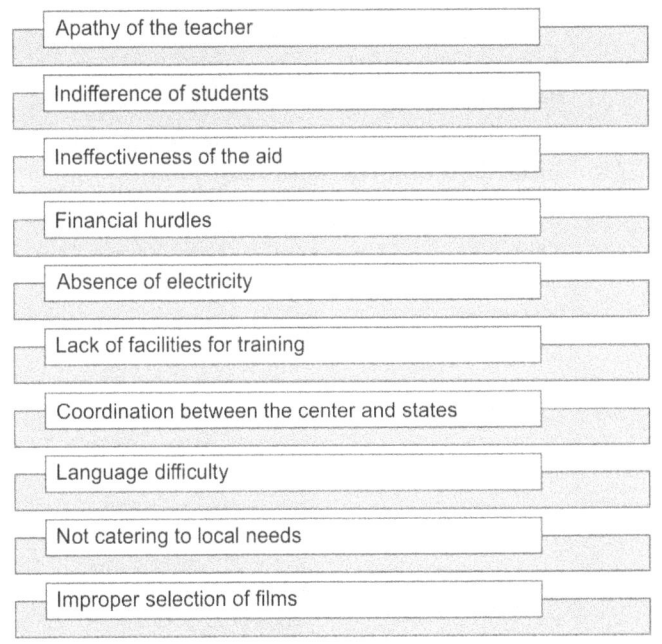

Fig. 9.4: Common issues needs to considered in selecting AV aids.

- **Teacher indifference:** Teachers are generally still not convinced that teaching with words alone is very boring, wasteful and ineffective.
- **Student indifference:** Judicious use of aids intrigues, but improper use loses meaning and importance.
- **Ineffectiveness of aids:** Due to lack of planning and laziness on the part of teachers, and lack of proper preparation, correct presentation, proper application and discussion, and necessary follow-up work, aids are ineffective. plug. The movie is like a good lesson in the different steps of preparation, presentation, application and discussion.
- **Financial obstacles:** The central and state governments have launched an interesting program to disseminate educational materials with the audiovisual education commission, but lack of funds prevents it from doing its best.
- **Lack of power:** Most radio and TV projectors cannot function without power, which is not available in many schools.
- **Lack of training facilities:** Colleges or institutions should make special arrangements to train teachers and workers in the use of these tools.
- **Coordination between the center and the state:** Excellent film libraries audiovisual educational museums fixed and mobile exhibitions and educational melas should be organized both centrally and nationally.
- **Language problems:** Most educational films are in English. I need to display these in Hindi and other major Indian languages.
- **Local needs are not considered:** Little attention is paid to local sociological, psychological and educational factors in the production of audiovisual materials.
- **Inappropriate movie selection:** Movie not selected as required for class.

CLASSIFICATIONS OF TEACHING AIDS

Classification 1

Projected and non-projected aids. *See* **Table 1**.

Classification 2

Audiovisual material, visual materials and audiovisual materials. *See* **Table 2**.

Classification 3

Big medias and little medias:
- Big medias include computer, VCR, and TV.
- Little media include radio, film strips, graphic, audio cassettes and various visuals.

Table 9.1: Classifications of AV aids.

Projected aids	Graphic aids	Display boards	3-D-aids	Audio-aids	Activity aids
Films	Cartoons	Black board	Diagrams	Radio	Computer-assisted instruction
Films strips	Charts	Bulletin	Models	Recording	Demonstration
Opaque projectors	Comics	Flannel board	Mockups	Television	Dramatics
Overhead projectors	Diagrams	Magnetic board	Objectives		Experimentation
Slides	Flash cards	Peg board	Puppets		Field trips
	Graphs		Specimens		Programmed instruction
	Maps				Teaching machines
	Photographs				
	Pictures				
	Postures				

Table 9.2: Types of audio, visual and audiovisual aids.

Audio material	Visual material	Audiovisual materials
Language laboratories	Bulletin boards	Demonstration
Radio	Chalk boards	Films
Sound distribution system sets	Charts	Printed materials with recorded sound
Tape and disco recording	Drawings etc	Sound filmstrips
	Exhibits	Study trips
	Film strips	Television
	Flash carts	Video tapes
	Flannel boards	
	Flip books	
	Illustrated books	
	Magnetic boards	
	Maps	
	Models	
	Pictures	
	Postures	
	Photographs	
	Self-instructional	
	Silent films	
	Slides	

Classification 4

Three dimensional aids:
1. Models.
2. Mock-ups.
3. Specimens

Three dimensional aids are the replicas or substitutes of real objective.

CONE OF EXPERIENCE

Edgar Dale: A major proponent of audiovisual materials in the classroom is the originator of cone of experience. All learning experiences that can be used for classroom instruction are presented by Edgar Dale in a pointed form of paint called the cone of experience. Climbing up from the root, you can see that each tool is arranged in order of increasing abstraction or decreasing directness. In simple terms, we can say that the cones are ranked according to the communicative effect of the audiovisual aid (most effective at the base of the cone). Relative effectiveness diminishes over time.

At the top of the cone is a direct, goal-oriented experience. The top of the cone has a word symbol.

The experiences included in the cone are as indicated below:

- **Direct purposeful experience:** The experiences gained through the senses are direct and purposeful. It has been amply observed an ounce of experience is better than a tonne of theory simply because it is only as an experience that any theory has vital and verifiable significance. This direct experience is gained through the aids mentioned at the base of the cone.
- **False experience:** When we cannot perceive reality directly, we need to simplify it. A fictional experience is like a working model of reality that differs from the original in size and complexity. Real objects can be too small or too big, cluttered or covered. In such situations, imitation is preferred for better comprehension.
- **Dramaturgical participation:** In dramaturgy, certain real-life events are represented through acting (usually a form of drama based on local history), pantomime (actors do not speak, but move), and table-to-table (scene lines) is represented. Characters are stationary, the play represents a puppet.

THE IMPORTANCE OF AV AIDS IN EDUCATIONAL COMMUNICATION

- Audiovisual aids and devices stimulate our senses and provide a better way to learn. It is rightly stated that the senses are the gateway to all knowledge.

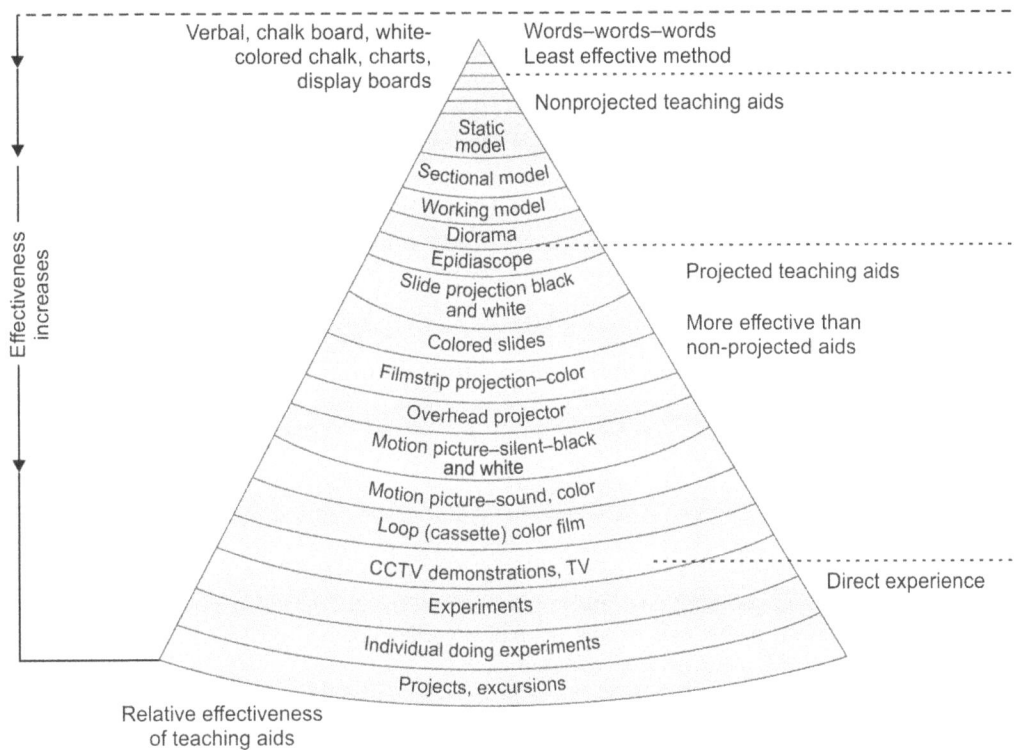

Fig. 9.5: Cone of experience.

- Audiovisual materials can improve information perception and learning retention due to their sensory appeal.
- Audiovisual materials bring the reality of our world into the classroom and make learning more purposeful.
- Audiovisual materials organize abstract ideas and make them easier to understand.
- AV aids accelerate learning in the era of knowledge explosion.
- AV materials are economical in the long run as they are highly reproducible and reach a large number of students
- Audiovisual aids are used to complement teachers and supplement regular classroom instruction, enhancing spoken and written language.
- AV aids help break down language barriers between students and teachers and streamline learning.
- AV tools offer a variety of teaching methods, sometimes motivating children to learn independently of their teachers.
- AV aids reduce vocabulary in the classroom. Hence Bourdon by students.

THE ROLE OF EDUCATIONAL MEDIA IN TEACHING

- Educational media help introduce the subject matter itself and provide an overview of what is being taught
- Ideas, facts, principles, or to help explain the main points
- Summarize the lesson
- It also helps motivate learners
- Encourages more students to participate in learning
- Provides more tangible experiences that provide a basis for thinking, reasoning and problem-solving
- Large amounts of current information (e.g., facts, ideas, principles, data, etc.) in a short period of time
- Increase the amount of initial learning and increase the persistence of learning.

PSYCHOLOGICAL BASIS FOR AV-AIDS

Psychological studies on learning and retention show that 80% of information and its retention occurs through hearing and sight. Because of their sensory appeal, audiovisual aids increase the span of learning and memory.

- **Motivation:** The sensory appeal of audiovisual materials motivates and stimulates students to facilitate learning in an appropriate atmosphere.
- **Curiosity:** Student curiosity is aroused by the novelty and variety of classroom materials.
- **Engagement:** Many AV tools give students the ability to manipulate their learning environment and sustain their interest in learning.

- **Real and imaginary experiences:** Using AV tools, students directly experience real-life situations or imaginary situations that resemble reality. Such direct experience makes learning meaningful for students.
- **Concreteness:** AV aids make learning concrete by reducing the abstraction of spoken and written language.
- **Note:** AV aids make learning an enjoyable experience and capture the attention of students.

Psychology also emphasizes multisensory experiences in learning. Psychologists advocate a maximum of "learning more, learning faster, longer" that can only be achieved by awakening every possible sensory or gateway to knowledge acquisition.

CONCLUSION

Audiovisual aids are sensory objects or images that initiate, stimulate and reinforce learning. Audiovisual materials are valuable when used properly. Teaching materials are classified into projected and nonprojective materials, audiovisual materials and teaching materials. Image material big media, little media, and 3D tools. A variety of audiovisual materials include graphs, charts, maps, posters, cartoons, and flashcards. Audiovisual aids or diving are additional aids that help instructors clarify, coordinate, and coordinate precise interrelated concepts.

REVIEW QUESTIONS

Long Essays
1. Define educational media, explain the categories and importance of educational media.
2. Enumerate the classifications of teaching aids, explain cone of experience.
3. Describe the importance of AV aids in educational communication.

Short Essays
1. Important values of AV resources.
2. Teaching material functions.
3. Principles for the use of materials.
4. Selection of AV materials.
5. Advantages of the teaching aids benefits.
6. Role of educational media in teaching.

Short Answers
1. Audiovisual aid.
2. Audiovisual media.
3. Audiovisual communication.
4. Need for teaching materials.
5. Characteristics of good teaching materials.
6. Classification of teaching aids.
7. Edgar Dale.
8. Psychological basis for AV-Aids.

Chapter 10

Still Visuals

Learning Objectives
- Benefits of Still Images
- Visual Learning Strategies
- Non-projection Media: Chart, Graph, Poster, Cartoon, Blackboard/Whiteboard, Bulletin Board, Flannel Sheet, Flipcharts, Flashcards, Still Image/Photo
- Print Materials: Handouts, Newspaper, Magazines
- Projected Aids
- Filmstrip Principles
- Microscope, Powerpoint Slide, Overhead Projector, Opaque Projector, LCD Panels, Slide Projector and Slides

INTRODUCTION

Visual learning is one of the best types of learning styles to help you see the information you are learning. Capture images of what you see based on spatial awareness imagery, color brightness, or other visual information. Therefore, the classroom is the perfect place for students to learn visually. Today, teachers are adopting visual teaching methods using whiteboards, handouts, pictures, videos and presentations for effective learning. Visual learners can improve their confidence and performance in school.

DEFINITIONS

Still images/visual aids are an effective tool that teachers can use in the classroom to enhance the understanding of students' interests and improve retention of information and concepts.

BENEFITS OF STILL IMAGES

Visual aids help teachers explain, connect and associate ideas and concepts to make the learning process more interesting, enjoyable and effective. Here are just some of the benefits that visual aids bring to teaching and learning:
- Helps encourage students to learn more effectively
- Helps students retain information longer
- Give examples for thinking about concepts
- Increase students' vocabulary
- Help students put the topic and concepts in perspective
- Give students hands-on experience
- Creative atmosphere interest.

VISUAL LEARNING STRATEGIES

Visual learning is one of the most effective learning styles for students. The emphasis is on learning by reading and observing rather than by listening. There are several ways to learn through visual aids, e. g., images, videos, various color themes, charts and maps. Images, videos, charts, maps, documents, charts, and more can be used to teach students in the classroom. Students with a visual learning style are said to perform better academically. They pay attention to your slides, whiteboards, PowerPoint presentations, handouts, graphs, maps, charts, and more.

Following strategies to get your students' attention in classroom:
- Make a presentation using handouts, diagrams, photographs, maps, tables, etc.
- Using color themes in presentations and handouts
- Providing notes to students
- Engaging students in learning activities, assignments, group activities, etc.
- Using videos and still images in presentations
- Concepts through demonstration play and outdoor and indoor activities

- Get more assignments from the syllabus
- Draw pictures to help illustrate new concept
- View web pages with graphs, pictures, charts, etc. related to the syllabus
- Education
- Storytelling helps visualize concepts
- Create flashcards with concepts and images
- Use color coding in paragraphs to help students understand topics
- Tell students, encourage writing

Learners imagine things to remember information. When your teacher shows you some kind of picture, the information sticks in your mind. As a student, it can help you improve your academic performance.

Following strategies for better learning outcomes:
- Use color coding for notes, words, textbooks, etc. This helps you remember information
- You can read pictures, diagrams, photographs, and maps to keep concepts in your mind longer.
- Take notes with different colored pens. It helps you easily identify the theme.
- Organize your notes by highlighting headings and subheadings.
- Watch informative videos to deepen your understanding and learn quickly.
- Organize the information you want to study into graphs, charts, and tables. Excel spreadsheets can help you draw graphs and create tables to better understand your information.
- Draw a mind map of a topic you want to remember for a long time
- Draw a picture on a topic that is simple and easy to understand.
- Create a descriptive topic image. You can draw pictures to remember things effectively.
- Use more symbols to represent information to make it easier to understand. Videos and pictures are better than words. In this case, practical knowledge will help you retain information for the long term.

NON-PROJECTION MEDIA

Non-projection visuals are tools used without projection. As such, it transforms abstract ideas into more realistic forms. They allow lessons to move from an oral presentation to a more concrete level.

Heinich (1996) states that nonprojected media can make teaching more realistic and engaging. Many of the media and materials are so general that teachers tend to underestimate their educational value, Acts as a reminder, provides clearer structure and contribute to speaker credibility.

Use of Non-projected Images
- Educators, scientists, and students should use projected images in relation to lectures or presentations in their fields. No images can be used or displayed.
- Motivate students
- Presenting matter symbolically
- Presenting abstract ideas in visual form
- Producing problems and stimulating thought.

Benefits of Non-projective Visualization
- Abundant and are easily obtainable
- No electricity required
- Suitable for low budgets
- Less artistic skill is required when using these visual aids.
- Versatile for all education and discipline levels
- Used to inspire creative expression.
- Many of these can be converted into projection aids.
- Some can be projected with opaque projectors.

Disadvantages of Non-projection Images
- It may be out of date.
- Our ability to utilize all our senses for a complete learning experience is so limited that we are unable to effectively present our motor materials.
- Copies may wear out from overuse. Picture quality may diminish overtime.
- They are difficult to revise and update if produced in a hardbound format.
- Easy to damage.
- Non-interactive.

CHART

A chart is a combination of pictures, graphs, numbers or vertical material that provides a clear visual summary. The most common types of charts include outline charts, table charts, flowcharts, and org charts. Other types of diagrams include technical diagrams and process diagrams. Flip charts and flowcharts are also used. There are readymade diagrams available for classroom use in almost every area of every subject. More useful, however, are the diagrams created by the teacher himself, inputting his own ideas and approaches to a particular subject.

Chart Purpose
- Use facts, numbers and statistics to show relationships.
- A symbolic representation of the material.
- Summarize the information.
- Indicates process continuity.
- Visualize abstract ideas.

- Indicates the unfolding of the structure.
- Provoking problems and stimulating thought.
- Promote the use of other communication media.
- To motivate students.

Use of Charts Effectively

- Graph should be preferred.
- Students should be involved in creating the diagrams.
- The chart should be sized so that all students in the class can see all the details shown no matter where they are sitting.
- The chart should only show information about a specific area of the topic.
- Chart should not contain too much text.
- Do not include too much detail in the diagram.
- A chart should give a neat appearance.
- When a chart is to be used in the classroom the teacher should make sure that there is provision for hanging the chart at a vantage point.
- The teacher should have a pointer to point out specific factors in the chart.
- Straight pin staple. Pegboards, clips, rubber hangers, paper clips, and folded construction tape can all be used to mount charts without damaging them.
- Diagrams should be carefully saved and retained for future use.

Types of Charts

The following is a list of basic types of charts in term of arrangements and the kinds or ideas which they may express:

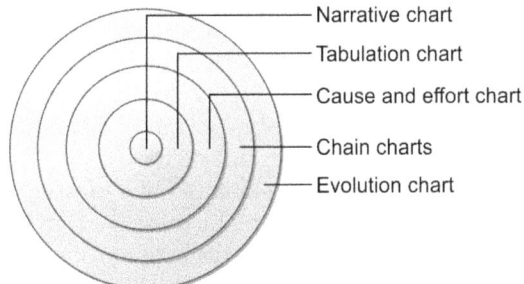

Fig. 10.1: Types of chart.

- **The narrative chart:** An extended left to right arrangement of facts and ideas for expressing:
  - The events in a process such as shoemaking, oil cracking or the like.
  - The events in the development of a significant issue to its point of resolution or to present status (sometimes a time limit). Examples: The events leading to the separation of the Bangladesh from Pakistan, the events leading to the establishment of the ideas that an individual should be free and that be should have a voice in his own government and events leading to increasing regulation of business by government.
  - Technological improvement over a period of years such as improvement over a period of years such as improvement in transportation, communication, manufacturing etc.
- **The tabulation chart:** A left to right, top to bottom arrangement of facts and ideas for expression:
  - Numerical data for making compartments.
  - List of products, mountains, rivers, or the like in selected areas.
- **The cause and effort chart,** usually a limited left-to-right arrangement of facts and ideas for expressing.
  - Relationship between standard of living and such factors as economic system, availability of natural resources, level of technological advancement.
  - Relationship between a culture and neighboring cultures.
  - Relationship between rights and responsibilities.
  - Relationship between a complex of conditions and change or conflicts.
  - Relationship between the elected and electors
  - Relationship between community workers and the community which support them.
- **The chain charts:** A circular or semicircular arrangements of facts and ideas for expressing:
  - Transitions, such as transition from raw materials to useful products.
  - Cycles, such as the water cycle.
- **The evolution chart:** A left to right arrangement of facts and ideas for expressing:
  - Changes in specific items from beginning to data to data, perhaps with projections into the future. For example: origin of the automobile and its subsequent development early basic homes and changes in basic homes to date.
  - Change in standard in food consumption, length of work, weak purchasing power of a rupee, or the like.

Other Types of Charts

There are many varieties of charts. Some common types of charts are briefly discussed below for your understanding.
- **Bar chart:** Bar charts are made of a series of bars along a measured scale. They are used to compare quantities at different times, or, under different circumstances.
- **Pie chart:** Pie charts are in the shape of circles, and are used to show proportions and percentages.
- **Tabular chart:** Tabular charts are used to bring together mass related data in compact form. Example: time-table.

- **Tree chart:** Tree charts are used for showing development or growth of a program or project. The origin is shown in a single line, or as a tree trunk, and various developments are shown as branches.
- **Flowchart:** Flowcharts show organizational structure of departments, institutions, resources with lines and arrows.
- **Pictorial chart:** A pictorial chart gives the viewer a vivid picture, and creates a rapid association with the use of graphic messages, such as cartoons, and illustrations. Each visualized symbol indicates quantities. This type of chart is more useful for illiterate audience in extension work.
- **Overlay chart:** Overlay charts consist of a number of sheets which can be placed, and Audio Visual Aids one over the other, conveniently. On each individual sheet a part of the whole is drawn. This enables the viewer to see not only the different parts, but also how they appear when one is placed over the other. After the final overlay is placed, it shows the full view of the whole picture. This type of chart presentation is dramatic and effective.
- **Pull chart:** A pull chart consists of written messages on a large sheet. Messages are hidden by strips of thick paper held in position by the slits provided on either side. The messages can be shown to the viewer one after another, by pulling out the concealing strips. The same strip can be replaced in the slits after showing the message. This type of chart presentation is dramatic and creates suspense for the viewer.
- **Strip tease chart:** They are similar to the pull chart, however, messages are concealed by strips of thin paper instead of thick paper. The ends of thin paper strips are pinned or pasted at both ends of the message. Whenever the message is to be exposed, one end of paper strip is stripped off. This has the advantage of surprise and anticipation.
- **Flip chart:** A flip chart is a series of visuals drawn into large sheets of paper or cardboard, fastened together at the top. These are turned over or flipped, one at a time by the extension worker. This kind of chart exposes the audience to segments of the subject in sequence, and holds attention remarkably well.
- **Window chart:** In this, flaps cover the messages and when the message is to be shown, the presenter open the flaps like windows. It creates suspense in the audience.

Preparation

While preparing any type of chart, consider the following points:
- Keep it simple.
- Promote a single idea or message with important details.
- Maintain logical order.
- Use symbols, words, or colors to explain the chart.
- Use lines and bars in only one dimension.
- Compare units and avoid comparing unrelated units.
- The chart title must emphasize certain parts of diagrams.
- The title for 8" × 10%" sheet and for 30" × 40" charts, the height should be about 2%".

Other Types of Charts

There are different types of charts. For better understanding, some common types of charts are briefly described below:
- **Bar chart:** A bar chart consists of a series of bars along a measured scale. They are used to compare quantities at different times or under different circumstances.
- **Pie charts:** Pie charts are shaped like circles and are used to show ratios and percentages.
- **Tabular charts:** Tabular charts are used to summarize mass-related data in a compact format. For example: Time-table.
- **Tree diagrams:** Tree diagrams are used to show the development or growth of a program or project. The origin is represented by a single line or tree trunk, and various developments are represented by branches.
- **Flowchart:** Flowcharts show the organizational structure of departmental resources with lines and arrows.
- **Picture Boards:** Picture boards convey vivid images to the viewer and create quick associations using graphic messages such as cartoons and illustrations. Each symbol visualized indicates a quantity. This type of chart is more useful for illiterate people in counseling work.
- **Overlay charts:** Overlay charts consist of multiple sheets that can be conveniently stacked on top of each other, as well as audiovisual material. Each individual sheet depicts a part of the whole. This allows the viewer to not only see the different pieces, but also how they look when placed on top of each other. It shows, this type of chart presentation is dramatic and effective.
- **Pull chart:** A pull chart consists of a message written on a large piece of paper. The message is hidden by a thick strip of paper held in place by slots on each side. By pulling out the cover strip, you can cycle through the messages to your audience. After displaying a message in the slot, you can reinsert the same strip. This type of diagram presentation is dramatic and gives the viewer a sense of tension.
- **Strip charts:** Similar to pull charts, but the message is hidden in a strip of thin paper instead of thick paper. The edges of the thin strip of paper are pinned or glued to each end of the message. Whenever a message is revealed, one end of the strip is pulled out. This has the advantage of surprise and anticipation.

- **Flipchart:** A flipchart is a series of drawings on a large sheet of paper or cardboard that is fastened at the top. These are individually turned over by the extenders. This type of chart exposes the audience to topical segments one at a time and is very well-attended.

When creating various charts, keep the following in mind:
- Keep it simple.
- Promote a single idea or message with important details.
- Maintain logical order.
- Describe the chart using symbolic words and colors.
- Use lines and bars in one dimension only
- Compare units and avoid comparing irrelevant units.
- The chart title should emphasize a specific part of the chart.
- The 8" × 10%" sheet title should be about W high and the 30" × 40" chart should be about 2% high. Defined as a visual representation of numerical data, charts are essentially tools for representing numerical relationships and are much slower to visualize when statements are made up of words and numbers only.

GRAPH

A graph is a flat image that uses dotted lines or images to visualize numerical and statistical data to represent relationships or statistics. A chart defined as a visual representation of numerical data. Diagrams are basically tools for representing numerical relationships, and they are much slower to visualize than if you made a statement with just words and numbers.

Graphs help you present quantitative data in a visual format. Charts are very effective at covering complex facts and showing comparisons and contracts. There are area charts, bar charts, pie charts, line charts, and pictograms.

Definition
- A Graph is a flat image that uses dotted lines or images to visualize numerical and statistical data to show relationships or statistics.
- A Graph defined as a visual representation of numeric data.

Use Graphs
- Capture students' attention and thoughts.
- Provide compressed information.
- Present information effectively.
- Concrete abstract ideas.
- Intriguing.

Different Graphs
- **Bar graph:** A graphical representation in which the scale expands horizontally along the length of the bar. The vertical dimension does not have a scale, it has space for multiple items and a bar to measure each.
- **Column graph:** Looks like an inverted bar chart. It has two scales, one measure across the graph (usually time) and one measure above or below (usually volume). This means that all points in such diagrams are measured on both scales. A line Graphor is a form of chart in which the

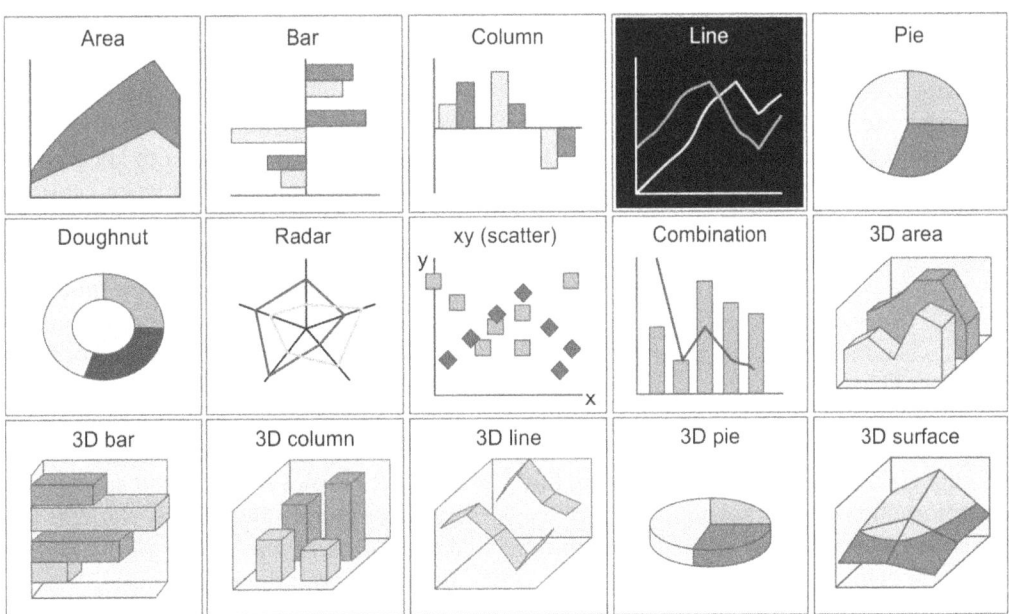

Fig. 10.2: Graphs used as AV aids.

plotted points are connected to each other rather than to the base, creating curves that give the chart its name. Line charts represent data using simple lines drawn horizontally or vertically. Line charts sometimes use pictorial illustrations or cartoons to increase the interest and readability of the concept.
- **Pie graph:** A circle divided into wedges. A scale is a range divided into appropriate scale units, such as percentages.
- **Surface graph plot:** Connect each plotted point to the next. Connect each point to the base, like a column chart.

Advantage

Visually summarize large data sets. Just compare two or three data sets. Make trends clearer than tables. You can estimate key values at a glance.

Cons

Additional written or verbal clarification required. It can be easily manipulated to give the wrong impression.

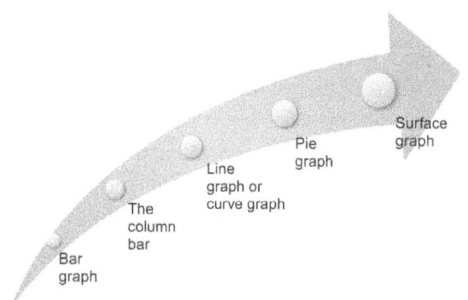

Fig. 10.3: Different types of graphs.

POSTER

Posters are a great way to extend your ideas to an audience. An image that needs to grab the viewer's attention and convey a simple message at a glance. Your guide should be aware of the event practices and ideas you want to convey. The poster should be bold in design, easy to understand, and in attractive colors.

Purpose

- The purpose of a poster is to promote a particular idea with a few words and illustrations.
- A good poster is expected to guide learners through her first two steps of public education.
- Attention and interest. Not expected to enlighten, but expected to inspire action—now or eventually.
- This requires strong ideas that are strongly presented through the content of the poster.
- It should always be part of other teaching methods. Campaign Meetings Demonstrations, etc.

Use Posters

- Make an immediate appeal.
- Convey one or more ideas.
- You can tell at a glance.
- Wide range and clear enough from a distance.
- Suitable for educating patients on scientific facts, safety precautions and many other health aspects.

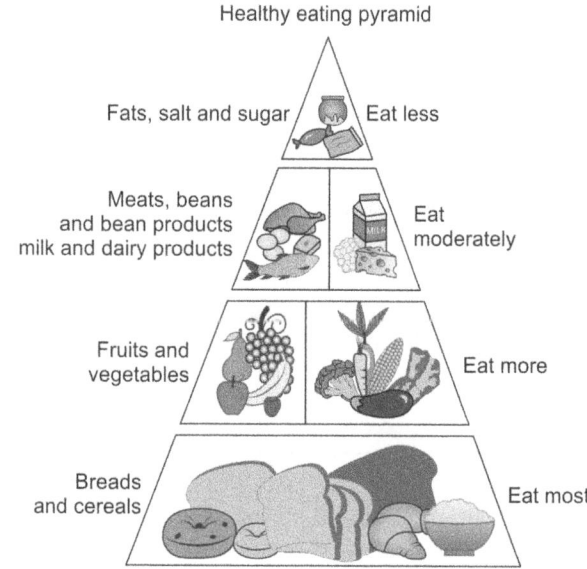

Fig. 10.4: Poster used to explain balanced diet.

Poster Components

- **Image or illustration:** Must be self-explanatory. A drawing should boldly highlight what is actually being expressed. Avoid unnecessary details so as not to confuse your audience's attention. When using photos, avoid unnecessary surroundings and leave immediately.
- **Verbal captions:** It is best to keep all five captions as small as possible. Do not write captions vertically. It becomes difficult to read. Because captions don't break.
- **Colors:** Use bright and attractive colors. Intermediate cores can be highlighted with a more prominent color. Captions can also have different colors for prominent words. Do not use more than 3 colors. Otherwise, it can get confusing. Do not use strange color combinations.
- If the poster is packed with pictures and words, the viewer will get lost, so make sure you have enough space.
- **Layout:** Should be balanced so that the viewer's eye moves smoothly and quickly through the captions and illustrations. You need to grab your audience's attention and clarify your message.
- Once the rough is done, show it to a few people at viewer level. Please remove any misunderstandings or

ambiguities. Contributors should recommend an action. It should be installed in places where people pass by or where they gather. Only ideas exist, details should be provided through other mediums.

In areas with short exposure times (such as streets), the message of the poster should be short, simple, direct, instantly comprehensible, and immediately comprehensible. where people have time. Bus Station Train Station Hospital Health Center The right amount of materials should be in the right place at the time. Stances typically have a short lifespan and need to be changed frequently.

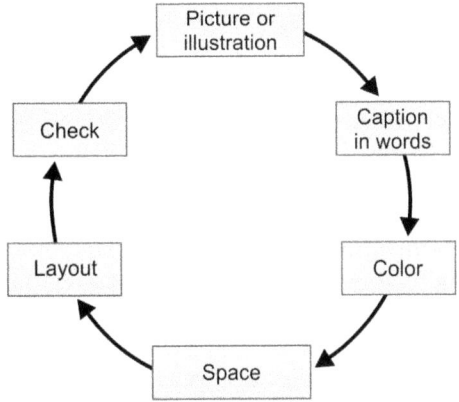

Fig. 10.5: Poster design rules.

Poster Design Rules

- Do a special job.
- Promote points.
- Support local demonstrations and local exhibitions.
- Target audience.
- It should stop people and show them.
- Get your message across at a glance.
- Use bold (20" × 301)
- Use simple words to convey your ideas.
- Use pleasant colors.
- You must arrive on time.

Restrictions

- Posters only give a first impression and cannot provide detailed information.
- Need help by other means or methods for more information. Flyers and demonstrations.
- Creating a good poster is a technical task, requiring skill and time.
- Cannot be repeated. I have to create a new poster each time.
- Please remove the poster after shipping or once it has served its purpose.

Benefits of Posters

- It attracts the attention of the audience.
- File an immediate appeal.
- Convey one or more ideas.
- At a glance.
- Wide range and well defined distances.
- It presents scientific facts and is suitable for patient education, demonstrating safety measures and many other aspects of health.

CARTOON

Cartoons are humorous caricatures that convey the right message. In cartoons, features of objects and people are exaggerated along with generally accepted symbols. Cartoons have visual appeal and evocative messages. Newspaper cartoons are often sarcastic and ridiculous. The main source of information for comics is magazines.

Definitions

- A metaphor for reality. It makes learning more interesting and effective because it has a strong emotional appeal.
- Cartoons are interpretive illustrations that symbolize opinions, scenes, or situations.

Comic Source

- The main source of comics is magazines.
- Newspapers publish daily cartoons that are political or social in nature.
- Special periodicals and magazines feature comics on science management, economics and education

Learning Benefits of Cartoons

- Cartoons can be used effectively to introduce a particular lesson.
- Cartoons can be used to motivate students to initiate discussions.
- Cartoons can be used to make lessons lively and interesting.

Using Cartoon

- Cartoon makes learning more interesting and effective because of their strong emotional appeal.
- Cartoons are straightforward and tell the story without too much explanation.
- Cartoons are a great way to grab attention and motivate students to learn.
- Cartoons help provide students with opportunities for self-expression and creativity.

- Cartoons help learners develop an interest in behavior change and positive attitudes.

Preparation/Techniques for Using Cartoons

- Be simple.
- Must provide information and pertinent knowledge on various topics and current affairs in an interesting way.
- Teachers should create cartoons for classroom needs.
- Students should participate in the preparation process to maximize their learning experience.

Humor

- Personal humor
- Fantasy
- Uncomfortable
- Satire
- Exaggeration

Principles

- The quality of drawings should be high, mainly for visual impact.
- It should be clear what the story is telling without much explanation.
- Symbols should be familiar, representing concepts and ideas to which students can respond intelligently.
- Teachers should evaluate the perspectives presented.

Strengths: Can be used for judgment, interpretation and emphasis.
Cons: Time consuming.
Board devices

BLACKBOARD/WHITEBOARD

Blackboards and chalk are very helpful for students to visualize concepts and ideas. These can be used for drawing such as diagrams and sketches. The blackboard is a simple and unique tool that, despite new devices and technologies, remains irreplaceable and indispensable in the classroom. An old friend of the teacher. A mirror in which the student visualizes everything the teacher thinks for a while. It is the cheapest material and is still the end of our entire educational system. The most universal tool. Writing on clay and sand was the archetype of chalkboard writing. It helps to summarize and confirm the main points.

Main Uses of the Board

- Teachers can use the board to explain the main points of the lesson.
- You can clarify abstract statements in the description stage and summarize salient features in the summary stage.
- Questions and problems can be posted on the bulletin board.
- Writing and drawing on the blackboard can increase students' interest in the lesson.
- Teachers can use boards for graphics, sketches, maps, statistics, and more.
- Teachers can erase what they have written or drawn and start over.
- Different abilities and perceptions of students are taken into account.
- It helps teachers to draw students' attention to the lesson.
- Teachers can use the blackboard to review the entire lesson for the benefit of the entire class.

Board Type

- **Fixed chalkboard:** Fixed on the wall facing the class, usually made of wood or concrete cement.
- **Chalkboard on easel:** A portable, adjustable chalkboard mounted on a wooden easel that can be taken out of the classroom during outdoor classes.
- **Rolling board:** Made of thick canvas, rolled into rolls, mainly used for teaching in upper grades.
- **Graphic board:** It has graphic lines and is used for teaching mathematics, science and statistics.
- **Magnaboard:** A board that allows the teacher to place objects in a vertical plane to demonstrate her three dimensions. When placed on this vertical surface, small magnets are used to hold the appropriate items in place.

Chalkboard of Different Colors and Color Chalks

S. No.	Color of the blackboard	Color of the chalk
1.	Green chalkboard	White or yellow chalk
2.	Gray board	Yellow
3.	Red chalkboard	Green, yellow
4.	Orange chalkboard	Blue or light green
5.	Yellow chalkboard	Blue
6.	Rose chalkboard	Purple, dark blue
7.	Black chalkboard	Any color

Chalkboards in Various Finishes

- Lacquered pressed wood
- Matte plastic finish
- Glazed steel surface
- Frosted glass board

Effective Use of the Board

- Blackboard should be kept clean so that writing on it could be easily read by the student from all parts of the room.

- Any writing on the board must be readable.
- Letters and pictures should be large enough to be seen from anywhere in the room.
- Writing must start from the upper left corner.
- Write in straight lines.
- Do not use the bottom corner of the chalkboard as it is difficult to read.
- Materials on the board must be hidden by standing in front of the board.
- Write only the main points of the subject on the chalkboard.
- A visual presentation with pictures involves many processes that need to be prepared before starting the lesson.
- It should be ensured that the panel is well lit by natural or artificial means.
- Everything needed for the blackboard should be collected before class begins.
- When writing on the whiteboard, the teacher should make sure the class is paying attention.
- Use a rag to clean the board, not a hand towel or handkerchief.
- Occasionally students are asked to write or draw diagrams on the board.
- Teachers should develop the ability to draw freely on the blackboard. A map or chart that grows in front of a student is far more useful and valuable than a well-made map or chart.

Techniques for using the Board Use it Effectively

- Check the visibility of the board from several positions in the room to ensure the surface is glare free.
- Plan what you are about to write.
- Save time and improve the quality of your drawings with drawing aids like rulers and stencils.
- Pretty print instead of using scripts. For a 32 foot classroom, letters should be 3 to 3.5 inches high and the lines forming the letters should be 1/4 inch thick.
- Hold the chalk or marker at an angle to avoid scratching or squeaking.
- Highlight with color. Two or three different colors are fine.
- Set guidelines to help you write in straight lines. A water-soluble felt-tip pen will suffice. Please don't talk on the message board. Face the class when you speak. Move so as not to block what is written on the board.
- The board should be completely wiped after each use. Do not leave markers on board overnight. It can be erased immediately by tracing with an erasable black pen.
- For general cleaning, wipe the board with a damp soft cloth.
- Cap erasable markers tightly and store horizontally to prevent drying.
- Change your presentation technique. Don't overuse the board or rely entirely on it.

BULLETIN BOARD

The bulletin board display is one of the inexpensive instructional devices used for teaching. It may be sued for informational and educational purposes. It can be used effectively in connection with every learning situation and it properly used can motivate supplement and enrich learning. It is a board with a background of colored cloth. It can be covered with glass or a flat plate. Exhibits include news sheets, announcements, brochures, newsletters, newspaper networks, cartoons, photographs, charts, posters, maps, diagrams and topical sketches. They can serve useful educational functions at all levels and in all areas of secondary and higher education. They can be used in industry, commerce, government education and communications.

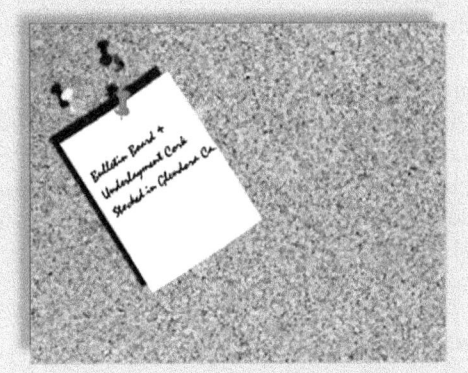

Fig. 10.6: Bulletin board.

Purpose

- Can be used to motivate learners, for example, to reduce the learning experience in a study project by a group of students.
- Extend the learner's sensory experience and provide an experience beyond the learner's environment.
- Adds variety to classroom activities.
- To facilitate information.
- Unit planning allows you to use materials as an integral part of the curriculum to complement and tie together instruction.
- Materials that cannot be presented during class can be used on the bulletin board to save time.

Bulletin boards are available for nursing training. As a classroom aid for posting unit plans in hallways, lounges and libraries for educational purposes. Appropriate use of bulletin boards can facilitate patient information in outpatient clinics. The clinic's clinical conference room as a correlation between the classroom and the clinical learning experience.

Bulletin Board Details

- There are certain items that are of interest only for one day and should be removed from the bulletin board at the end of the day.
- Results of sports extends new projects undertaken individually or collectively should always be put on the bulletin board.
- Achievement of the individual pupil and that the school may be advertised.
- New arrival in the library may be exhibited on the notice board.

How to Use Bulletin Board

- Teacher must collect suitable instructions for instructional projects.
- Teacher must also classify and file the material beforehand.
- Arrange the material in an interesting manner.
- Teacher must put a title and give a brief description.
- Use color harmony.
- Teachers should observe the bulletin board and encourage students to post on the bulletin board.
- Consistently serve as a showcase for outstanding student work.

General Due Diligence

- You should choose carefully the materials you post on the bulletin boards.
- Materials posted on the bulletin board must relate to regular classroom activities.
- Exhibit materials must be changed frequently and in a timely manner.

Bulletin Board Features

- The bulletin board should be placed in a location that is easily visible to most people.
- Different types and sizes are used depending on the application.
- The length of the board should be slightly longer than the width.
- The highest point of the board should be slightly higher than the eye level of the average person.
- Different types of bulletin boards can be used depending on the purpose and available funds.
- The fixed type can be attached to the wall, and the movable type can be removed and light enough to be carried from room to room.

The items used in the bulletin board are:
- Photo
- Cutouts
- Illustrations
- Publications
- Drawings
- Samples
- Posters
- Newspapers
- Posting announcements, tasks, awards and achievements.

Bulletin Board Usage Principles

- Bulletin boards should be kept separate from bulletin boards for current events and research.
- The proposed plan for placing the bulletin boards is to place an additional third group near the library in each clinical conference room of the clinic and a fourth group in the bulletin board classrooms near the educational administration office. arranging groups.
- Board content should be organized around a central content theme. Materials should be dated so that they do not remain longer than necessary.
- Appearance should be neat and tidy and attractive.
- Materials must be changed frequently and systematically.
- Contributions must be properly labeled. It's hard to fix a wrong first impression.
- Student contributions should be encouraged and utilized.
- She should be the only one editing the board. Appoint a bulletin board committee to provide materials
- Everyone must be responsible for reading and knowing the contents of the tablet
- All materials should be properly sorted and labeled for future reference.
- The plaque should be left uncovered for 1-2 days to arouse interest.

Bulletin board use in nursing practice: As a teaching aid for posting unit diagrams in corridors, lounges, and libraries for educational purposes. Appropriate use of bulletin boards can facilitate patient information in outpatient clinics. The ward clinical conference room is a correlation between the classroom and the clinical learning experience.

Bulletin Board Usage

- For informational purposes.
- Communicate your ideas.
- Motivate learners.

- Add variety to classroom activities.
- I can explain how to make a particular object.
- Follow-up instructions on what ideas are presented and emphasized.
- To save time, materials that cannot be presented during the lesson can still be posted on the bulletin board.
- Complement and correlate lessons.

FLANNEL SHEET

A type of cloth sheet in which flannel is tightly stretched over a surface and glued to matchwood or very thick cardboard. Pieces of flannel stick together so that letters, shapes or symbols cut from the same material can be attached to a flannel board without the use of adhesive tape, pins, pictures, cards or other similar materials.

Flannelgraph can be described as picture drama. The story should be simple and not have too many characters. It should start well on the topic and end with a concrete proposal. Place the board on a sturdy table or in a place where it can be easily seen by those listening. Number and organize your various goals.

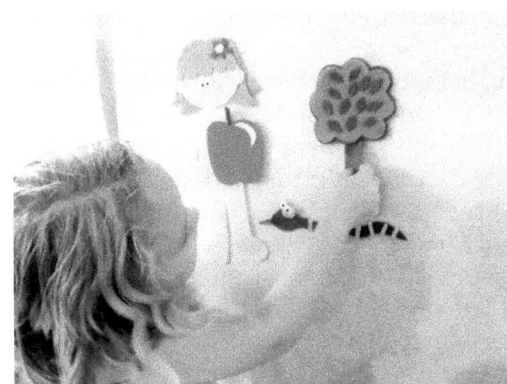

Fig. 10.7: Flannel sheet preperation.

To aid your memory, take quick notes on a piece of paper and identify them with a picture or cloth glued to the flannel sheet. Do not block the view and allow enough time for your audience to see and understand each part.

Purpose

- To save time in presenting lessons.
- Encourage the visual expression of ideas.

Benefits of Flannel Boards

- You can prepare in advance.
- Quick fore/aft adjustment.
- Various visual elements are available.
- Promotes attentional factors.

Cons

- The exact look of your board should be planned in advance.
- Take a washcloth and occasionally need to clean and roughen it.

Use of Flannel Box

The preliminary plan should include answers to the following questions:
- What are you preparing?
- Are the cut materials ready and ready to use?
- Why use flannel boxes?
- How is the information presented?
- What does the audience get out of it?

Selection Tool

Attach flannel terry cloth or felt to a hard surface and glue or line the cut fingers with flannel or felt, sandpaper or cotton.

FLIPCHARTS

Flipcharts are useful teaching aids. You can buy readymade or blank flipcharts, or create your own. A flipchart is a piece of stationery consisting of a large pad of paper. It is usually mounted on the top edge of a whiteboard and is usually carried on a tripod or four-legged easel.

A collection of charts on a single subject, arranged in sequence and pinned to the top (like a calendar). It can be used step by step for teaching.

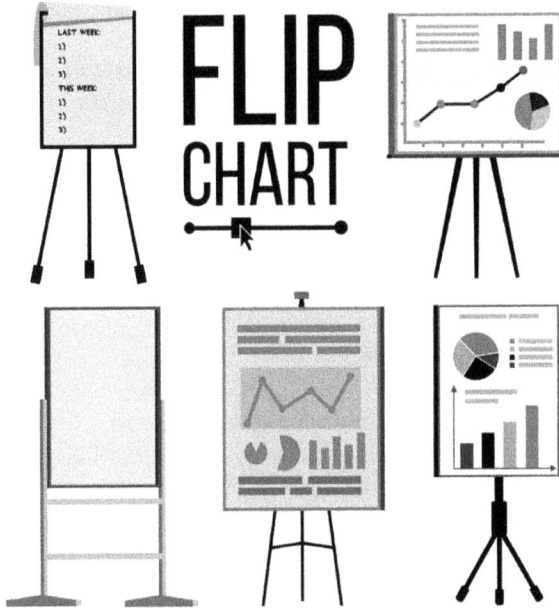

Fig. 10.8: Different types of flipcharts.

These are the types of chart:
- A teacher has to prepare by incorporating his own ideas and lines of approach of the specific topic are more useful.
- The flip charts are a set of charts related to specific topic.
- These are labeled together and hung on the support stand.
- Each graph contains a series of related messages in sequence.
- A gist of a particular topic is presented.

Steps of Preparation
- Select the charts 20" × 20"
- Select the topic
- Prepare the content
- Select pictures
- Organize a set of materials
- Prepare blueprints
- Pretest materials
- Audiovisual materials
- Complete diagrams
- Clip them up and flip them one by one.

Instructions for Use
- Place the flipchart on the table and turn it over one by one during the discussion
- Make it visible to the audience
- Summarize the topic
- Reuse charts as needed.

Flipchart Benefits
Flipcharts are both static display tools (like slides and props) and dynamic creation tools (like whiteboards and the ubiquitous napkin backs).
- Writing and drawing on a flipchart is a positive process that energizes the speaker. My energy level goes up every time I look at the flip chart.
- The audience asks more questions. I'm not sure why, but maybe it's because flipchart doodles and sketches are less permanent (than electronic slides) and feel more open to questions and dialogue.
- Writing takes time, so provide your audience with healthy pauses to absorb information or take notes.
- Flip charts and brainstorming go together like peanut butter and bananas (yummy!). One of my favorite training techniques is using a flip chart to record brainstorming sessions. I ask questions and then speedily record responses shouted out by my audience.
- Flipcharts are lowtech and analog. No need to worry about passwords, projector lamps or extension cords. (I am not saying it is better than slides, but I think speakers should master both options).

Pros
Using flipcharts has the following advantages:
- Flipchart does not require electricity. Never worry about a burnt out light bulb or forgetting an extension cord.
- Flipcharts are economical. You do not need to use special film or printers to create it.
- Adding color is easy—a box of cheap flipchart markers gives you all the creativity you need.
- Flip charts allow for spontaneity and are easy to accommodate last minute changes.

Tips for Effective Use
Flipcharts are lowtech, but reliable and require no special skills to use. Here are some tips for using it effectively.
- The best flipchart stand has a clamp on top that can hold most types of flipchart pads. Most flipcharts can be hung, but some can only stand. Do not wait until the last minute.
- Make sure the Flipchart you are using matches the Flipchart Stand you are using. Some have holes at different intervals on the top.
- Flipchart pads are usually sold in packs of two and are available either plain or with grid lines. Using the pad with grid lines makes your job easier for drawing straight lines and keeps your text aligned. Also make sure the pad has perforations at the top to allow easier removal of sheets. I have seen many presenters struggle to tear off a sheet evenly.
- When preparing your charts it is best to first design your charts on paper first before drawing them on the actual flip chart pad.
- First, lightly pencil the text before using the actual flipchart markers. This allows you to adjust the spacing of the text and the shapes you draw. Do not use all block letters (uppercase). Using upper and lower case makes it easier to read. I like to use the 7 × 7 rule. No more than 7 words per line and no more than 7 lines per sheet. Using the 6 × 6 rule works even better.
- Use flipchart markers instead of regular magic markers. Flipchart markers do not bleed through the paper. Also, it doesn't smell as strong as regular markers. You can also find scented markers. They are usually found in various fruit scents.
- Avoid yellow, pink and orange. These are very confusing to the audience. Do not let your audience strain their eyes to see your point. Avoid too many colors. Using dark and accent colors works well.

- You can 'pencil lightly' next to any key points you need. The audience cannot see them. You can also write what is on the next sheet. Knowing this will help you properly introduce your next hand.
- If you make a mistake, you can use the 'whiteout' to correct minor mistakes. For larger areas, cover the error with a double layer of flipchart paper and correct the error.
- Place a blank piece of paper between each text sheet. This will prevent the written material from other sheets to peek through.
- Properly store and transport your flip charts in a case or the cardboard box that some come in. This will protect your flipcharts and keep them fresh and ready to use each time. Take great care of your flipcharts. I have some flipcharts that have been used over 100 times and they still look like new.

FLASHCARDS

This is a set of cards that can be presented to the audience in the correct order tell the full story. Flash cards are 10" × 12" in size and contain an image or chart. Individual cards are flashed in front of the audience, and a counselor or student who wants to use thins flashes the cards one by one to give a verbal commentary.

Using Flashcards

- Have your audience watch, listen and learn.
- There is information on the topic.
- Get the audience's attention.
- It makes learning interesting and informative.
- Promote/develop knowledge.
- Inspire curiosity.
- Increases and maintains alertness and concentration.

Preparing Index Cards

I need to write a short story. The story should end with a lesson that leads to suggestions and actions. You should choose a title that fits your story. The story should be divided into several scenes that should be presented on several individual cards.

Cards are numbered consecutively and each set of cards must have a title. Write comments on the back of each card so that the person presenting the card at the time of the accident can easily read the comments from the back. Attractive captions enhance the impact of your index cards.

To use the flash card:
- They should be well known to the student or person presenting the card.

- You should use simple language and local expressions.
- Hold the card so that the audience can see the body and point out the image on the card.
- Some key points may be highlighted on the back of the card to aid storytelling.
- The cards must be stacked in order, as the finished card can be pushed behind the other cards. Then you'll be fine next time.

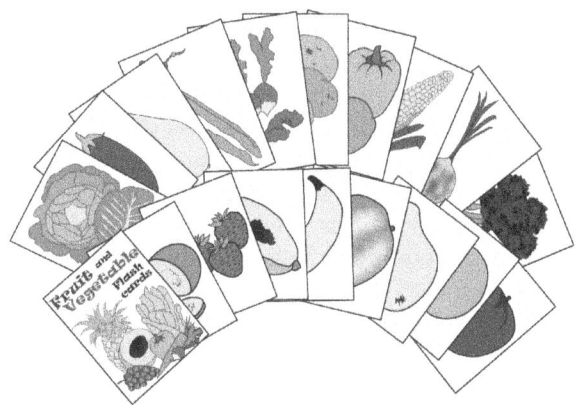

Fig. 10.9: Flash cards.

Teacher Instructions for Using Flashcards

To successfully teach using flashcards, teachers need to keep in mind the following points.
- You must know the story of each card.
- Simple language and local terminology should be used.
- Hold the card at chest level where people can clearly see it, do not lift your body, face different parts of the group and show everyone the card.
- When you are ready to explain, look at the card to make sure you have the correct information.
- Use pointers. Do not cover objects with your hands.
- Demonstrate enthusiasm and joy when explaining problems.

STILL IMAGE/PHOTO

An image is a graphic, pictorial, or photographic representation that conveys a precise idea of an object. A good picture can tell a story without using a single word. Images can be black and white or color. Color images and enlarged photos are more attractive. A good 35 mm lens for extended shots. A single lens reflex camera with necessary accessories such as flash, lens hood, filters, and close-up lens is useful.

Definition

Images and photographs are visual aids used to engage learners. Properly selecting and adapting them will help the reader understand and remember the content of the accompanying oral material.

- Provides an accurate visual record of an object or person. Photos are more accurate than paintings because they do not reflect the skill or prejudices of the artist. Example—a photo of her woman accurately represents her, but a portrait of her can make her look younger and more beautiful than she actually is.
- Summarizes both inanimate and animate objects.
- Can be used for student personal study. This is especially useful for slow learners.
- Cover various topics. You can take pictures or draw pictures of almost anything. Teachers should collect as many of them as possible and create their own image/photo files instead of wasting time looking for specific images only when needed. Example—pictures of traditional wedding attire from different religions and states.
- Compact, laminated and cared for years of storage. This is useful for conducting historical research on the past. Examples—costumes, architecture, lifestyle vehicles, etc.

Use of Images and Photos

Images and photos are used in a variety of promotional activities such as training programs, publication campaigns, exhibitions, slides, filmstrips, films, television, newspapers, displays, etc. used in the method. Such synthetic adhesive cardboard cut to shape with a ferret machine can produce excellent 3D effect display materials.

Restrictions

However, there are some restrictions on photos and pictures. May be misleading among students about the size and color of time:

- **Time:** A picture of a child growing up - it may have taken him 12 years to actually develop.
- **Size:** Elephant painting—children who have never seen an elephant may think it is as big as the painting. Or a close-up photo of a mosquito can give you an idea that it's actually that big. Adding other objects that students are familiar with to the diagram helps them estimate the size of the new objects.
- **Colors:** Students may be misled about the color of flowers when the pictures of flowers and the actual color of the flowers are different.
  - The cost of camera development and printing is increasing, so photos can become more expensive. Make sure your camera film and processing costs are within budget. Cameras range from fully automated to simple autofocus models to complex ones. A camera that is easy to use and convenient is desirable.
  - Drawn images, not images collected from print, require artistic skill.
  - These tools cannot represent ideas that rely primarily on motion. Example—the function of a sewing machine.
  - Both images and photos can fade or crack if not stored properly.

PRINT MATERIALS

Print advertising is a form of advertising that uses physical print media such as magazines and newspapers to reach consumers, business customers and prospects. Advertisers also use digital media such as banner ads, mobile ads, and social media ads to reach the same audience. The proliferation of digital media is reducing advertising costs in traditional print media.

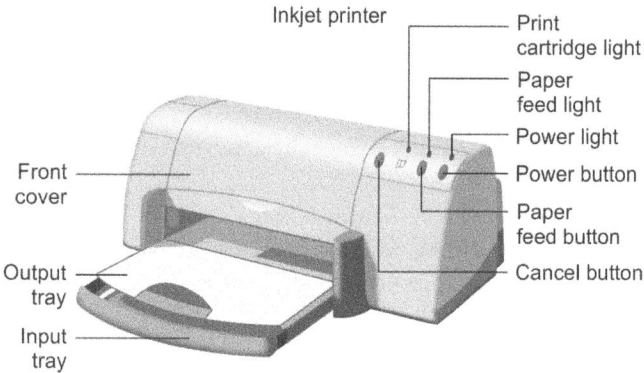

Fig. 10.10: Printing material.

Print media are materials used to inform, motivate, or guide learners. Kemp and Dayton (1985) classify printed media into his three types:

- **Training material:** Handout study guide instructor handbook.
- **Information materials:** Brochures, newsletters, reports. Lewis and Paine (1986) list the advantages: They contain informative and entertaining content of general or special interest. They may appear once or daily, weekly, biweekly, monthly, bimonthly or quarterly. Its competitors include electronic broadcasting and Internet media. Today, many books, newspapers, magazines, and newsletters publish digital electronic editions on the Internet.
- Easy to use, generate, modify and update.
- Inexpensive, especially if the media is black and white. color is more expensive.

Print Media Disadvantages

- **Brochure:** A small booklet or pamphlet containing information or discussion on a single subject.
- **Leaflet:** A printed paper containing information or advertising, usually distributed free of charge.

HANDOUTS

Handouts are printed materials distributed to students prior to the presentation. It is mainly used to reduce the time students spend copying notes and diagrams off the blackboard or screen.

Fig. 10.11: Handouts.

Multiple Uses

- Directly related to lesson content
- As a fact sheet—presenting complex, rare or hard-to-find information
- As a reading list
- As a worksheet/quiz sheet/proforma/workbook
- As a permanent reference.

  Whatever type of handout you use must be well organized, well designed, and strictly errorfree. Must be checked. I would also recommend asking a colleague to confirm this. It is a good idea to make the handout interactive with space for annotations and let students know that it is helpful to comment on the information as the session progresses. The layout and content of handouts is largely up to the individual teacher.

Handout Preparation Guidelines

A well-designed handout looks like this.
- Use 12 point or larger font
- Use headings and page numbers consistently
- Use bullets instead of body text
- Use spacing appropriately
- Left justify lines with a jagged right margin
- Do not use excessive capitalization or underlining
- Leave enough space between columns of text
- Do not start sentences at the end of a line
- Avoid using glossy paper

Handout Preparation

Handouts should not be repetitions of material provided in the textbook or in live lectures. Effective use of handouts requires careful planning. The required information should be written neatly and concisely.

Instructions for Creating Handouts

- Determine the type of handout. To provide variety, each lecture may differ in type and purpose.
- Write only items directly related to the lesson topic and intended goal.
- Identify keywords and taglines and highlight them to emphasize in handout
- Use simple, clear language. Make short sentences.
- Draw sketches and diagrams with or without annotations. Remember that "a sketch is worth a thousand words".
- Draw a diagram. Write as accurately as possible.
- Provide an appropriate title and subtitle.
- Use visual symbols and easily recognizable nomenclature.
- Use appropriate colors whenever possible. Or have students color in a black and white handout.
- If possible, provide enlarged slides for handouts. Teachers can project slides to fill in blanks and label parts. This is a very effective method.

Distributing Handouts

Teachers should explain the purpose and use of handouts. Handouts can be distributed to learners at any of the following times:
- Well before the presentation.
- Just before the session starts.
- As needed during the session.
- Right after the session ends. Handing out a lot of handouts in advance is like a textbook. This is useful if you do not have a book available or need some prior reading/work before attending the course. Handouts distributed at the beginning of the lesson draw the class's attention to the lesson objectives and content. This is generally satisfactory.

  Handouts will be provided in due time. Maintain a high level of attentional motivation and interaction at multiple points in time, either immediately before the discussion, possibly immediately after some points have been raised, or just after watching the video.

Distributing handouts immediately after a lesson leaves a record of the lesson and teacher follow-up determines whether students read it.

NEWSPAPER

Newspapers have many examples that you can use to introduce your lessons. Health messages can be published in local languages that are easily accessible to the general public. Information is provided in a language that is inexpensive, easy to read and understand. People can learn to read and interpret the content along with the pictures (use good enough good pictures).

Newspapers carry a big mass appeal for educating and influencing the opinion of the masses. Being a source of latest information and treasure of knowledge on the local and global issues related to each and every aspect of the social life a newspaper can potentially become an effective aid in the process of teaching-learning.

In its simple meaning newspapers are known as the papers or written documents containing the news of varying general and specific interests concerning people and places. Their scope and area of circulation may be too limited as happens in the case of local newspapers related to the lives and interests of the people belonging to a community village town city or region or it may be too wide covering the national and international boundaries and touching the lives and interests of the people from all over the world. The newspapers one often comes across at home and libraries thus may be categorized as local daily, local weekly regional daily and national daily, etc.

Using newspapers for educational purposes requires reading them and understanding the information and ideas they contain. As such, it is a visual device that requires prior reading and comprehension skills from the user. But readers can also refer to and learn from the use of newspapers as teaching materials.

Educational Benefits

The educational benefits of using newspapers as educational tools can be summarized as follows. It can also help develop children's interest in specific readings related to specific topics and issues from an early age. It helps to properly develop basic language and communication skills such as writing, summarizing, reporting, editing, commenting, critically evaluating and criticizing.

Extensive knowledge of personal, social, local and global issues. As such, it has proven to be an extensive source of information and knowledge for students of all ages and grade levels in all areas of the school curriculum.

- Newspapers as a lowcost educational tool also help strengthen and develop advanced cognitive abilities and skills such as thinking skills, reasoning and problem-solving skills, analysis, synthesis and evaluation, and application skills.
- Creative skills and forms of expression can also be well nurtured and developed with the help of newspapers as teaching materials.
- Newspapers can be a source of endless learning experiences that can be applied to any subject in the school curriculum.

MAGAZINES

Magazines offer advertisers a wide range of readership and frequency options. Consumer magazines cover a wide range of interests including sports, hobbies, fashion, health, current affairs and local issues. Many business and trade publications report on specific sectors such as finance and electronics. Some cover cross-cutting topics such as communications and human resources, while others focus on specific jobs, such as publications for executives, marketers, and engineers. Publication frequency is typically weekly, monthly, or quarterly. Similar to newspapers, advertisers can use a variety of advertising spaces, from classified ads to black-and-white or color full-page ads.

PROJECTED AIDS

Projected aids are those that require the proper presentation of audiovisual equipment. Tools in this category include slides, filmstrips, transparencies (VU graphics), and movies. It is important to remember that most nonprojection aids can be adapted for use as projection aids. For example, diagrams can be photographed and processed into slides

Projected Aid Value

- Makes learning more fun
- Promotes faster learning
- Increased retention: Higher percentage increases retention
- Educational situation is more adaptable
- Gets attention
- Increase or decrease the actual size of the object
- Filmstrips that bring the distant past and present into the classroom:
- Filmstrips are continuous filmstrips made up of individual still images or images, usually arranged in a row with a descriptive title. Each strip contains 12 to 18 or more images. This is a fixed sequence of related still images on a roll of 35 mm or 8 mm film.

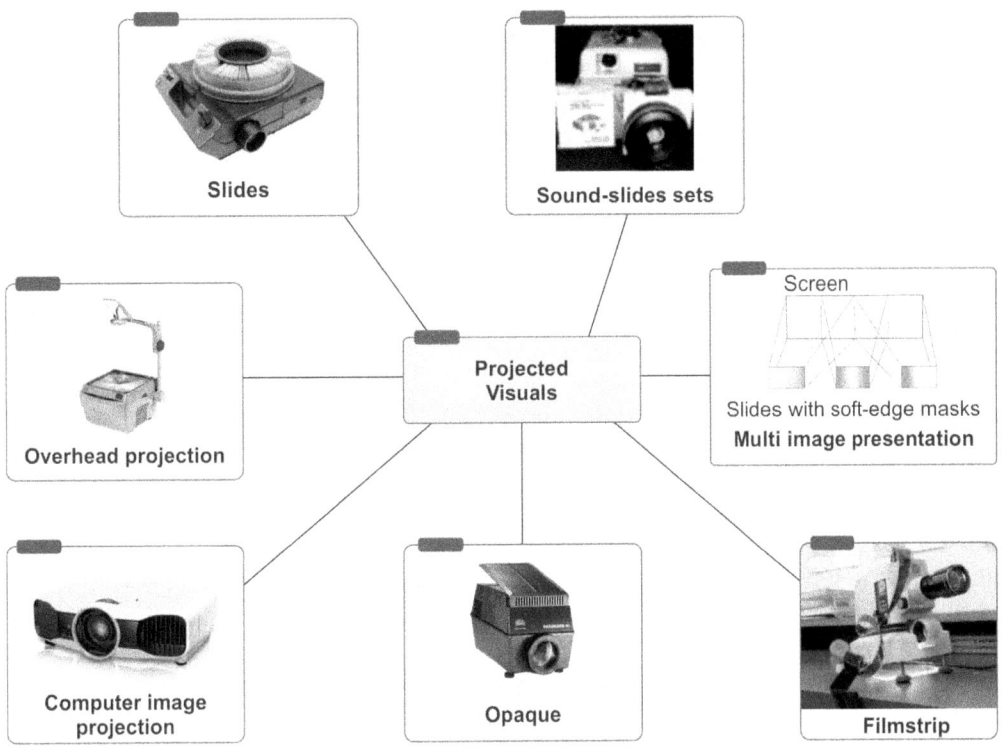

Fig. 10.12: Types of projective aids.

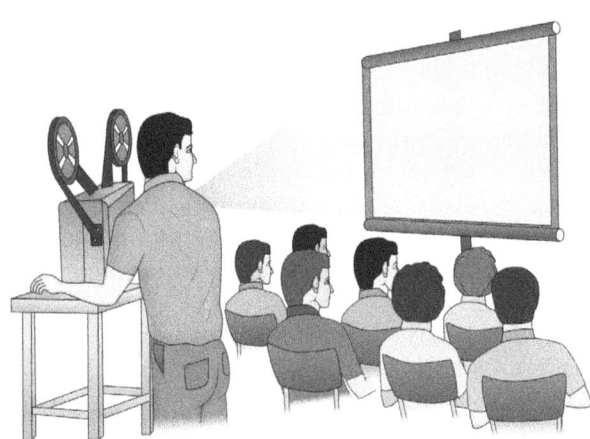

Fig. 10.13: Teaching with projective aids.

Benefits

- Inexpensive visual aid.
- Easy to manufacture, convenient to handle and carry.
- It does not take up space and can be easily stored.
- Makes the lesson flow logical and keeps individual images on the strip longer in students' minds.
- Filmstrips can be projected onto screens, walls or paper screens depending on requirements and teaching situation.

FILMSTRIP PRINCIPLES

- See and carefully select a filmstrip that meets the needs of your subject before use.
- Identify the portion of the filmstrip that needs closer inspection.
- Use filmstrips to evoke emotions, build attitudes, and point out problems.
- Proper introduction and exploration of relevance to the research topic.
- Use the pointer to draw attention to specific details on the screen.

Filmstrip Types

- **Discussion filmstrip:** A continuous filmstrip consisting of a series of frames, usually with a descriptive title. A recorded description of the discussion is meant to be heard in sync with the images.
- **Sound slide film:** It is similar to filmstrip but instead of explanatory titles or spoken discussion recorded explanation is audible, which is synchronized with the pictures.

Instruction to be followed while using filmstrips:

- Use filmstrips to inspire emotions, build attitudes, and point out problems.

- Properly introduce and clarify the relationship to the research subject.
- Students should be interested in critically viewing and discussing the movie screen.
- Teachers and students should learn how to operate the projector.
- Use the pointer to draw attention to specific details on the screen.

MICROSCOPE

Science teachers want their students to make accurate observations and draw correct conclusions from what they see. Live insects and specimens on microscope slides may need to be viewed by a small group of students.

Usually a microscope can be used for this. Using this technique, the teacher can draw the student's attention to the features of the picture. But since only one student can see through the microscope at a time, the teacher is not sure he is seeing what he is saying. In such situations, microprojection with a simple dissecting microscope or a compound microscope can be used.

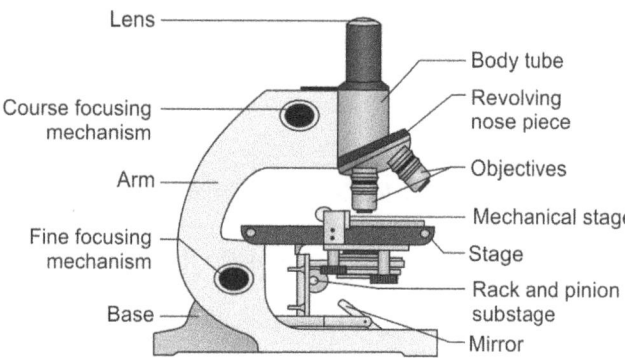

Fig. 10.14: Structure and parts of microscope.

Microprojection is a technique that allows a real microscope slide or small object to be magnified and projected onto a screen for viewing by a small group.

As a dissecting microscope, organisms such as mosquito larvae and tadpoles can be clipped into the watch glass. When using a compound microscope, a few drops of water may be placed on the glass slide to dislodge microorganisms such as Paramecium.

POWERPOINT SLIDE

PowerPoint slide show (PPT) is a presentation created with Microsoft's software that allows users to add audiovisual and audiovisual features to their presentations. Considered as a multimedia technology, it also serves as a collaboration and content sharing tool.

Meaning

Sometimes abbreviated as "PP" or "PPT" PowerPoint is a presentation program developed by Microsoft that creates slide shows of key information charts and images for presentations. Most commonly used for business and school presentations.

Definition

A combination of various slides presenting graphical and visual interpretations of data in order to present information in a more creative and interactive way is known as a PowerPoint presentation or PPT.

Items that can be added to slides:

The following items can be added to PowerPoint slides:
- Clipart
- Charts
- Table
- Photos
- Charts
- Media clips
- Videos

MS PowerPoint Features

The same is discussed below.
- **Slide layout:** Several options and layouts are available to base your presentation on. This option is available in the Home section and allows you to choose from multiple layout options provided.
- **Insert—clip art video, audio etc:** Under the Insert category several options are available that allow you to choose which features to insert into your presentation. This can include images, audio, video, headers, footers, icons, shapes, etc.
- **Slide design:** MS PowerPoint has different themes to add background colors, designs and textures to your slides. This makes your presentation more colorful and grabs the attention of your audience.

  This feature can be added using the "Design" category mentioned on the homepage of MS PowerPoint. Although there are existing design templates available in case someone wants to add some new texture or colour the option to customize the design is also available. Apart from this slide designs can also be downloaded online.
- **Animations:** During the slide show the slides appear on the screen one after the other. If you want to add animation to how your slides look, you can browse the animation category.

Use PowerPoint Presentations

- PowerPoint presentations are useful for both personal and professional use. Below are some of the main areas where PPTs are very useful, survey modified.
- **Marketing:** PowerPoint presentations can be very important in the marketing field.
- Graphs and charts can make it clearer which numbers your audience ignores when reading resume—create a digital resume using MS PowerPoint.
- Various sample photos can be added to CV
- **Demonstrate growth:** Use PPTs because both graphics and text can be included in presentations that demonstrate growth, such as business student grades.

PowerPoint Benefits

- Considered the standard for presentation software. When you create a PowerPoint presentation, people are more likely to find it easy to open and view.
- It includes many optional presentation features such as slide transitions, animations, layout templates, and more. Windows Media Video and PowerPoint XML.

OVERHEAD PROJECTOR

The overhead projector is a projection medium that allows group lessons to be conducted using transparency film or overhead transparency film (transparencies). Teachers can maintain eye contact with students while using the OHP. It can be used in bright rooms. You can make foil using acetate foil with a special marker pen. Complex graphics can be transferred from the original material to acetate by Xerox.

Definition

Overhead projectors are very simple but reliable tools used to display images on screens and walls. It consists of a large box with a cooling fan and a very bright light with a long arm outstretched to the side. There is a mirror at the end of the arm that catches the light and directs it towards the screen.

Points for Using OHP

- For OHP, you can easily obtain an A4 size plastic sheet on which information can be written.
- Then use the slides with an overhead projector to display the written material on the screen.
- This resource may be next to a board or handout that you use frequently.
- OHPs are used to create information to visually illustrate key points, illustrate figures, highlight issues, teach and support other methods of visual communication.
- Transparencies can be created with the transparencies pen. There are basically two types of pens,
  - A spirit-based pen with an image that lasts.
  - A water-based pen that can be erased with water.
- Use large, bold type and clear, simple graphics with as few lines and tables as possible.
- In addition to pens, copiers, laser printers, matrix printers and plotters can also be used to create transparencies. These can be black and white or inkjet colored.
- The principle applies here that text or graphics can be transferred from paper to paper in different ways.
- Instead of paper, information is transferred to slides used for presentation in lectures, seminars, conferences, or workshops.

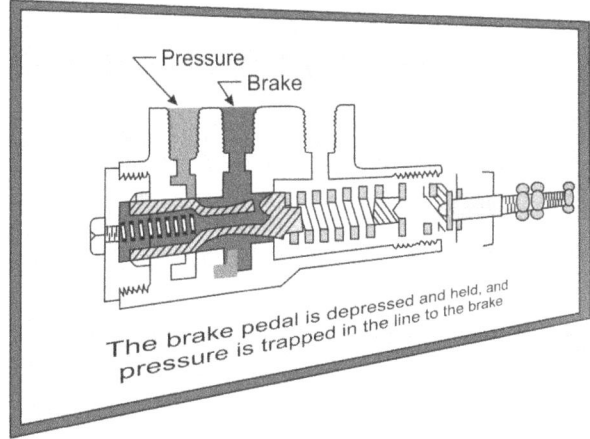
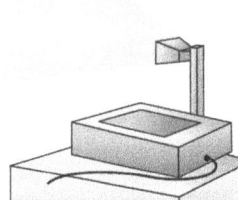

Fig. 10.15: The overhead projector is self-contained, portable and adaptable to large and small classrooms.

Transparencies Useful Instructions for Preparing Transparencies

- Leave a margin from top to bottom of the slide. This allows you to view all the information at once.
- Plan your text and graphics carefully. Try to summarize.
- Teachers should not attempt to broadcast the entire lecture on OPH

Advantages

- You can synchronize the projection with the lecture by facing the audience and observing their reactions.
- Presenters can also write, sketch, and erase while projecting.
- It is helpful to cover part of the slide with paper and overlay the charts gradually revealing them.
- Make your presentation dynamic and engage your audience.
- I can present complex ideas clearly. Save time when giving lectures.
- Easy to prepare and plan materials.
- Transparent materials are inexpensive and readily available.

Cons

- The image is not clear due to wrong projection location selection, power cut or wrong angle.
- It does not make sense without white walls and screens.
- This is expensive and cannot be used if the project is stopped.

Important Notes on Use of OHP

- Transparencies are readily available A4 size plastic sheets on which information can be written.
- Then use the slides with an overhead projector to display the written material on the screen.
- This resource may be next to a board or handout that you use frequently.
- OHPs are used to create information to visually illustrate key points, illustrate figures, highlight issues, teach and support other methods of visual communication.
- Transparencies can be created with the transparencies pen. There are basically two types of pens:
  - A spirit-based pen with an image that lasts.
  - A water-based pen that can be erased with water.
- Use large, bold type and clear, simple graphics with as few lines and tables as possible.
- In addition to pens, copiers, laser printers, matrix printers and plotters can also be used to create transparencies. These can be black and white or inkjet colored.

- The principle here is that text or graphics can be transferred from paper to paper in various ways.
- Instead of paper, information is transferred to slides used for presentation in lectures, seminars, conferences, or workshops.

OPAQUE PROJECTOR

The opaque projector is the only projector that can project a wide variety of materials such as: An opaque projector simultaneously projects and directly magnifies the original print, any kind of written or visual material in any order made by the teacher. A dark room is required because the projector is large and practically unmovable.

A very useful tool that allows you to capture images using reflected light or magnify flat images or drawings and project them onto the screen for viewing by the whole group.

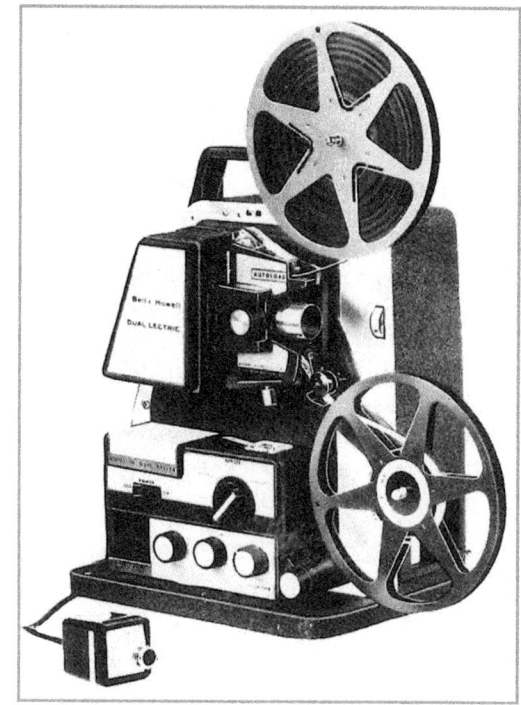

Fig. 10.16: Opaque projector.

Opaque projector simultaneously projects and magnifies any kind of written or visual material directly from the original print in any order specified by the teacher. A dark room is required because the projector is large and cannot be easily moved.

Uses

- Regular lesson on the big screen.
- Approach to reading.

Advantages

The Opaque Projector is a great teaching tool, capable of vividly magnifying and projecting objects from postage stamp size to practically a quarter page. In a regular classroom, everyone can see the projection, even those sitting in the far corners or on the back benches.
- Attract attention and arouse interest.
- If you have a copy, you can project a wide range of materials such as stamps, coins, and patterns.
- Can be used to enlarge drawings, photographs and maps.
- No written or typed material required, handwritten material can be used.
- Help students retain knowledge over time.
- Review the lesson questions.
- Test your knowledge and ability.
- Easy operation.

Disadvantages

- Expensive equipment.
- Should be used with caution.
- The projector requires a dark room.

Classroom Opaque Projectors

Opaque projectors serve many educational purposes. The procedure allows teachers to use it for the following purposes, depending on their needs and teaching situation:
- Charts, graphs and graphs can be projected onto a large screen for regular teaching.
- Picture stories from any source are projected and used as a reading approach.
- The young artist in charge was overjoyed when the original picture was projected on the screen.
- Written works—stories, poems, essays, letters—may be projected. It is an effective system for sharing students' doubts. The darkness of the room stands out.
- Demonstrate the basics of arithmetic handwriting, spelling, and composition using an opaque projector.
- You may plan out a written or typed outline for your new unit of study.

LCD PANELS

This tool has been largely superseded by data projectors. Since many small classrooms and training rooms may not be equipped with data projectors, the following guidance is provided. By connecting a liquid crystal display (LCD) to the computer and placing it in an overhead projector, computergenerated images can be projected onto the screen and read by the entire class. To display an effective LCD, you need to set up an overhead projector with a much more powerful lamp than the normal type of projector.

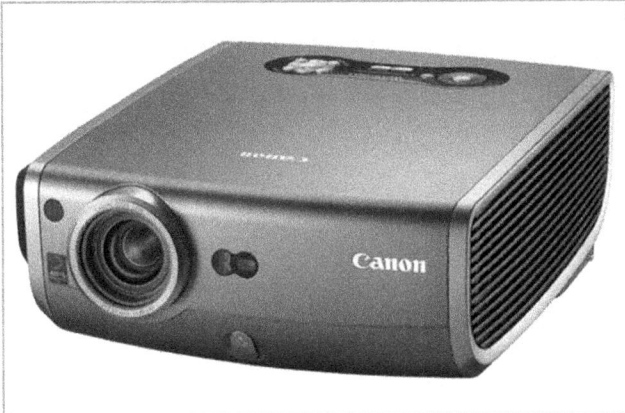

Fig. 10.17: LCD projector.

PowerPoint Presentation Guide

PowerPoint is a very popular presentation that allows you to create interesting and visually appealing presentations instead of using overhead slides.

A major advantage of using PowerPoint is the flexibility in both the content of the presentation and the way the information is presented. Graphs, tables, and org charts add interest to presentations, but they usually keep presentations simple and clear. PowerPoint is best used to emphasize the main features of your topic.

Here are some guidelines for PowerPoint presentations:

- Limit the number of slides to 12 or fewer in a 10-minute presentation.
- Make the text stand out against the background, but avoid patterned Background.
- Use only 1 or 2 animations or transition effects.

Advantages

- List search steps that can potentially throw content out of order.
- Less prone to technical issues and last minute surprises.

Disadvantages of PowerPoint Presentations

- Teacher cannot manipulate content to illustrate points raised by students.
- PowerPoint can take up to 1 minute to load presentations.
- For teachers who take longer to prepare.
- Technical failures are possible and if the computer is not supported by a UPS, it cannot be used in the event of a power failure.
- The floppy disk may not open or the file may have been corrupted by a virus.

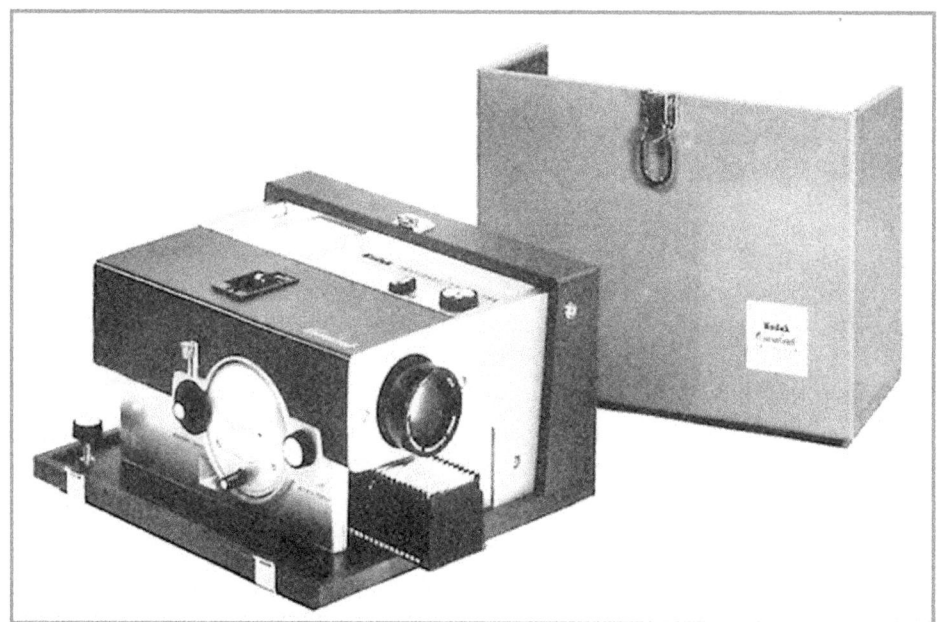

Fig. 10.18: Slide projector.

THE SLIDE PROJECTOR

A slide is a small piece of transparent material on which a single image, scene, or graphic is photographed or reproduced. Molded slides are 2" × 2" or 4.5" × 4". Allows teachers and students to take pictures and snapshots when going on excursions for historical, geographical, literary or scientific excursions to create slides from photos and images. Arranging the slides in the correct order according to the topic covered is an important aspect of teaching with slides.

Teachers must use their imagination and creativity to make the most of them.

Benefits of Transparencies

- Helps students remember what they are teaching
- stand out
- Intriguing
- Support educational development
- Test the student's understanding
- Read the instructions
- Encourage student and teacher participation.

SLIDE

A slide is a transparent image that is projected by passing light through it. Commonly used slide sizes are 2' × 2' and 31%. Slides can be created from photographs and images taken by teachers and students when they go on historical, geographical, literary or scientific excursions. Arranging the slides in the correct order according to the topic being discussed is an important aspect of teaching with them. This is a layered image. You can project onto a screen or a white wall. 35 mm film slides mounted in individual cardboard or plastic frames are widely available and are often used for extended work such as training programs, seminars, workshops, group meetings, campaigns and trade shows.

Benefits of Slides

- Get attention
- Intriguing
- Support educational development
- Test the student's understanding
- Read the instructions
- Encourage student and teacher participation
- Help in retention of the material taught in the minds of the pupils.

CONCLUSION

From this chapter students will be able to classify and understand about nonprojected – drawings and diagrams, charts, graphs, posters, cartoons, board devices, chalk/white board, bulletin board, flannel board, flipcharts, flash cards, still pictures/photographs, printed materials-handout, leaflet, brochure, flyer about, and about projected – film stripes, microscope, PowerPoint slides, overhead projector and widely utilize them in clinical practice.

REVIEW QUESTIONS

Long Essays
1. Define visual aids, explain the benefits of visual aids.
2. Describe nonprojection visuals, explain the benefits and disadvantages of nonprojected aids.
3. Define chart, explain the purposes, types and uses of charts.
4. Define bulletin board, explain the features and usage of principles.
5. Define print materials, explain handout preparation and instructions for creating handouts.
6. Define projected aids, explain filmstrip types and principles.

Short Essays
1. Visual learning strategies.
2. Graphs: Types and uses.
3. Posters: Purposes and components.
4. Cartoons: Uses and learning benefits.
5. Preparation/techniques for using cartoons.
6. Main uses of the board.
7. Effective uses of the board.
8. Techniques for using the board use it effectively.
9. Flannel sheet: Purposes and benefits.
10. Flipchart benefits.
11. Preparing index cards.
12. Use of images and photos.
13. MS PowerPoint features.
14. Use and benefits of PowerPoint presentations.
15. Important notes on use of OHP.
16. Classroom opaque projectors.
17. Benefits of transparencies.

Short Answers
1. Still images.
2. Use of nonprojected images.
3. Chain charts.
4. Cause and effort chart.
5. Tabulation chart.
6. Strip tease chart.
7. Pictorial chart.
8. Flowchart.
9. Poster design rules.
10. Bulletin board use in nursing practice.
11. Flashcards uses.
12. Print media disadvantages.
13. Newspaper.
14. Magazines.
15. Microscope.
16. LCD panels.
17. Benefits of slides.

Chapter 11

Moving Visuals and Audio Aids

Learning Objectives

- Moving Visuals/Moving Images
- Video Learning Tools
- Video Cassettes/Videotapes
- DVD (Digital Versatile Disk)
- Blu-Ray
- USB
- Realia and Models/Three Dimensional Aids
- Puppets, Models, Mockups, Object and Specimen, Moulage and Diorama
- Audio Aids/Audio Media: Tape Recorder
- Use of Tape Recorders for Educational Purposes, Radio, Compact Disk, Public Address System and Digital Audio

MOVING VISUALS/MOVING IMAGES

Simultaneously conveying sound and vision, moving images influence children's minds by mixing images, words, objects, movements and even colors. Viewers can see reproducible movements. You can control the time factor and scale your objects up or down in a series of events. I can now see the process that was a mystery until now. By using direct shots and special effects, videos can take the viewer into another world. This medium can therefore give students a realistic representation of the exam.

Definition

Motion picture film (also called motion picture or film) is a series of still images, typically 8 mm or 16 mm film material, taken in rapid succession and projected by a motion picture projector to provide a visual effect to the viewer. Gives the illusion of convey movement.

The educational value of movies:

- Enrich the learning process and increase overall achievement.
- Modify the beliefs directly in the desired direction and encourage the student to seek additional information on the subject of study.
- It helps improve educational outcomes in a variety of subjects.
- Call attention.
- Bring the experience closer.
- An edited version of reality.
- Animation can control timing factors for each process/sequence of events.
- Video can soften the distant past and present of the classroom.
- Video can easily provide a reproducible record of an event or operation.
- Provide a common denominator of experience.
- May affect and even change settings.
- Moving images help students understand abstractions by stimulating thought and encourages them to think more about relationships.
- Movies add variety to the teaching material.
- Movies provide a satisfying experience.

Motion Picture Film Applications

- Film can effectively convey factual information about a wide range of audiences, ages, abilities and conditions of use.
- Movies are effective in teaching perceptual motor skills.
- Video can be made more effective as a learning tool by using a variety of teaching techniques.

- Films can change motivations, interests, attitudes, and opinions if they are intended to stimulate or reinforce beliefs in existing audiences. Characteristics are greatly affected.

What films can be used for:
- To provide a backdrop for a sensory experience.
- How to provide a concrete experience as a basis for thinking, reasoning and problem solving.
- Provide an easily accessible knowledge base that stimulates student interest and motivates further study and learning activities.
- Presents a large amount of information in a short amount of time.
- Increase initial study volume and study period.
- Cultivate an attitude of gratitude and better social relationships.
- Promotes consistent learning.
- For verification purposes.
- Introduce the unit by presenting the student with an entire set of problems.
- Demonstrate the process.
- Emphasize and stress the underlying principles of nursing procedures.
- Supplement laboratory instructions.

Applications
- Attract attention
- Have a personal experience
- Reality compilation
- Makes the distant past and present real in the classroom
- Can control the time factor
- Provides a common denominator of experience
- Influences and transforms attitudes you can even change
- Bring variety to the lesson.

Teacher's Role
- Selecting the right film
- Checking everything before showing the film
- Previewing the film
- Presenting the film.

The educational role of the film:
From the above, we can add the following features of the educational role of the film:
- Moving images call attention. If the physical conditions in the classroom are comfortable, you can't help but watch a movie. The 'magnetic' appeal of sounds and images ensures an intense experience with an illusion of reality and sometimes a high emotional quality.
- The film uses a variety of techniques to bring a near-direct reality to the students' experience.
- This movie is a compilation of reality. Augmented reality is the main feature of the film. Like many other audiovisual materials, video can enhance realism and its stereoscopic effect makes it the most effective teaching tool.
- Movies can bring the distant past and present to life in the classroom. For cinema cameras, the distant past is only happening in the present.
- Movies can control timing factors for each operation or sequence of events. Timing is a great feature of movies.
- Films can provide an easily reproducible record of an event or operation.
- The film offers a common denominator of experience. Reading opportunities vary from student to student.
- Film can affect and even change settings.
- The film helps students to understand abstractions and thoughts, thereby encouraging them to think more about relationships.
- The film diversifies material that might otherwise remain mundane. The aesthetics I experience are the result of the work the film does. Using color makes the whole process interesting and imaginative. This becomes a means of satisfying the aesthetic experience.

Benefits
- Specific meanings of movements are best conveyed through video. This makes it easier to describe certain ongoing processes, such as plant growth or the functioning of bodily systems.
- This movie needs attention. A dark room creates an enchanting atmosphere for watching movies.
- Film enhances reality.
- Films can control temporal facts or arbitrary manipulations or sequences of events, showing various sporting achievements, embryonic development, etc.
- This film can bring the distant past and present into the classroom. All historical films capture the past from the present.
- Film can readily provide a reproducible record of events and operations."
- Film can magnify or reduce the actual size of an object.
- Videos can be used to demonstrate processes invisible to the human eye. Animation drawing techniques can be used to show the working of the human heart, the physiological processes of the eye, the working of motors, etc.
- The film represents the common denominator of the experience within the group. The basic details of the film are captured through the subtle differences that may exist in the clarity and quality of interpretation.

- Videos can influence certain settings for emotional quality.
- This film can promote an understanding of abstract relationships. The film contains various visual and auditory means such as charts, diagrams, sound effects and background music to analyze a point.
- Movies are often a satisfying aesthetic experience. Harmony of intellectual and emotional experiences is commonly created through the use of various cinematic techniques of photography, action, color, or sound. Because all aesthetics are personal, they are easy to learn and retain forever.
- Motion picture can record an event as it occurs and make it available again.
- Combine seeing and hearing to affect two senses at the same time.
- Movies break down the illiteracy barrier.
- Through the process of microphotography, film can push the boundaries of human vision by combining the properties of a microscope with a film camera.
- By using the concept of one frame at a time, an artist can create drawings shot with a motion picture camera to create an animated film. This technique allows the conceptualization of ideas that do not exist in concrete form, such as: As a vivid explanation of jet propulsion and flight theory.

Disadvantages

- Since motion pictures are somewhat expensive it is necessary to purchase prints and place them in libraries which serve a large number of teachers. Since copies are limited teachers have to request them far in advance. This type of limited access has prevented optimal use of film. Lower costs have made 8 mm films more available thus helping to alleviate this problem.
- The cumbersome and confusing machinery that teachers often face when trying to use film is a major impediment to its widespread use. The use of film is also limited, as projectors usually have to be shared by many teachers. Again, simple projectors such as cartridge loading and self-threading can help overcome this limitation.
- We often complain that the moving images available are not appropriate for the subject or audience. Educators must rely on filmmakers' products. These materials are usually not manufactured for very specific purposes. This problem will decrease as more movies become available.
- Films and projectors require transportation and maintenance.
- Movies are seen as entertainment rather than educational.
- The projector relies on power, either mains power or a mobile generator.
- The audience must be notified in advance of the time and place of the film showing.

Movie Usage

Movies Selection

- Movies are expensive and should be produced for as many different target groups as possible.
- Particular attention should therefore be paid to the quality and suitability of the film chosen.
- Educational films must be specifically selected and used.
- Movies should not be used primarily for entertainment purposes.
- Obtain Catalog from the film library.

Use of Movie Film

Successful use of educational films requires preparation and follow-up planning.

Preparation

- Upon receipt of the film, a preview of the film should be arranged to ensure that the film is suitable for the intended audience.
- Read the instructions that came with the film, if any. Write down key lesson points, key sequences, and difficult words your audience might not understand.
- Write 3 or 4 questions that the movie can answer. Ensure proper physical environment and correct projection settings.
- Before showing the movie to an audience, make sure the projector is working and that the room is dark enough if you plan to show the movie during the day.
- Run the film through the projector before the audience arrives.

Presentation

- With the right motivation and preparation, audiences can learn a lot from movies. A basic guideline, therefore, is to provide motivation and maintain the intensity of interest.
- You need to tell the viewer the title of the movie and, in general, what the movie is about.
- You should explain why the material is important. Relate the lessons to your interests.
- Ask them to call attention to important scenes in the movie. Define all difficult words. Ask questions and explain that those questions can be answered in the film.
- They are expected to understand and learn from watching educational films. If possible, the film should be shown without breaks in a quiet environment without distractions.

Debriefing Activity
- Immediately after the screening, the trainer should invite the audience for discussion.
- Questions should be asked to the audience. It is easy to tell if the movie is fully understood. After a short discussion, show the movie again. Practice the skills demonstrated in the film, if applicable.
- Allow your audience to critique freely and even encourage criticism of your film.
- If the film requires the use of other audiovisual aids—models, mockups, charts, recordings, these may be included. Follow-up care can be provided through home visits or small group meetings.

Note
Videos have special educational benefits:
- Three sources to rent movies for free.
- Videos must be carefully selected and used for a specific purpose.
- Proper use of film requires planning and preparation.
- Choose the well-illustrated teaching aid.
- Do not use film when you have access to equally effective but cheaper teaching tools.
- Don't confuse your audience about time and size.
- Movies should not replace teachers.
- Do not use film alone. This should be part of your overall communications program. It should be integrated with other activities and media.

VIDEO LEARNING TOOLS
Video-assisted learning is a growing strategic teaching method in many modern classrooms. Educational videos have never been more accessible, and teachers are increasingly taking advantage of this readily available resource. But as screen time increases, so does controversy and debate. While video is great for social emotional learning, cognitive skills, inclusivity, and more, video can do just that if not used properly in the right environment.

Definition
Video-assisted learning (VAL) is an educational tool to enhance students' cognitive understanding or social emotional skills. or conceptually defined as a strategic educational approach to using video.

Meaning
- Video-based learning literally refers to learning experiences enabled by video. You can combine camera footage, animation, graphics, text, and audiovideo to create a multi-sensory learning experience unlike any other e-learning format.
- With that in mind, it is no surprise that video-based learning is fast becoming the dominant standard for online training.

Examples of Video-based Learning
Video-based learning comes in many different forms that serve their own purposes. Here are some real-life examples of video-based learning today:
- **Animated explainers:** Apart from being visually appealing animated videos are also effective for illustrating complex or abstract topics that would otherwise be harder to convey. This makes it easier for learners to process the information as well.
- **Expert-led explainer videos:** Expert advice is always valuable. But when delivered in the form of instructional videos by the experts themselves, it creates an engaging experience modeled after lectures and one-on-one lessons.
- **Interactive video:** Video-based learning does not have to be a passive experience. Adding interactive elements allows you to create immersive experiences that allow learners to influence the content based on their choices.

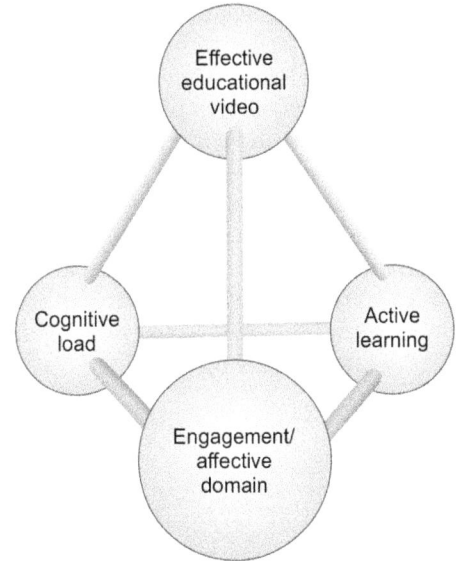

Fig. 11.1: Video-assisted learning.

Benefits of Video-based Learning
In addition to knowing what video-based learning is, it is important to understand why video-based learning is so beneficial.

The main advantages of video-based learning are:
- **Improve learner engagement:** Videos consist of a variety of elements, from visual and audio effects to interactive activities that require users to click on or enter answers. I'm here. As such, videos can engage learners through multiple senses, creating a more engaging experience as well as improving memory.
- **Enable microlearning:** Videos do not have to be long. In fact, they are an ideal format for facilitating a micro learning strategy.
- **It makes content widely accessible:** As more and more learners are becoming mobile first users it's important for e-learning professionals to optimize their content for small screens and keep up with the trend of mobile learning. Video is a format learner can easily access outside desktop devices including tablets smartphone and even smart TVs.
- **It enables on demand learning:** Employees need widely accessible learning content that's also available anytime they find themselves stuck on the job. Videos are a great format for providing performance support resources that meet your workplace needs.

VIDEO CASSETTES/VIDEOTAPES

Videos introduce your students to a topic in a whole new way and help them understand the material they are reading or working on. The impact digital video has on our everyday culture is undeniable. Online video sharing sites such as YouTube Vimeo and Metacafe have millions of monthly viewers. As digital video grows in popularity, it seems only natural that this familiar and widely used platform will be extended to the educational system.

The potential of videotape is to provide a foundation for learning a wide range of motor, intellectual, cognitive, interpersonal and emotional skills. These are important aspects that are not adequately addressed in print. Facilities is especially useful for distance learning programs to update field workers' skills and techniques.

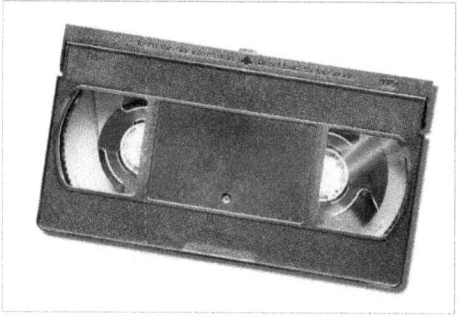

Fig. 11.2: Video cassettes/videotapes.

Types of Tutorial Videos

- **Tutorial videos:** Video tutorial exercises are various media objects explicitly created to help the viewer learn about a particular point. A video teaching exercise is a guide to visualize step by step how a client can achieve something.
- **Training videos:** Training recordings are short in nature, and if not targeted to a specific audience, the videos will quickly disappear. Fertile is brief, and he has one undeniable reason. This is to convey the product evaluation in the shortest possible time. The explainer video style is meant to grab individual attention.
- **Screencast video:** Screencast is his one of the educational videos available today. A screencast is an advanced video recording of your PC screen, usually including an audio presentation. Screencasts are just one type of educational recording. Screencasting does not just save you time answering similar inquiries over and over again.
- **Animated lectures:** Animated videos are drawing tools that help you tell more of your story. Animated infographic videos are short tutorial videos that convey business ideas in a simple and direct way.
- **Presenting with simple slides:** Simple slide organization allows you to get your message directly to your audience without interruption. People love records and 75% are glued to them through reports, articles and other types of media. This is why more and more organizations use them for their business tasks. One of the more common types of videos is the video introduction.

Ideas for Using Videos in the Classroom

- After watching a film clip, have the student, in pairs or small groups, develop her five questions about the film and answer them to her classmates. I will ask you, you should make sure your question reflects your choice of different levels of Bloom's taxonomy or Q & A.
- Students select 3 to 4 videos of literary works produced by professional actors, other students, or educational institutions and note the differences between different video versions.
- Which version do you prefer and why? Did the students notice any perspective distortions or differences in cultural attitudes? Let them brainstorm and write down the context and meaning of the words based on the clip.
- Students write a press release for a movie being released soon. It does not need to be an "official" movie.
- For homework have students find video clips related to the topic taught during the day's lesson.

Student Benefits

- Video creates a more engaging sensory experience than using print alone. Learners can actually see and hear the concepts being taught and process them the same way they process everyday interactions.
- A onestop shop for browsing from anywhere with an Internet connection. Videos can be accessed on a variety of devices including laptops, tablets and smartphones. This allows students to view from anywhere at their convenience.
- Videos can be paused and replayed as many times as needed to improve knowledge retention. You can also review it after the first lesson.
- Very useful for learning all subjects, but especially those that are complex and very graphic (e.g. mathematics). Step-by-step instructions for solving problems or scientific and mathematical formulas.
- Improve digital literacy and communication skills, critical skills of the 21st century.

Benefits for Teachers

- Videos increase student engagement and help improve performance as a result. If students are interested in the material, they are better able to process and remember what they have learned.
- Provides flexibility to pause rewind and skip videos to facilitate lesson discussion or review specific areas.
- This allows teachers to create flipped classrooms and "mixed" learning environments. However, videos are also beneficial for teachers teaching in traditional classrooms.
- Digital video facilitates distance learning opportunities, enabling teachers to reach students around the world.
- Many videos now include analytics so teachers can track student engagement and attendance while watching. Companies like Next Thought also offer platforms that allow you to track how long videos are watched and what percentage of videos are watched. This allows moderators to determine the validity of the video.
- Provide opportunities for student feedback and video support. This is useful for students who are unable to attend class or need tutoring.
- The video aims to change the role of the lecturer from lecturer to facilitator. Please note that the videos are intended to enhance course materials and lectures, not replace them.

Agency Benefits

- Great potential to improve marketing and communication. Digital video can help you grow your audience by reaching more people. These can be published on the institution's website, linked in e-mails and digital advertisements, or published on social media.
- More flexible training for teachers and staff. Schools often find it difficult to get all staff together at the same time, resulting in piecemeal information gathering. Using digital video as a training delivery method ensures equal access to information for faculty and staff. Providing this option not only improves retention and memory, but also acts as an archive that you can review at any time.
- Ability to record campus events for live or ondemand viewing. When parents, students and alumni feel closer to what is happening at school, they feel more engaged and are more likely to have positive referrals and interactions with new and old students. .
- Opportunity to expand online course offerings. Online college programs are very popular due to the diverse student population. Expanding an institution's online programs can greatly increase its appeal to potential online students.
- Digital video can be integrated into your institution's learning management system (LMS). Easily upload video clips to your LMS to provide additional resources for your students and teachers.
- Improving campus accessibility through video instills a positive public relations attitude among parents, prospective students and alumni. This can attract potential students and is a powerful recruitment tool.
- The use of video in education shows a high return on investment (ROI) for institutions using tools to measure it. This includes higher grades reported when a video review module is provided and viewed prior to the exam.

Benefits

In addition to the benefits of educational television, there are other benefits:

- Machine control and the learning process are put in the learner's hands by controlling the mechanics of the machine.
- The ability to order a sequence of events controls learning speed and facilitates sequence practice.

Cons

- Equipment costs cannot always be kept low by using inferior equipment.
- Educational video production requires new technology that is different from entertainment mode. Producers, screenwriters and directors need knowledge of teaching and learning.

DVD (DIGITAL VERSATILE DISK)

- DVD technology is beginning to expand the amount of information in different areas that can be manipulated and transmitted with relative ease. Multimedia possibilities are just emerging for general use. But to get a clear picture of how DVD technology came about, we need to briefly discuss compact disk (CD) technology. Compact disks) are becoming more popular than compact discs because they can store vast amounts of data and information.

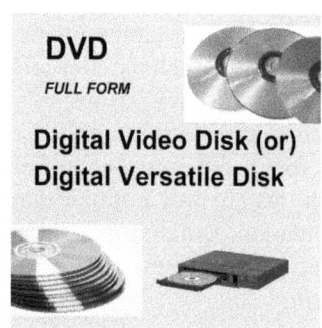

Fig. 11.3: DVD (Digital Versatile Disk).

- A normal CD stores about 640MB of data, while a single layer DVD has 4.7GB of storage capacity and a dual layer DVD has almost 8GB to 18GB of storage capacity.
- This optical disk is inexpensive and can handle large amounts of data efficiently. Data can be stored permanently. Doublelayer hard drives are used because they can store large amounts of data.

Benefits of Learning through Educational DVDs

- They provide a good overall experience for children.
- Preschoolers can easily learn pre-reading skills with the help of these digital tools.
- School going children can easily understand the concepts through various graphical representations and illustrations.
- Practice sessions with the tools can greatly improve your knowledge on various topics.

DVD Advantages

- **Large capacity:** DVDs (Digital Versatile Disk or Digital Video Disk) have enormous capacity for storing data. The need to store or process large amounts of data and information has led manufacturers to produce high quality DVDs with enormous storage capacities.
- **Availability:** Due to mass production by manufacturers, DVDs are readily available in the market and high quality DVDs are flooding the market at low prices. DVDs have become a household item these days and are available in small stores.
- **Low cost:** The raw materials used to make DVDs are very cheap these days. Therefore, mass production greatly reduces manufacturing costs. The computer peripherals industry is considered to be the most competitive industry in the world.
- **Quality:** DVDs were used to store images, audio and video. It has grown in popularity due to the quality it maintains when accessing and generating results. DVDs are high quality and can store data permanently.
- **Portable:** The main advantage of DVDs is that they are portable and can be easily transported from one place to another. DVD data can be easily copied to another location.
- **DVD-RW:** Data on DVD can be read and accessed using DVD-RW. DVD-RWs are also inexpensive and can be purchased from local stores. DVD-RWs are readily available in the market, and various manufacturers offer products at competitive prices.

DVD Disadvantages

- **Dependencies:** If you have a DVD-RW disk installed in your computer or laptop, this DVD may be read-only. Therefore, this hard drive has significant limitations, which in my opinion is one of the main drawbacks of DVDs.
- **Storage capacity:** DVD storage capacity is excellent, but the amount of data and information that users play is enormous. As such, DVDs do not have storage space to store data. Modern games and software are so huge that modern DVDs cannot handle this data. As such, modern storage devices such as hard drives and USB flash drives have conveniently replaced them.
- **Read-only:** Regular DVDs are inherently readonly. This means that once data is recorded or written to DVDs, they cannot be replaced, erased or updated. These DVDs are very expensive and not for everyday use.
- **Data security:** This is considered to be the main drawback of DVDs as the data present on the disk can be easily copied and you can make as many copies as you like. Losing a disk can lead to a data breach.
- **Fragile:** DVDs are made of a thin, plasticlike material that breaks easily. After long-term use, the surface of these disks may become scratched, making it impossible to read data correctly.

BLU-RAY

Blu-Ray Optical disc data storage format, most commonly used for HD (high definition) video playback. Bluray represents the third generation of compact disk (CD) technology after audio CDs and digital video disks (DVDs). All three technologies store data on a 120 mm (4.75 inch) diameter plastic disk. Data is encoded in pits that form a spiral track on the disk. A blueviolet laser emitting at a wavelength of 405 nanometers reads pits.

A single tier hard drive (25 GB) can hold about 4 hours of high definition video or about 12 hours of standard definition video. This huge capacity is very useful for storing training sessions in video format.

Advantages of Blu-Ray	Disadvantages of Blu-Ray
• Very large storage capacity 25–50 Gb • Sound and picture quality is excellent, making them ideal for storing HD films • Blu-Ray disks are now mass produced so they are relatively cheap • A hybrid Blu-Ray/DVD disk can be read in both a Blu-Ray and DVD player	• Blu-Ray does not work in DVD or CD drives • They can be easily damaged by breaking or scratching • Using a Blu-Ray for backup means that up to 50 GB of data is stored on disk, which may then break. That is a lot of data to lose. Perhaps splitting it into several DVD is less risky.

- Blu-Ray (not Bluray), also known as Bluray Disk (BD), is the Blu-Ray Disk Association (BDA) of PC and media for consumer electronics. Developed by a group of the worlds leading manufacturers (including Apple Dell Hitachi HP JVC LG Mitsubishi Panasonic Pioneer Philips Samsung Sharp Sony TDK and Thomson).
- This format offers more than five times the storage capacity of traditional DVDs, holding up to 25 GB on single-layer disks and 50 GB on dual-layer disks. This additional capacity combined with advanced video and audio codecs will provide consumers with an unprecedented HD experience.

Properties of a Blu-Ray

Data access	Direct access
Cost of storage	Blu-Ray cost more per byte of storage than hard disks or magnetic tapes
Capacity	25 GB (single layer) to 50 GB (double layer)
Speed	Slower than a hard disk or flash memory, faster than magnetic tape
Portability	Fairly portable. Too large to fit into a pocket, but will easily fit inside a bag. Can be carried between home/school/office
Durability	Easily scratched by general wear and tear or by not protecting it in a plastic case. Scratches on the disk surface can damage the data being stored Needs to be protected from extremes of heat. Has a limited number of read/write cycles
Reliability	If scratched, the data might not be able to be read. Needs a computer with a Blu-Ray drive in order to read the disk. Cannot be read by a CD drive or DVD drive

USB

Universal Serial Bus (USB) is a type of flash memory that stores information for viewing on a PC. Compared to other storage devices such as CDs and floppy disks, USB is much smaller. But the purpose of all devices remains the same. For data backup and storage.

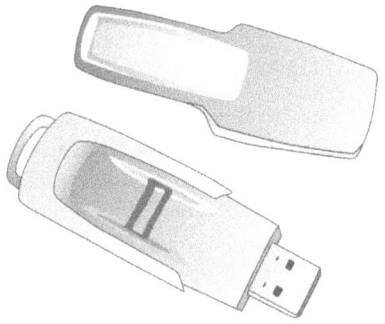

Fig. 11.4: Universal serial bus (USB).

USB drive, also known as a flash drive or memory stick is a small portable device that plugs into your computer's USB port. USB drives are widely used for backing up storage data and transferring files between devices. USB drives come in different storage capacities and different connectors, each with their own shape. Using a USB drive may vary depending on the type of computer you connect it to. Read on to find out how to use a USB drive with Windows.

USB drives serve as a very portable option for data storage and transport for student assignments and everyday requirements to turn work in on time. They can also be easily loaded with information that serves to help students to learn.

Flash Drive Tips

- Purchase a reliable brand name drive. Some of the cheaper brands don't properly test their chips. You only get what you pay for.
- Avoid bumps while connected to the computer.
- Keep it clean and dry. Drives with protective caps or retractable ends help keep your device clean.
- A drive with clip, key ring loop, or lanyard is beneficial for users who tend to lose track of their device.
- Flash memory is expected to wear out over time. Therefore, use it only as a backup. Don't keep all your important files in one place.
- Confirm with the students the correct way to remove the USB flash drive from the computer. Do not pull the drive out of the slot until it is safe to do so. It may not be finished writing and pulling it out too soon can damage the drive.

- Get your students to put their name on the outside of the drive. If lost it can (fairly easily) be returned.
- It is difficult for students and parents to determine whether virus software on family computers is up to date. Instruct students how to run a quick virus scan on a document before opening it on the network. Most new programs will automatically scan your device when it is plugged in, but check with your system administrator.

Advantages of USB Flash Drives

- **Cost:** USB flash drives can be easily scaled up, making them very inexpensive to manufacture. USB drives are relatively inexpensive compared to most external storage devices. Prices may vary depending on storage capacity. Therefore, even people with a small budget can easily use it.
- **Speed:** USB drives do not require an Internet connection, so transfer speeds are relatively fast. However, speed is determined by several factors, including the USB version of the hardware bus and the USB controller device.
- **Capacity:** In the early days, USB drives did not support much storage capacity. So far, there are USB drives that support storage capacities up to 2 TB. Therefore, users do not have to bear the burden of carrying external hardware due to the large storage capacity.
- **Physical size:** All USB drives are small and lightweight, making them highly portable. It can be properly placed in your pocket or pocket without too much inconvenience. A perfect alternative to hard drives and tablets that take up a lot of space.
- **Compatibility:** Today there are many operating system platforms and devices that support USB drives. Everything has a USB port, whether it's a desktop laptop or a game console. However, you need to make sure these devices share the same port as your USB drive. Otherwise you will not be able to connect.
- **Durability:** Unlike hard drives, which lose all data when exposed to frequent mechanical shocks, USB drives have little chance. Also, no data loss due to scratches, dust, or exposure to magnetic fields.
- **Automatic configuration:** When you connect a USB peripheral for the first time, you only need to install the device driver software once. The host operating system loads the configurations automatically, so you don't have to reinstall them.

Disadvantages of USB Flash Drive

- **Corruption:** A USB drives tends to be used in different computers. If in case one of the computers happens to be malware infected it could easily transfer them on to the drives since it is not malware-free. This could result the files unreadable making them useless.
- **Lifespan:** The lifespan of USB drives is not unlimited. The number of read and write cycles is limited. Roughly speaking, this is about 100,000 cycles. After this period of time, the USB drive may fail.
- **Security threats:** Some USB drives contain security holes in the form of encryption. This type of vulnerability can pose a security threat as it exposes all sensitive data. To overcome this, most flash manufacturers have developed updated software that all users should check out.
- **Loss risk:** The physical size of the USB stick can also cause loss. Due to its large size, it can be easily misplaced or stolen. For example, it can slip out of your pocket or be snatched without your knowledge.
- **Broadcast:** No broadcast function between USB and host computer. Only one message can be sent during that time.
- **Build quality:** Some manufacturers produce low priced, poor quality USB drives. However, the overall quality remains questionable. Printed circuit boards are always integrated with metal chips in the soldering process. Poorly soldered parts can lead to weak stress points.
- **Mechanical damage:** However, USB drives are less susceptible to mechanical damage. Not completely free. USB drives contain retractable USB connectors that can become worn or bent. In this case, the drive becomes completely unusable.

REALIA AND MODELS/THREE-DIMENSIONAL AIDS

Both realia and models are three-dimensional materials; these materials are visual instructional materials which give some accurate representation of real life specimens or first-hand experience. Realia provides first-hand or direct experiences for learners.

- Three-dimensional aids serve as good substitute for the real objects. There is no doubt that an encounter with real objects serves as an unmatchable sources of learning. However, for a variety of reasons, it may not be possible to bring real-world objects into the classroom.
- Sometimes the physical objects are too large to move or store in the classroom. With depth or thickness, height and width, her three-dimensional material (called 3D) is an excellent means of providing students with an experience that is superior to direct experience in the real world.

Important for 3D Tools

- It may be too small for a group of students. In fact, it can be too complicated to understand.

- Sometimes the movement is too slow to fully examine. It may be too expensive to purchase from an educational institution.
- Teachers disabled in such situations should look for suitable substitutes for the real object.

Advantages of 3D Tools

Direct realworld experience, and the disadvantage of being an invented experience edited by such editing. Students can get to the heart of the matter by removing offending and distracting elements.

How to Use 3D Tools

How to Use 3D Materials

- **Students should have handson experience:** Using various 3D materials to communicate with students through direct personal contact provide a first experience for. This helps students see and feel items/objects. The more direct the experience, the more likely it is to be beneficial.
- **Teachers and students should have specific goals:** Teachers should have specific goals for using sensory aids. Similarly, students must learn to recognize and understand the purpose of assistive devices. It is the teacher's responsibility to guide students in developing awareness of their ability to observe specific objects. Observation alone is not pedagogical, so teachers need to make students think about whether learning takes place.
- **Students are encouraged to explore:** Research into orthopedic aids is aimed at meeting the immediate needs of students. It is not enough for students to gain experience by seeing how a tool is used and how it is generalized. All of these experiences should be integrated with past, present, and future considerations of the material presented in each class.

Using 3D Tools

Using 3D Materials

- Provide students with correct initial concepts when they first learn about an object or process.
- Clarify the concept in the student's head. Seeing an object creates a unique image and gives meaning to the words that name the object.
- Strengthens and energizes objects in the student's mind. The presence of three-dimensional media can transfer attributes such as shape, size, color movement, and other properties into the student's mind, thereby enhancing the object being viewed.
- Share a specific experience. The use of 3D materials reduces the tendency of teachers to become too abstract in the classroom.

PUPPETS

Puppets come from the Latin puppa, which means doll. The word puppet today means a figure that fits snugly in the hand and is manipulated with the fingers from behind.

Types of Puppets

- **Hand puppets:** These are the simplest of all puppets. They are operated from below by fingers.
- **Rod puppets:** These are operated from below the stage by a combination of rods and springs. These have jointed bodies made with stiff wires or wooden sticks attached to arms and legs.
- **Gloves and hand puppets:** This is like a threefinger glove that fits over your hand. Stick your index finger in your hand and move it around as you tell the story. The middle finger and thumb fit the hand and can be moved.
- **Thread puppets:** Fingers with movable hands and feet that are operated with strings from above.
- **Shadow puppet:** Hand and puppet shadows are used as puppets against a lit screen.

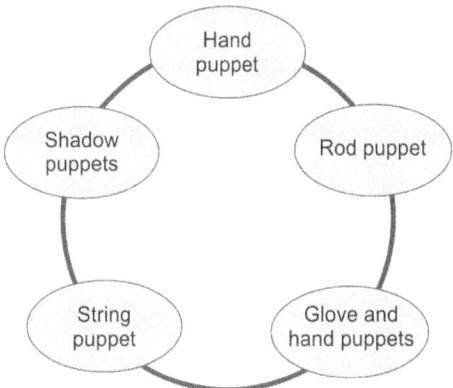

Fig. 11.5: Types of puppet.

To Prepare the Hand Puppet

Materials needed: Used postcard old newspaper glue 2 strings ink paint box pin brush scrap pad and scissors needle and thread.

Instructions

- Wrap a used postcard around your finger and tape it to a tight, finger-fitting tube.

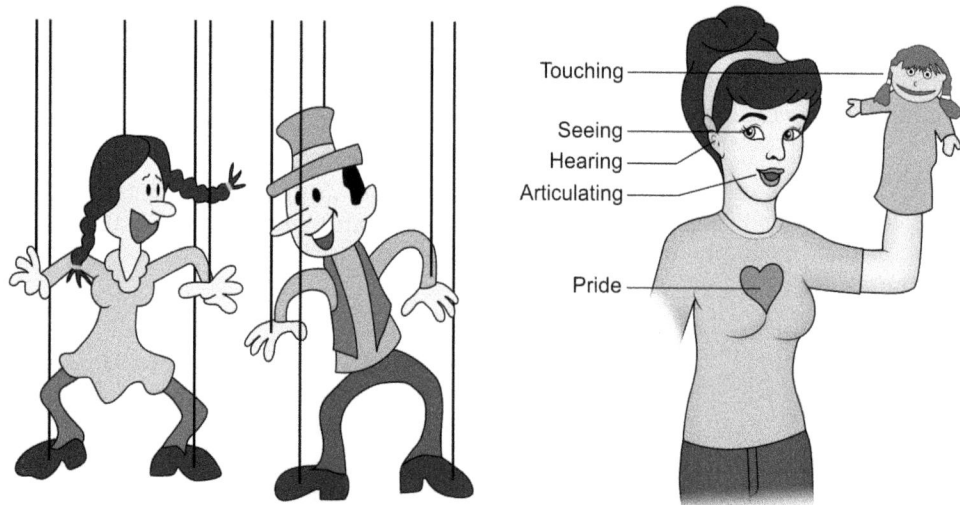

Fig. 11.6: String puppet presentation.

- Crumple a piece of paper into a finger-sized ball, press the ball against your finger over and around the tube, and bend the tip.
- Tie plain paper and draw eyes, hair, nose and lips with ink. Apply red and black colors as needed to create an attractive look.
- Take a piece of bright colored cloth and sent it into a long tube and tie the cloth on the neck and then turn it.
- Some puppets may be prepared to play roles of females some of males or children. They may have moustaches turbans salwars kurtas, etc. A representation of the life and characters you want to show the audience.
- A wooden frame, two chairs, a crib and two porch posts can be used to stage an additional puppet show.
- Puppets must not be viewed by the puppeteer's hands or body. A song or speech from behind or a recorded dialogue is used. Normally, he has two puppeteers behind the scenes, so he can only be on stage with up to four people at a time. It can imitate real-life voices of men, women and children.
- There is a brief explanation of the dialogue before the show. Silent pauses should not occur. Dialogue should be fast and speeches and scenes should be short. There should be a lot of action with wit and humor.
- Everyday people and familiar situations related to village issues should be used.

Puppet Principles

- Theatrical puppets be implemented equally well by other dramatic means.
- Keep the game short.
- Puppets require skillful manipulation.
- Do not miss the music and dance possibilities of a puppet show.
- Customize your puppet show in every way possible for your audience. The student's age background and challenges should be related to the type of puppets used and the game itself.
- Don't hesitate to embrace the puppet show. It's not worth sticking to the text. If you deviate from this, you can add interest and points to the game.

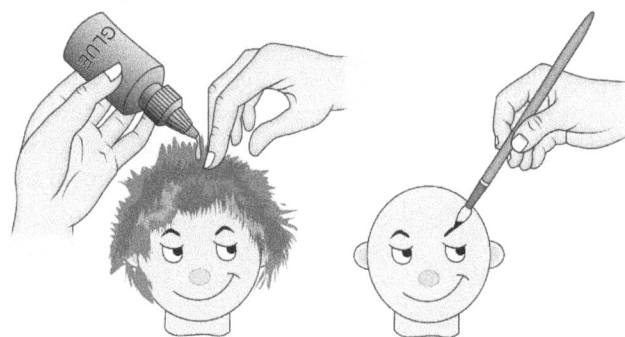

Fig. 11.7: Puppet preparation.

Hand Puppet Benefits

- The craft of puppetry is an effective aid to learning.
- It develops cooperation among children.
- Children develop their imagination by providing the puppets wit speech.
- Children increase their manual dexterity through manipulation.

- Puppet playing helps timid children express themselves more freely because they are separated from the audiences by a screen.

Disadvantages

- Communicating ideas requires special training in working with puppets and puppets.
- The ideas conveyed in a puppet show can be misinterpreted by the audience.
- The student's age background and duties should be considered.
- Puppets plays with too much action take away the attention of the audience.

MODELS

Models are the replicas or copies of the real object. Models are usually of three types: solid cross-sectional and working. Models are concrete objects some considerably larger than the real object. A cross-sectional model clearly describes the original structure or function. In some cases, the original working model is used when certain features of the original are duplicated and can be easily explained.

Main features of the model:

- The model can be simplified easily.
- A model embodies an abstract concept.
- The model allows you to shrink or enlarge the object to an observable size.
- The model provides a correct conception of an industrial unit, a bridge or a dam such as the Bakhla Dam.
- Working models describe various processes of objects and machines.
- Creating models from project work topics. This is very helpful in getting students interested in creative activities. Box plastic Paris gypsum from Paris thermocouples and metals can be used for modeling.

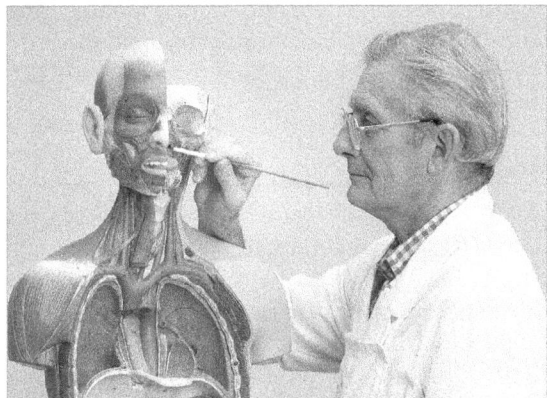

Fig. 11.8: Model preparation.

Key Features of the Model

- Accuracy
- Simplicity
- Usability
- Robustness
- Ingenuity
- Useful

Model Features

- Simplify reality.
- Concrete abstract concepts.
- You can shrink or enlarge the object to observable size.
- Provides correct conception of real objects such as dams/bridges.
- The working model describes the various processes of objects and machines.
- Encourage creative interests in students.

Model Type

- **Scale model:** Allows you to see the correct representation of the object.
- **Simplified model:** Represents the ideal shape of an object. For example, animal fish. For example, fetal circulation.
- **Cross-section model:** Inside of an object in visible immense value will be observed in sciences. For example cross-section of blood vessel.

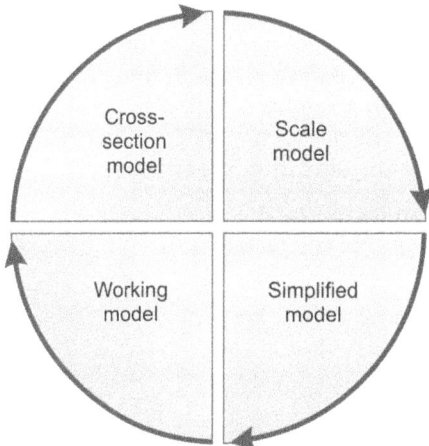

Fig. 11.9: Types of models used in teaching.

MOCKUPS

- A mockup refers to a specialized models or working replica of the object being depicted.
- Mockups emphasize or accentuate certain elements of the original reality to make them more meaningful for

the lesson. A mockup is a recognizable limitation of an object (whether larger or smaller than the original), but the mockup may or may not be similar.
- Models of airplanes, automobile engines, bridges, ships, tunnels, etc. Demonstrations can be made to illustrate their structure and actual behavior.
- Mockups are often used in technical guides for training purposes.

Advantages

- Recreate things from the past or future.
- Reduce the size of things.
- Models of things are too small to examine.
- Making models of distant objects.
- Explain difficult concepts.
- View the working parts.
- To attract interests attention.
- To promote increased learner participation.
- Always show selected aspects of the whole in a simple way.
- Instant sensation.

OBJECT AND SPECIMEN

A pattern is part of an object. It may be a sample that shows quality or structure. Examples would be a section of a long bone a dissected lens from an animal's eye a sample of a crude drug. An object is the thing itself in its entirely brought from its natural setting into the classroom to supply the type of sensory experience that will make instruction meaningful. An object might be a thermometer a splint a forceps a calf's heart or any such thing which pertains to the subject being taught.

Sources of Objects and Specimens

- Local market
- Manufacturers and factories

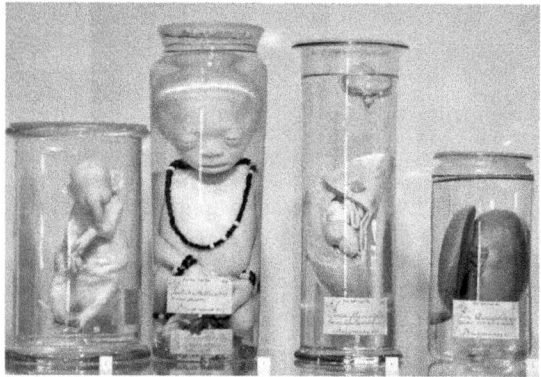

Fig. 11.10: Specimen used in teaching human anatomy.

- Discarded materials from homes
- Students can collect specimens found in nature on excursions and nature hunts
- Purchase plaster models
- You can also get wildflowers, leaves, shells, stones, butterflies, moths, and insects.

Benefits of Objects and Samples

- The collection of objects and samples by students requires interaction with others and leads to the development of social skills and values.
- Students who collect and display objects and specimens are happy to provide something of value to schools and teachers.
- Through the collection of objects and specimens, students' observational skills and first-hand experience are enhanced.
- Collecting objects and specimens can be an interesting educational activity for both teachers and students.
- Stimulates student interest in learning.
- Objects and patterns that use all five senses in the learning process.
- Increases classroom realism.
- Energizes teaching.

General Notes

- Samples are of actual objects or materials.
- **Using objects and preparations:** When using preparations and objects as teaching tools, teachers should keep in mind the following:
  - Plan your teaching with certain simple and direct observations of the object or specimen being referred to.
  - Ask questions from the students to elicit more details of the features of the object or specimen under observation.
  - Clarify and emphasize important structural details of the object or specimen under observation.
  - Provide review and practice to make learning permanent.

MOULAGE

- A moulage is a mold made of plastic (one of a diverse group of plastics suitable for this purpose) for stimulating living things. A part of the body showing signs of trauma, infection, surgery, or disease.
- Phillips describes an excellent mold developed by the medical Illustration Service of the army institute of pathology that will be of great use in teaching nursing students.

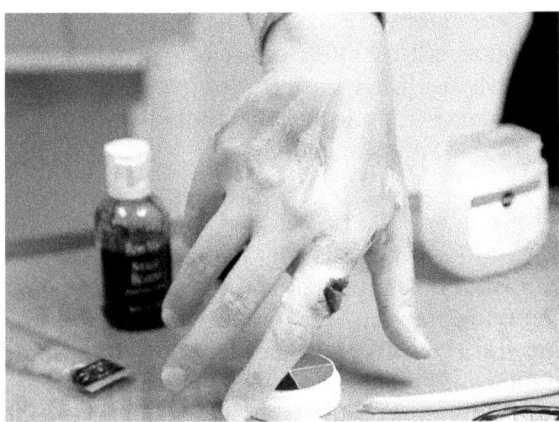

Fig. 11.11: Moulage preparation.

- Colostomy kit, 2 barrel and 1 barrel colostomy with skins that can be attached to a chase mannequin or live model to teach colostomy care.
- The moulage application should function in a way that contributes to realism. Therefore, it is important to consider accuracy and reliability when using this technique. If used incorrectly, it can confuse the learner and cause the simulated patient's actual diagnosis to solve the simulated her scenario.
- As with techniques for increasing simulation fidelity, educators should keep learning goals and objectives in mind.
- The safety and comfort of the person wearing the mulrage must also be considered. Injury patterns may look intriguing, but add no value to the goal and are uncomfortable for the SP. This can also affect performance.
- Typical materials include wax latex petroleum jelly tissue paper stage blood charcoal powder and eye shadow along with common household cooking ingredients such as corn syrup cocoa powder and food coloring. For example a burn can be made with tissue paper and petroleum jelly while corn syrup and food coloring can be applied near the mouth of an SP to simulate blood.
- Cocoa powder and charcoal powder can be a standing for dirt. Moulage also involves constructing and attaching prosthetics to a person, rather than using makeup directly on the skin.

DIORAMA

A diorama is a three-dimensional visual aid that helps you depict and depict reality on a smaller scale. Desire for realism, learning by observing real objects and real situations is commonly abundant among learners, and dioramas have proven to be a valuable means of fulfilling this desire.

Definition

- Michaelis (1976) activities at the airport, life in the Sahara desert, etc. Therefore, with the help of suitable dioramas, small objects, modeled characters and backgrounds can be placed in perspective to the appropriate environment. By using , you can easily draw authentic real-life scenes.
- SL Ahluwaila (1967) a diorama can therefore be defined as his three-dimensional visual representation of a scene in miniature form, rendered in real perspective using a background using miniature objects.

Diorama Type

- Objects such as people, trees, humans and animals that appear in the diorama are displayed in miniature. However, all necessary measures should be taken to give the displayed diorama the necessary liveliness and realism.
- For example, buildings and trees at the far end are scaled down to show that they are further away.
- Thus, the emphasis is on creating the illusion of depth and distance just right for the relatively small space of the diorama on display.
- Lighting effects may be used to achieve diorama display purposes.

Instruction Purpose

- Dioramas can represent reality in miniature form, they are a very useful visual aid for teaching and learning many concepts related to the school curriculum. Take, for example, the lessons "Village Festival Scenes", "Social and Religious Festivals" or "Station". Such themes can be conveyed emotionally through the presentation of appropriate dioramas depicting all that is usually seen on such occasions.
- Various dioramas are available depicting historical, social and geographical aspects such as life in ancient cities such as Harappa, life in a modern Indian village, and Eskimo life, such as the distribution of natural wealth in the countryside.
- Concepts related to the physical environment and economy that require a three-dimensional representation of place, such as: Developments produced by humans or nature, material or human resources, stages of processes, functions of systems, historical evolution, inventions, and fictional situations can be very well explained to students with the help of useful and appropriate dioramas.
- For maximum educational effect, these dioramas are made in collaboration with student groups to quickly collect cardboard, pieces of wood, paper, poster paint, brushes, sewing tools, staples, scissors, faucets, etc. It

should be made using cheap materials that are available, etc., glue to build.

AUDIO AIDS/AUDIO MEDIA

Tape Recorder

The Tape Recorder records audio onto magnetic tape so that it can be played back over and over again. Tape recordings are scratch resistant and can be played back over and over again. Scratches and stains can be repaired on the spot.
- You can listen and listen to previous recordings.
- Have students hear their own voices and what is happening in their school.
- Use tapes to facilitate language learning.
- Classes can record and listen to their own songs and discussion programs for later improvement.

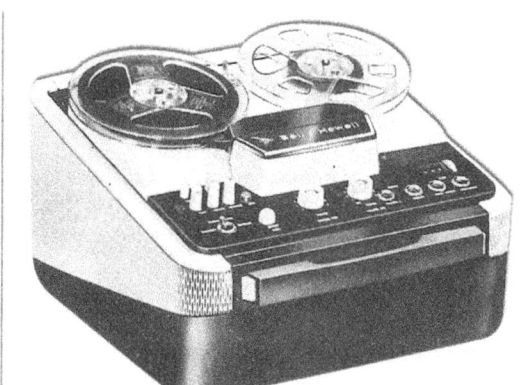

Fig. 11.12: Audio tape recorder.

Use Of Tape Recorders for Educational Purposes

- May be used to record educational broadcasts and play them back at appropriate and convenient times.
- Tape recorders can be used to record music and other sound effects for use in school plays and cultural performances.
- Can be used to record important visitor conversations to the facility for later use.
- Tape recorders are often used in language labs for voice training and correcting pronunciation errors.
- It can be used for listening to music and teaching.
- Provide feedback necessary for discussion to improve teaching.

Tape Recorder Functions

Tape recorder has two functions when running AV programs. and record a "live" interview. filmstrip. Playing the cassette allows planners to recognize what it sounds like and decide where they want more or less emphasis. The planner may want to bring her tape recorder to the scene and record live interviews to hear people›s opinions on topical issues. Later, the recorded interview can be used when the image is projected along with the subject photo of the speaker and their comments.

Radio

Characteristics of the radio and record listening experience:
- **Immediacy:** Radio can describe events as they happen.
- **Emotional impact:** The combined impact of sound and music in a conversational environment arouses student interest and stimulates the imagination.
- **Reliability:** Professionals can access any classroom at any time (via audio media). A student's knowledge of a topic is enriched by listening to experts. Talk about lack of study on the radio. In this way, radio can bring the outside world into the classroom.
- **Conquest of time and space:** Through simulated programs, audio media can really transcend the boundaries of time and space.
- **One-way communication:** No possibility of feedback from students.
- **Auditions:** You cannot audition to determine educational value.

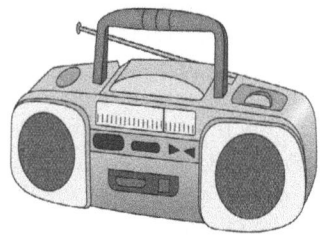 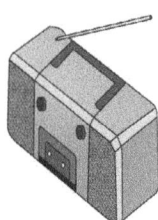

Fig. 11.13: Radio used as teaching aid.

Purpose

- To improve listening participation and assessment skills.
- Set the stage for student discussion by presenting outside expert opinion from distant sources.
- Provide new knowledge interests and diverse sources of information to support the development of values and attitudes.
- This keeps nurses up-to-date on all sources of information relevant to health maintenance and education, so that nurses are not only well-informed, but also useful in patient health education.
- Radio helps caregivers have background knowledge and listen attentively.
- Obtain information on the cultural backgrounds of many different ethnic groups.

- Better understand the patient's likes, dislikes, and characteristics.
- Social factors of religion that nurses must consider in their work. Through radio, students can learn the teachings of major religions and receive personal and inspiring value from religious programs. She can help patients meet their religious needs.
- To call attention to social problems which frequently involve health.
- To build attitude appreciation and understandings of the great medical and nursing personalities their struggle in bettering man's health and lengthening his lifespan.
- They familiarize students with the social implications of scientific discoveries.
- To maintain a good knowledge of literary history and current affairs, and to develop a complete and balanced personality that enhances their understanding and appreciation of them.
- Put the school in timely virtual contact with the outside world. Present and interpret events as they occur, keeping students up-to-date with what is happening around the world.
- He is one of the mass media that can be used to inform the public of the goals and needs of nursing education.
- The public should be informed and encouraged to participate in maintaining and improving health standards.
- Enhancing school programs.
- Develop critical thinking, interest in recreation, and gratitude.
- Broadcasting is an effective means of presenting musical drama and discussion for study and appreciation.
- These are actually team teaching demonstrations.

COMPACT DISK

- A compact disc (CD) is a multimedia storage disk that stores various data types, such as text, graphics, audio, animation, photos, and video in digital form, and can be used by computers (and CD player) can be accessed. (Types based on media format and data storage).
- CD-RW (rewritable media)
- VCD (video compact disk)
- SVCD (super video compact disk)
- Photo CD
- Improved Music CD
- School, college and university use

Use of CDs

- Beneficial to all learners and all subjects
- Data storage and use as a playback device-learning process

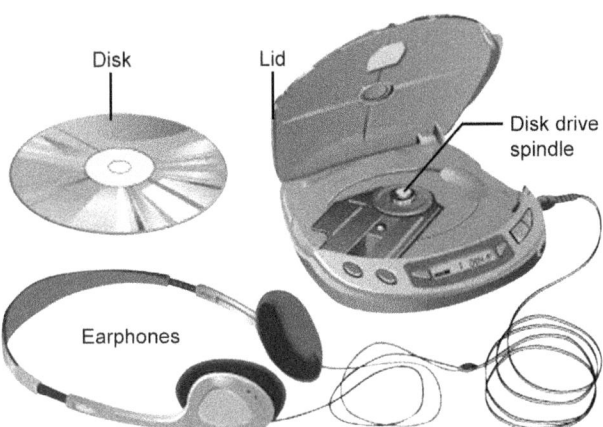

Fig. 11.14: Compact disk accessories.

- Educational CDs serve as reference materials for scientists and students.
- Used as an aid to improve a learner's computer literacy, reading comprehension, and critical analysis skills.
- VCDs can be a source of entertainment.

Benefits

- Beneficial to all learners and all subjects.
- Can perform some of the teacher's duties and assist learners without a teacher.
- Plays an important role in computer-assisted learning.
- The CD acts as a tutor.
- The CD is an audiovisual learning resource.
- Provides inexpensive access to quick and easy retrieval mechanisms for data in various formats.
- Encourages robust concept development, influences various strategies and fosters networking.
- Engage learners with animated audio-video and other graphics.

Cons

- Poorly designed animations are dangerous for learners to comprehend.
- The use of CDs as learning resources is still under development.
- CD cannot used effectively.

PUBLIC ADDRESS SYSTEM

Public address system has been the standard communication device in schools across the country for decades, from grade school to college. One of the functions of the public address system is to enable schoolwide announcements in the event of an emergency. The PA system is also useful for school

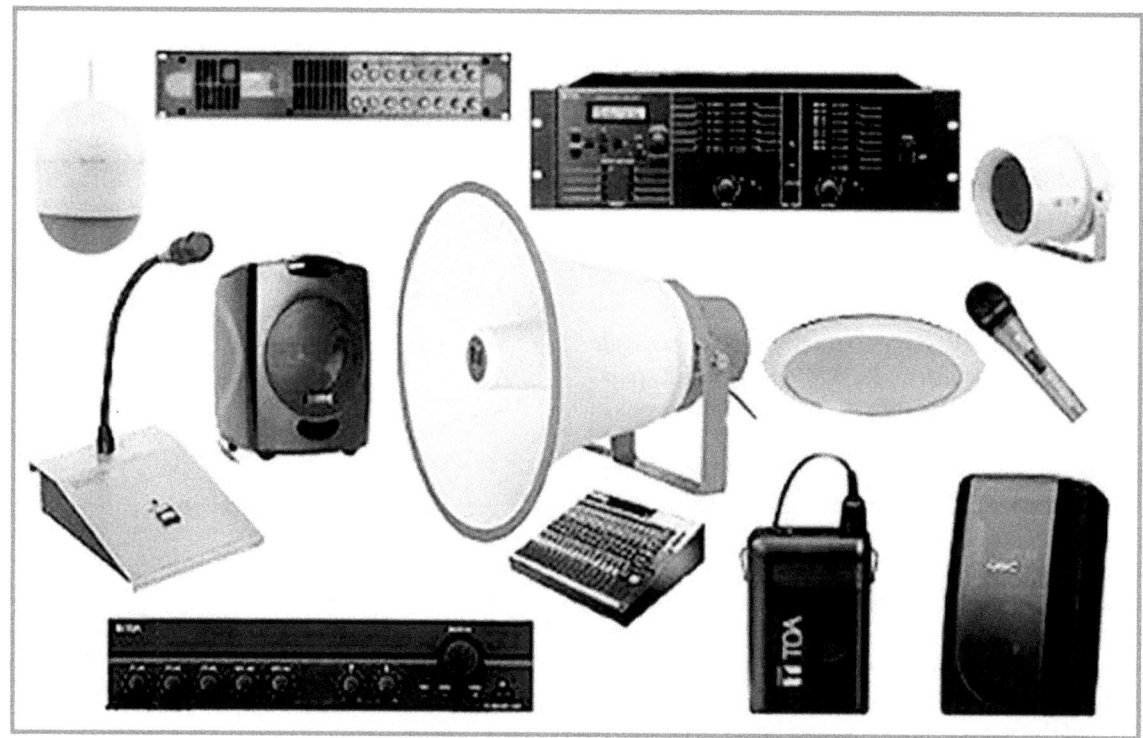

Fig. 11.15: Public address system.

administrators to make regular schoolwide announcements or to direct staff and students to report to her one location if their current whereabouts are unknown.

Early PA systems: Early PA systems were not high tech. They consisted of loudspeakers placed in each classroom and microphones for the speakers in locations of his choosing. The audio signal was wired to speakers in each room and was not of high quality.

Modern public addresses: There are wireless and digital devices that make deploying and maintaining public addresses easier than ever before. With these audio systems, sound quality devices have also become affordable and convenient.

PA system options currently include:
- Wireless microphone
- Amplifier
- Mixer
- Digital signal processor
- Telephone paging interface
- Ceiling speaker
- Wall loudspeakers
- Horn loudspeakers
- Industrial cluster loudspeakers
- Modern multimedia possibilities.

More Speakers
- Requires 50 to 2000 watts of power. It is mainly used in small venues such as school buildings, churches, shops and hotels.
- **Large systems:** The largest PA systems require 1000 to 3000 volts of power. It is mainly used for the construction of industrial sites on campus or entire outdoor complexes.
- **PA over IP:** PA over IP refers to PA paging and intercom systems that use the internet protocol (IP). Used to distribute audio signals to paging locations located throughout a building or campus, or elsewhere within IP network range. Requires 6 watts of power.
- **WMT PA system:** Wireless mobile telephony PA system refers to a system that incorporates PA paging and a wireless mobile telephony system. Use GSM networks. It is used to distribute audio signal to paging location across building campus or anywhere else.
- **Long line PA:** A long line Public Address System is any public address system with a distributed Architecture normally across a wide geographic area. It is used mainly in rail, light rail and metro industries from one or more locations.
- **Small venue systems:** Primarily used in small clubs, bars and coffeehouses, using a fairly simple setup with

FOH speaker cabinets facing the audience and monitor speaker cabinets primarily facing the performers. So you can hear songs and instruments.
- **Large venue systems:** Large systems are far superior to other SR systems. Portable sound systems are recommended to drive large, high power speaker amplifiers.

Public Address System Requirements
- Howling should be avoided
- Spread the sound intensity evenly
- Reduce reverberation
- Correct speaker orientation must be used
- Select correct microphone and speakers
- PA system must provide a sense of direction
- Speaker impedances must be properly matched
- Proper grounding must be provided
- Use closed area connection for loud speakers.

Components of Public Address System
- Speaker: Main speaker subwoofer and monitor
- Amplifiers: It needed only if using passive speakers
- Audio mixer: Analog or digital
- Speaker processors
- Microphones: Dynamic or condenser
- Effect: Only used if needed
- DI box: Direct injection box
- Cables and accessories.

Function
The main function of PA system is to increase apparent volume of a human voice musical instruments other Acoustic sound source recorded sound or music.

Factors to be considered before buying any PA System
- The output power of the PA system should be sufficient for a giving application
- The number of microphones are given that can be connected at the input
- Provision to connect a tape recorder or CD player at its input
- Equipped with tone control graphic equalizer circuit
- PA system with DC battery during power outage
- Individual amplitude control for each input microphone
- Number of speakers supported by PA. Always buy lightweight, low cost PA system.
- Reliable operation guarantee and after-sales service.

Advantages of Active PA Speakers
- Integrated power amplifiers provide the best performance for each speaker.
- Loudspeakers can be easily added or reconfigured into the system without load calculation.
- Each speaker's built-in DSP allows you to adjust the tone of each speaker individually.
- A built-in front mixer allows some speakers to play multiple roles in different settings (main amp or return).
- Some DSPs offer automatic delay adjustment and network control functions.

Disadvantages of Active PA Speakers
- Built-in amplifiers can add weight to a single speaker.
- Total power consumption can be much higher than traditional systems.
- Improper operation of independent voice control or electronic devices can cause discrepancies and increased noise.
- Active power is generally more expensive than passive power.
- Each horn speaker in a PA system should have its own power cord, sometimes connected by a chrysanthemum chain.

DIGITAL AUDIO
Digital audio recordings are media in CD format to improve students' listening skills. Digital Audio Recording was created with the understanding that many students have been studying English for several years and are still hesitant to speak. The process of using the digital voice recordings began with a listening session that provided contextual examples of dialogue and expressions that could be used. Expressions were everyday situations students encountered when speaking English on a daily basis.
- The next step was to create her own language, which is also included in the listening material, and record her voice in digital form by recording it on a computer.
- Digital audio recordings were used to create an atmosphere in which students could begin speaking in English after becoming familiar with the audio material.
- Students can use their own recordings to hear what was said again.
- Digital voice recording is the electrical or mechanical recording and duplication of sound waves, such as spoken words.
- In this study, digital audio recordings were used as listening materials and student projects.
- Digital audio recordings can be stored for ever unless they are corrupted by viruses. Another advantage of digital audio recording is the ability to track exactly all the parts the listener needs. This made it easy for teachers to see which parts needed to be repeated many times.

- Listening activities are easier than analog, and the sound quality is clear.

Advantages of Audio Technology

- **Inexpensive:** All voice/speech technologies are relatively cheap.
- **Easy access:** Almost every household in the United States has a telephone. Additionally, most students have access to a tape recorder at home or in their car.
- **Easy to use:** Most people are familiar with telephones and audio cassettes. With voice technology, there is no software to install and no hardware to configure.

Audio Technology Disadvantages

- Planning may be required. Some language technologies (such as audio conferencing) are synchronous. In other words, it should be scheduled at a time that is convenient for students and teachers.
- Do not encourage visual information. Many students find it difficult to concentrate and learn using only voice input. Additionally, audio-only formats limit the content that can be conveyed (abstract concepts are very difficult to convey audibly).
- Can be inhuman. Voice only interaction has no eye contact or body language. Students can be 'turned off' by the talking box.

Audio Technology Integration Guidelines

- Predistribute visuals. If an audio conference is planned, handouts or other visual materials that may be of value during the presentation should be distributed well in advance.
- Specifies the communication protocol. Because participants cannot see each other, it is important to agree on a protocol for identifying speakers in an audio conference. In most cases, it is a good idea to tell all speakers to name them before commenting. Example: This is Maria. I have something to say..."
- Encourage interaction. Audio conferencing requires dialogue to be built into the format. For example, teachers should encourage certain students, direct students to take turns asking questions, and ensure that no one student can dominate the conversation. Both conference calls and tapes require students to use email, fax, or voicemail to communicate with each other and with the instructor.
- Audio conference recording. Recording an audio conference is very easy. This allows you to distribute tapes to students who were unable to attend the meeting or who want to review the content.
- Get along with your students. If possible, look for ways to get to know students, such as visiting remote locations, gathering students in one place, and exchanging photos and videotapes.

CONCLUSION

From this chapter students would have gained knowledge about the moving visuals: Video learning resources—videotapes and DVD, USB, flash drive and motion pictures/films, realia and models, real objects and models, audio aids/audio media.

Such as audiotapes/compact disks, radio and tape recorder, public address system and digital audio, with this knowledge student can easily apply these aids to improve their communication skills in educational and clinical practice.

REVIEW QUESTIONS

Long Essays

1. Definition motion picture film, explain the educational value of movies.
2. Describe the benefits and disadvantages of educational films.
3. Define video-based learning, explain with examples of video-based learning.
4. Define video cassettes/videotapes, explain the types of tutorial videos.
5. Define blu-ray optical disc, explain the properties, advantages and disadvantages.
6. Define universal serial bus (USB), explain the properties, advantages and disadvantages.
7. Define puppets, explain the types and techniques to prepare puppet.

Short Essays
1. Motion picture film applications.
2. Educational role of the film.
3. Role teacher in educational films.
4. Benefits of video-based learning.
5. Ideas for using videos in the classroom.
6. Benefits of videos for students and teacher.
7. DVD advantages and disadvantages.
8. Realia and models/three-dimensional aids.
9. Puppet principles.
10. Mockup advantages, explain benefits of objects and samples.
11. Object and specimen.
12. Use of tape recorders for educational purposes.
13. Compact disc (CD): Uses and benefits.
14. Public address system: Components and functions of public address system.
15. Advantages and disadvantages of audio technology.

Short Answers
1. Uses of educational films.
2. Use of movie film.
3. Expert-led explainer videos.
4. Interactive video.
5. Animated explainers.
6. DVD (digital versatile disk).
7. Benefits of learning through educational DVDs.
8. Important for 3D tools.
9. Advantages of 3D tools.
10. Hand puppet benefits.
11. Features of the model.
12. Moulage.
13. Diorama type.
14. Audio aids/media.
15. Tape recorder functions.
16. Characteristics of the radio and record listening experience.
17. Advantages of active PA speakers.

Chapter 12

Electronic and Telecommunication

Learning Objectives
- Electronic Media
- Telecommunications
- Computer, Internet, Web-based Video Conferencing
- E-Learning
- Smart Classroom
- Cable TV
- Types of Educational Television Programs
- Satellite Transmission
- Video Conferencing
- Telehealth
- Telenursing
- Mobile Technologies

INTRODUCTION

Electronic media refers to materials, devices, and processes that use electronic technology to convey information, knowledge, and ideas to members of society. For example, radio, television, computers, e-mail, and projectors can be used by teachers to teach students effectively. Digital media in education refers to the use of interactive multimedia in the classroom. These media may include the integration of digital software across multiple devices and platforms as a learning tool. Today, the use of digital media in education is growing rapidly, competing with books as the primary form of communication. This form of education is slowly fighting against the traditional forms of education that have existed for a long time. The advent of virtual education has necessitated further integration of new digital platforms into the online classroom.

ELECTRONIC MEDIA

Media appeal to visual, auditory, and kinesthetic learners. Students can watch movies, listen to music, and interact with digital media using great teaching tools like custom touchscreen tablets and her SMART Board, which is essentially an interactive whiteboard. The most effective teachers use a variety of methods to reach as many students as possible rather than relying on a single teaching style. By providing a rich learning experience through classroom media, students stay focused and engaged in learning.

Using media in the classroom makes students aware of the everchanging world of electronic communication. Familiarize yourself with these resources now to prepare for future success. Students not only learn how to use the Internet to access instructional videos and search digital journals for information, but they also learn the value of respecting and protecting expensive media tools. Additionally, you will learn how to value media and get familiar with creating your own media.

TELECOMMUNICATIONS

Telecommunications is the transmission of signs, signals, letters, words, sounds, messages and images by radio, optical or other electromagnetic systems. Telecommunication occurs when information is exchanged between participants using technology. The role of telecommunications in education is already evident when students only attend school during normal school hours. However, with the development and introduction of communications, the situation has changed significantly.

The Internet, which is part of telecommunication services, allows students to do socalled e-learning or distance learning. This process allows students to pursue higher education in the course of their choice. Nearly all types of methods are available at these distance learning institutions, and there are faculty members who provide students with notes and lessons, just as they do in traditional schools.

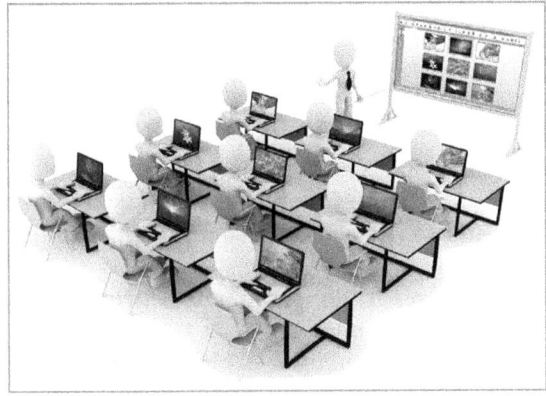

Fig. 12.1: Communication through electronic media.

Contains many services. As far as distance learning is concerned, critical steps are carried out more efficiently. The only communication product required is a computer connected to the Internet. Students can then begin coursework. Additionally, students have the option of not leaving home to attend courses and institutions. Instead, these institutions use telecommunications to offer multiple courses that students can take from home. This saves a lot of money that would otherwise have been spent on airfare and other hostel room charges.

COMPUTER

Computers are used as teaching materials in the classroom and are unique in that they personalize the lesson. Computer-assisted instruction (CAT) in the form of tutorial modes, drill modes, stimulation modes, and animation techniques offer great possibilities for teaching.
- Computers are used in classrooms as teaching tools and are unique in their individualization of instruction.
- Computer Aided Instruction (CAI) in the form of Tutorial Modes, Drill Modes, Stimulation Modes, and Animation Techniques provide numerous teaching opportunities.
- In this method lessons are mechanized and reused. A teacher is required only for the preparation of the software program.
- The computer can also be used for a large number of questions and objective test items on a hard disk/CD that acts as a question bank.

Purpose of Computers in Education

Computers are one of the most valuable resources in the classroom because they perform so many useful functions. Students today have a wealth of information at their fingertips thanks to computers and the Internet. This information will help her develop her research and communication skills while preparing her for future careers in an increasingly technology-dependent work environment.

Benefits of Computer Instruction

- Enables students to interact in learning situations.
- Computers can also greatly personalize learning.
- You can also increase your student's self-esteem in a number of ways.
- The computer can answer the student's answer with a statement.
- Computers' nonjudgmental nature and endless patience are also important advantages.
- A record of a student's performance in a simulation or practice test can be saved on the computer.
- Computers can also be used longer by students than by teachers.
- The computer can also be used for a large number of questions and objective test items on the hard disk/CD that act as a question bank.

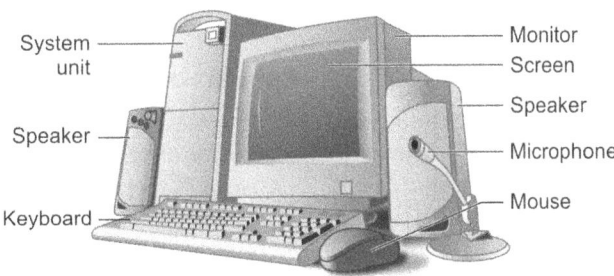

Fig. 12.2: Teaching with computer.

Role of Computers in Education

Computer education plays an important role in the modern educational system. Students find it easier to look up information on the Internet than to look for it in a thick book. The learning process goes beyond just learning from a prescribed textbook. The Internet is a much larger and more accessible repository of information. Computers are easier than handwritten notes when it comes to storing the information you retrieve.

- **Computers are ingenious helpers in the classroom:** Online education has revolutionized the education industry. Computer technology has made the dream of distance learning a reality. Education is no longer confined to the classroom. Thanks to computers, it became widespread. With the spread of the Internet, physically distant places have become closer. Students and teachers can communicate with each other very well even if they are not in the same facility.
- **Computers have boosted distance learning:** Computers make it easy to present information effectively. Presentation software such as PowerPoint and animation software such as Flash can be very helpful for teachers to give lectures. Computers facilitate the audiovisual presentation of information, making the learning process interactive and interesting. Computer-assisted instruction adds an element of fun to teaching. Chalk and blackboards are rarely used by teachers today.
- **Computer software helps us better present information:** The Internet can play an important role in education. Since it is a huge information base, it is possible to search for information on a wide range of themes. You can get information on various topics using the Internet. Both teachers and students benefit from the Internet. Teachers can find additional information and references on the topics they teach. Students can browse web sources for additional information on topics of interest. The Internet helps teachers create test papers, create homework questions, and define project topics. In addition to academics, teachers can also use her web sources to get ideas for sports competitions, afterschool activities, picnics, parties, and more.
- Computers provide access to the Internet, which holds literally all information. Computers save paper by allowing data to be stored in electronic form. The storage capacity of computer storage devices is measured in gigabytes. This allows you to store large amounts of data. Moreover, these devices are compact. They take up very little space and still store a lot of data. Both teachers and students benefit from the use of computer technology.
- Computer hard drives and storage devices are great ways to store data. This was about the role of computers in education. However, computers have not only impacted education. They are of great help in all areas. Life without a computer is unimaginable. This emphasizes the importance of computer education. Computer skills can steer your career in the right direction. Today computers are part of almost every industry. No longer confined to a particular field.

Applications of Computers in Education

Computers assist teachers in:

- **Classify students:** Computers help classify children according to their abilities and evaluate their performance.
- **Timetable preparation:** Computers can help you create timetables and so on.
- **Management of progress charts:** The computer maintains progress charts, keeping them efficient and confidential.
- **Tutorials and interactions:** Computers can act as tutors. This helps teachers engage students in their tutoring work. There are tutorial interactions and dialogues.
- **Instant feedback:** Computers help teachers provide instant feedback to students to improve interaction and motivation.
- **Problem solving and creativity:** Computers can be used to develop students' problem solving skills and creativity.
- **Laboratory and internship work:** Computers can complement laboratory and internship work, especially in scientific and technical subjects.
- **Training with stimulation techniques:** Computers can be used to train students through stimulation and game techniques.
- **Education for people with disabilities:** Computers can be used to provide education for people with disabilities, such as those who are deaf or mute.
- **Repetition:** Lessons that were once incomprehensible can be fully understood by the average student after a few repetitions. The computer can work at the pace of the student.
- **Guidance:** Computers assist teachers in providing guidance and reference information/data.

Benefits of Computer Education

- It increases the thinking ability.
- Provide an efficient and comfortable environment. Better use of IT technology.
- Proven to be favorable for career aspirations.
- Improve research work. Helps communicate with various educational providers.
- Provides instant information on any topic with one click much more.

Computers in Education

- **Organized information storage:** Vast memory is another important feature of computers. Students and teachers can download many educational materials, books, presentations, lectures and address notes, surveys, etc., and save them on their computers. Students can find different ways to solve a given problem. Through computers, you can interact with people who have the same problem.
- **Processing data:** Fast speed is a fundamental characteristic of computers. With one key press he can easily find the information.
- **Audiovisual guidance in educational processes for sustainable learning:** One of the main uses of computers in education is to "get on the internet" for information retrieval on any subject.
- Parents can track charging progress. Parents can browse the school's website and know that they are checking their children's progress every minute via computers and Internet. You can view various evaluation results, attendance reports, participation in subjects and extracurricular activities, etc.
- **High speed communication and response:** Another major advantage of using computers in teaching is to improve the quality of teaching and learning processes and communication between students and teacher. Prepare electronic presentations for lectures using Microsoft PowerPoint.

INTERNET

The Internet is a new computer-based communication system that opens up tremendous possibilities for knowledge transfer and enables direct and immediate communication worldwide via e-mail and online chat made it possible. It is a rapidly growing medium of communication and has great potential to become an important health education tool. There are already so many people using these media in India and the number is increasing day by day. Most of the health-related literature from WHO and other health authorities is available online. It is health information of health and welfare division of India is also available on another of his websites.

Internet Usage

Below is a list of common internet usages. Number two.

- Today, we can use e-mail functionality for better communication. Chat with your loved ones for hours. There are many messenger and e-mail services that offer this service for free. With the help of services like this, it has become very easy to build a kind of global friendship where we can share ideas and explore other cultures of different ethnicities.
- **Information:** The greatest advantage of the Internet offering is information. The Internet and the world-wide web have made information easily accessible to everyone.
- **Economy:** Global trade has experienced a huge boom with the help of the Internet as it has become easier for buyers and sellers to communicate with each other and promote their sites. Today, most people use online advertising sites to buy, sell, or promote products and services.
- **Social networking:** Today, social networking sites are an important part of online communities. Almost all users are members and use it for personal and business purposes. A great place to network with the many entrepreneurs who come here to start building their own personal and business brands.

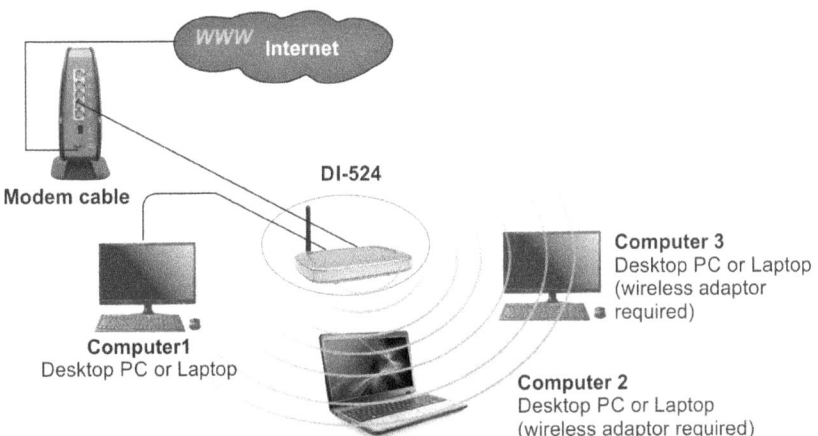

Fig. 12.3: Internet based learning.

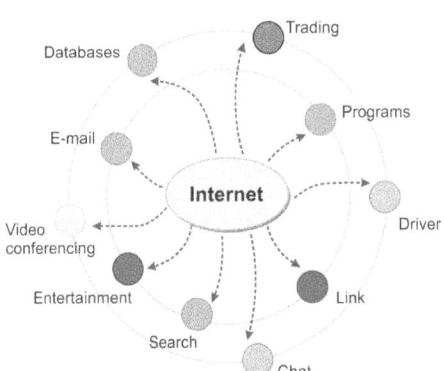

Fig. 12.4: Applications of internet in communication.

- **Shopping:** In today's busy life, most of us are interested in online shopping. These days, you can buy almost anything online. In countries like the United States, most consumers prefer to shop at home. There are many online shopping sites such as amazon.com, Dealsglobe.com. You can also use the Internet to auction items. There are many online auction sites where you can sell just about anything.
- **Entertainment:** You can find all forms of entertainment on the Internet, from watching movies to playing online games. Most people can find entertainment that works for them. When people surf the Internet, they find out many things. You can find news about your music tastes and more and share it on the Internet. There are many games that can be downloaded for free from the Internet.
- **E-commerce:** E-commerce is the term used for any type of commercial or commercial transaction in which information is transmitted worldwide via the Internet. It has become a phenomenon associated with nearly every kind of shopping. From home essentials to entertainment, we have a truly amazing range of products.
- **Services:** Many services are now offered over the Internet. Online banking, job search, buying tickets to your favorite movie, consulting services on various issues in all fields, hotel bookings, paying bills. Often these services are not available offline and can cost more. Job Search: The Internet makes life easier for both employers and job seekers as there are many job boards that connect employers and job seekers.
- **Dating/personal advertising:** People use the Internet to connect with others and find life partners. The internet not only helps you find the right person, but it also helps you keep the relationship going.

The Importance of the Internet in Education

The importance of the Internet in Education is illustrated by the following points:
- Media apps and online learning platforms that provide realtime support, allowing teachers and students to engage in dynamic interactions whenever they need them.

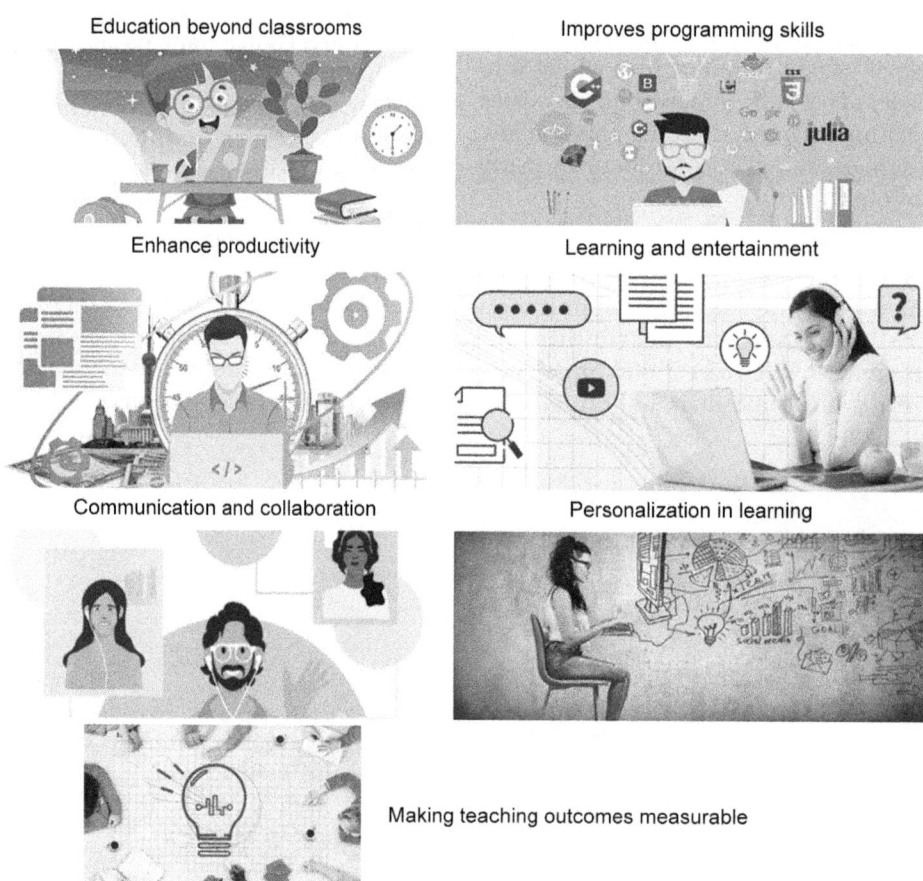

Fig. 12.5: Importance of the internet in education.

- **Learning flexibility:** The resource and location limitations of traditional forms of education do not apply to online learning and its platforms. With access to the Internet, you can study your own study materials online, remotely and at your own pace. It also serves as a 24/7 support system for student-teacher interactions. Adults can also enroll in classes that fit their schedule.
- **Economics:** Purchasing books and study materials is usually expensive. However, online courses and other sources of information have made accessing learning materials online more cost-effective.
- **Dynamically and proactively updated:** Numerous online websites and data archives can receive realtime updates. This allows users to download information that is up-to-date and ready for distribution.
- **Multimedia integration:** Research shows that we tend to consume data faster and more efficiently through audiovisual formats. These formats include multimedia infographics, slide shows, and more. These multimedia formats can be actively used in courses and classes due to the use of the Internet.

The Role of the Internet in Education

The Internet plays an important role in the educational process by providing excellent development opportunities.
- **Distance learning:** A major advantage of the Internet in education is the development of online distance learning. When available, you can enroll in short courses that include lectures, face-to-face classes, exams, and receive university support. One of the main advantages of distance learning is the accessibility to people from any part of the world who wants to get knowledge on various subjects full courses and so on.
- **Use of helpful resources:** The Internet provides a great opportunity to use various resources such as essay helper that offer high quality online essay writing services. This will help you save time and get everything done before a certain deadline.
- **Student interaction with classmates and teachers:** The pandemic has significantly impacted education systems around the world. Distance education has become a lifeline for students and teachers. Parents can also check their child's progress at any time.
- **Effective tools for teaching and learning:** The Internet has become an important tool for effective teaching and learning. A teacher can use it as a teaching tool by posting educational materials (notes and videos) on her website or forums at the institution.
- **Mobility:** Convenient online learning: at your convenience, from anywhere. Video is now 100% mobile platform adapted so you do not need a computer to do this.

Anyone can organize their education space and create a convenient schedule. It would not be a bad thing if he had to leave in a hurry half an hour after the lecture started. Just pause the video.

Benefits of Online Learning

- **Efficiency:** Online learning provides an efficient way for teachers to deliver lessons to students. Online learning has a variety of tools such as videos, PDFs, and podcasts that teachers can use as part of their lesson plans. By extending lesson plans from traditional textbooks to online resources, teachers can become more effective educators.
- **Easy to access time and place:** Another advantage of online education is that students can attend classes from anywhere they want. It also allows schools to access a wider student network without being constrained by geographic boundaries.
- **Affordability:** Another advantage of online learning is the low financial cost. Online education is much cheaper than physical learning. This is because online learning eliminates student transportation costs, student meals, and most importantly real estate expense items.
- **Increased student participation:** Students are less likely to miss classes because online classes can be taken from home or from any location.
- **Accommodating different learning styles:** Every student has a different learning process and learning style. Some students learn visually, while others prefer to learn by audio.

Drawbacks of Online Learning

- **Inability to concentrate on the screen:** For many students, one of the biggest challenges of online learning is the difficulty of concentrating on the screen for long periods of time. With online learning there is also a greater chance for students to be easily distracted by social media or other sites. Therefore, it is imperative for the teachers to keep their online classes crisp engaging and interactive to help students stay focused on the lesson.
- **Technology issues:** Another key challenge of online classes is Internet connectivity. While internet penetration has grown in leaps and bounds over the past few years in smaller cities and towns a consistent connection with decent speed is a problem. If students and teachers are not consistently connected to the Internet, children may lack continuity in their learning. This harms the educational process.

- **Isolation:** Students can learn a lot from their peers. However, online classes have minimal physical interaction between students and teachers. This often leads to students feeling isolated. In situations like these, it is imperative that schools allow other forms of communication between students and teachers.
- **Teacher training:** Online learning requires teachers to have a basic understanding of how to deal with digital forms of learning. However, this is not always the case. Teachers often have a very basic knowledge of technology. In some cases, they may not even have the resources and tools necessary to run an online course.
- **Manage screen time:** Many parents are concerned about the health risks of their children staring at screens for hours on end. This increased screen time is one of the biggest concerns and drawbacks of online learning. Students may also develop poor posture and other physical problems from slouching in front of the screen.

WEB-BASED VIDEO CONFERENCING

Web-based conferencing (or web conferencing) is an online service that allows businesses and individuals to hold remote meetings. Web conferencing software can provide an online environment for holding virtual meetings. You can usually join a web conference from your desktop or mobile app.
- Video conferencing software enables online communication of audio conferences, video conferences, and seminars with built-in features such as chat screen sharing and recording.
- These applications are implemented to enable long distance or international communication, improve collaboration, and reduce travel costs.
- Employees at all levels within an organization can use video conferencing tools to host or join virtual meetings with colleagues, corporate partners or customers, regardless of where the participants are physically located.
- Web conferencing solutions can be used for audio conferencing, video chat, or both. Web conferencing software offers an alternative to face-to-face meetings or dialing in to a conference call from a landline or mobile device.
- This means you no longer have to attend every physical meeting. One of the benefits of using online meeting software to attend meetings is that you can join from anywhere with Internet access.
- This means meeting attendees no longer need mobile or landline phones to participate in these meetings and important decisions.

Web Conferencing Need

Web-based video conferencing is the use of video conferencing discussions through an online platform to perform many common tasks such as:
- Live meetings
- Conferences
- Presentations
- Trainings

Video Conferencing Platforms
- Zoom
- Google hangouts
- Dialpad meetings
- TrueConf online
- Skype
- Free meeting
- Go life size
- Slack video call
- Facebook live
- YouTube live

Zoom

Zoom is great for people who work remotely or have team members far away. Zoom is also popular among virtual teachers. Zoom makes it easy to set up meetings and recurring meetings in your personal conference room. Quickly create and share private meeting links with individuals or teams to connect remote team members with video.

Top free features

- Host up to 100 participants
- One-on-one group meetings
- Unlimited meetings
- HD video and audio
- Screen sharing
- Scheduled meetings
- Private and group chats
- Host controls

Google Hangouts

Easily connect with your Google contacts (or people outside your network) Google Hangouts make it private. You can also use it for business reasons. This tool can be used for one-on-one conversations, team meetings, recorded demos, and more.

Top free features

- Up to 25 video participants
- Messenger discussions

- Record video meeting
- Join calls with Google calendar
- Screen sharing

Dialpad Meetings

The free version of dialpad meetings is perfect for teams of 10 or less. The free version limits video calls to 45 minutes, making it ideal for short meetings. With unlimited video conferencing, you can use this video conferencing tool for regular meetings such as one-to-one meetings or monthly team briefings.

Free top features

- Up to 10 participants
- Unlimited meetings
- Call recording
- HD audio
- Screen and document sharing
- Mobile app.

TrueConf Online

TrueConf offers a free plan that allows up to 3 people to join a video call. This solution is perfect for small teams and individuals who want a simple tool for hosting video calls and collaborating with small groups. Collaboration features such as remote desktop control are useful for support staff who need to help resolve customer issues.

Free top features

- Up to 3 participants in a team call
- HD video
- Collaboration tools (screen sharing, remote desktop control, call recording, file transfer, shared virtual whiteboard).

Skype

Skype free The edition is excellent for small teams with less than 10 total members. It's a good tool if you want an easy way to video chat from your computer phone or tablet and tend to have small group meetings or his one-on-one conversations. Skype also offers a tool called Skype in the Classroom specifically designed for online education.

Top free features

- Up to 10 people on video calls
- HD video calling
- Screen sharing
- Video call recording
- Interactive video chat
- Location sharing

Free Meetings

Free meetings, ideal for small teams or meetings with 5 or fewer participants. The main advantage of this video conferencing tool is its ease of use. No download required to use. In addition, moderator controls help video conference organizers keep the meeting on track.

Key free features

- Up to 5 online meeting participants
- Screen sharing
- Document sharing
- Moderator control
- Text chat.

LifeSize Go

LifeSize Go can be used by remote workers, remote freelancers, or clients who rarely host large group meetings. They have plans to include solutions for large teams, but the free version offers features suitable for individual and small group conversations. Up to 8 participants, Unlimited meeting length has Screen sharing.

Slack Video Calls

Slack users can use the command or click the phone icon at the top You can use the call function only. This of a conversation with another of her Slack users is an easy way to call a teammate directly from Slack when you need to ask a quick question. When you start a call from a channel, you can also use Slack with up to 15 people and allow the rest of the channel members to join. This tool is suitable for teams looking for a complementary video calling solution for smaller teams.

Facebook Live

Facebook Live is perfect for business or individual influencers who want to broadcast demo videos or showcase their company culture while live streaming. Facebook followers can comment and chat live. You can select a custom audience for your video. You can also schedule videos in advance to increase excitement.

Top free features

- Transfer up to 4 hours
- Advanced scheduling
- Custom audience

YouTube Live

Like facebook live, youtube live is a platform for product demonstrations with live Q & A that hosts training sessions and screen sharing to engage viewers. or use a whiteboard or host to explain. Live conversations with team members.

Top free features

- 3D stream quality options (normal latency, low latency, ultra low latency)
- Delay added
- Raw questions from viewers
- Private live stream (only accessible via link)
- Advanced scheduling
- Automatic live captions
- Location tags

Effective Video Conferencing Tips

This is a list of tips to help staff think about how web and video conferencing can be used for teaching and learning.

- Web and video conference lessons are different than face-to-face lessons. Teachers may need to change their teaching methods.
- Careful planning is essential for effective teaching and learning using web and video conferencing.
- Prepare and upload materials before the web conference begins.
- Gain confidence in technology by learning how the technology works before the session begins with guidance and advice from experienced users.
- Provide students with a practice run as a guide to demonstrate how to use the technology.
- Provide resources, guides and instructions for students to refer to before and during the session.
- Create engaging activities that encourage discussion and interaction among students and with teachers.
- When using presentations such as PowerPoint slides, allow at least every 5-8 minutes for student interaction and discussion.
- During the Q & A session, ask individual students a few questions to emphasize that all students are expected to participate.
- Provide students with a session agenda listing the items or topics for the session. Include factors such as session objectives and student expectations for learning activities.
- Stay close to the microphone so the sound is clear. Test your microphone and sound before starting your session.
- Review student questions before answering to make sure all students understand the context of your answer.
- Keep students engaged by direct contact with all locations connected for video conferencing.
- Hire volunteer meeting organizers at each location to facilitate discussions from that location.
- Contrasting clothing and colors may be applied during video conferencing
- Use the meeting tool to facilitate meetings with subject teachers in other locations.

Overcoming Barriers with Video Conferencing for Education

Teachers and students alike can benefit from using online conferencing software as part of their daily classroom activities. Educators can broaden their horizons by making it available to more students, and students can meet guest her speakers and experts even on the other side of the globe. However, this is just the tip of the iceberg. There really are no limits when it comes to video conferencing for distance learning.

- Students participate in excursions to the other side of the world without actually stepping out of a classroom or auditorium.
- A modern, virtual twist on the idea of the oldfashioned handwritten pen-pal helps students connect with other like minded students living thousands of miles away.
- Teachers can contact and give individualized attention to students who are struggling in a particular course or subject.
- Students now benefit from endless sources of knowledge as schools can combine educational resources.
- Teachers can use her webbased video conferencing software to connect with students when students are isolated by weather or location.
- You do not have to leave your home to attend music classes or other courses.
- Teachers and staff can further develop their skills by participating in online webinar workshops, seminars, and other professional development events.
- Increasingly, professionals and professionals are being able to participate in classroom presentations and discussions. Because such presentations don't require you to travel, you just need to be "virtually" in the classroom with your students using online meeting software.
- Students can ask questions of experts remotely, regardless of location, creating the basis for more in-depth research.
- Distance learning video conferencing allows interpreters to be present in the classroom and language is no longer the daunting barrier.

E-LEARNING

E-learning has proven to be the best tool in the corporate sector. In particular, multinational companies run training programs for professionals around the world, enabling employees to learn key skills while sitting in or holding a conference room. A seminar that brings together employees of the same or different organizations. Schools using e-learning technology are a step ahead of those using traditional learning approaches.

E-Learning Meaning

E-learning is a formalized, instruction-based learning system but aided by electronic resources. Teaching can take place inside or outside the classroom, but the use of computers and the Internet form the main components of e-learning. E-learning can also be described as network-based transfer of skills and knowledge. Educational deliveries are made to multiple recipients at the same time or at different times. Previously, the system was not fully accepted as it was thought to lack the human element necessary for learning.

Definition

- E-learning is a learning method that uses electronic technology to access the curriculum outside the traditional classroom.
- E-learning, also known as online learning or e-learning, is the acquisition of knowledge through electronic technology and media.
- Simply put, e-learning is defined as "electronically enabled learning".
- E-learning is the use of technology to enable people to learn anytime, anywhere.
- E-learning includes training on just intime information delivery and export methods.
- E-learning includes different types of media that provide text, audio, images, animations and streaming video, audio or video, tap satellite TV, CDROM and computer-based learning, local Intranet/extranet. It includes technology applications and practices such as and web-based learning.
- E-learning uses technology to enhance the learning experience. These technologies are used to create and deliver personalized, immersive and dynamic learning content that facilitates learning anytime, anywhere.

E-learning Function

- All e-learning courses are created because you need to learn.
- E-learning courses focus on one or more learning objectives.
- E-learning courses are created with specific students and their needs in mind.
- The e-learning is produced with the help of subject matter experts.
- E-learning is self-paced and reaches a wider audience.
- E-learning is linked with electronic media.
- Every e-learning course has an exam.
- E-learning development follows streamlined process.

E-Learning Strategies

There are millions of e-learning worldwide. Today's e-learners come from many different backgrounds and ages. Most professionals are trying to educate themselves and improve their chances.

- E-learning requires motivation and self-discipline.
- Define goals and plans for success.
- Integrate work life and other educational experiences into the learning process.
- Willingness and ability to devote sufficient time to the e-learning process.
- Access the devices you need and create your personal space.

The Importance of E-Learning

- E-learning was introduced to help learners get basic education and improve their skills. You can even earn a diploma without actually attending a school, university, or other institution.
- Great source of income for tutors as they can teach at any time and from anywhere.
- The use of e-learning at all school levels helped students to understand the lessons properly and quickly.
- According to psychology, audiovisual teaching methods lead to a disciplined learning environment. There is effective tutoring and student engagement.
- One of the implications of e-learning in education is that both teachers and participants can develop advanced learning skills. For example, the creation and sale of e-books is one such advancement.
- E-learning has worked to bring learners, tutors, professionals, practitioners and other stakeholders together in one place. Therefore, there are knowledge-sharing best practices to follow on various online platforms. This is important in this age of increased competition and a growing world. Therefore, quick information helps individuals grow better.

Types of E-Learning or E-Education

Digital and self-initiated learning can be taken wherever you want. E-learning education is versatile and well-resourced for all learning styles, so you do not have to walk around looking for learning completed online - no need to meet in person.

Communication—Different Formats

- **Synchronization:** Communication between provider and recipient is direct, like a chat room or video audio conference.
- **Asynchronous:** Information is shared through forums, email, wikis, etc.
- Self-study is also encouraging.
- Web-based learning is another great option
- CD-ROMs provide in-depth study relevant to the subject.

Benefits of E-Learning in Education

An analysis of the benefits of online learning prompts us to think about how teachers, students and institutions today want to receive relevant and easily accessible content. This is achieved with online learning methods as students can study at their own convenience and need.

Benefits of E-learning for Students Unlike traditional blackboard and chalk teaching methods, e-learning is enriched with online learning modes that allow students to learn ondemand. Let's take a look at the benefits of e-learning for students.

- Unlimited access to study materials.
- Study the course anytime, anywhere.
- Students have access to updated content at any time.
- Unlike traditional teaching methods, e-learning has a rapid implementation method. This indicates that the learning time is shortened.
- E-Learning provides scalability to help deliver training.
- All students receive the same type of curriculum learning materials and can be trained through e-learning
- E-learning saves time and money and reduces travel costs. Therefore, e-learning is cheaper than traditional learning.
- Because e-learning is delivered online, it does not require the paperwork of traditional learning. This helps protect the environment.

You can link different resources in several different formats.

- Web-based learning promotes active and independent learning.
- College students, housewives YouTubers and coaching agencies can use e-learning education.
- One of the greatest advantages of the Internet or e-learning is that you can study and graduate from the comfort of your own home.

These are some impossible things that are only possible through technology.

- Another advantage is that e-learning is based on convenience and flexibility. All your student and teacher resources are available in one place.
- Everyone can continue their education every day. This can be on weekends or when you have free time.
- E-learning also benefits companies. Because employees also need to be informed about the new skills. It helps them improve their efficiency and is fruitful for the future direction of education in the times.
- There is an easy way to clear your doubts through discussion forums and chat boxes. Tutors can easily answer students' questions. So it leads to better interactions.
- Global level education: Tutors can offer online classes in multiple languages to people in different time zones.

E-Learning Benefits

Below are some e-Learning benefits you should not miss.

- Online learning for all needs
- Lessons can be taken from anywhere and at the time of the student's or teacher's choice.
- Provides access to exclusive, productive and updated content, accessibility is open, secure and uninterrupted.
- E-Learning allows you to keep up with the latest learners and stay abreast of current trends.
- We guarantee prompt delivery of orders. Traditional classrooms come with some kind of delay. E-learning provides fast and unique instruction. There is no procrastination in e-learning. It is a fast way to learn.
- The scalability and duration of consumption of learning content is reasonably measurable. Beneficial for those who feel nervous in groups and isolated. It helps you learn without sacrificing the comfort of your environment. We are pleased with the consistency of the input results and the alignment of the e-learning. This allows teachers a higher level of coverage to deliver content on a regular basis. This ensures consistency in learning.
- This method becomes available at a significantly reduced cost. The importance of e-learning education is that it is quick and inexpensive. Long training periods, infrastructure, stationery and transportation costs are reduced.
- The effectiveness of transferred or transmitted knowledge and learning is high and powerful. Information gathering and assimilation becomes easier. Audiovisuals help you retain knowledge longer. The courses prepared by the tutors are also well planned.
- Mobility assured is a very convenient and affordable option. It's not so easy to iterate and practice different courses in a traditional class. In contrast, missed lessons can always be made up online. This makes it easier for tutors to convey the right information.
- It facilitates a self-directed learning process.

E-Learning Restrictions
- **Computer skills and access to devices:** Learners must have basic equipment and minimal computer skills to be able to perform the services required by the system.
- **Some subjects are not suitable for e-learning:** Certain subjects that require exercise or practice, such as sports and public speaking, are not suitable for e-learning.
- Students themselves may be restricted to e-learning:
  - A high degree of personal responsibility was required of students.
  - Successful e-learning students must be well organized, self-motivated and have good time management.

SMART CLASSROOM
Smart classroom allows teachers to tailor their teaching style to the needs of their students. Using a variety of technologies and intelligent classroom management, teachers can support the educational and supplementary needs of students and tailor learning and teaching to each child's individual learning plan.

Based on the equipment available, smart classrooms can be categorized as:
- **Basic smart classes:** The classrooms with basic smart technology include gadgets like laptops or computers, projector, DVD or VCD player and a viewing screen etc.
- **Intermediate smart classroom:** The intermediate smart classrooms are one step ahead of the basic technology smart classrooms. They include gadgets like a smart podium with the control panel in addition to a laptop, projector, screen and DVD or VCD player etc.
- Advanced smart classroom goes a step beyond the basic technology smart classroom. This includes devices such as laptop projector screens and DVD or VCD players, as well as smart podiums with control panels,die features are very advanced and use the latest.

Equipment Installed in Smart Classrooms
- **Computer or laptop:** A computer or laptop is a basic and necessary requirement for a smart classroom. Instead of writing on a board with chalk or markers, the educational process takes place through presentations, photos, or multimedia in smart classrooms.
- **Projector:** Optical equipment. Project stationery or moving objects onto the screen. They create images by shining light through clear lenses or lasers.
- **Screen:** The surface used to display the image projected by the projector. Screens can be either rigid wall-mounted screens, pulldown screens, fixed frame screens, motorized screens, switchable projection screens or mobile screens.
- **Microphone:** Commonly called microphone. A device that converts audio signals into electrical signals. These signals are amplified and transmitted or recorded.
- **Amplifiers and Speakers:** These are electronic devices used to increase the volume of sounds.
- **Pedestal:** A pedestal, usually wooden, that lifts a standing person into view from the entire audience.
- **Document camera:** Also known as Visual Presenter Visualisers Digital Overheads. They are used to show objects to a large audience. The document camera magnifies and projects an image of his 3D object as well as a 2D object. Simply place the object under the document camera. The camera records that image and produces a live image through a projector.
- **Smart podiums:** Also known as Smart Boards or Smart LCDs. An interactive pen display that can be externally connected to a computer or laptop via USB or RGB port. It can be said that it is an external monitor that has the potential of digital coloring. Smart podium allows you to open documents, presentations and multimedia files and write on them with your digital pen. You can also save your work.
- **DVD or VCD player:** Although there are many videos on the Internet, some videos are copyrighted and must be purchased, so a VCD or DVD player is still required. These are often in the form of DVDs or CDs.
- **Overhead projector:** A device that projects an enlarged image on a screen with a transparent acetate sheet spread on a pedestal. This device was very popular a few years ago, but has now been superseded by computer-based projectors.

Smart Classroom Targets
Here are some of the targets for the smart classroom application.
- Help teachers take on new challenges and develop student skills and achievements.
- Enable teachers to access multimedia content and information to teach students more effectively. Educationally sound and visually engaging curriculum resources.
- This allows teachers to voice their opinions and ensures that each child understands the concepts being implemented, ultimately impacting grades.
- Provide a clear understanding of concepts. Making abstract concepts real.
- To have interactive and live teaching to elaborate and compare different objects and perceptions towards the particular concepts
- Design smart class modules that allow students to visualize concepts far better than static images. Graphics and animations that students will never forget.

- Take steps toward student achievement-focused growth.
- Make learning an enjoyable experience for students. Activities and games to facilitate the learning process.
- To effectively connect technology to the classroom and notify teachers of classroom events
- Teach remote and local students at the same time.
- Enhance creative thinking in the learning process to visualize concepts and practices using models and demonstrations.
- Optimize the use of electronic resources through e-books, e-journals, minutes, lecture notes, documents, etc.
- Provides the ability to customize and update content according to school work plans.

Smart Classroom Features

- **Adaptive learning:** Every class will always have students with different learning abilities. Our modern approach to adaptive learning gives students the freedom to learn at their own pace and in the way they are most comfortable.
- **Collaborative learning:** Collaborative learning is one of the most effective forms of learning. Teaching and learning in isolation is highly restrictive and impedes progress. Studying in groups expands learning and develops critical thinking. Colearning activities include joint writing group projects, joint problemsolving discussions, and more. Collaborative learning is redefining the traditional student-teacher relationship in the classroom.
- **Computing devices:** Computers are readily available in modern classrooms as they are essential tools for 21st century students, replacing pen and paper. They give teachers the opportunity to improve their teaching and help them.
- **Mutual respect:** Teachers and students should always respect each other. The role of the teacher is no longer that of a sage, and students must always remember the value of receiving guidance from them. Teachers should also encourage students to speak confidently and respect their opinions.
- **Performance related assessments:** Regular performance related assessments are conducted by teachers through a variety of methods, not limited to tests. This can be done by conducting quizzes and surveys.
- **Student centered:** In intelligent classrooms, teachers play the role of facilitators. They help students think critically. Students discover and master new concepts. Our student-centered classroom environment puts student interests first and focuses on each student's needs, abilities and learning style.
- **Students take responsibility for their own learning:** Students take responsibility for their own learning when they are encouraged to actively participate in their learning.
- **Students understand and follow rules and procedures:** The learning environment is carefully planned and well organized.

Suggested Features for Smart Classroom

Smart classroom must have some of the following features:
- Redecorated interiors
- Enhanced lighting controls
- A gyro wireless mouse to control the computer and projector from anywhere in the classroom.
- Toggle control to easily switch projector output between PC laptop document camera and DVD/VCR.
- New projector.
- Laptop plug that allows you to bring your own computer and instantly connect.
- Document camera that allows you to project transparencies and small objects and even take snapshots of them.
- A smart Sympodium. You can view electronic memos and images.
- The classroom performance system (CPS) uses wireless multiple-choice response devices to get real-time responses from students in the classroom.

Smart Classroom Components

- Smart Board (6 × 4)
- Smart LED TV high (Panasonic 42 Inch 2 USB Viera connect)
- Short throw projector (panasonic PT-VX400)
- Video 4: Video conferencing equipment
- Laptop with Internet connection (using public IP)
- Document camera/visualization (12 × optical zoom and 8 × digital zoom)
- Podium (with ITC 6236B 60W amplifier)
- Life-size express 220) and Screens
- Library intelligent classroom architecture

Intelligent Classroom Principles

Below are intelligent classroom principles for placement and educational organization. It is generalizable and should be considered transforming formal learning spaces into smart classrooms.

- **Principle of adaptability:** Based on the idea that every teacher and class is different and spaces can be adjusted to suit their needs, the intelligent classroom concept includes the principle of adaptability to the type and needs of the teacher and each student.

- **Connectivity principle:** The concept of connectivity has two characteristics. On the one hand, to be able to optimally exploit the potential of mobile devices, the study room should have good network connectivity, both locally and globally. Connectivity should be wireless. This is fundamental to maximizing comfort in physical mobility and technology use in space.
- **The comfort principle:** According to this principle, this well-being enabler should be integrated into the study room for different learning tasks. Sofas, cushions, carpets, and comfortable chairs. A smart classroom is a place where you can conveniently carry out various activities such as reading, watching videos, playing games, listening to music and audio, writing, talking, discussing, and experimenting.
- **The principle of physical placement flexibility:** The placement of intelligent classrooms and their elements allows for flexible and easy variation of activities allowing student groupings to change the types of resources used. It's like doing. Use different kinds of resources at the same time. Non-ICT for different students to perform different tasks. Looking for information. Talking while watching her video, etc.
- **Diversity principle:** This principle refers to intelligent classrooms with features that enable the use of different types of resources and stimuli. Between teaching and learning, this arrangement allows opportunities for creativity, reasoning, reasoning, etc., and can be as close as possible to the different needs and learning styles of learners.
- **Order/organization principle:** This is an important principle, but it is not easy to design and implement sustainable layout, storage arrangement and usage rules of available space and resources. For this reason, the teacher carefully considers the order and placement of rooms and resources to best suit the learning activities that take place in her smart classroom.
- **The openness principle:** This principle refers to the erroneous and deeply rooted belief that learning occurs only in the formal space of the traditional classroom, where teachers present information and teach lessons in a figurative way. Since learning takes place outside the classroom, both physically and virtually, the activities proposed for the smart classroom are these extended learning places and hours for learning beyond the classroom, and traditional should take into account.
- **Principles of personalization:** Intelligent classrooms allow students and teachers to personalize the environment according to their preferences and needs.
- **Security principles:** Intelligent classrooms are arranged to prevent physical accidents for users, and access to information and communications on the Internet from the classroom is also safe. Therefore, security systems are considered in the conception and design of smart classrooms.

Usage

- Using the e-class is as easy as controlling your TV with a remote control. Just like the E-Class, you get an E-Box that needs to be connected to your TV, and you can use the E-Box remote control to navigate the learning materials loaded into the E-Class.
- Students have access to learning materials so they can plan their studies the way they want. Reviewing has never been more fun by switching to an e-class and just sitting down and learning with audio-video learning.
- E-classes let you learn at your own pace and focus on your weaknesses.

Benefits of Smart Classes

- Improved interaction and communication between students and teachers
- Blending teaching and learning in real-time
- Helping students understand concepts better
- Introducing teaching technology to students and teachers
- Enhancing visualization and creativity
- Provide students with a better educational experience
- Encourage e-learning and virtual classrooms
- Improve students' academic performance and thereby enhance their mental and physical development
- Web-based online learning
- Students learn in their own phase tendency to learn
- Ease of learning use and accessibility.

Disadvantages of Smart Class

- Difficult to create presentation videos and programs
- Expensive and complex to implement
- High maintenance costs
- Computers, digital boards, and other equipment are fragile and difficult to use
- Depends heavily on current
- Requires proper network connection such as LAN WAN Internet.

CABLE TV

Cable TV in the classroom is a form of distance learning. Many local school administrators have become converts because of the benefits of distance learning. Through communications satellites, local schools can access cuttingedge courses for students and teachers while maintaining a local character and personal touch. Regarding urban and sub-urban schools, Schlosser (1991) suggests that satellite television globalizes the classroom by exposing students to world events and cultures other than their own.

- A system for distributing TV programs on a reservation basis.
- A TV system that uses cables to transmit signals instead of radio waves.
- A system for broadcasting television programs over cable.
- Transmission of television programs in the home or office over coaxial cable.
- Broadcasting of television programs over coaxial cable to paying subscribers.

According to Wayne Coy, described television as an "electronic bulletin board"

- ETV combines both sensory and auditory experiences. This is an extension of the broadcast.
- Provide consistency in communication.
- A versatile teaching tool.
- Stimulate and reinforce ideas.
- Provides live coverage of 'onsite' events. Provides a powerful visual medium.
- It is a means of recreation.

TYPES OF EDUCATIONAL TELEVISION PROGRAMS

Educational television (ETV) programs are offered to students in different modes. Some of his ETV programs of the main types are listed below:

- **Monologue:** A narrator tells a side story and interweaves it with images and illustrations.
- **Dialogue:** A conversation between people.
- Interview
- Panel discussion
- Telephone program
- Quiz
- Drama
- Simulated classroom
- Virtual classroom

Benefits

- Cable TV services are often very stable and don't shut down during storms or thunderstorms.
- Users can easily select packages and bundles, resulting in a lot of savings. For example, you can choose cable TV and phone or Internet service.
- Cable TV service prices are much more affordable than competitors.
- Users can choose the services of local companies that can provide as many channels as they want.
- Service is fast and local technicians will solve your problem.
- Most people prefer cable TV because of its ease of use. You don't have to learn new tricks to do the same thing.
- Cable TV is still the preferred option for many families facing problems due to mountain ranges.
- A great option for those looking for a very simple and straightforward entertainment solution.
- Unlike Internet streaming services, cable TV does not require data streaming, making it easy to reduce the additional cost of Internet streaming.
- Many cable operators also offer free channels
- Do not worry about the signal being blocked.
- Perfect for the technically minded.
- No additional equipment required.
- A great option for sports enthusiasts.

Disadvantages

- Cable TV is stable, but it takes a long time to start working if the cable breaks.
- May be very expensive in some countries.
- I can only watch the program at the reserved time.
- New age Internet services are much cheaper and offer more features.
- Lack of flexibility.
- Most cable companies have blackout periods.
- No custom display options.
- Sudden price increase.
- Most programs on cable television contain commercials.
- Past episodes and seasons cannot be viewed.
- Some programs are not available in HD.
- Pricing packages are often confusing.

SATELLITE TRANSMISSION

Satellite communication is an effective teaching tool, helping language teachers to successfully communicate in the target language with their students. In addition to audiovisual components, it provides authentic, contextualized input to realworld situations. These features of teaching materials are essential to improve a student's communicative skills and cultural awareness, two very important aspects of achieving the very goal of language teaching.

Meaning

A satellite is a spacecraft that receives signals from transmitters on Earth, amplifies those signals, changes the carrier frequency, and then sends the amplified signals back to a receiver on Earth. The space age and satellite launches began in 1957 with the launch of Sputnik by the former Soviet Union. Since then, numerous satellites have been launched for various purposes, including communications, weather, remote sensing, disaster warning, and defense.

Satellite Type and Satellite Characteristics

- **Energy:** An active satellite requires no normal energy to maintain its position in space, except for a small amount of energy required to occasionally correct its position. The energy for sending and receiving signals is supplied by solar cells onboard the satellite. These batteries are charged. Solar panels are used to operate satellite systems and convert sunlight into electrical energy.
- **Long range:** Satellite-based communications are distance independent and serve rural and urban centers and peripheries simultaneously. It can simultaneously feed very widely dispersed populations. This property of satellites is especially useful for distance learning. The space scientist claims that her three satellites in geostationary highaltitude orbit could provide fulltime communications service to the entire planet, except for the polar regions, which are out of sight from that orbit.
- **Versatility:** Satellites can be used simultaneously for mobile phones, TV and data traffic. There are various combinations of multipurpose satellites. Besides communications, satellites are also used for remote sensing, such as soil surveys, flooding (evaluation of sea level, etc.), forestry (tree resources, tree disease, etc.), and oceanography, if necessary.
- **Cost:** The initial investment in satellite development and launch is very high, especially in third world countries. Building and launching multipurpose satellites like INSAT required huge amounts of money. However, when INSATIB was launched and put into operation, all communication requirements were met without the need for new investments. Meanwhile, terrestrial systems, including microwaves, required additional infrastructure to meet the country's growing information needs.
- **Planning:** Implementation of satellite-based communications requires preliminary planning. It takes longer lead time than terrestrial communication. Therefore, the use of satellites should be tied to the country's overall socioeconomic and educational development. It (satellite communications) is closely related to the country's educational development and economic growth, so it should have a basis for long-term planning.
- **National and region-specific communications:** Satellite-based communications can serve both the national and region specific needs of a country. It can also be localized to provide regionally specialized services.
- **Satellite life:** The use of solar panels/cells represents the life of the satellite. The electrical energy output of solar cells decreases with age. After 8 to 10 years, the solar cell's electrical output drops by about 20%. Communications satellites are usually replaced after 10 to 12 years of continuous operation.

VIDEO CONFERENCING

Simply put, a conference call is a meeting between one or more people in the same city or in different cities, states or countries over a telephone or network connection. Realtime information exchange between people. People can have meetings, trainings, demonstrations, data transmission, etc. Educational conference calls are a valuable vehicle for distance learning. It uses multiple media and uses two-way transmission to enable interactive group communication. Today, we are becoming more and more dependent on this technology. Interest in the use of audio and related visual data that can be transmitted over normal telephone lines appears to be relevant to increasing distance learning.

Teleconferencing Benefits

Teleconferencing support is primarily due to the following benefits:
- The number of learners in the center is sparse, for example, less than 10 students in a particular course or program.
- **Cost effectiveness:** Compared to other available methods of teaching remote learners, the cost of starting and running an audio conferencing system is relatively low.
- **Flexible system:** The system used can be quickly adapted to suit large or small groups.
- **Familiar education mode:** The education mode is similar to a seminar where the instructor is responsible for discussion and can stimulate interaction between sites.
- **Easy scheduling:** Scheduling is almost as easy as a classroom on campus.
- **Intercampus access control:** Access to classes within the program may be controlled by a limited number of off-campus entities.
- **Quality education:** The quality of teaching materials can be kept high due to careful and early preparation.
- **Immediate feedback:** Teleconferencing systems provide learners with an opportunity for immediate feedback and allow tutors to communicate their responses.

Satellite Education Project

- **Secondary Education Television Project (1961):** Aims to improve education standards given the lack of laboratories, space equipment and qualified teachers in Delhi. This project was experimentally started in October 1961 to teach Physics, Chemistry, English and Hindi to students in Class XI.
- **Delhi Agricultural Television (DATV) Project (Krishi Darshan) (1966):** The project is called Krishi Darshan was started on 26 January 1966 to provide farmers with agricultural information in 80 selected villages of the Union Territory of Delhi through communities. provided on a trial basis to send TV and other conversations to each other.
- **National Satellite Project of India (INSAT) (1982):** The main objective of the INSAT project was to draw the attention of the local people to the latest developments in agricultural productivity, health and hygiene. It was originally intended for villagers and school children in selected villages in Orissa, Andhra Pradesh, Bihar, Gujarat, Maharashtra and Uttar Pradesh.
- **UGC Higher Education Television Project (HETV) (1984):** College students were beneficiaries of this project. The Commission on University Grants, in partnership with INSAT, initiated an educational television project commonly known as "Nationwide Classroom" on August 15, 1984 to update and improve the quality of education and to expand its reach.
- **IGNOU Doordarshan Television Broadcast (1991):** Intended to provide remote counseling to college students in remote areas. Due to strong audience response, the frequency of this project was increased to five days a week. This program is very popular.
- **Gyan Darshan Educational Channel (2000):** Human Resources Development Information and Ministry Broadcast Prasar Bharti and his IGNOU jointly announced on 26 January 2000 that he made Gyan Darshan (GD) dedicated to education in India. Launched as a TV channel.

Teleconferencing Limitations

Teleconferencing has inherent limitations and is not widely used in education. Some of them are:
- Teleconferencing requires a nationwide, highly efficient telephone and television network.
- Very likely technical failure.
- Telephone charges are very high and not all educational institutions can afford them.
- Teleconferencing is a costly technique of instruction. It requires sophisticated technology and expert human power.
- Teleconferencing is a mode of group communication so the willingness of each participant is an essential requirement but this is generally lacking especially among distance learners
- Organization takes time.

TELEHEALTH

Telemedicine is the use of digital information and communication technologies to access medical services and manage medical care remotely. Technologies include computers and mobile devices such as tablets and smartphones. This is technology that you can use at home. Alternatively, telemedicine can be provided by nurses or other medical professionals from clinics or mobile vans. Locally, for example. Telemedicine is also a technology that healthcare providers use to improve or support their healthcare services.

Definition

- Telemedicine is defined as the use of technology to provide medical services remotely. This includes everything from conducting a doctor's visit to a computer to remotely monitoring a patient's vital signs.
- **Telemedicine technology:** Several technologies are used in telemedicine, including m-Health (or mobile health), video and audio technology, digital photography, remote patient monitoring (RPM), and store-and-forward technology.
- **Telemedicine and telemedicine:** Although the terms telemedicine and telemedicine are often used interchangeably, telemedicine has evolved to encompass a wider range of digital health activities and services. To understand the comparison between telemedicine and telemedicine, it is important to first define telemedicine.

Types of Telemedicine Care

Telemedicine can be delivered in three ways:
1. **Synchronous:** When the doctor communicates with the patient in real time via computer or telephone.
2. **Asynchronous:** When data, images, or messages are recorded to share with the doctor later.
3. **Remote patient monitoring:** When measurements such as weight or blood pressure are sent to the healthcare provider.

Objectives

- Promote access to healthcare for people living in remote and rural areas.
- Protect yourself and others if you get an epidemic like COVID-19.

- Provides primary care for many medical condition.
- Make services easier or more convenient for people with limited time or means of transportation.
- Provide access to specialists.
- Improve communication and coordination of care between members of the health care team and caregivers.
- Provide advice on health care autonomy.

Telemedicine Service

Telemedicine allows all of the following activities and services:
- Take measurements such as weight, food intake, blood pressure, heart rate, blood sugar, and Record via mobile device. and send them to your doctor.
- You can visit doctors and nurses virtually from your computer or smartphone.
- Review test results using the online portal. Request a prescription refill. Message your doctor or make an appointment.
- Share information about lab results, diagnoses, medications, drug allergies, etc. with providers you see.
- Coordinating care between GPs and visiting specialists—including sharing lab notes and lab results between clinics in different locations.
- Receive e-mail or SMS reminders when mammograms, colonoscopies, other tests, or routine immunizations are due.
- Monitor older people at home to make sure they are eating, sleeping, and taking their medications as planned.

Patient Benefits

Telemedicine can help treat many conditions. Seeing a qualified doctor and providing clear information about your symptoms is most effective. Other benefits of telemedicine include:
- Shorter commutes also mean less ancillary costs like childcare and gas bills.
- **Improving access to care:** Telemedicine makes care more accessible for people with disabilities. It can also increase access to other populations, such as those who are geographically isolated or incarcerated.
- **Prevention:** Telemedicine makes it easier for people to access preventative measures that improve their health in the long run. This is especially true for people with economic or geographic barriers to quality care. For example, a 2012 study of people with coronary artery disease found that preventative telemedicine improved health outcomes.
- **Convenience:** Telemedicine allows people to receive care from the comfort and privacy of their own homes. This may mean that a person does not need to take time off from work or organize childcare.
- **Slowing the spread of infection:** Going to a clinic often means meeting with potentially ill people in a confined space. This is especially dangerous for people who have had previous illnesses or who have a weak immune system. Telemedicine eliminates the risk of infection in the clinic.

Healthcare Provider Benefits

Healthcare providers who offer telemedicine services enjoy several benefits, including:
- **Reduced overhead:** Providers of telemedicine services may experience reduced overhead. For example, front desk support fees may be lower, or you may be able to invest in office space with fewer labs.
- **Additional revenue sources:** Clinicians may find that telemedicine allows them to treat more patients, thereby increasing their income.
- **Less susceptible to illness and infections:** When healthcare providers see patients remotely, they don't have to worry about transmitting pathogens they may carry.
- **Patient satisfaction:** Patients may be happier with their provider if they don't have to drive to the clinic or wait for treatment.

Disadvantages for Patients

Telemedicine is not suitable for all patients. Some drawbacks of this type of care are:
- **Insurance coverage:** Insurance companies are currently required to cover or reimburse telemedicine costs. However, these laws are constantly changing.
- **Protecting medical information:** Hackers and other criminals can gain access to patient medical information. This is especially true when patients are accessing telemedicine over public networks or unencrypted channels.
- **Delayed treatment:** When a person requires urgent care, initial access to telemedicine can delay treatment. Especially since doctors can't provide life-saving treatments or lab tests digitally.

Benefits

- Many patients feel uncomfortable going to hospitals and clinics. This system creates communication between patients and doctors. Healthcare professionals engaged for convenience and convenience.
- Save lives in emergency situations when you do not have time to take the patient to the hospital.

- In many rural and remote areas, or in postdisaster situations, ongoing medical care is not available. Telemedicine can be used to provide emergency medical care in such places and situations.
- This system helps patients living in inaccessible or remote areas. Patients can receive clinical care at home without the hassle of going to the hospital.
- Modern information technology innovations such as mobile collaboration make it easier to share information and discuss important medical cases among medical professionals in multiple locations.
- Telemedicine has reduced the number of outpatient visits by facilitating patient monitoring via computer, tablet or telephone technology. Doctors can now check prescriptions and monitor medication monitoring. In addition, home-based patients can receive medical assistance without having to drive an ambulance to the clinic. This has reduced medical costs.
- The system also facilitates health education, as basic medical professionals can observe the working procedures of medical professionals in their respective fields, and experts can supervise the work of novices.
- Telemedicine eliminates the possibility of transmitting infectious diseases between patients and healthcare workers.

Disadvantages for Healthcare Providers

Healthcare providers may also face some disadvantages associated with telemedicine.
- The state in which the license and the patient live.
- **Technology concerns:** Finding the right digital platform can be difficult. Even weak connections make it difficult to provide quality care. Clinicians should also ensure that the telemedicine programs they use are secure and fully compliant with data protection laws.
- **Unable to screen patients:** Providers must rely on patient self-reports during telemedicine sessions. This may require clinicians to ask more questions to ensure a comprehensive medical history. Treatment can be compromised if important symptoms that patients notice during face-to-face care are missed.

TELENURSING

Telenursing is the use of information when providing care services when there is physical distance between the patient and caregiver, or between any number of caregivers. It refers to using technology. As an area of expertise, it is part of telemedicine and has many interfaces with other medical and nonmedical applications such as telediagnosis, teleconsultation and telemonitoring. Telecommunications technology to improve patient care. It involves the use of electromagnetic channels (e.g. wire radio and optical) to transmit voice data and video communications signals.

Types of Technology-based Services

Telehealth can be divided into four types of technology-based services:
1. **Video conferencing:** Utilizing Internet technology video conferencing allows healthcare providers such as nurse practitioners to speak "face-to-face" with patients. Video conferencing is best used for consulting conducting mental health evaluations and diagnosing basic ailments.
2. **Digital transmission:** Internet technology allows healthcare providers to read scans, view prerecorded patient videos, and view medical charts from virtually anywhere.
3. **Remote patient monitoring (RPM):** RPM is a technology designed to monitor patient medical problems such as blood pressure, blood sugar and heart rate. This allows healthcare providers to track patient health data without the need for numerous appointments.
4. **Mobile health:** Smartphone and tablet technology allows patients to use apps to provide health information and track health decisions such as calorie intake and exercise.

Types of Telecare Services

There are different types of care services that can be provided remotely. The basics of the nursing process still apply, including assessment planning, interventions, and outcome evaluation. The only difference is that care is provided remotely rather than in person.

Telecare offers the following services:

- **Triage:** As mentioned earlier, telecare is widely used in call centers to triage patients to determine the severity of their condition and provide appropriate counseling.
- **Preoperative:** Preoperatively, the nurse can complete the portion of the patient assessment that does not require physical presence, including personal information and a complete medical history. Based on the information you receive, you can order additional laboratory and other tests and plan for special needs in advance after the patient's admission.
- **Home care during illness and recovery:** Patients who do not require hospitalization or who are recovering at home after illness or surgery can be monitored, counseled and educated through remote nursing. For example, through video calls, nurses can assess wound healing and teach wound care.

- **Counseling of minor illnesses:** Many minor illnesses for which patients routinely visit a clinic can be successfully diagnosed and treated through remote consultations, especially when video conferencing is available. Examples include common childhood conditions, uncomplicated allergic skin reactions, and minor injuries.
- **Chronic disease care:** An important growth area for telenursing is the care and monitoring of older people with chronic diseases. Caregivers can monitor the health of these patients through regular video conferencing and digital monitoring devices. Nurses also address additional healthcare service needs, such as: They play the role of nutritionist, physiotherapist, or optician and act as a coordinator between patients and various medical services.
- **Mental healthcare:** Telemedicine services are often used for crisis intervention and suicide prevention. Through telenursing services, patients with mental health and substance abuse problems can be screened regularly. A nurse can also standby if the client encounters a problematic situation. This is of particular value in areas where mental health resources are in short supply.

Telemedicine Nursing Benefits

- **Better access to quality care:** Telemedicine care provides 24/7 access to healthcare, especially for patients in older communities and rural areas.
- **Ability to better manage chronic diseases:** Chronic diseases such as diabetes and CPOD are better managed with regular monitoring. Remote patient monitoring facilitates communication between patients and caregivers.
- **Reduced risk of infection:** Patients do not come in contact with other people in clinics and medical facilities, eliminating the risk of infection from sick people.
- **Save time:** Patients can have their questions answered. Telemedicine eliminates travel time, waiting room waits, and waiting times for appointments.
- **Save money:** Inperson visits to clinics, emergency centers, or emergency rooms cost travel and time for medical billing. Telemedicine significantly reduces these costs.
- **Reduce trips to hospital:** Provide telemedicine access in communities where older people live to connect patients with doctors, nurses, or specialists in real time, reducing unnecessary hospital visits. can be avoided. Trips to hospitals from these communities are frequent because there is not always a doctor on site. Telemedicine provides 24/7 medical access.
- **Convenience:** Telemedicine provides convenient access to medical professionals for nonemergency situations that occur at inconvenient times, such as nights, weekends and holidays.
- **Helps keep caregivers connected:** Allows distant family members to be involved and informed in the care of their loved ones. Technology can be used to monitor patient health, ask questions, and virtually participate in meetings with healthcare providers. This improves safety for everyone involved.

Cons of Telemedicine Care

- **Not suitable for all situations:** Telemedicine is a tool that can improve individual care, but it cannot replace face-to-face care for all. A healthcare provider may need to perform a physical examination to check for fractures, listen to the patient's heart and lungs, or take a throat swab to check for strep throat.
- **Technology barriers:** The technology required for telemedicine is not universally available. Reliable Internet connections are often lacking in rural areas, and not all patients have smartphones or computers.
- **Reduced continuity of care:** Patients using telemedicine may be connected to different providers each time, making it impossible for patients to arrange in-person visits. This can lead to gaps in care and lead to untreated medical problems.
- **Patients may experience barriers to care:** Older adults may find it difficult or uncomfortable to communicate with healthcare providers via technology rather than face-to-face.
- **Potential inconsistency in reimbursement/insurance issues:** Insurance plans are not widely accepting telemedicine with consistent coverage and reimbursement rates.

MOBILE TECHNOLOGIES

Mobile technologies are technologies that allow users to move anywhere. It consists of portable two-way communication devices, computing devices, and the network technology that connects them. Mobile technology is now embodied by Internet enabled devices such as smartphones, tablets and watches. These are the latest in trends including interactive pagers, notebooks, mobile phones (fold phones), GPS navigators and more.

Definition

- Mobile technology is a type of technology that allows users to use mobile phones to perform communication-related tasks such as communicating with friends,

family, and others. Used to send data from one system to another. Portable two-way communication systems, computing devices, and accompanying network devices constitute mobile technology.
- **Mobile learning:** The use of portable computing devices (such as iPads, laptops, tablet PCs, personal digital assistants [PDAs], and smartphones) with wireless networks enables mobility and mobile learning. Teaching and learning are extended beyond traditional teaching and learning. You can expand your classroom.

Types of Cellular Networks

- **Cellular network:** A cellular network with distributed cell towers that allow mobile devices (cell phones) to automatically switch frequencies and communicate uninterrupted over large geographic areas. The same basic switching functions allow cellular networks to serve many users on a limited set of radio frequencies. It uses packetswitching techniques to organize data into parts or packets for transmission and reassemble the information at the destination.
- **G network:** The 'G' of the generation, is said to be 10 times faster than 3G, but 5G is still on the way. 5G uses various aggregated frequency bands to free up bandwidth and is about 20 times faster than 4G.
- **WLAN:** Radio waves that connect devices to the Internet through localized routers called hotspots. Abbreviation for Wireless Fidelity A WiFi network is like a cell phone tower for Internet access, but without establishing a WiFi connection, it does not automatically traverse the service. Most mobile devices can automatically switch between WiFi and cellular networks based on availability and user preference.
- **Bluetooth:** A telecommunications industry specification for connecting devices over short distances using shortwave radio waves. Bluetooth allows you to quickly connect or pair devices such as headsets, speakers, phones, and other devices.

Use of Mobile Radio Technology

- The incorporation of mobile technology into business has supported telecollaboration. People can now use mobile technology to connect from anywhere and access the papers and documents they need to collaborate.
- Work is being redefined by mobile technology. Employees are no longer tied to their desks. Work from anywhere in the world.
- Mobile technology helps businesses save time and money. Employees working from home routinely save thousands of dollars. Mobile phones eliminate the need for expensive technology such as landline providers. Cloud-based services are more costeffective than traditional systems. Technology can also help businesses become more flexible and productive.
- Mobile technology has the potential to greatly improve productivity. Mobile application integration saves an average of 7.5 hours per employee per week. Employees can also be more productive using smartphones and mobile his devices.
- Cloud-based services are becoming more and more popular these days. Cloud-based mobile technology applications are proving to be more convenient than any smart phone, especially regarding available storage space.

Benefits of Mobile Technology

- Today, various applications allow us to stay in touch with friends and family at any time. You can now communicate with anyone you want or make a video visit simply by using your mobile phone. That said, portables keep us up-to-date with the world.
- Today's mobile phones have made our daily activities more natural. Now you can call up current traffic conditions on your mobile phone and make the right decisions to arrive on time. Weather also plays a role.
- Advances in mobile technology have brought the entire gaming world under his one roof. When you are tired from monotonous work or taking a break, you can listen to music, watch movies, watch your favorite shows or watch videos of your favorite songs.
- Mobile phones are used for a variety of legitimate tasks, such as scheduling meetings, sending and receiving documents that introduce yourself, alerts, and applying for jobs. Mobile phones have become an indispensable tool for all workers.
- Mobile phones are now also used as wallets for payments. You can now use the utility to send money to friends, relatives and others.

Disadvantages of Mobile Technology

- Modern families have become dependent on mobile phones.
- Either way, when I do not have to travel, I surf the Internet and play around, making me a real addict.
- With the proliferation of mobile devices, there is a significant risk of loss of protection. Anyone can easily retrieve data by efficiently browsing web-based social networking accounts.
- The price of mobile phones is increasing according to their value. People today spend a good amount of money

on their mobile phones, but that would be better spent on something more beneficial, like education or something that helps us in our lives.

Mobile Learning Issues

Researchers point to common mobile learning issues such as:
- Physical characteristics of mobile devices such as small screen size, heavy weight, lack of memory, and short battery life.
- Content and software application limitations, such as lack of built-in functionality, difficulty adding applications, challenges in learning how to operate mobile devices, differences in applications and usage conditions.
- Network speed and reliability.
- Excessive screen brightness issues when using physical environment devices outdoors; personal safety issues; potential radiation exposure from devices that use radio frequencies; need for rain cover when raining or damp. There are issues such as gender.

CONCLUSION

From this chapter students will be able to understand about the electronic media and its learning resources such as computers, web-based videoconferencing, E-learning and smart classroom, also learn the trends in telecommunication using the cable TV, satellite broadcasting, video conferencing, telephones-telehealth/telenursing, mobile technology its advantages and limitations in educational and clinical settings.

REVIEW QUESTIONS

Long Essays

1. Define electronic media, explain in details about tele communications.
2. Define computer, explain the purposes and benefits of computer education.
3. Define internet, explain internet usage in education.
4. Describe overcoming barriers with video-conferencing for education.
5. Define e-learning, explain functions and types of e-learning.
6. Define smart classroom, explain equipment installed in smart classrooms.
7. Define satellite communication, explain satellite type and satellite characteristics.
8. Define telehealth, explain types, objectives and services.
9. Define telenursing, explain the types of technology and services provided.

Short Essays

1. Role of computers in education.
2. Applications of computers in education.
3. Benefits of computer education.
4. Using computers in education.
5. Importance of the internet in education.
6. Role of the internet in education.
7. Benefits of online learning.
8. Web-based video conferencing.
9. Effective video conferencing.
10. Importance of e-learning.
11. Benefits of e-learning in education.
12. Smart classroom targets.
13. Smart classroom features.
14. Intelligent classroom principles.
15. Cable TV in the classroom.
16. Types of educational television programs.
17. Teleconferencing benefits.
18. Satellite education project.
19. Telehealth benefits for the patient and healthcare provider.
20. Telemedicine nursing benefits.
21. Mobile technologies: Types of cellular networks.
22. Benefits of mobile technology.

Short Answers
1. Social networking.
2. Multimedia integration.
3. Drawbacks of online learning.
4. Web conferencing need.
5. Video conferencing platforms.
6. Google hangouts.
7. Dialpad meetings.
8. TrueConf online.
9. Skype.
10. Slack video calls.
11. E-learning benefits.
12. Smart classroom components.
13. Benefits of smart classes.
14. Disadvantages of smart class.
15. Video conferencing.
16. National Satellite Project of India (INSAT).
17. Gyan Darshan Educational Channel (2000).
18. Teleconferencing limitations.
19. Cons of telemedicine care.
20. Disadvantages of mobile technology.
21. Mobile learning issues.

Unit 6

Assessment/Evaluation Methods

Chapters

13. Assessment/Evaluation Methods/Strategies
14. Assessment of Knowledge
15. Assessment of Skills
16. Assessment of Attitude and Higher-Learning

KEYWORDS

Accountability: The demand by a community (public officials, employers, and taxpayers) for school officials to prove that money invested in education has led to measurable learning.

Achievement test: Standardized test designed to measure the amount of knowledge and/or skill a person has acquired. Such testing evaluates the test-takers learning in comparison with a standard or norm.

Alternative assessment: Used to describe alternatives to traditional, standardized, norm- or criterion-referenced traditional paper and pencil testing. Portfolios and instructor observation of students are also alternative forms of assessment.

Analytic scoring: Evaluating student work across multiple areas of performance rather than from an overall impression (*See:* Holistic scoring). In analytic scoring, individual scores for each area are scored and reported.

Anchor: A sample of student work that exemplifies a specific level of performance. An anchor would be used to score student work, usually comparing the student performance to the anchor.

Assessment: The process of observing learning, describing, collecting, recording, scoring, and interpreting information about courses/programs/services undertaken for the purpose of improving the institution, services, programs, and student learning and development.

Assessment activities (methods): Mechanisms by which achievement of an outcome is determined. Examples include: Surveys, interviews, standardized tests, portfolios, juried performances, research data from outside sources, peer review, etc.

Assessment for accountability: This involves the summative assessment of units or individuals to satisfy external stakeholders.

Assessment for improvement: This type of assessment feeds directly, and often immediately, back into revision of the course, program, service or institution to improve student learning, programs, or services. Assessment for improvement can be formative and/or summative.

Authentic assessment: Involves asking students to demonstrate the behavior the learning is intended to produce. Rather than choosing from a set of responses, students are asked to accomplish a task or to solve problems.

Benchmark: A description of a specific level of expected performance. Benchmarks for student learning are often represented by samples of student work.

Capstone experience: Holistic activities designed to assess students' knowledge, skills, and problem-solving abilities using concepts learned at the end of the program.

Classroom embedded assessment: Activities used by an individual instructor to determine if students are meeting the outcomes in a single class meeting or a small number of consecutive class meetings. The instructor evaluates the results to decide if changes are needed to help improve student learning.

Criteria: Measures or characteristics that are used to determine or verify student knowledge, attitudes and performance.

Criterion-referenced assessment: Assessment comparing an individual's performance to a specific learning outcome or performance standard and not to the performance of other students.

Cohort: A group of individuals whose progress is tracked by examining identified measurements at specified points in time.

Competencies: Knowledge, skills, or behavior that a student can perform or demonstrate.

Competency test: A test used to determine if a student has met established minimum standards of skills and knowledge.

Course-embedded assessment: Assessment methods that are integrated into the teaching-learning process as part of the coursework.

Curriculum mapping: The process for documenting the link between course learning outcomes and program goals and outcomes.

Curriculum-embedded or course-embedded assessment: Assessment that occurs simultaneously with learning and as a natural part of the teaching-learning process. These would include activities such as projects, portfolios and assignments. The assessments occur in the classroom setting, where tasks or tests are developed from the curriculum or instructional materials.

Cutoff score: Minimum score used to determine the performance level needed to pass a competency test.

Dimensions: Desired knowledge, attitudes or skills to be measured in an assessment as represented in a scoring rubric.

Direct assessment of learning: Assessment activities that gather evidence of student knowledge and skills based upon student performance, rather than perception.

Educational objectives: Objectives that describe the knowledge, skills, abilities, or attitudes students are expected to acquire as a result of completing the academic program. Objectives are sometimes treated as synonymous with outcomes.

Evaluation: The use of qualitative and quantitative descriptions to judge individual, course, program and institutional effectiveness. Depending on the level, evaluation information is used for making decisions about individual performance review, student grades and course, program and institutional changes for improvement.

Evaluation of faculty and staff: A process where employee performance is measured at an institution.

External assessment: This uses criteria (i.e., rubric) or an instrument developed by an external source and is usually summative, quantitative, and standardized.

Formative assessment: Specific assessments identifying what individuals know or are able to do and not do when a given learning task. This is a specific focus of student learning assessment within a course.

Norm-referenced assessment: An assessment where student performance or performances are compared to a norm group.

Objective test: A test for which the scoring procedure is completely specified and not subjective, enabling agreement of the correct answer among different scorers.

Outcome: An observable act that can be measured, usually a culminating activity or product.

Outcome (student): A measurable activity, product, or performance that involves students.

Outcome (student learning): Descriptions of what a student should be able to know, think, or do when they have completed a course or program.

Performance-based assessment: Direct observation and rating of an individual's performance of an educational objective. The assessment may be conducted over a period of time and usually includes the use of a rubric or scoring guide to provide for objectivity. A test of the ability to apply knowledge in a real-life setting is an example of performance-based assessment.

Performance criteria or standards: Specific descriptions of what individuals must do to demonstrate proficiency at a defined level.

Portfolio: A collection of work, usually drawn from students' classroom work. Portfolios can be designed to assess student progress, effort and/or achievement, and encourage students to reflect on their learning.

Portfolio assessment: Reviewers assess student work on meeting outcomes by use of a portfolio and established criteria of performance. Each item in the portfolio may be individually scored, or a holistic scoring process may be used to present an overall impression of the student's collected work.

Program assessment: Processes identified by faculty and staff members of an academic or non-academic program to measure identified outcomes as a result of participation in the program or service. The result of the assessments should be used to decide if changes are needed to improve the program or service.

Qualitative assessment: Provides data that is analyzed by interpretive criteria and does not lend itself to be analyzed by quantitative methods.

Quantitative assessment: Provides data that can be analyzed using quantitative methods.

Rating scale: Qualities of a performance on an assessment that is based on descriptive words or phrases that indicate levels of achievement.

Reliability: The measure of consistency for an assessment indicating that the assessment yields similar results over time when applied to similar populations in similar circumstances.

Rubric: A scoring guide that defines the criteria of how an assignment or task will be assessed. A rubric typically provides an explicit description of performance characteristics corresponding to a point on a rating scale.

Sampling: Method to obtain information about characteristics of a population by examining a smaller, randomly chosen selection (the sample) of the group members.

Standardization: Procedures for designing, administering, and scoring an assessment in an effort to assure that all students are assessed under the same conditions and scores are not influenced by extraneous conditions.

Standardized test: An objective test that is given and scored in a uniform manner, often with scores being norm-referenced. Standardized tests are often accompanied by guidelines for administration and scoring in an effort to reduce influence on the results.

Standards: Statements of expectations for outcomes, which may include content standards, performance standards, and benchmarks.

Student learning outcomes assessment: The systematic collection, examination, and interpretation of qualitative and quantitative data about student learning and the use of that information to document and to improve student learning.

Subjective assessment: An assessment where the impression or opinion of the assessor contributes to the determination of the score or evaluation of performance.

Summative assessment: Provides a summary at the culmination of a course, unit, or program.

Unit: The designation used for the instructional and non-instructional departments, programs, and college services under the MVCC Institutional effectiveness process.

Validity: The extent to which an assessment measures what it is designed to measure and that the results are used to make appropriate and accurate inferences. An assessment cannot be valid if it is not reliable.

Chapter 13

Assessment/Evaluation Methods/Strategies

Learning Objectives

- Evaluation Principles
- Scope of Assessment and Scope Assessment
- Rating Types and Features
- Teaching Measurements Function
- Evaluation Tools
- Assessment Methods
- Choosing an Assessment Method
- Types of Tools Used in the Evaluation
- Evaluation Methods
- Assessment Issues
- Case Study, Achievement Tests, Standardized Tests, School Performance Test and Interpretation Items

TERMINOLOGY

- **Validity:** Relates to the degree to which a stated dimension can be correctly assessed in the participant being measured.
- **Reliability:** Refers to the consistency of results even when testing on the same group at frequent intervals/staggers.
- **Psychological testing:** This is a self-report study in which responses are measured and combined to give an overall score.
- **Norms:** Psychological test norms refer to the typical level of performance for a particular group of people.
- **Test:** A test is a specified set of consistent tasks that students must complete. These tasks are a good selection of knowledge or skills in a broader substantive area.
- **Scoring:** Scoring is the determination of the value of event items or individuals against specified criteria. Educators assess student progress by comparing student performance to success criteria based on teaching objectives.
- **Ability testing:** Performance testing is a systematic procedure for measuring a representative sample of learning tasks.
- **Paper and pencil performance:** Paper and pencil proficiency tests differ from more traditional paper and pencil tests in that they focus on applying knowledge and skills in a simulated environment.
- **Discrimination tests:** Discrimination tests include a number of test situations with varying degrees of realism.
- **Student performance:** Student performance focuses on proper practice. Students are typically expected to perform the same movements that would be required to perform the task in real life, but the conditions are simulated.
- **Checklist:** A prepared list of descriptions of properties to be evaluated, performance, etc.
- **Social metrics:** This is a method of assessing the social relationships that exist within a group.
- **Analysis:** To decompose into separate parts and discuss, investigate, or interpret each part.
- **List:** List some ideas, aspects, events, things, qualities, reasons, etc.
- **Ratings:** Give your opinion or cite expert opinion. Include evidence to support your assessment.
- **Compare:** Look for similar qualities and characteristics. It emphasizes their similarities, but sometimes also mentions their differences.
- **Contrast:** Emphasizes differences, differences, or differences in things, properties, events, or issues.
- **To criticize:** Express a judgment about the value or truthfulness of a stated element or belief. We provide

an analysis of these factors and discuss their limitations and benefits.
- **Definition:** Gives concise, clear and authoritative meaning. Do not go into details, but be sure to indicate the limits of your definition. Shows how what you define differs from that of other classes.
- **Description:** Retell, characterize, sketch, or narrate in order or story form. Figure—provides a graphical scheme or graphical answer. Graphs usually need to be labeled. In some cases, add a short description or description.
- **Discuss:** Investigate, carefully analyze, and justify the pros and cons. Fill in all the required fields and enter your details.
- **Enumerate:** Write in a list or summary format, stating the main points individually and concisely.
- **Evaluation:** Evaluate the problem carefully and identify both advantages and limitations. Emphasize the authority's assessment and, to a lesser extent, your personal assessment.
- **Description:** Clarify, interpret, and spell what you are proposing. They try to justify differences in opinions and results and analyze their causes.
- **Illustrations:** Use illustrations, diagrams, or specific examples to explain or clarify the problem.
- **Interpreter:** Translate a topic, give examples of solutions, comment, and usually give your opinion on it.
- **Justification:** To prove or justify a decision or conclusion, taking care to make it persuasive.
- **List:** Writes a series of detailed succinct statements, similar to List.
- **Summary:** Organizes the description into major and minor points, omitting details and emphasizing the placement and classification of things.
- **Prove:** Prove that something is true by providing factual evidence or clear logical reasons.
- **Related:** Shows how things are related or related, how one causes the other, or what the other is like.
- **Review:** Critically consider a topic, analyze and comment on key statements to make about it.
- **Sketch:** Means "decompose into components".
- **Status:** Presents the main points in a concise and clear order. Detailed diagrams and examples are usually omitted.
- **Summary:** Presents the main points or facts in a condensed form, like a chapter summary, without details or figures.
- **Tracks:** In narrative form, describe progress, development, or historical events from a particular starting point.
- **Identify or characterize:** Means to distinguish this term or person from all other similar terms or persons. Both are explicit commands to be as specific as possible.
- **Illustrated or clarified:** Means "to give an example" to demonstrate understanding of a concept, not a definition.
- **Logbook:** A validated record of learner progress, documenting acquisition of required knowledge, skills, attitudes, and/or competencies.
- A portfolio is a summary of a learner's progress in tasks and competencies, A portfolio is evidence of events recorded in a logbook.
- **Activity:** This term refers to a predefined task performed by a learner that contributes to the achievement of a specified goal or ability.
- **Remediation:** Remediation is a deliberate activity aimed at correcting deficiencies that prevent learners from achieving their intended results.

INTRODUCTION

Evaluation involves a number of steps. Various assessment methods are available to measure teaching and learning outcomes. Evaluation methods are divided into qualitative and quantitative methods. It can also be classified according to the behavioral aspect to be evaluated and the evaluation method.

DEFINITION

- Score is a relatively new term introduced to indicate a broader concept of measurement than is implied in traditional tests and surveys. —**Wringhtone**
- Evaluation is essential in the never-ending cycle of setting goals, measuring progress along the way, and determining new goals as a result of new alerts.
 —**Clara M Brown**
- Evaluation in education is the process of assessing the effectiveness of educational experiences through careful evaluation. —**LE Hidgerken**
- Evaluation is the process used to determine what happened during a particular activity or within a facility.
 —**John W preferable**

PURPOSE OF ASSESSMENT

- Assessment procedures help students identify desired behaviors to achieve, desirable behaviors to achieve and what to learn.
- Helps students identify difficulties and problems in their learning and track their progress.
- Guide teachers and students in the selection of future learning content.
- Provide instruction and advice on learning to students.
- Evaluate the adequacy and feasibility of the set goals.

- Provide guidance to teachers on the effectiveness of curriculum teaching methods and the effectiveness of the learning experiences provided.
- Determination of promotion, placement, etc.
- Report student performance to parents.
- Diagnose each student's strengths and weaknesses and suggest improvements.
- Motivate and encourage students to learn.
- Determine the level of knowledge and understanding of students at various levels.
- To collect information necessary for operations such as the selection of students for the Honors Course. Placing students in higher qualifications and assessing completion of graduation requirements helps administrators determine the effectiveness of the curriculum, its strengths and weaknesses, and communicate the school's goals and achievements to the public.

EVALUATION PRINCIPLES

- The purpose of the evaluation must be clearly stated prior to conducting the evaluation.
- The evaluation method should be chosen according to the objectives pursued.
- Comprehensive evaluation requires different evaluation methods.
- Appropriate use of valuation techniques requires recognition of their limitations and strengths.
- Evaluation is a means to an end, not an end in itself. Evaluation processes are linked in terms of decisions made.
- The evaluation process should contribute to improved policy and managerial decision-making.
- Appropriate assessment methods are necessary because assessment is about obtaining evidence of targeted behavior as an educational goal.
- Scoring ensures that a student's typical reactions can be estimated by collecting sample evidence of student reactions (behavior).

SCOPE OF ASSESSMENT AND SCOPE ASSESSMENT

- Value judgment
- Effectiveness of assessment or instructional methods
- Providing a basis for instruction and counseling
- Employment and promotion
- Determining the extent to which educational goals have been achieved.
- Development of attitudes, interests, skills, creativity, originality, knowledge and skills, etc.
- Development of tools and techniques
- Curriculum development and revision
- Interpretation of results.

RATING TYPE

- **Contextual assessment:** Explores the political, social, financial and other contexts of programs and evaluations.
- **Needs assessment:** To identify, justify and design program needs can be used.
- **Process evaluation program monitoring:** Determines whether the program is implemented as promised and how the program was delivered and received.
- **Formation evaluate:** Use information collected in the early stages of the program to modify later stages. .
- **Performance evaluation:** Summative Evaluation: Determines whether the program objectives have been met. The data collected comes directly from the purpose of the program.
- **Efficiency evaluation cost efficiency cost-benefit analysis:** Compare program costs and benefits.
- **Usage:** Evaluate if the evaluation itself was used. Many good ratings are not considered for reasons unrelated to the rating itself.

EVALUATION STEPS

According to L Heidgerken
- Starting goals.
- Define the expected change in behavior as a result.
- Describe and describe the circumstances that give you the opportunity to express the behavior described.
- Development of appropriate and systematic means of selecting actions implicit in the goals being assessed.
- Consider how behavior is recorded and summarized (scored, rated, or described) as a basis for the evidence gathered.
- Verification of the effectiveness, reliability and difficulty of the measures used.
- Create an environment in which students can perform at their best.
- Score based on the steps above.
- Development of interpretation methods.

Evaluation tool or device selection criteria: The most important criteria in the selection and development of evaluation tools is:
- Goal example.
- Content tasting.
- Validation of effectiveness, reliability, practicality, usefulness.

Evaluation method: There is a specific method for evaluation. The backbone of education as painted by Gilberto is: This consists of his four steps.
1. Define your goals.
2. A project evaluation system.

3. Prepare.
4. Run the evaluation.

This process is repeated to provide feedback, reassess goals, and make necessary changes to the education system (program). Evaluation is an ongoing process, the results of which are used in Gilbert's educational spiral.

RATING FEATURES

Rating has the following features.
- Placement function:
  - This assessment helps to examine all aspects of children's entry behavior.
  - This helps in the implementation of special educational programs.
  - To allow individualization of lessons.
  - It also assists in the selection of students for further study in various professions and specialties.
- Teaching functions:
  - Planned assessment helps teachers determine and develop teaching methods and techniques.
  - Assist in the formulation and redefinition of appropriate and realistic teaching goals.
  - Help to improve teaching and plan appropriate and appropriate teaching technique
  - It also helps improve curriculum.
  - Evaluation of various teaching practices.
  - Determine the extent to which learning objectives have been achieved grams.
  - Improving the educational process and the quality of teachers hours plan a good and good learning strategy.
- Diagnostic function:
  - The assessment should diagnose not only the weaknesses of the student, but also the weaknesses of the school's program.
  - Relevant Relief Program Suggestions.
  - The talents, interests and intelligence of each individual child must also be recognized so that they can be motivated in the right direction.
  - I adapt my lessons to the different needs of my students.
  - Evaluate the progress of underperforming students in terms of performance, abilities, and goals.
- Prediction function:
  - Discover potential learner skills and talents.
  - In this way you can predict the future success of your children.
  - It also helps children choose the right electives.
- Administrative functions:
  - Introduce better education policy and decision-making.
  - It helps to separate students into different suitable groups.
  - For promotion of students to the next advanced class
  - Evaluation of supervision practices.
  - Have proper placement.
  - Compare and describe the performance of different children grams.
  - Make a solid plan, it helps test the effectiveness of a teacher in delivering the right learning experience.
  - Mobilize public opinion and improve public relations.
  - Helps develop comprehensive reference tests.
- Administrative functions:
  - Assisting in decision-making about majors and careers.
  - Help learners identify their learning pace and learning gaps.
  - Help teachers get to know children in detail and provide them with the educational, professional and personal guidance they need.
- Motivational functions:
  - Motivate, guide, inspire and engage students in learning.
  - Reward and motivate their learning.
- Development functions:
  - Provides reinforcement and feedback to student-teacher and instructional-learning processes.
  - Help change and improve teaching strategies and learning experiences.
  - Helps achieve educational goals and objectives.
- Research functions:
  - Helps provide data for generalization of research.
  - This evaluation clears any doubts for further investigation and research.
  - Contribute to the development of action research in education.
- Communications:
  - Communicate progress results to students.
  - Report progress to parents.
  - Communicate your progress to other school.

TEACHING MEASUREMENTS FUNCTION

- **Assessment improves teacher quality:**
  - Through teaching, teachers can see how well they have achieved their educational goals.
  - Teachers can evaluate how successful their teaching has been.
  - Assessment helps teachers adopt appropriate teaching strategies.
- **Assessment helps clarify objectives:** Teachers gain greater insight into different aspects of the subject under consideration.

- **Assessment motivates learners:** Students are more likely to learn a subject when teachers continuously assess their learning.
- **Ratings can be used as a guide:**
  - Ratings clarify individual differences.
  - Assessment acts as a guide, as through assessment we can identify the learner's specific difficulties.
- **Assessment helps change the curriculum:**
  - Educational inquiry presents principles and strategies.
  - Educational assessment provides direction for bringing about such change.

About the students:
- During the selection process, the strengths and weaknesses of the students are diagnosed and the classification of the students is established.
- To check the student's current status.
- Determine individual student progress (through regular assessment).
- Knowing aptitudes of students.

In relation to teachers:
- Knowing how successful teaching and effective methodologies are.
- To find individual differences.

Regarding teaching methods:
- Assessment includes objective teaching and continuous assessment of student progress.
- It enhances teaching and learning.

About the school program: Evaluation is important to give a comprehensive evaluation of the entire school program.

To improve practice: Student assessments also serve as the basis for reporting to parents to improve public relations and mobilize public opinion.

EVALUATION TOOLS

The word "tool" literally means "device for mechanical manipulation". However, in education, assessment tools can be defined as tools for gathering evidence of student performance. The main tools of evaluation in forming theories and frameworks are achievement tests, case records, cumulative records, checklists, rating scales, questionnaires, etc. The method of evaluation depends on the situation and purpose. For example, personality tests use your responses to discover personality traits, and financial assessments measure how much you know about concepts like saving and investing.

Evaluation Tool Characteristics

- **Reliability:** A good evaluation tool will deliver the same results over time. Therefore, these results are consistent or accurate. Here you should consider whether the results are reproducible in your tests each time you use them. For example, assessments are considered reliable if students perform the same task at the same time.
- **Validity:** Validity of an assessment depends on how well it measures the various criteria tested. In other words, the idea is that testing measures what you want to measure.
- **Equality:** A good assessment tool is fair, meaning no one participant wins or loses. Fair assessment means that students are assessed using the methods and procedures that best suit them. Each participant must be familiar with the context of the test to perform satisfactorily.
- **Standardization:** Standardization means consistency in testing methods. For example, if you send out a survey, it should contain the same questions for all participants and all responses should be graded according to the same criteria.

Other features of the assessment tool include:
- A good evaluation tool should provide a window for quality feedback.
- This is doable and equivalence is considered.
- Intended to encourage participants to participate in the test.
- Be transparent, non-discriminatory and meet expectations.

Test Design

Test development or test design refers to the science and art of planning, preparing, managing, evaluating, statistically analyzing and reporting test results. This article highlights the systematic process used to develop tests in order to maximize the evidence of validity of the results obtained from the tests.

Steps in Construction of Test

Test Building Steps

- **Complete planning:** A systematic plan that guides all other test development activities: Articulates test objectives and defines structure. Desired interpretation or conclusion of test results. Proof of planned effectiveness. validity of the test format. Psychometric model time planning, safety, quality control plan.
- **Defining content:** Precise sampling plan related to articles and domains, rational or empirical basis. Primary source of content verification.
- **Test specification:** Content that is operationally defined and specific to definition of document content. Provides content validation proof for score inference on the domain.

- **Item development:** Creating effective test stimuli or item formats. Principles of effective article writing. Article author training. Content and editorial review to reduce bias.
- **Test design and structure:** Test form design and administration. Selection of items or prompts. Operational sampling according to planned design. Pre-test trial item.
- **Create test form:** Publish or create a test. Security effectiveness and quality control issues.
- Management effectiveness issues related to standardization fairness issues. Security timing issue monitoring.
- **Response score validity issue:** Psychometric model. quality control, key verification, item analysis.
- **Determining passing scores:** Defining reasonable cut points or passing scores. Relative and absolute methods, validity issue, comparability of standards and consistency of scales.
- **Report test results:** Validity issues—accuracy, quality control, regular, cheating issues.
- **Item banking:** Effective item banking with safety and flexibility.
- **Documentation:** Technical reports process documentation: Thorough detailed documentation.

Selection of Evaluation Tools

The evaluation process requires careful selection of evaluation tools. There are some guidelines to keep in mind when choosing an assessment tool. The following points should be kept in mind when choosing an assessment tool:

- **Good:** Your tool should be able to measure what you want to measure.
- **Suitable:** The tool must be suitable for the area to be measured.
- **Comprehensive:** The tool must be able to evaluate all variables it examines.
- **Effective and reliable:** Tools should be pretested to be reliable and effective
- **Inexpensive:** Using this tool should not be too expensive.
- **Save time:** This tool should not be too cumbersome.

Principles of Test Design

- **Measure all instructional objectives:** Objectives communicated and taught to students.
  - Designed as operational controls to control learning and experience.
  - Synchronous with teacher's instructional objectives.
- Consistent with the teacher's teaching goals. Covers all learning tasks. Measures a representative portion of the learning task.
- Appropriate testing strategies or items.
  - Items assessing specific learning outcomes.
  - Area based measurements or tests.
- Enable the test and enable the test.
  Reliable: Reliable if it produces dependable, consistent, and accurate results.
  - Useful for measuring what it claims to measure.
  - Tests that are written clearly and clearly are more reliable.
  - Tests with significantly more items are more reliable than tests with fewer items is higher.
  - Well-planned tests cover a wide range of goals and objectives.
- **Use testing to improve learning:** Testing is not only an assessment, it is also a learning experience.
  - Scanning through test items helps teachers find items they forgot.
  - Discussion and clarification of the right choices to enable further learning.
  - Changed instructional practices with elaboration and revised explanation exam.

ASSESSMENT METHODS

Refers to the various methods and tools used to assess and document educational needs.

Definition

Evaluation methods define the nature of investigator behavior and include interviews and tests. A research methodology is the process of investigating, testing, observing, studying, or analyzing one or more evaluation objects (that is, specification mechanisms or activities).

Type

- Formative assessment techniques monitor student learning throughout the learning process. The collected feedback is used to identify areas where students are struggling, so teachers can adjust teaching and students can adjust their learning. These are lowstakes (that is, low scoring) assessments that are often taken early in the semester.
- Assess student learning using summative assessment techniques. These are high stakes assessments (i.e., high point values) given at the end of a lesson or course that measure how well students have achieved the desired learning outcomes.

Formative (Low Stakes) Evaluation
Informal Techniques

- **Reflections:** Also called "minutes" or "most obscure points," these common evaluation techniques are

used immediately after a learning opportunity. Prompt students to respond to reflect (e.g., at the end of a lesson or after completing an exercise) (classroom activity). Answer one or two basic questions such as:
- What is the most important thing you learned today?
- "What is important?" using the response system at school) or outside of class are collected. This can show not only the student's engagement with the material, but also misunderstandings and misunderstandings of prior knowledge.
- Checking for comprehension: By pausing every few minutes to check if the student is : embedded quiz) can also be useful for splitting and coordinating multiple quizzes. More digestible sips.
- Wrapper: A wrap-up activity with a series of reflective questions helps students develop skills to monitor their own learning and adjust as needed.
- Exam 5: Wrapper includes questions on preparation strategies, surprises, and remaining questions on learning objectives for the next unit. This helps students reflect on their study strategies to find out how best to prepare for future exams.
- Homework: The wrapper contains questions about the student's confidence in applying their knowledge and skills both before and after completing the task. This gives students immediate feedback on the correctness of their perception.
- Lectures: The wrapper contains opening lesson questions about what the student expects from the lesson and/or closing lesson questions about the main points of the lesson. By having students compare their own key points with the teacher's key points, students develop active listening skills and can identify key information.

Formal Techniques
- **Classroom activities:** When students work in pairs or small groups to solve problems, this creates space for effective peer learning and engaging class discussion. While students are working, teachers and TAs can roam the classroom, helping students who are stuck or pointing them in the wrong direction.
- **Quiz:** Assess a student's background knowledge, assess progress mid-unit, and create a friendly in-class competition briefing before testing. Quizzes are great tools that do not necessarily have to be based on student performance. Using quizzes at the beginning of each lesson is also a fun way to assess what students already know, clear up misunderstandings, and demonstrate how much they will learn.
- **Online assessments:** Many online learning modules have built-in assessments that allow students to solve problems and answer questions on the fly. This allows you to analyze student reactions and class performance, so you can customize lessons to meet individual learning needs.
- **Classwork outcomes:** Classroom activities are designed so that students, usually in groups, are asked to submit their work to the grade level. Of the various techniques that can be used, the most effective are balancing individual and group responsibilities and requiring students to think about genuine and complex problems. In team-based learning, he uses four criteria when designing collaborative application exercises.

Summary (High Stakes) Rating
- **Exams:** This includes midterm, final and end of course exams. The best tests include multiple types of questions, such as short-answer multiple-choice questions, true-false questions, and short essays, so students can fully demonstrate their knowledge.
- **Lectures, projects and presentations:** These give students the opportunity to delve deeper into the material to apply the knowledge they have learned or to create something new out of it. This level of application is a very important but often overlooked part of the learning process. Projects like this gives under performing students a chance to shine.
- **Portfolio:** Submitting a portfolio at the end of the course is a powerful way for students to track their progress. A good portfolio includes not only a student's semester accomplishments, but also reflections on their learning. Asking students to explain the concepts and techniques used in each piece, the themes covered, and the obstacles covered also brings a sense of completion to the learning process.

CHOOSING AN ASSESSMENT METHOD
The main objective is to choose the method that most effectively assesses the objectives of the unit of study. Furthermore, the choice of assessment method should be aligned with the overall goals of the program, whether it is the development of disciplinary skills (such as critical evaluation or problem-solving) or the development of professional competencies (such as specific communication and teamwork skills, etc.).
- Critical thinking and judgment (argument development, reflection, evaluation, judgment)
  - Essay
  - Report

- Journal
- Letter of recommendation to (on a matter of public health policy)
- File a lawsuit against an advocacy group
- Prepare a briefing for a committee for a specific meeting
- Book reviews (or articles) for specific magazines
- Writing newspaper articles for foreign newspapers
- Commenting on the theoretical aspects of articles
• Posed, problem definition, date analysis, experimental design, application of information
  - Problem scenario
  - Group Work
  - Work-related issues
  - Drafting a review board report
  - Drafting a research proposal with realistic challenges
  - Analyzing cases
  - Conference papers (or conference paper notes and annotated references).
• Performing procedures and demonstrating techniques (calculations, instrumental measurements, following laboratory procedures, following protocols, following instructions)
  - Demonstration
  - Role play
  - Video creation (script creation and video production/creation) video
  - Developing posters
  - Examination reports
  - Developing illustrated manuals on how to use the equipment for specific target groups
  - Observing actual or simulated professional practice
• Working collaboratively, working independently, learning independently, self-determining, managing time, managing tasks, organizing.
  - Journal
  - Portfolio
  - Study contract
  - Group worksource
    - Annotated references
    - Projects
    - Papers
    - Application tasks
• Demonstrate knowledge and understanding (remember, explain, report, retell, recognize, identify, relate, relate)
  - Written test
  - Oral test
  - Essay
  - Report
  - Make encyclopedia entries
  - Make A to Z.
- Write answers to customer questions
- Short-answer questions: True/false/multiple-choice questions (paper-based or computer-assisted assessment)
• Portfolio, performance, presentation, hypothesis and project
• Communication (one-way and two-way communication). Within groups, verbal, written and nonverbal communication. Discussion, explanation, assertion, interview, negotiation, presentation, specific written use).
  - Written presentation (essay report, reflection, etc.)
  - Oral presentation
  - Group work
  - Discussion/debate/role play
  - Participation in the "investigative court"
  - Presentation on camera
  - Observation of actual or simulated training.

TYPES OF TOOLS USED IN THE EVALUATION

Many tools and equipment are used in the evaluation process. Some tools are briefly described here.

Achievement Tests

- The most commonly used tool by teachers is achievement tests. An assessment approach should understand the term 'performance' in relation to instructional goals that lead to behavioral change.
- The same learning points could have been learned by different students at different levels.
- The teacher is interested in knowing each student's proficiency in each subject and assesses them against the given lesson objectives. A test aimed at this purpose is called a performance test.

Questionnaire

- The most commonly used assessment method is the paperbased questionnaire. This is generally self-administered and you complete the survey yourself and follow the instructions.
- Considered to be the most cost-effective assessment tool from an administrative perspective.
- When developing, teachers should ensure that it is simple, concise and clearly expressed. Questionnaire evaluations are quantitative.

Interviews

- Interviews are her second most important assessment method of asking questions of students participating in the assessment.

- Interviews are useful for obtaining quantitative and qualitative information. Interviews can be conducted in groups or individually.
- This is a lengthy process. Therefore, it should be designed according to the wishes of the interviewer and the interviewee.
- It can also be used to evaluate the program upon student acceptance, known as the final interview.
- The interview will be conducted in a quiet room and the information obtained will be treated confidentially. An interview guide can be created to provide objective guidelines for interviewers to follow.

Findings

- Observation is the direct visualization of an activity performed by a student. Knowing how many skills a student has mastered is very useful when evaluating student performance.
- Observations should be recorded at the same time if the delay could cause important points of the observation to be lost.
- Observation is subjective, but this can be overcome by developing objective criteria.
- Students should also be aware of standards so that they can prepare accordingly and control their anxiety levels. Teachers also need to be prepared to promote fair assessment.

Rating Scale

- A grading scale is another assessment tool that continuously measures student performance.
- The rating scale ensures the objectivity of the rating. Grades may then be awarded to students based on their performance on the grading scale.

Checklist

- A checklist is her two-dimensional tool for evaluating student behavior in terms of attendance or absence.
- Teachers can assess student performance using detailed checklists containing items and clearly defined and developed criteria.
- Checklists are an important tool for evaluating student performance in clinical areas.
- The sequence of steps taken to complete a step can be arranged in an order that makes it easier for the teacher to check if the required actions have been taken.
- This is an important tool used in both summative and formative assessments.

Attitude Scale

- The attitude scale measures how a student feels when answering a question.
- The Likert scale is the most common. Attitude scales contain a series of statements (usually 10–15) that reflect opinions about a particular topic.
- Participants (students) are asked how much they agree or disagree with the statement.
- A 5-point Likert scale is commonly used to assess student attitudes.
- Contains an equal number of positively and negatively formulated statements to avoid distortion of any kind.

Semantic Difference

- Another measure used to measure student attitudes is semantic difference. This tool includes bipolar scales (adjectives) such as good-bad, rich-poor, positive-negative and active-passive.
- The number of spaces between two adjectives is usually 5 or 7, so the number in the middle represents a neutral attitude.

Self-Report or Diary

- A self-report or diary is a narrative record in which students reflect their critical thinking after careful observation.
- It does not matter if it is a onetime order or a recurring order. Recurring tasks are stored in spiral notebooks and can be assessed daily, weekly, monthly or semester.
- Self-reports or diaries help improve existing programs or create new ones based on self-reports submitted by students.

Anecdotal Notes

- Anecdotal notes are that teachers keep about student performance and behavior during clinical experiences.
- This has proven to be a very valuable tool for both formative and summative assessment of student performance.
- It is maintained immediately after the event occurs. This is a continuous assessment and allows us to assess our students fairly. It is the teacher's duty to give feedback to the students.

EVALUATION METHODS

Tests, observations, interviews, case studies, sociometry and projection methods are the main evaluation methods in education. Of these tests, this is the most common one. Other techniques are described below:

Observation

- Continuously observing individuals and measuring various aspects of their behavior in relation to teachers is one of the most effective techniques for assessment.
- This behavior has relevant characteristics and should be recorded as objectively as possible.
- There are different types of observations, including controlled and uncontrolled observations, and observations by participants and non-participants.

Interview

- Here the teacher observes the child's behavior directly and tries to gather information orally.
- Here you can hear each other and understand each other's language.
- Questionnaire interviews help gather information. A diagnostic interview is conducted to understand the child's problem.
- Treatment interviews are used to plan appropriate treatment and counseling sessions are used to resolve individual educational or professional problems.

CASE STUDY

- The most reliable method of examining an individual child as a whole is the case study method.
- In this method, the teacher collects data related to the individual's socioeconomic status, family background, study habits, health and mental state, etc.
- Case studies attempt to use data collected from multiple sources. We then use a variety of methods to interpret the data in turn to study children's problems.

Sociometry

- This is a method developed by JL Moreno to assess social relationships between members of a social group. Helps teachers identify stars, isolates, and cliques.
- Orphans are people who have not been chosen by any organization, and cliques are small groups who have only close relationships with each other. A graphical representation of sociology is called a sociograph.

Projection Techniques

Abnormal cases in which behavior is often controlled by the unconscious are particularly susceptible to such direct techniques. In such cases, by unconsciously projecting the client's inner state, it is possible to provide a stimulus that prompts the client's reaction. Then you can interpret these answers. Examples: The Rorschach Inkblot Test, The Thematic Apperception Test (TAT) are examples of projection methods.

ASSESSMENT ISSUES

Lack of Time

- Nurse teachers often complain and apologize for lack of time because they do not assess students regularly.
- Time shortages can be caused by poor time management skills, so teachers should try to overcome this hurdle. However, if that is not manageable, outside consultants can be hired to ensure that the core activity of education is not jeopardized.
- Assessment should be considered as important as lectures and skill demonstrations to nursing students.

Lack of Skills to Conduct Assessments

- Some teachers may not be competent enough to plan and carry out assessment plans.
- These teachers must be nominated by the university director and corrective action must be taken. For those who need it, we can plan a refresher course during your tenure.

Errors in Measurement and Evaluation

- There are many sources of measurement errors. One of the main measurement errors is the respondents themselves. He may not be able to express his true feelings well.
- The style of operation of the knife and the appearance of the person measuring the phenomenon also contribute to errors that can distort the measurement process.
- Another factor that can contribute to measurement error is the context factor.
- Poor test quality and meter defects are another factor contributing to measurement errors.

ACHIEVEMENT TESTS

Achievement tests are an important school assessment tool and are very important in measuring student progress in the classroom and subject areas. Accurate performance data is critical for curriculum planning, teaching, and program evaluation.

For Administrator

- Tests can be used to assess how well educational goals are being achieved.
- Tests help classify school goals.
- The test identifies the type of learning experience that achieves these goals with the best possible results.
- Evaluate, revise and improve the curriculum based on these results.

- Identify background children in need and plan outreach activities for these students.
- We select excellent students to take special classes and courses.
- Determine proper student placement.
- To better understand students' needs and abilities.
- Selection of students with excellent grades or scholarships.
- Group the students within the class so that individual differences are as small as possible.
- It helps parents identify their child's strengths and weaknesses, focus their energy only on appropriate goals, and avoid placing excessive demands on their child.
- Judge the efficiency of one school in comparison to another.
- Determine the overall performance level of the class and assess the teaching effectiveness of the teacher. Class achievement can be assessed based on class performance at the beginning and end of the school year.

Teacher's Role

- The teacher learns about the general abilities of the students in the class.
- Based on the above, select the appropriate materials so that everyone can get the maximum benefit from teaching.
- Teachers identify and diagnose student weaknesses in various subjects.
- Teachers recognize good and underdeveloped children.
- He evaluates the group's progress on a particular subject over a particular period of time.
- Teachers determine whether students are performing to their maximum potential by reviewing student achievement and intelligence test results.

Performance Test Classification

Performance Test

- Oral exam.
- Written test (common test).

Written Exam

- Essay test.
- Objective testing performance testing can be categorized according to its function.

Proficiency Tests

- **Proficiency tests:** Proficiency tests measure the knowledge skills and other learning outcomes each student needs to master.
- **Poll tests:** Poll tests compare individual student scores to overall performance scores.
- **Diagnostic tests:** Diagnostic tests are designed to identify specific faults and performance deficiencies through subscores and responses to individual items. Helps identify specific faults.

STANDARDIZED TESTS

Tests and scales that meet the test criteria are called standardized tests.

Written exam: There are two types.
1. Common test.
2. A test made by the teacher open-ended type includes:
   - Essay type.
   - Short answer

Corrected answer

- Very short answer
- Lens type
  - Yes, no, true or false type
  - Multiple choice type
  - Suitable type
  - Transfer type.

Communication skills

- Direct observation
- Indirect observation.

Observation techniques: Observation techniques are systematic methods of recording student observations for assessment purposes. This category includes anecdotal notes, rating scales, and social measurement technique checklists.

SCHOOL PERFORMANCE TEST

Academic Performance

- Written exam
- Oral exam
- Practical exam
- Daily work
- Skill achievement.

Written Exams (Classroom Tests)

Written exams are the most commonly used type of assessment by teachers as they are used to develop administrative and assessment tests. However, it cannot measure all learning outcomes expected of students, and primarily only knowledge or intellectual areas.

Classroom testing: Classroom testing plays a central role in assessing student progress. The purpose of creating a class test is to develop a tool for evaluating student performance.

Principles of classroom testing—Von Groulund (1971) building:

- Test building procedures should consider the purpose of the test.
- The type of test you use depends on the specific learning outcome you want to measure. For example, knowledge sets principles.
- Test interviews should be based on a representative sample of course content and the specific learning outcomes being measured.
- Inter requires moderate difficulty.
- Interpretation should be constructed in such a way that external factors do not interfere with student responses.
- Exam tasks should be designed so that students can only answer them correctly if they achieve the desired learning outcomes.
- Tests should be structured to contribute to improving the teaching and learning process.

Steps to Create a Class Test

- Identify and define goals for desired behavior change and specify learning outcomes as the first step in assessment.
- Provides an overview of the content of the theme.
- Create a specification table that relates objectives to topic content.
- Create specific test questions according to the specification.

Common Drawbacks of the Written Exam

- **Obviousness:** It is important that all questions are important and useful.
- **Second error:** Question wording, especially multiple choice questions.
- **Evidence:** Examiner's preference for answers given alternative or correct answers.
- **Complicated instruments:** Make comprehension difficult, especially when using a non-native language.
- **Ambiguity:** Use of language that may result in spending more time understanding questions than answering them. It is said to be a vague question. As a result, students will give appropriate answers to the questions asked.
- **Collusion:** Students are expected to answer very difficult questions that even the brightest of students could answer.
- **Obsolescence:** Students are forced to answer using the examiner's outdated ideas, and this prejudice is often reinforced by traditional teaching methods.

Scoring the Answer Sheet

There are two ways to score the answer sheet—absolute rating and relative ranking.

1. **Absolute grading:** This is a grading system that gives students a grade for their response based on how well they meet the requirements of the example response, expressed as a percentage.
2. **Relative performance:** Grades tell students how their responses compare to others taking the same test by indicating whether the average is above or below average.

Grading System

- This system marks the answer sheets and assigns a number from 0 to 100 to indicate the percentage of grade achieved by the student.
- Candidate positions in lectures and university exams can be precisely defined in the scoring system, making it easy to identify top performers.

Advantages of Grading System

- In this system, a student is assessed and graded using her 5 or 7 scale pattern. Example: A plus A minus B plus B minus and C, etc.
- Excellent grades, based on criteria set by school teachers ranging from 10 to 100 O. 81-100 A plus - very good and so on.

Types of classroom tests: Classroom tests are generally of two types—objective type and essay type.

INTERPRETATION ITEMS

Interpretation exercises consist of a set of objective items, documents, tables, diagrams, graphs, maps and photographs. Students are presented with a shared dataset and are asked to identify relationships within the data to identify valid conclusions and evaluate assumptions and conclusions. Interpretation exercises measure complex performance (according to Groulund).

Helps assess higher levels of cognitive domains to apply principles and identify assumptions and conclusions.

Test Evaluation

After recording an objective test, you can evaluate the effectiveness of the test elements. The effectiveness of each item can be determined by analyzing student responses to that item. This is item analysis data that contributes to the overall improvement of classroom instruction by providing hints on classroom weaknesses and how to improve them.

Item Analysis Procedure

Item analysis: The teacher must determine the ranking. Work from highest score to lowest score. About a third of this work he divides into three groups, with the highest score being one-third and the lowest score being one-third depending on the rank of each test item. Tabulate the number of students in the upper and lower groups who selected each option. Estimate the difficulty of each item. Percentage of students who answered the item correctly. Respect the individuality of each element. This is the difference in the number of students who answered the question correctly in the upper group and the lower group.

CONCLUSION

From this chapter student can clearly understand about different assessment, evaluation methods and strategies, purposes, scope and principles in selection of assessment methods and types learn the barriers to evaluation and understand the guidelines to develop assessment tests.

REVIEW QUESTIONS

Long Essays

1. Define evaluation, explain the purposes and principles.
2. Describe teaching measurements function.
3. Define evaluation tools, explain the characteristics of evaluation tools.
4. Enumerate types of tools used in the evaluation.
5. Define achievement test, explain the types and role of teacher.

Short Essays

1. Scope of assessment and scope assessment.
2. Evaluation steps.
3. Rating features.
4. Steps in construction of test.
5. Selection of evaluation tools.
6. Principles of test design.
7. How to choosing an assessment method.
8. Evaluation methods.
9. School performance test.
10. Common drawbacks of the written exams.
11. Item analysis procedure.

Short Answers

1. Reliability.
2. Features of the assessment tool.
3. Test design.
4. Formative assessment.
5. Informal techniques.
6. Classroom activities.
7. Quiz.
8. Online assessments.
9. Portfolio.
10. Achievement tests.
11. Questionnaire.
12. Rating scale.
13. Checklist.
14. Attitude scale.
15. Semantic difference.
16. Self-report or diary.
17. Anecdotal notes.
18. Sociometry.
19. Projection techniques.
20. Assessment issues.

Chapter 14

Assessment of Knowledge

Learning Objectives
- Essay Type Test
- Short Answer Questions
- Multiple Choice Questions
- Objective Tests
- Matching Type

INTRODUCTION

Assessments play an important role in the learning and motivation process. The types of assessment tasks we ask of our students determine how they approach learning tasks and what learning behaviors they adopt.

Well-designed assessment methods provide valuable information about student learning. It tells us what our students learned, how well they did, and where they ran into difficulties. A good rating will allow you to answer question.

ESSAY TYPE TEST

Essay tests are one of the oldest types of tests, with a long history dating back over 4,000 years. Gilbert Sachs believes that "An essay test is a test containing questions that require the student to answer in writing." The essay test emphasizes recall rather than recognizing the correct choices. Essay tests may require relatively short or long answers. They are used so often that everyone seems to know what they mean.

Definition

An essay test is a test that requires students to write an answer, usually spanning multiple paragraphs.

Essay Test Features
- The length of responses required varies by grade and time.
- Subjective judgment required. Judging means making a judgment or evaluation, while subjective means not fair enough. It depends on the person.
- **Best known and most widespread:** Essays have become an important part of formal education. Middle school students are taught a structured essay format to improve their writing skills.

Basic Type Test Preparation Principles
- Do not ask too long questions.
- Avoid formulations, brief discussion.
- Questions should be well-structured, each addressing a specific purpose.
- Wording should be simple, clear and careful.
- Do not have too many choices.
- Elements should be selected based on the difficulty and complexity of the student.

Scoring Task
- For each question, strike through the items you think should appear in the answer scoring system.
- After grading all student responses to a question, proceed to grade another question.
- If more than one teacher scores the same test, they must agree on the scoring procedure and prepare an answer script before the test.
- The time allotted and grades awarded will serve as a guide for students to answer the questions.

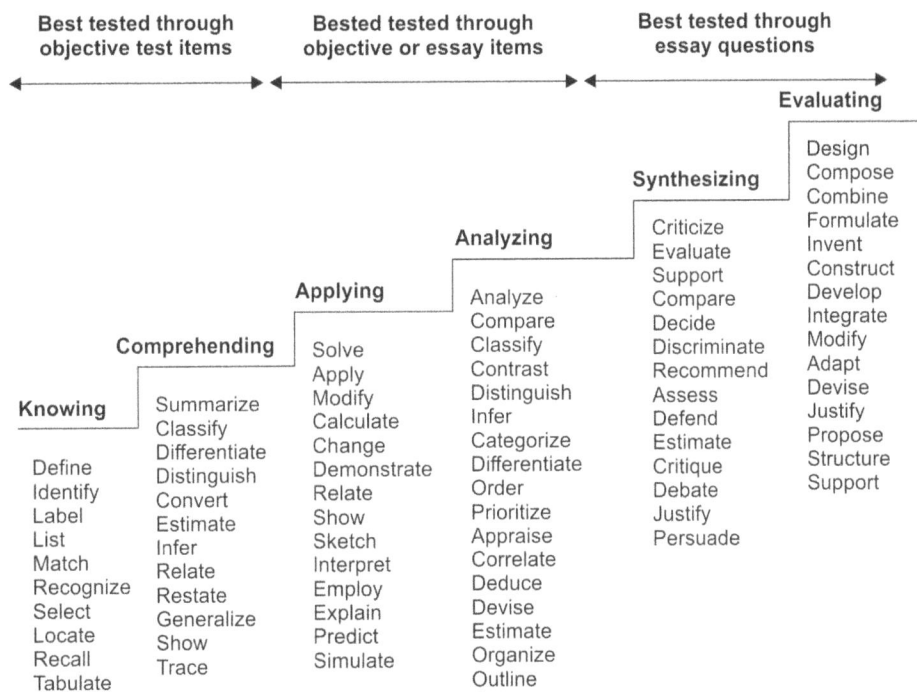

Fig. 14.1: Bloom's taxonomy for framing questions.

Questions with Limited Answers

- Restricted answer questions are usually restricted in both content and answers.
- Content is usually limited by the topic being discussed. Answer format limitations are usually stated in the question.

Extended Answer Question

- Expanded answer questions allow students to select factual information that they believe is relevant to order their responses using their best judgment, while synthesizing and evaluating ideas that they believe are relevant.
- This freedom gives you the ability to select, integrate and evaluate ideas.
- On the other hand, this freedom makes extended response questions inefficient in measuring more specific learning outcomes and creates assessment difficulties that greatly limit their use as a measurement tool.

Written Advantages

- It is relatively easier to create and administer.
- This is the only way to assess a candidate's ability to organize and present their thoughts in effective prose in a logical and coherent manner.
- Skills such as logical thinking, critical thinking, and systematic presentation are most valued in this type.
- Works well in virtually all subjects.
- It helps to encourage and develop study habits, such as writing summaries and organizing arguments for and against a topic.
- Grading the thesis exam takes relatively little time.
- This type eliminates guesswork.
- Freedom to react gives you the opportunity to free your mind and free your imagination.
- Gives test takers a wide range of latitude to answer and can measure student counter thinking.
- Spend less time typing, duplicating, and printing. You can write on the board even if the number of questions and the number of students are not so large.
- It is more economical to use essay tests than objective tests.
- It can measure complex learning outcomes that cannot be measured by other means.
- Emphasis is placed on the integration and application of thinking and problem-solving skills.
- Can be used as a tool to measure and improve a candidate's language skills.
- More useful for assessing the quality of the educational process.
- Students focus on learning general concepts and articulating relationships, comparisons and contrasts.

- Greater standards are set for teacher professional ethics, as more time is required for evaluation and evaluation.
- Less room for unfair means to be used.

Essay Type Disadvantages

- Essay questions generally test long-winded enumeration of memorized facts.
- Poor or limited selection of content, especially for advanced response types.
- Less effective and less reliable due to the following factors:
  - Limited content selection
  - Subjective evaluation
  - It is polluted by irrelevant factors such as spelling, good handwriting, colored ink, neatness, grammar, and length of answers.
  - Halo effect based judgment based on preimpression
  - Good language skills when there are no relevant points
  - Examiner mood
  - First impressions
  - Hours inappropriate comparison of bright and dull student responses
  - Ambiguous wording of questions.
- Inconsistent judgments even among competent examiners.
- Essay questions have a "halo" effect. This means that an examiner's judgment in assessing one trait is influenced by another trait. Well-behaved students are likely to get higher grades because of their behavior.
- Essay questions have a "carry over effect between questions". The student with the best answer at the beginning of the answer sheet is more likely to score more points on the next question and vice versa.
- The essay question is "Candidate". This means that certain students receive grades based not only on what they have written, but also on previous students' responses.
- Examiners may be influenced by the candidate's language. A candidate's handwriting, whether good or bad, can influence the examiner. The length of the answer, not the depth of content, can also affect the rating.
- Some examiners are too lenient in their evaluations, others too strict.
- In some cases, the examiner's mood also affects the assessment. An immediate happy event in the family at work may motivate the examiner to be more generous. Disputes within the family can result in poor grades being given.
- May not accurately represent test taker's understanding. Some students do well on exams by answering and writing in the same way.
- Writing exams for students and marking answer tables by teachers takes time for both examiners and candidates.
- Writing speed can affect student performance. Speed can cover the answers to all questions.

Misconceptions

- Assess higher order skills or critical thinking regardless of how it is written.
- Essay questions are easy to create.
- With essay questions, guessing problems are gone.
- Essay questions are useful for all students as they emphasize the importance of written communication skills.
- Essay questions encourage students to prepare more thoroughly.

Limitations of Essay Tests

- One of the main limitations of essay tests is that these tests do not allow a large content sample size.
- Such tests encourage selective reading and emphasize cramming.
- Additionally, scores can be affected by spelling, good handwriting, colored ink, cleanliness, grammar, length of answers, and more.
- Long answer questions have lower predictive value due to lower validity and reliability.
- Writing takes a lot of time from students. On the other hand, reading and judging essays is very time consuming and tedious.
- Assessments can only be done by teachers or qualified professionals.
- Inappropriate and vague language affects both students and values.
- A reviewer's mood affects the score of a response script.
- There is a biased judgment of the halo effect based on pre-impression.
- Scores can be influenced by personal prejudices and biases towards particular points of view, how the question is understood, the weighting of different aspects of the response, favoritism and nepotism.

SHORT ANSWER QUESTIONS

Short answer questions ask students directly and expect them to answer the question with words, sentences or numbers. Questions are expected to be answered quickly and should be formulated so that they can be expressed in a variety of ways. He accepts only one answer.

Definitions
- A short answer question (SAQ) is an open-ended question that requires the student to compose an answer rather than selecting from alternative answers.
- These are often used in exams to assess basic knowledge and understanding of a topic before more detailed assessment questions.

SQA Creation Principles
- Easy to create and manage.
- Create a task that requires an answer.
- Do not take descriptions directly from books and use them as the basis for short-answer questions.
- Express your answer in numerical units. Indicates that units are expected in the response.
- When using complementary elements, there should not be too many spaces.
- Create a space in the right margin or top of the survey to record your responses.
- The guidelines for answering each test item should be very clear.
- Each question weight should consist of written questions.

Mini Essay Question Type
- **Clear answers:** Use direct questions. For example: What is the function of a cell?
- **Draw a diagram:** Draw a diagram as instructed in the question.
- **Completion type:** In this case the student is given an incomplete sentence and asked to complete the answer by entering the correct word.

Short Answer Format
- Designed to help you remember specific names, facts, and basic knowledge.
- Focus the question so that there is a finite number (or only one) of possible correct answers to distinguish performance.
- Use the word element to make the required answer short and specific.
- When using complementary elements, there should not be too many spaces.
- Emphasize the underlined negative word or phrase when negative elements are used.
- Some applications capitalize or italicize *"did not."*
- They work best when there is no disagreement about acceptable answers.

How do you design a good answer question:
- Design short response items that provide a good assessment of learning objectives.
- Make sure your short answer questions assess knowledge that corresponds to your desired learning objectives.
- Formulate questions clearly in language appropriate to the student population.
- Make sure each question has only one correct answer.
- Make sure the item clearly states how to answer the question (e.g., ask the student to give a short answer and give a concise answer in a single word or short phrase). Are questions given a certain number of spaces for students to answer?)
- Consider whether item space placement facilitates efficient scoring.
- Rephrase the instructions clearly to specify the specifics of the knowledge and actions required.
- Be clear and precise with your question.
- Direct questions are better than questions that require complete sentences.
- For numeric responses, tell whether students will receive grades for presenting a piece of work (process-based) or for outcomes (product-based). The importance of units is also pointed out.
- Share with your students what your assessment style is. Is bullet point format acceptable or does it have to be in essay format?
- Prepare a textured marker sheet. Assign grades or partial grades for acceptable responses.
- Willing to accept other equally acceptable answers.

Benefits of Short Answer Tests
- Short answer tests are easy to create and manage. Short answer tests are essentially direct questions aimed at low cognitive ability. Based on knowledge and understanding. Evaluation of such tests is therefore relatively quick and easy.
- Candidates must present answers as required by an objective test and cannot select the correct answer from the choices given. So you cannot guess at all.
- Short answer tests cover a wide range of content and allow more questions to be included in the test/exam.
- Short answer exams minimize the impact of handwriting and spelling errors on your score.
- Short answer tests can be used as part of both formative and summative assessments. Traditional school and university exams generally use short questions. This will make the student more comfortable with the practice and reduce anxiety.

Disadvantages of Short Answer Exams
- Short answer tests are not suitable for measuring the complex learning outcomes of test takers.

- Short answer tests are not suitable for assessing candidates' analytical and reasoning abilities.
- Short answer exams are usually used to measure basic knowledge. This encourages candidates to memorize. Appropriate questions are required if raters want to use short answer questions to assess deeper learning.
- Time management can be a problem when answering shortanswer questions
- Tests with short answers can be difficult to score. If the question is not properly crafted, this will result in different answers to the same question.
- The examiner's handwriting and mechanics (accuracy of grammar and spelling) may affect the score.
- Short answer exams are primarily openended exams, where candidates are free to answer in their own way, so graders are not completely sure of the expected answers.

MULTIPLE CHOICE QUESTIONS

Multiple choice questions consist of a list of questions and suggested solutions. Problems can be formulated in the form of questions or incomplete statements called "item stems". Each question consists of his three parts. What matters is the correct answer or the alternative, and what gets in the way or the wrong answer. At least three options should be specified to reduce the chance of guessing. A question may require only one correct or best answer.

Definition

A multiple choice question consists of a stem, a correct answer, and a distraction. A stem is the beginning of an item, presenting it as a problem to be solved, a question, or an incomplete description that needs to be completed. The options are the possible answers you can choose, the correct answer is called the key and the wrong answer is called the distractor.

Example

Strain 1: Vitamins necessary for wound healing are.........
Intruder (wrong response)
- Vitamin A
- Vitamin B
- Vitamin C (correct)
- Vitamin D

Legend: Correct.

Components of Multiple Choice Questions

Multiple choice questions and answers are made up of several important parts.
- **Stem:** Stem is the main question or statement. The stem should be clear, simple and written in plain language.
- **Saboteurs:** Saboteurs are false choices intended to distract and challenge the respondent. You have to choose your distraction carefully so that it doesn't stand out too much.
- **Answer:** This is the correct answer to the tribe or question. In some cases, there may be more than one correct answer and the respondent may choose more than one answer.

Types of Multiple Choice Questions

There are two main types of questions: Single choice and multiple choice questions.
- Single choice multiple choice question
- Multiple choice question
- Drop down menu for multiple choice question
- Multiple choice with star ratings
- Multiple choice with text slider
- Multiple choice with number slider
- Multiple choice with thumb up/down
- Multiple choice with matrix table
- Ranking multiple choice questions
- Image-based multiple choice questions
- Simple choice multiple choice questions

How do I write good multiple choice questions?

Article authors should consider the following suggestions and guidelines when writing good multiple choice articles:
- Stems must be clearly worded and presented in the form of direct questions.
- Do not use spaces at the beginning or between sentences of multiple choice completion elements.
- Remove superfluous, irrelevant information from stems.
- Include words in the stem that can be repeated in each choice.
- Use negative stems only when significant learning outcomes are expected.
- Make all distractions believable and equally engaging.
- Ensure that all alternate characters are approximately the same length. The relative length of the choices should not indicate the answer.
- Unless you are using a partial credit score, make sure each multiple choice item has only one correct or best answer.
- Remove the hint from the answer. Word associations, grammatical discrepancies, or connections between stems and answers. Make all options in the structure grammatically parallel and avoid repeating words that occur within the stem.
- Minimize the use of "all of this" and "none of this" as options.

MCQ Tips

- Use simple sentence structure and precise wording
- Make all choices plausible
- Make all possible answers the same length
- Avoid double negatives
- Make the number of choices consistent
- Please do not deceive test takers. They should test knowledge, not reading comprehension.
- Get the correct answers out of order (to test your knowledge).

Advantages

- High quality and workability.
- Effectively measure learning outcomes.
- Objective tests are more reliable.
- No ambiguity or ambiguity.
- Computer correction saves teachers time.
- Consists of multiple questions and may be used from time to time.

Limitations

- MCQ creation takes a long time.
- Higher intellectual abilities are difficult to test.
- MCQs are limited to language level learning outcomes, but cannot determine how students will behave in real-world situations.
- Not suitable for measuring ability to organize and present ideas.
- Writing good multiple choice questions requires some experience.
- It is hard to find enough false but plausible distractions.

MCQ Components

- An MCQ consists of a base or stem enabled by a series of four or five suggested answers or alternatives.
- A stem consists primarily of statement questions, case studies, situational diagrams, diagrams or photographs.
- Suggested answers that are not a single correct answer or alternative are called distractors. These fake alternatives get their name from their intended function.
- The key is correct.

Guidelines for Creating MCQs

- Item roots should be self-explanatory and avoid inherent problems.
- Articles should contain relevant content and no irrelevant content. The entire alternative must grammatically match the stem of item.
- The item must contain exactly one correct answer.
- All distractions that fail the learning outcome should be removed from the correct answers.
- In a well-constructed MCQ, each disaster is chosen by the student, and if the distraction is not picked by someone, it is not eliminated.
- For each item, enter a space for the number or letter of your answer.
- Do not use MCQ items when other item types are more appropriate. Correct answers must appear in approximately the same number of items in random order in each alternate part.
- If you use more than one type of MCQ in your paper, you can group them.
- Use statements inside elements. If repeated information is used within an element, it should be underlined.

OBJECTIVE TESTS

Objective tests are tests in which there is only one fixed correct answer. Candidates write an answer or select an answer from the choices given. In other words, an objective test is one that is scored by the examiner in a way that leaves no room for subjective judgment. Answers to objective test items are either true or false and do not require interpretation or judgment on the part of the evaluator as is required in subjective tests such as essays. Also called novel test or limited response test.

Objective Test Meaning

- Objective questions are highly structured and require students to select the correct answer from a limited number of choices.
- Students must demonstrate the specific knowledge, understanding, or ability required for the subject.
- This allows for fast, easy, accurate and objective assessments.
- Covers a wide range of topics and may contain details on the topic.
- Ratings do not contain personal opinions, which makes them more reliable.
- They are effective testing tools because they save time and provide more reliable, valid, unbiased and meaningful results.
- The evaluation can be easily done by machine or computer.

Benefits of Objective Testing

- Objective task grading is more objective than essay task grading. Ratings do not change from time to time or from examiner to examiner. Such tasks are free of personal bias and the examiner's mood does not affect the grade.

- Objective testing provides highly reliable test results. Plus, it is quick and easy to score.
- Objective test assessments are performed using answer keys. Evaluation of objective type tests can be both electronic evaluation by machines and manual by humans.
- Objective tests are more comprehensive. It can cover a large amount of content. Therefore, a teacher can cover a large number of course materials with her one test.
- An objective test eliminates superfluous (irrelevant) factors such as speed of writing, fluency of expression, style of writing, good handwriting and cleanliness.
- Objective tests can be standardized by applying them to a large number of students of the same age group before the actual test. Results from this standardized test can be used to compare a student's performance with that of other students of the same age and grade.

Disadvantages of Objective Tests

- Objective tests (especially good questions) take time to create. Configuring objective test items is difficult, but very easy to answer. Multiple choice tasks make it difficult to prepare good decisions and choices. However, matching items take longer to answer than other target items.
- All objective test items have an option to guess. For items with alternative responses, the estimated range can increase to 50%.
- Some form of cheating is possible in any objective test if the supervisor is lenient. Candidates can easily answer many questions correctly by cheating.
- Objective exams limit the number of candidates. The examiner must select an answer from a list of choices. Candidates do not have the opportunity to prove their ability to express their ideas and thoughts.
- It is often said that objective tests cannot verify stuffing. Candidates concentrate on memorization work even if they do not understand.
- Objective type testing results can be misleading if elements are not properly standardized. Many respondents may have received the same score.

Goal Type Test

All goal elements can be divided into her two broad categories: Constituent elements and choice elements.

Constructed Item (Recall Item)

This format requires candidates to provide a one word response or a complete statement. Construct type items can be expressed in two ways in the form of direct questions or partial sentences. Both formats are almost similar, but display differently.

- **Very short answer elements:** Very short answer elements are given in question form and the candidate provides the correct answer in the form of her single word numbers or phrases.
- **Completion task:** The completion task requires the candidate to enter an answer (in one or two words) to complete the statement. This is also called "blank padding".
- **Correction task:** This form asks the candidate to correct the task by providing the correct answer. The wrong part of the item is usually underlined, colored, or written in italics, and the candidate must replace it with the correct answer.

Choice Items (Cognitive Items)

Another important category of objective items are multiple choice items in which the test taker selects the correct answer from a number of given choices or alternatives. Contains items that match multiple choice choices.

- **Alternate response items:** Alternate response items are items from which the test taker must select the answer they believe is correct. For simpler alternative response items, two responses are provided for one item and the test taker must choose between these two:
- Statements are expressed in the form of declarative statements that are either entirely true or entirely false. For example, essay tests measure a student's higher cognitive abilities (true/false).
- **Yes/No:** This is a form of objective factor expressed in the form of a question. For example, are you apprenticing to a good job? (Yes/No)
- **True-false:** The objective element of this form is labeled as true or false depending on whether the statement is true or false Expressed in the form of simple sentences. For example, the sun revolves around the earth (Yes/Wrong).

Classification of Objective Type Tests

S. No.	Supply type	Selection type
1.	Short answer	True or false (alternative response type)
2.	Completed type	Matching type Multiple choice Interpretive items (complex achievement)

Supply Type

Short Answer Type

1. Who is the father of our nation? (Mahatma Gandhi).
2. Who was the first prime minister on India? (Pandit Jawaharlal Nehru).

Completion Type

Example:

The formula for ordinary common salts is ----------- (Nall).

Choice Type

True or false (alternative response item).

Example—indicates whether the following statements are true or false.

Water boils at 120°C—these determine whether the learner is true or false, true or false, true or false, true or false, yes or no, fact or opinion, agree or disagree. It is a description that must be judged. There are only two possible answers from the ground at once.

Uses

- Measures the ability to check the accuracy of statements of fact, definitions of terms, etc.
- Measures the student's ability to distinguish principles.

Restrictions: Limited to more basic learning outcomes in knowledge domains.

MATCHING TYPE

A matching exercise consists of two parallel columns, with each word number or symbol matched to a sentence or phase in the other column. Items in the column for which a match is sought are called premises, and items in the column where the selection is made are called answers (ground).

A matching question consists of two consecutive lists of related words, phrases, pictures, or symbols. Each item in one list is paired with at least one item in the other list. Matching can be viewed as a variant of multiple choice where more than one choice is correct.

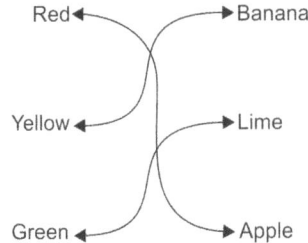

Fig. 14.2: Matching types questions.

Matching Question Characteristics

- Used to identify relationships and make associations.
- Can be used for a wide range of topics.
- Conforms to:
  - Terms and definitions
  - Symbols and names
  - Questions with answers
  - Part with function
  - Method with operation
  - Principles with situations in which they apply.
- Good matching items can easily be converted to multiple choice items
- The premises and answers should be uniform.

To Create a Matching Item

- Hold the matching test item and place the short answer to the right.
- Shorten the list for consistency. A quick test also helps students read long premises and quickly review a list of answers.
- Place all elements of the matching question on the same page.
- When writing matching items, the number of choices should always be greater than the number of statements to reduce guesswork.
- Students should identify matching pairs of items based on their meaning.

Advantages

These questions are easy to create.
- Easy to write.
- Easy to score.
- Effective in assessing definitions and relationships.
- A space-saving, objective, and compact way to assess learning objectives.
- Can be developed for use with images, maps, graphics, etc.

Disadvantages/Limitations

Item matching is limited to measuring factual information based on simple associations, the ability to perceive relationships between two things, and facilitate memorization.
- It is not well suited for assessing higher order thinking. It does not measure interpretation, judgment or application of any kind.
- A correct match may indicate a guess rather than an understanding (make sure there are more definitions than elements to eliminate this).
- If the list contains the same number of choices, the last choice may be given.
- Students can answer these exercises by memorization, especially since typical matching questions involve the

assessment of everyday associations such as names and dates.
- Creating uniform assumptions and answers can be difficult.

Examples

S. No.	Column A	Column B
1.	Citrus fruits are rich sources per this vitamin	Vitamin A
2.	Fish and cold liver oil are the source	Vitamin B
3.	Seen in yellow fruits and vegetables like papaya, carrots	Vitamin C
4.	Found in parboiled rice	Vitamin K
5.	Helps in clotting of blood	Vitamin B_{12}

General Principles

- Terms used should be clearly stated.
- More choices are listed in the right column.
- Terms within a column should not refer to answers for aspects of other columns.
- Each item in the right column can be used multiple times in an answer.
- Keep the list and answers relatively short.
- Provide clear guidance explaining the intended basis for observations.
- Alphabetize both answers so as not to imply the answer.
- If the answers are of numerical quality or quantity, rank them from lowest to highest.
- Use long and short sentences in your answers.
- Choose uniform promises and responses for each matching cluster.

How Do I Write Good Articles

Item authors should consider the following suggestions and guidelines when writing good matching items.
- The number of alternative answers should be greater than the number of stems in each matching exercise. This is done to reduce the chance of guessing through the erasing process.
- The basis on which the comparison is made must be clearly stated or specified. Here, for example, Listing I shows author names and Listing II shows book titles. Match the author's name with the title of the book.
- All elements of one matching exercise must be on the same page. Otherwise, matching will be difficult.
- Only homogeneous or related materials should be used in each exercise.
- The types of stems and the number of possible answers should not be too short or too long.
- Figures can also be used for comparison. Avoid grammatical or other clues in the correct answer.

CONCLUSION

From this chapter student will understand how to prepare multiple choice question, essay type questions, short answers and matching types how to set the questions, advantages and disadvantages to learn how to assess the gained knowledge.

REVIEW QUESTIONS

Long Essays

1. Define essay type test, explain the features and preparing procedures.
2. Define short answer questions, explain creation principles.
3. Define multiple choice questions, explain the components and types of MCQs with examples.
4. Define objective tests, explain goals and disadvantages of objective test.
5. Define matching the types, explain create a matching item.

Short Essays

1. Bloom's taxonomy for framing questions.
2. Essay type disadvantages.
3. Limitations of essay tests.
4. Short answer format.
5. Benefits of short answer tests.
6. Guidelines for creating MCQs.
7. MCQs advantages and disadvantages.
8. General principles of matching items.

Short Answers
1. Extended answer question.
2. Written advantages.
3. Mini essay question type.
4. Disadvantages of short answer exams.
5. MCQs components.
6. Classification of objective type tests.
7. Completion type.
8. Short answer type.

Chapter 15

Assessment of Skills

Learning Objectives

- Clinical Evaluation
- Objective Structured Clinical Examination
- Observation
- Checklists, Rating Scale, Videotape
- Written Communication
- Progress Notes
- Care Plan
- Process Record
- Written Assignments
- Oral Test (Viva)
- Practical Exam
- Simulation
- Objectively Structured Clinical Examinations
- Anecdotal Notes
- Performance Evaluation in Nursing Self-assessment
- Clinical Portfolio
- Clinical Log

INTRODUCTION

Competence evaluation is the performance of a competency under the conditions specified in the standard, compared to the actual performance of the competence against the specified standard, to assess whether performance meets or exceeds the requirements. Evaluation of skills should adhere to the four principles of effectiveness, reliability, fairness and flexibility. Assessment uses a variety of tools and techniques to gather information about student learning progress. It is a systematic process of analyzing and interpreting student performance and progress in educational and noneducational areas with the aim of providing a basis for improvement.

DEFINITIONS

- Proficiency assessment definitions are tests designed to assess an individual's competence in a particular skill or set of skills. Competency tests ask you to demonstrate your knowledge of a specific topic or issue. Then compare this to what you should know based on relevant guidelines.
- Skills assessment is the process of gathering data that evaluates individuals against specific criteria to learn more about their abilities and abilities to perform various skills.

CLINICAL EVALUATION

A clinical evaluation is an examination of a person's body for disease or injury and a review of the person's laboratory test results.

Definition

Clinical evaluation is the evaluation and analysis of clinical data using science-based methods to determine the safe clinical performance and/or efficacy of a medical device when used as intended by the manufacturer. A series of ongoing activities that validate.

Concept of Clinical Assessment

- Knowledge is tested in theoretical tests and skills are assessed in clinical or practical tests.

- Various methods of assessing student nursing skills include traditional or traditional practical exams, case studies, observational checklists, viva voce, OSCE rating scales, etc.
- None of these methods can independently assess student performance with great validity, objectivity, or reliability.
- A meaningful combination of these methods is absolutely necessary for overall competence assessment.

Clinical Evaluation Criteria

Communication

- Build relationships with clients and other key people.
- Use therapeutic communication skills when dealing with clients and other important people.
- Determine the relevance and accuracy of oral and written communications.
- Report and document progress towards assessment interventions and client outcomes.
- Determine which communication channels drive the most positive customer outcomes.
- Use information technology to develop personalized care plans.
- Present a case study at a clinical meeting.

Collaboration

- Build relationships with healthcare teams to achieve positive outcomes for clients.
- Collaborates with client key figures and members of the medical team to provide a protective, supportive and corrective environment for clients with altered survival and functional needs.
- Analyze critical thinking behavior in making decisions about customer care.
- Work with members of the medical team to help manage customer care.
- Use problemsolving techniques to create an environment in which you can achieve positive results for your customers.

Rating

- Integrate knowledge and skills gained from communication arts, information technology, social and life sciences, and previous nursing courses.
- Identify clinical manifestations associated with complex changes in survival and functional needs.
- Assess the client's mental health by taking a medical history and performing a physical examination.
- Collect developmental, social, cultural and spiritual assessment data from referral clients with complex changes in survival and functional needs.
- Determine customer's ability to utilize available community resources.

Clinical Decision-making

- Use assessment data to plan care for clients with complex and changing survival and functional needs.
- Create nursing diagnoses based on the NANDA classification for clients with complex changes in survival and functional needs.
- Identify outcome criteria for clients with complex changes in survival and functional needs.
- Use critical thinking skills to prioritize care plans for clients whose integration needs have changed.
- Apply evidence-based practice concepts to planning nursing interventions to promote a protective, supportive, or corrective environment for clients with complex changes in survival and functional needs.
- Identify clinical judgments and management decisions to ensure safe care.
- Integrate cultural, social and spiritual values into healthcare plans for clients with complex changes related to survival and functional needs.
- Evaluate client outcome criteria.

Care Interventions

- Implement client-centered care for clients with complex and changing survival and functional needs.
- Show compassionate behavior when dealing with clients.
- Demonstrate the ability to implement technical skills for clients with complex and changing survival and functional needs.
- Meets standards for safe drug delivery.
- Discuss the importance of achieving JCAHO's National Patient Safety Goals when caring for clients-teaching and learning.
- Determine your customer's willingness to learn.
- Design curricula containing desired learning outcomes specifically tailored for clients with complex and changing survival and functional needs.
- Implement the curriculum under supervision.
- Involve family members and loved ones in the lesson plan.
- Evaluate the learning success of clients and key personnel based on the fulfillment of outcome criteria.
- Revise the curriculum based on the evaluation of the results.

Professional Conduct

- Practice under the New York State Nurses Practice Act.
- Observe the spirit III Bill of rights.

- Demonstrate responsibility for the care provided.
- Get proper guidance from your instructor and health team member.
- Identify legal and ethical responsibilities in providing care.
- Maintain client confidentiality and privacy.
- Report unsafe behavior to appropriate personnel.
- Dress appropriately and arrive at the hospital area on time.
- Satisfies the written test criteria.
- Submit your written assignment by the deadline.
- Assess your nursing skills and knowledge.

Care Management

- Adapt customer care delivery to changing healthcare environments and management systems.
- Prioritize care when assigned to multiple clients.
- Identify opportunities to coordinate implementation of individualized care plans.
- Arrange appropriate referrals based on evaluation and diagnosis.
- Discuss available resources and services with customers and other important people.
- Select nursing strategies to ensure cost-effective nursing care.
- Recognize the value of using quality improvement measures in the clinical setting.

Type of Clinical Evaluation

Case Study/Presentation

- Students, with the help of a clinical supervisor, select one of the patients for a focus study that they find interesting.
- Through learning counseling and experimentation, students solve problems and determine care strategies that meet patient needs.
- Students should be given the opportunity to care for patients over the long term, understand patient behavior, gain confidence, and recognize the effectiveness of care interventions.
- Students will learn to recognize the impact of personal and social factors on illness and recovery, organize information, and identify problems.
- Students will also learn about problemsolving approaches in nursing. The report will serve as a reference for other students.
- Finally, students can present their papers in front of the group. The report should be evaluated for content organization, clarity of thought, presentation skills, and interest.
- Oral presentations help students speak in front of groups.

Traditional or Traditional Practical Examination

- This system in nursing usually describes detailed procedures or processes of nursing for one or two patients and then requires students to demonstrate their nursing performance to the patient. It involves observing.
- Observing student performance in a clinical setting is the most commonly used assessment method in the medical field.
- Used to assess all three areas of her including knowledge, attitudes and relationships as well as competence.

Benefits

Practical exams provide an opportunity to assess the skills and abilities that students have acquired.
- Practical exams provide examiners with an opportunity to assess the student's use of articulated knowledge in an integrated manner while providing comprehensive care to the patient.
- Evaluators are given the opportunity to assess the student's communication and interpersonal skills as well as their clinical competence in carrying out the nursing process.

Cons

- Practical exams are not considered standardized assessment practices when assessing students while working with patients.
- Not considered an objective evaluation method. It may contain subjectivity and prejudice.
- Time consuming process.
- Not considered a practical method for assessing large groups of students.
- It may be considered unethical to expose a patient for examination by a student.
- Emergencies and complex station processes can interfere with the smooth conduct of the practical exam.

Observation Checklist

- The observation checklist is the most commonly used performance evaluation tool.
- This is an approach to monitor the performance of specific skills, behaviors, or dispositions of individual students.
- How to record whether a feature exists or an action has been performed.
- This is simply a list of actor actions related to a particular nursing intervention in space, allowing the rater to confirm or check whether that particular action occurred.
- Examples of writing skills, speaking skills, action-based skills, and procedural skills.

Advantages

- Allows comparison between individuals.
- Provides an easy way to record observations.
- Adaptable to each subject area.
- Checklists help you assess anticipated learning activities.
- Helps evaluate process work.
- Properly constructed checklists allow observers to limit direct observation.
- Be objective when evaluating traits.
- Helps evaluate processes that are divided into a series of actions.
- Reduce the possibility of errors.

Cons

- Checklists are of limited usefulness because they do not indicate quality of service.
- Allows only a limited assessment of overall clinical performance.
- You can only assess the presence or absence of postural movements and performance parameters, but you can also assess the degree of correctness of the performance.
- Limited use for qualitative observations.
- Preparation is not easy.

Rating Scale

- Rating is a term used to express an opinion or judgment about the performance of a person, object, situation, or character.
- Rating scales contain qualitative descriptions of a limited number of aspects of things or characteristics of a person.
- When using rating scales, you rate objects in absolute terms against certain criteria.
- You can use a 3-, 5-, or 7-point rating scale.
- For example, a student's overall performance in oral care treatment—excellent, very good, good, bad, average.

Advantages

Easy to manage and evaluate measured attributes.
- Widely applicable to the evaluation of nursing education.
- Graphical rating scales are easy and fast to create.
- Rating scales are easy to use for large groups.
- Also used for quantitative methods.
- Also used to assess interests, attitudes and personal characteristics.
- Customizable and flexible assessment tool.

Cons

- It is difficult or dangerous to determine ratings for different aspects of a person.
- May lose objectivity if misused.
- Subjective assessments can occur, making the scale unscientific and unreliable.

Rigolosum/Oral Exam

- Rigolosum is an integral part of the traditional practical exam.
- Oral exams are designed to assess a student's specific qualities, such as depth of knowledge, attitude, self-confidence, ability to work under stress, and professional competence.
- The focus of the oral exam should be on testing the student's problem-solving skills, ability to develop rational responses, and to make decisions quickly. Do not put too much emphasis on remembering facts during the exam.
- Viva voce also provides an opportunity to clarify incorrect answers.

Benefits

Direct contact with candidates to assess communication presentation skills and overall impression.
- Provide the ability to mitigate the account situation.
- Allows flexible movement of candidates from strengths to weaknesses.
- Possibility of simultaneous assessment by two or more examiners.

Cons

- Costly in terms of professional time.
- Suffers from the undue influence of extraneous factors.
- Favoritism is allowed and cannot be used for future reference.
- Lack of standardization and objectivity.

OBJECTIVE STRUCTURED CLINICAL EXAMINATION (OSCE)

- Objectively structured laboratory testing is a modern type of testing widely used in various specialties, including nursing.
- Designed to test the performance of clinical skills such as communication, laboratory testing, medical or nursing procedures in clinical areas where students are asked to perform specific tasks on patients and assessed by an examiner.
- Usually consists of 8 to 12 short stations, in which candidates move around these stations in a prescribed manner, spend a specified amount of time (5–10 minutes) to complete the task, move to next station.

- There are two types of stations. Treatment stations and response stations at treatment stations, students are required to perform a random task (taking a medical history), which is observed and scored by an examiner.
- In the answer room, students write answers to questions on answer sheets.

Advantages

- More meaningful than traditional clinical laboratory approaches
- Allows researchers to decide in advance what to test.
- Reviewers have better control over content and complexity.
- You can shift the emphasis from testing factual knowledge to testing a broad range of skills, including advanced clinical skills.

Cons

- Students' knowledge and skills are tested in subjects, but not their ability to see things holistically and patiently.
- Challenges for inspectors and patients.
- Not always able to maintain consistent difficulty.
- Examiners should pay close attention to students who repeat the same task multiple times.
- Exams take longer to prepare than traditional exams.

OBSERVATION

Many complex psychomotor skills also involve a student's cognitive and emotional abilities. Skills observations often refer to assessment goals as competencies in health professionals, where students progress from novice to expert over the course of the program. One framework for assessing skills and competencies, known as the Mirror Pyramid, provides examples of constructively calibrated assessments for each level.

Ability Observation Assessment Benefit

- Enable students to be assessed against real, contextual assignments.
- Allow students to give immediate feedback.
- Identify specific areas where the student excels and needs improvement.

Skill Observation Assessment Challenge

- Can be time consuming to administer.
- Can be resource intensive if multiple reviewers are required.
- It should be noted that timed exams generally create more stress independent of a student's mastery of the material.

Principles

- Understand the need and purpose of the exam.
- Make sure it is appropriate for children the process makes sense.
- Consider ethical issues.
- Validate the results.
- Use proper observational methods.
- Consider the timing of your observations, morning to afternoon, Monday to Friday, as your child may behave differently in different situations.
- Ensure that there are sufficient staff to assist observers if additional liability relief is required.
- Clarify what the result will be?

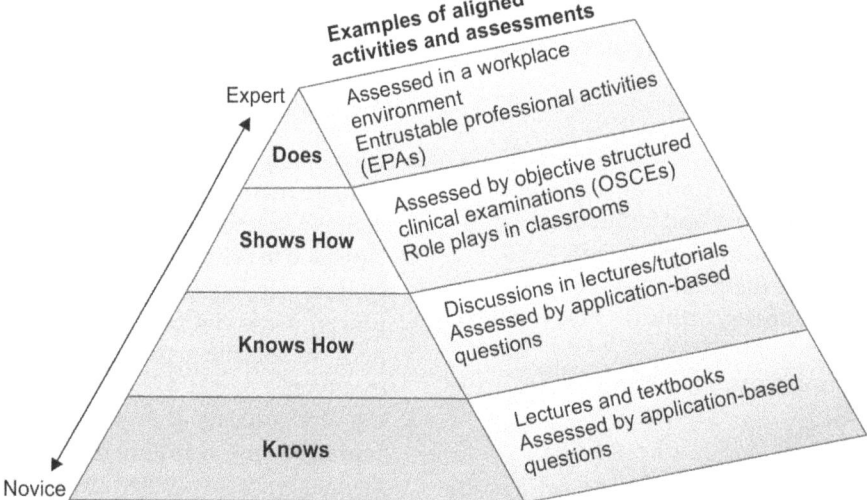

Fig. 15.1: Ability observation assessment.

Procedure

- Determine need and purpose.
- Plan the process.
- Clarify ethical issues.
- Start the evaluation
- Think about the results.
- Use the results to decide how to proceed.
- Adjust your plans accordingly.
- Monitor progress.

Create Skills Observational Assessments

- Make assessments in simulations, role plays, case studies, standardized patients, or ideally real-world clinical settings as authentic as possible.
- Create a checklist or rubric and share it with your students ahead of time to ensure your standards are clear to them.
- Recognize that cognitive and implicit biases and impression formation can influence the inferences made during observation.
- Observe skills over time, if possible, to allow learners to integrate feedback.
- Add descriptive comments in addition to the quantitative rating.
- Whenever possible, use existing validated tools rather than creating new tools for observation.
- When using multiple observers, use common criteria and train the observers in making observations.

Student Preparation

- Clarify goals, expectations, criteria and outcomes of the assessment in advance.
- Use formative skill observation activities to provide opportunities for practice with feedback.
- Create a culture that encourages learners to practice authentically and welcomes feedback.
- Have students practice using the assessment checklist or rubric and consider giving each other feedback.

Performance Observation Assessment

- Give students clear instructions about the criteria for evaluation.
- Focus feedback on observable behavior.
- Observe the student without interrupting the encounter.
- Give feedback on student performance as soon as possible.
- If multiple observers are used, provide standardization information and training so that observers can use the same standards.

Skills Observation Test Scoring

- Create and use a checklist or rubric to give to students in advance.
- Frame feedback with future direction. Instead of indicating that the student is not proficient in the skill, it indicates that the student is not yet proficient.
- Consider the possibility of allowing full or partial unit retesting.
- Recognize that the formation of cognitive and implicit biases during observation can influence conclusions.

CHECKLISTS

Checklists are lists of behavioral characteristics, achievements in a particular field or practice, or descriptions of the deliverables or works of art of achievements.

Checklist Procedure (by Groulund)

- Identify and articulate each desired action within the performance.
- Add actions that represent common errors to the list if they are limited in number and can be clearly identified.
- List the required actions and possible errors in the approximate order in which they are expected to occur.
- Provides an easy way to number actions sequentially and see each action in action.

Advantages

- Easy to evaluate
- Increased content effectiveness.

Cons

- Time consuming
- Recognized need for training
- Individual checklist required for each candidate.

RATING SCALE

Rating is the measurement of properties of an object or person through judgments on a continuum. For example: Grades or grades. Performance evaluation of employees within the organization. A rating scale is a device for systematically recording an observer's judgment of quality or the extent to which an imprint is present, and should indicate how strongly or to what extent the property is imprinted.

Definition

- Evaluation is a term used to express an opinion or judgment about a particular situation. Opinions are usually expressed based on values.

- A rating scale is a tool used to qualify a judgment or analyze an opinion about a trait. A rating scale is a tool for one person to simply check another person's level of achievement.

Principles of Effective Assessment (from Groulund)
- Only learning outcomes that can be clearly assessed and reported should be matched against the rating scale.
- The property evaluated must be directly observable.
- Features and points on the scale must be clearly defined.
- Reviewers should refrain from reviewing if they feel they are not qualified to do so.
- Reviews from multiple observers should be combined where possible.

Rating Scale Quality
- Transparency
- Trust
- Accuracy
- Versatility
- Objectivity
- Uniqueness.

The sociometric method is a method of assessing the social relationships that exist within a group.
- Each member of the group is asked to identify someone they would like to collaborate within a group work or group situation, or who they would like to pick as a leader with certain qualities.
- The number of choices given to each person serves as an indicator of this social acceptability. Analysis of social measurements provides information on leadership potential, social adaptation and personality traits.
- Social metrics are particularly useful for modeling personality triads.

Rating Scale Type

Numeric rating scale or NRS
- Numeric scales use numbers to identify items on the scale. However, not all numeric values need to be assigned attributes.
- For example, you can ask your audience to rate your product on a scale of 1 to 5. You can enter 1 as "completely dissatisfied" and 5 as "completely satisfied".

Verbal rating scale or VRS
- Verbal rating scale is used to rate pain. Also known as the verbal pain score and verbal descriptor scale, the scale is a compilation of a series of descriptions that describe the intensity and duration of pain.
- For example, when you go to the dentist and are asked how bad your tooth pain is. A scale is then displayed with items such as none, low, moderate, severe, and very severe.

Visual analog scale (VAS) or slider scale
- The idea behind VAS is to allow the viewer to choose any value from the scale between her two endpoints. In scales, only endpoints have attributes associated with numeric values, the rest of the scale is blank.
- Often simply called sliders, viewers can rate what they like without being limited to a particular attribute or rank.
- For example, a scale rating from "very easy" to "very difficult" with no other value specified on the scale.

Likert scales
- Likert scales are useful tools for effective market research to obtain feedback on various psychometric characteristics. Agree/disagree scales are particularly useful for gathering likelihood information such as frequency, grade, and quality.
- The Likert scale is a good tool, for example, to assess employee satisfaction with company policies.

Graphic rating scale
- Imagine using images such as stars or smileys instead of numbers to ask your customers or viewers to rate you.
- Stars and smileys can generate the same values as numbers.

Description scale
- Numerical scales may not be very useful for certain surveys or studies. The descriptive scale explains each option to the respondent.
- Contains detailed commentary for insightful information gathering.

Advantages
- Easy to administer
- Easy to assess
- Can be used for large groups of students
- Broad application
- Clear feedback to students.

Cons
Abuse can lead to loss of objectivity.

Rating scale limitations
- People vary greatly in their ability to make ratings.
- Different people have different credibility as evaluation targets.

- Immediate emotional reactions affect ratings.
- Self-ratings tend to be too high for desirable traits and too low for undesirable traits.
- Reviewers often fail to justify their reviews, or tend to provide absurd justifications.
- **The generous mistake:** Reviewers do not want to disrespect their users by giving them low ratings. As a result, almost all cases are highly rated. Raters also tend to be overly lenient in assessing aspects they could not observe.
- **Halo mistakes:** Evaluators find it difficult to eliminate the halo effect, which forces them to shift their qualitative judgments from one aspect to another. The halo effect often occurs when the assessor has to assess many factors, some of which there is no basis for judging.
- **Central tendency error:** Some observers tend to place most raters near the midpoint of the scale.
- **Stringency errors:** The opposite of leniency errors is called stringency errors. Some evaluators are so cautious and hesitant that they tend to underestimate everyone.
- **Logical error:** It is difficult to tell raters exactly which quality to rate. Adjectives and adverbs may not have universal meaning.

VIDEOTAPE

In a video assessment, an instructor or administrator uses a visual recording as evidence to assess a student's or teacher's performance. Video grading software streamlines this process by making it easy to record, upload, save, analyze grades, and provide feedback on student videos.

- Video-based assessment software is a tool that helps students develop demonstrable skills in areas such as nursing education, teacher preparation, clinical psychology, communication, and foreign languages.
- The most common use case in higher education is student presentations.
- The steps, students and teachers take to record upload assessments and provide feedback on student presentations using video assessments.
- Tools exist to assess indicators across a range of intraoperative factors, and their validity and reliability are supported by the literature.
- New evidence supports the use of retrospective assessment of surgical technique to ensure optimal patient outcomes.
- Educators use video analysis to identify aspects of surgery to practice and the role of coaching in surgery is greatly enhanced through case review.
- Identification of critical events related to safety and surgical technique is not always apparent in real time.
- Video analysis allows surgeons and instructors to assess intraoperative factors that affect surgical outcome and patient safety.
- Technical skills assessment extensive video recording and analysis techniques can lead to non-technical skills and surgical errors.

Benefits of Video-Based Grading

Since its inception, Bongo Lewis has discovered several key benefits of video grading.

- **Individualized feedback:** Lewis provides individualized responses in the video so he can speak to each student individually. This is easier and saves more time than written feedback. You can also add timestamped feedback to student videos to alert them to specific points in their presentation that could be improved.
- **Soft skills assessment:** Answering standard quizzes may tell you what a nursing student, for example, knows, but not how they behave at the bedside. Similarly, video assessments can be used for business training in areas such as sales to assess pitch presentations, responses to objections, and so on.
- **Beyond presentation skills:** Video assessments are great for improving oral presentation skills, but they can also be used to check how well students understand concepts. For example, a math class can capture and share desktops while students are working on a problem or have a discussion so teachers can assess students' understanding.
- **Practice makes perfect:** An unexpected result of these video presentations is that Lewis students recorded their presentations multiple times because they wanted them to sound good on camera, and through repetition and revision, they learned more, decided to strengthen. By looking at the recording log, Lewis was able to get data on how much he had rehearsed.
- **Accommodate different learning styles:** Not everyone learns the same way. Some people thrive on written communication, while others struggle with it. I have a niece with a learning disability who has been asked to answer questions in writing and she is struggling.
- **Show a higher level of engagement when presenting themselves:** Students are much more engaged because their faces are on the work and not just their names on the exam paper.
- **Faster grading:** Feedback is also video-based, so educators can complete grading in much less time while providing more content-based feedback to students, he says. "I can say more in 60 seconds than I can type in five minutes and the student gets something better because now it is a personal connection," he says.

WRITTEN COMMUNICATION

Written communication is the development and expression of ideas in writing. It involves learning to work in many genres and styles appropriately adapting to the conventions of different disciplines and/or professional contexts. Written communication can also involve working with many different writing technologies including mixing texts data and images with narrative. Written communication abilities develop through iterative practice with feedback across the curriculum and co-curriculum.

Skills of Competent Writing

Even though the style and conventions of writing assignments differ across the disciplines a review of written communication rubrics from multiple fields identifies several core elements of competent writing. They include:
- Easily identifiable thesis
- Continuous support of the thesis throughout the task
- Appropriate use of evidence to support the thesis
- Logical organization
- Relevance
- Clarity of ideas
- Depth of analysis
- Appropriate audience knowledge
- Proper integration of charts, tables and graphs (photos).

Elements of Written Communication

Consists of five main elements in which written communication skills are taught. Here are some examples of each of these items:
1. **Conciseness:** The purpose of written communication is to get the point across quickly. To effectively convey information, it is important to provide only relevant details.
2. **Clarity:** Clarity helps readers understand the message you are trying to convey. Clarity in writing reduces the occurrence of misinformation, misunderstandings and mistakes. Clarity comes from using simple language and avoiding complex words and sentence structures.
3. **Tone:** Tone is the voice of the writing, conveying emotion to the reader. For business correspondence, use a professional tone with the appropriate level of friendliness and formality.
4. **Active voice:** Active voice uses action verbs to make your writing clearer, easier to read, and more engaging for your readers. The active voice is preferred over the passive voice because it allows the reader to move quickly through the text.
5. **Grammar and punctuation:** Grammar and punctuation make text clearer, more interesting to readers, avoid misunderstandings, and communicate more effectively. In professional communication, grammar and punctuation help convey the correct information to the reader.

PROGRESS NOTES

Nursing progress notes are records kept by nurses and doctors during a patient's hospital stay. Nurses are often the professionals who spend the most time with patients, so add specific details about patient care and recovery progress.

Items to include in nursing progress notes:

When writing nursing progress notes, it is best to include as much detail as possible. This helps provide accurate and helpful context for other healthcare providers. Below is a list of some items to include in your care progress notes:
- Date and time of report
- Patient name
- Doctor and nurse name
- Patient summary
- Reason for visit
- Vital signs and initial health assessment
- Laboratory or blood test results
- Diagnosis and care planning
- Patient response to care
- Follow-up care instructions
- Additional observations.

How to Write Nursing Track Notes

Many healthcare professionals use the SOAPI method when creating nursing track notes. SOAPI stands for subjective objective assessment plan and intervention. Here is a list of steps that must be followed to create a care track record using the SOAPI method.
- **Collect subjective evidence:** After noting the date, time, your name and the patient's name, start the care tracking. By requesting information from the patient. This information is likely subjective and limited to the patient's knowledge and perspective. Subjective cues include the patient's pain level, reason for the visit, and patient concerns. If necessary, consider asking family members or friends who accompany the patient if they have noticed anything about the patient's condition
- **Record objective information:** After speaking with the patient and listening to their perspective, collect objective data to include in the progress note. This includes information such as the patient's vital signs, symptoms observed, and the results of blood tests ordered by you or your doctor. Objective information often supports the patient's subjective information, helps

provide context for the patient's concerns, and leads to the patient's diagnosis.
- **Record your evaluation:** In this section, record notes about the patient's condition based on the conclusions you and your GP draw from the patient's symptoms and objective data. The assessment also includes the drugs the doctor prescribed to the patient and the patient's response. Note any changes in the patient's appearance or symptoms since admission.
- **Create a detailed care plan:** Care plan section of the care progress note contains all the actions you and your doctor want to take for your patient's health. For example, if a patient has an upcoming MRI scan, a progress note can indicate that it is also important to detail all relevant information regarding the patient's response to the care plan. For example, if you and the doctor offered the patient a follow-up appointment, but the patient declined, note this in the progress note.
- **Identify the intervention:** Intervention section of the nursing progress note contains a variety of information. In most cases, this section of progress notes provides additional information about the care the patient received during the shift. Be sure to include details about when the patient was given medication, what the patient wanted, and any other observations you made about the patient.

Tips for Writing Nursing Progress Notes

Here are some tips to consider when writing your own nursing progress notes.
- **Ask for instructions:** Many nurses and doctors use the SOPAI method to create progress notes, but some hospitals and clinics may have their own templates and routines for progress notes. If you start a new job, be sure to ask your boss how to write and organize progress notes.
- **Be objective:** When writing progress notes, it is important to be as objective as possible. Include only facts and observations. This keeps your progress reports accurate and accessible to everyone who needs to see them.
- **Add details later:** Many nurses and doctors record a summary of information during a conversation with a patient and then return to add details to progress notes after the visit. It is important to complete the notes on one patient before visiting another. This way, you can remember the details of your visit. In situations where you cannot finish your notes before seeing another patient, at least write down the most important details.
- **Be concise:** Thorough notetaking is helpful, but you also need to be concise. To keep the report concise, please include only relevant details in your progress notes and try to explain in short terms. This allows other medical professionals to quickly see your progress. You can also reduce the time to take notes.
- **Write an end-of-day summary:** Some patients may need to add an end-of-day summary of the care received and other details. This helps professionals working the next shift track the patient's progress. The end of day summary allows you to review your notes for the day and make changes to your care progress notes.
- **Reading other nursing progress notes:** Most health professionals use their own opinion and style when creating nursing progress notes. Once you understand the format your manager prefers, consider reading other experts' notes and comparing your style to theirs. In some cases, it also encourages you to adopt better habits when writing your own notes. This convenient learning method also helps you become more familiar with your care progress notes.

CARE PLAN

Care plan is a formal process to accurately identify existing needs and recognize potential needs and risks. Care plans enable communication between caregivers, patients, and other healthcare providers to achieve health outcomes. Without a care planning process, quality and consistency of patient care are lost.

The care plan begins with the client's admission to the institution and is continually updated to address changes in the client's condition and assessment of goal attainment. The planning and delivery of individualized or patient-centered care is the cornerstone of good nursing practice.

Types

Care plans can be informal or formal. An informal care plan is a behavioral strategy that resides in the caregiver's mind. A formal care plan is a written or computerized guide that organizes a client's care information. Formal care plans are further classified into standardized care plans and individualized care plans. A standardized care plan specifies care for a group of clients with routine needs. An individualized care plan is created to meet the specific needs of a particular person or needs not addressed by standardized care plans.

Objectives

Goals and objectives in care planning are:
- Promote evidence-based care and create a comfortable and familiar environment in hospitals and health centers.

- Support holistic care, including physical, psychological, social and spiritual in the treatment and prevention of disease.
- Set up programs such as care pathways and care packages. The pathway of care requires teamwork to reach agreement on standards of care and expected outcomes. Care packages, in contrast, refer to best practices for the care of a particular condition.
- Identify and distinguish between goals and expected results.
- Review care plan communications and documentation.
- Take care measures.

Care Plan Goals

Goals and importance of creating a care plan are:
- **The nurse's role:** This helps them recognize the unique role of nurses in caring for the overall health and wellbeing of their clients without relying entirely on physician directives and interventions.
- Gives instructions for the individualized care of the client. This allows caregivers to think critically about each client and design interventions that are directly tailored to the individual.
- **Continuity of care:** Nurses in different shifts and departments can use the data to deliver the same quality and type of interventions when caring for clients, so clients get the most benefit from their treatment.
- **Documentation:** It should detail what observations should be made, what care should be provided, and what direction the client or family needs. There is no evidence that care was provided if it was not properly documented in the care plan.
- Used as a guide for assigning specific staff to specific customers. Client care may need to be entrusted to personnel with specialized and precise skills.
- Used as a measure of reimbursement. Insurance companies use medical records to determine how much to pay for a customer's inpatient treatment.
- Define customer goals. Engaging caregivers and users in treatment and care benefits them.

Components

Nursing care plans (NCPs) typically include nursing diagnoses, client issues, expected outcomes, nursing interventions and justifications. These components are described below:
- Medical results and diagnostic reports for client health assessment are the first steps in designing a care plan. Specifically, client assessment includes physical, emotional, sexual, psychosocial, cultural, mental/transpersonal, cognitive, functional, age-related, economic, and environmental domains and abilities. Related to Information in this area can be subjective or objective.
- Presents the outcomes the customer expects. These may be long term or short term.
- Nursing interventions are documented in nursing plans.
- Rationale for intervention as evidence-based care.
- Evaluation. This is a record of the results of the nursing intervention.

Nursing Plan Format

Nursing plan format is typically categorized or organized into four columns: (1) Nursing diagnosis, (2) Desired outcomes and goals, (3) Nursing intervention, and (4) Evaluation. Some agencies use a three-column plan with goals and scores on the same column. Other agencies offer 5-column plans that include a column for review notes.

PROCESS RECORD

A process record is a technique used to record verbal interactions between a caregiver and a client, or a written record of overall communication patterns between a caregiver and a client. Process records are written reports of verbal interactions with customers. These are verbatim reports (where possible) written by nurses or students to improve interpretation and communication skills.

Definition

- Process recording is the method by which a student records all verbal and nonverbal communication spoken and observed during an interview. **—Chris Jordan**
- A process record is a written record of everything that happens during and immediately after the caregiver-patient interaction.
- Records of conversations between nurses and patients in psychiatric facilities, conversations during interviews, and the nurse's conclusions.
- Process recordings are interactions or interviews conducted and recorded by caregivers using various communication techniques.

Meaning

Process recording is a tool used by students, trainers, and supervisors to study the dynamics of a particular interaction over time. Recording the process is a great educational tool for learning and honing your interviewing and intervention skills. Process recordings help students conceptualize and organize their ongoing activities using client systems, clarify the purpose of interviews and interventions, improve writing, identify strengths and weaknesses, and improve self-awareness helps.

Purpose
- To assist students in designing and organizing ongoing activities using the patient system.
- Improve your writing.
- To clarify the purpose of the interview or intervention.
- Identify strengths and weaknesses.
- To increase self-confidence.
- Separate fact from judgment.
- We examine the interaction of values between the student and patient systems by analyzing the filtering process used during session recording.

Goals and Targets
- Establish the treatment-patient relationship.
- Provide necessary health education to patients.
- To obtain patient identification information.
- Evaluate patient comprehension.

Process Recording Steps
- Preparation
- Record interactions between caregiver and patient
- Documented process records can begin with recordings during interviews
- Identification data
- Current complaint.

Types
- Verbatim dialogue.
- Emotions and reactions.
- Observation and analysis.
- Conclusion.

General Guidelines
- Record the conversation verbatim.
- Use the recording device and obtain permission from the patient. This helps validate the session if necessary.
- Note the nonverbal responses of the patient and caregiver as the session is recorded.

Process Record Format
- Name
- Age
- Gender
- Address
- Ward
- Bed number
- Marital status
- Language
- Religion
- Education
- Occupation
- Income
- Diagnosis
- Admission date
- Date of interview
- Brief medical history or patient illness
- Purpose of dialogue
- Timing and duration of dialogue.

Interview Details—Phases Process Record
- **Verbatim dialogue:**
  - Clarify interactions between nursing students and patients.
  - Dialogue allows clinical leaders and student nurses to consider client reactions to student leadership.
  - List the roles played by the students in the interaction.
  - This fact-based, objective interaction can be used to review patterns, themes, and useful information.
- **Emotions and emotional reactions:**
  - Shows the student's emotions and reactions.
  - Lists the student's emotional reactions to the interaction that took place.
- **Observation and observational analysis:**
  - Record the student's critical thinking about the patient's words and feelings.
  - A space where students can reference or interpret critical thinking behavior.
- **Critical thinking and reflection:** Students should record their critical thinking about their actions and motivations during the session.
- **Closing comments:**
  - Clinical trainers provide feedback and support for the learning process.
  - Comments are written about specific interactions and feelings.

Advantages
- Process recording helps distinguish between thoughts and feelings.
- Helps clarify the purpose of an interview or intervention.
- It will help you improve your writing expression.
- Helps identify strengths and weaknesses.
- Helps boost self-confidence.
- Helps separate fact from judgment.
- Analyzing the filtering process used when recording a session helps to investigate the interplay of values that operate between student and patient systems.

Cons
- This will take longer as clinical leaders may need more time to make assessments on individual students.

- Technical issues are common and can be frustrating.
- This process is cumbersome as it requires Handson observation and subsequent involvement of the clinical trainer during student and patient interviews.

WRITTEN ASSIGNMENTS

Written assignments on clinical practice combined with teacher feedback provide a powerful tool for developing a student's writing skills. Concepts, theory, and other content related to patient care.
- Assist students in understanding concepts, theories, and other content that relate to care of patients;
- Develop higher thinking skills.
- Examine your own feelings, beliefs, and values stemming from your clinical learning experience.
- Develop writing skills. Many types of writing tasks help reinforce clinical learning.

Types of Writing Tasks

Many types of writing tasks are suitable for assessment in nursing education. Some of these tasks indicate how well students have learned the content, but they don't necessarily improve their writing skills. For example, structured tasks involving short sentences or phrases, such as care plans or recording assessments or physical examinations, do not facilitate writing skill development nor provide sufficient data for writing assessments.

Other assignments, such as formal reports, can be used to assess students' comprehension and writing skills. Therefore, not all written assignments provide data to assess writing ability, and again teachers need to be clear about the outcomes the assignment is intended to assess. Many written assignments can be used in nursing courses. These include:
- Term papers.
- Research paper and research protocol development.
- Evidencebased exercise papers in which studentscritique and synthesize evidence and report on their use in clinical practice.
- Concept analysis and papers about its application in clinical practice practice.
- Papers comparing different interventions to their underlying evidence base.
- An essay about how what you have learned in class or read in textbooks or articles compares to your clinical experience and how it applies to patient care.
- Critical analysis reports in which students analyze problems, compare options, and develop arguments for work.
- Case study analysis with documented evidence.
- Reflective journals and writing assignments.

Assignment Objectives

Written assignments are an important teaching and assessment method in nursing courses. These provide many learning outcomes, but should be carefully selected and designed with the purpose of the lesson in mind.
- Written assignments allow students to critique and summarize the literature and report their findings.
- Seek critiques and synthesis of evidence against nursing practice.
- Analyze concepts and theories and apply them to clinical situations, improve problem-solving and high-level thinking skills.
- Gain experience in articulating your ideas and communicating them to others in a clear and consistent manner.
- Develop your writing skills. Many clinical course written assignments help students reflect on their care plan and identify areas that need further instruction.
- Some assignments, such as the reflection journal, encourage students to examine their feelings, beliefs and values and reflect on their learning in the course.

Written assignments for clinical study include:
- Concept map, a graphical arrangement of key concepts related to patient care. A written description of the meaning of the relationship.
- Analysis of clinical experience, student care, and alternative approaches that could have been used.
- Essays examining how measurements impact patient care.
- Mini-essays related to clinical practice.
- Curriculum.
- Nursing plan.
- Analysis of interactions with individuals and groups in clinical settings.
- Clinical observation reports.
- Reflective journals and other reflective writing activities.
- Projects and collections of materials that enhance student learning, an E-portfolio clinically demonstrated.

ORAL TEST (VIVA)

Viva voce is a Latin expression that literally means 'with a lively voice', but is most commonly translated as 'word of mouth'. Rigorosum is also called an oral examination, and is a form of dialogue between the examiner and the student, in which the examiner asks questions and the student answers.

Importance of Oral Exams

- Oral exams are traditionally used in conjunction with practical exams and specialized courses in clinical practice.

- This type of exam usually consists of a dialogue with the candidate asking questions of the student in a real or simulated situation.
- Oral exams should be marked by two examiners for greater confidence or disputes.
- Predetermined scores can be used by examiners. Each student's time limit must be respected.
- After the practical exam, a rigorous exam should be conducted with great care.

Purpose of PhD

There are many situations in which the use of a PhD is required. This is covered by academic and organizational regulations. There are several valid reasons for asking students to take rigorous exams, each of which can affect students differently. The main purposes of viva are:
- Assess the student's ability to communicate with others.
- To complement information obtained through other valuation techniques.
- Use stimulation methods such as role-playing and phone calls.
- Identify and analyze the existence of the student's mind.
- Assess student initiative and behavior.
- Gain in-depth knowledge through different types of questions.
- Diagnose students' limitations and weaknesses and take corrective action.

Principles for Conducting Viva Voce

- Viva should not be limited to a single topic, to avoid skewing Viva's results by the selection of topics to which candidates can exceptionally respond. In addition, a variety of topics should be covered. Well, or he/she doesn't know anything. All questions should be relevant to the purpose of your application.
- Do not make the introduction of the question too long. The examiner should speak as little as possible during the exam.
- Chairperson of the examiner must remain in charge of the session and respond appropriately to problematic candidates and difficult situations.
- When the final question is asked, have the student complete the answer to formally end the session.
- The Rigolosum test should normally not exceed 30 minutes.
- Candidates must be evaluated individually.
- Candidates should be notified in good time about the possibility of being invited to the PhD thesis. This usually takes 24 hours or more.

Viva Voce Benefits

- Contact candidates directly to assess their communication skills and overall impression.
- Provide an opportunity to mitigate the situation on your account.
- Provides flexibility in turning candidates from strengths to weaknesses.
- Have students construct responses without cues and observe responses to specific stimuli.
- Simultaneous evaluation by multiple examiners is possible.
- Provide examiners with an opportunity to solicit feedback on student and college performance.

Viva Voce Drawbacks

- Lack of objectivity in standardization and reproducibility of results.
- Favoritism is allowed and may not be used for future reference.
- Suffers undue influence from unrelated factors.
- It is costly in terms of professional time.

PRACTICAL EXAM

The practical exam is an integral part of the nursing exam. The purpose of the practical exam is to assess nursing competencies and practical skills. Practical exams are essentially a combination of testing methods such as rating scales and checklists.
- In addition to the practical exam, there is also an oral exam to supplement the knowledge gained.
- Students work through a series of "steps" to perform a variety of practical tasks such as assessing patients, developing nursing diagnoses based on priorities, planning care, administering care, and evaluating care.
- The evaluation sheet contains premade checklists and scales to increase the reliability of the evaluation. Therefore, all students are evaluated according to the same criteria by the same examiner.

Practical skills he can assess using two methods:
1. **Direct observation:** Examples of Handson testing in the clinical field using assessment formats.
2. **Indirect observation:** Project implementation.

SIMULATION

Simulation is an educational and training method for healthcare professionals intended to significantly improve the understanding and dissemination of knowledge, skills and attitudes for healthcare professionals at all levels. Through this technique, students experience and interact with a real hospital environment, greatly reducing the chances of making errors in completing assignments.

Simulation Concepts

Simulation is the process of trying to resemble real life, but not reality. Its realism is determined by the simulator's fidelity, environment and scenario description. Imperfect imitations of human systems will always exist, no matter how sophisticated the simulation model is. No matter how well trained a student is, when asked to use a skill in realtime under certain conditions, they may become very frustrated or "freeze" at not being able to successfully complete the process. So schools are trying to update their various simulation programs by investing in machines and having actors play the patient roles to add plausibility to the patient's reactions. Additionally, professors must be trained in simulation processes and technical issues.

Simulation Objectives

The objective of nursing training is to acquire solid theoretical knowledge as well as the clinical skills necessary for the timely integration of qualified nurses into the labor market. Integrated learning of critical thinking and optimal decision-making skills helps nurses deliver quality care. This can be achieved by incorporating simulation into the educational process. Advances in simulation and other teaching methods can be very helpful as students strive to become integrated and successful medical professionals.

Types of Simulation in Nursing Education

The use of simulation attempts to replace real patients with virtual standardized patients or techniques and methods that can reproduce real clinical scenarios for therapeutic and educational purposes. These processes include simple demonstrations of specific scenarios on a computer (cognitive tests), simulations of nursing competencies, or implementation of integrated processes. Basic types of simulation in nursing education include:

Use of Highfidelity Mannequins or Technology

- These are body blocks or body part blocks with life characteristics that may respond to actions or interventions by students.
- These represent the patient's clinical response/symptoms and are used to describe all circumstances surrounding the case, such as available tool stocks (such as bandaged syringes) and available time limits.

Low Fidelity Mannequin

Use of a low fidelity mannequin that can perform a few specific tasks or processes, for instance limb for catheterizing blood vessels or a mannequin for CPR training.

Subtask Simulator

- This category includes models (such as dexterity) used to implement clinical skill tasks that students can repeat.
- Typical examples include 'legs' for venous catheterization in the head of vessels, chest manikins for airway placement, and synthetic leather pads for practicing wound closure.

Virtual Reality

Virtual reality is increasingly being used as a simulation tool. For medical professionals, virtual reality simulations use computers and standardized patients to create realistic learning and assessment environments.

Standardized Patient—Volunteers Act as Patients

- These are trainees who behave in a specific way for realistic clinical interaction.
- These are widely used for teaching and evaluation in nursing education, especially for communication purposes and skill acquisition, and can provide feedback upon request.

E-learning (usually knowledge tests, multiple tests, etc.):

- A computer-generated simulator is a representation of a task or setting designed to facilitate learning.
- This includes a simple computer program that shows how the device works.
- An anesthesia machine or something highly complex, such as a detailed virtual reality environment where participants interact with virtual patients and other medical professionals.

Hybrid Simulation

- This type of simulation is defined as a type that combines two or more simulations to create a more realistic simulation experience.
- A typical example is the use of standardized patient wearable devices that allow students to perform specific procedures while interacting with a real person.
- For example, a standardized patient can have a suturing mannequin (pad) attached to the arm where the athlete sutures the wound. Therefore, we ensure that trainees can obtain informed consent, explain the process, etc.

Benefits of Patient Simulation in Nursing Education

- Simulation as an evidence-based training method and process first emerged when it became difficult for nurses working in hospitals to gain clinical experience. Simulation can help remove limitations associated with the clinical environment (including availability such as patient safety issues), promote teamwork and solidarity among students, and implement skill acquisition protocols.
- This is based on a scenario where learning becomes interactive, allowing feedback between the educator and other team members, and promoting clinical and critical thinking within the team.

Restrictions on the Use of Simulation in Nursing Education

Simulation is widely used in nursing schools and is becoming even more popular due to its enormous benefits. However, teaching nursing skills through simulation has certain limitations. The most important ones are:

- Simulation as a technique and holistic nursing as a philosophy represent her two distinct components of a nursing course integrated over time to acquire the knowledge and skills necessary for patient care.
- Simulation provides an opportunity to acquire and apply knowledge and skills through the use of simulators, standardized patients, and virtual environments. However, it is impossible to consider the patient as a whole as a biopsychosocial person. Simulation training takes place in a controlled environment supervised by educators who can stop and restart processes that are impossible in real life.

OBJECTIVELY STRUCTURED CLINICAL EXAMINATIONS

Objectively structured clinical examinations (OSCEs) are tests to assess clinical competence in which components are evaluated in a planned or structured manner. It is an approach that emphasizes the objectivity of inspections based on systematic planning framework. It consists of several stations around which students rotate and students perform specific tasks and are assessed.

OSCE Concepts

- The OSCE typically consists of a series of short (5–10 minute) stations in which each candidate presents one or two unbiased examiners and a patient (real or simulated or electronic patient simulator).
- Each station has a different examiner. In contrast, traditional clinical trial methods assign a candidate to her single examiner for the entire trial. Candidates alternate through stations and complete all stations in a round. All candidates are assessed at the same station.
- Ward unification facilitates comparison with other wards and allows evaluation of complex procedures without impacting patient well-being. The sum of the passing scores for all stations gives the overall passing score for the OSCE.

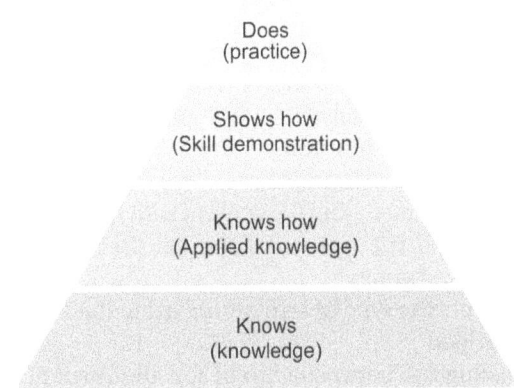

Fig. 15.2: Objectively structured clinical examinations (OSCEs) approaches.

Definition

Objective structure performance examination (OPSE) a new pattern of practical examination. OPSE is a consistent and objective test of each component of clinical competence for all students who take the practical exams in place.

OSPE provides a rational idea of each student's level of achievement in all relevant practical skills in a particular field. It can be used for formative and summative assessment. The main features of the OSCE are:

- Centralized inspection
- Short station
- Objective evaluation

The various functions accessible through the OSCE are:
- Clinical skills
- Communication skills
- Attitudes and ethics
- Critical thinking
- Decision-making
- Professionalism.

Various stations are carried out against it. It objectively assesses the various skills needed to implement an assessment plan and assess care.

Examples of different skills tested are:
- BLS—basic life support
- Medication administration
- Hand hygiene
- Wound care
- Partography
- NR—neonatal resuscitation, etc.

How do I organize an OSPE?

You should set goals for work experience in a specific field for example practical exam in medical surgical nursing.

- Each student must demonstrate practical skills. This can be done by assessing students to monitor and record their mouth temperature.
  - Convert 39 degrees to F
  - Attach the heart monitor to the patient
  - Tests urine for sugar
  - Begin patient infusion.
- Make an accurate and precise observation: This can be achieved by matching the student with her
  - Interpret the nature of the exotherm using the displayed graph
  - Identify the type of arrhythmia using the ECG graph provided
  - Distinguish between normal and abnormal ECGs.
  These questions may not require the examiner to observe the student's behavio,These questions are written on paper and can be collected later for evaluation.
- Data analysis and interpretation: This is one of the key competencies assessed for continuity of patient care. Nurses should perform this task when they may encounter normal and abnormal data related to patient lab reports. The student asked for an interpreter.
  - Hamogram: Normal or abnormal
  - Liver function test report
  - Report of renal function test
  - Lab report.
- Identify patient issues: To organize their work, nurses must identify and prioritize patient issues to address the patient's immediate needs.
  - Difficulty breathing according to their observations
  - Post-transfusion stiffness
  - Cone after lumbar puncture
  - CSF after head injury.
- Planning alternative nursing interventions in specific situations: To provide adequate care, nursing students need to plan alternative nursing interventions in the event of airway obstruction.
  - Keep in a supine position
  - Do oropharyngeal suction
  - Check and record vital signs

- Start oxygen inhalation as needed
- Prepare for endotracheal intubation
- Assists the physician in intubating the patient.

To assess specific practical skills, the OSPE is organized into stations and candidates are alternately passed through until they complete a full lap.

Types of Stations

S. No.	Stations	Questions	Method of scoring
1.	Procedure station	Check and record BP	Observed and scored by the examiner A using checklist
2.	Question station	List 5 factors which help in maintaining BP	Answer on a sheet provided
3.	Procedure station	Take oral temperature and record it	Observed and scored by the examiner B
4.	Question station	Convert 39°C to F by using formula	Answer a sheet provided
5.	Procedure station	Test the urine albumin and record it	Observed and scored by the examiner C
6.	Question station	List five causes of albuminuria	Answer on a sheet provided

How Do I Grade My Students on the OSPE?

- A checklist is created by assigning points to each step.
- Evaluation objectivity is achieved by having each component of a given station checked by the same rater, and students testing all of them in turn.
- The time allowed is the same for all stations. The time allotted for each station is 3–5 minutes.

Benefits

- Helps observe and assess students on a range of professional and technical skills in real-world situations.
- This gives you an overall picture of student performance.

Cons

- A student's score is subjective as it depends on the examiner's whim, imagination and mood.
- Time consuming and nonstandard bedside conditions affect student scores.
- Recognize the magnitude of the problems that exist when assessing students.

OSPE Instructions for Students

- Write down your role number. Please enter the number in bold and display it on your gown so that the examiner can identify you.

- Students are asked to report by a certain time. Everyone is assembled in a room or hall and the exam process is explained.
- The student may be instructed to cycle through the stations (numbered 1 to 6) and spend 3 minutes at each station.

ANECDOTAL NOTES

Anecdotal notes are factual descriptions of important events and occurrences observed by the teacher in the lives of students.
- Anecdotal records attempt to describe the most typical episodes of student behavior in the areas of personal or social adjustment. Reports may include negative, positive or outstanding performance or behavior.
- Incidents are recorded immediately after they occur.
- Conducted in a practical/clinical area to observe student behavior.
- The advantage of the anecdotal record is that it provides a description of the actual behavior in a natural setting.
- The downside is that it takes time to maintain a good record keeping system.
- Another drawback is that it is not inherently objective.

Advantages
- Adding and validating other structured means
- Provides insight into holistic behavioral incidents
- Uses formative feedback
- Economical and easy to develop.

Cons
- Carelessly recorded. purpose has not been met
- Subjectivity
- Lack of standardization
- Difficulty in assessing
- Time consuming
- Limited scope.

Self-report Techniques

Through interviews and surveys, individuals are asked how they feel about the specific situations and activities that are of most interest to them. Get information. HR issues have a lot in common with individuals. An interview is a personal relationship between the interviewer and the interviewee. Information is gathered through direct questioning, which may be structured or unstructured.

PERFORMANCE EVALUATION IN NURSING

Performance evaluation, or performance evaluation, is one of the oldest and most ubiquitous management practices. As a result, an evaluation system was born that classifies and evaluates employee strengths such as autonomy, reliability, and character in comparison with others. The trend today is to evaluate people for what they do (performance reviews) rather than what they are (performance reviews). The evaluation can be done by one or more of her supervisors, or by her subordinates and colleagues. There may also be a self-assessment system in which employees evaluate their performance.

Definition
- Performance appraisal refers to any formal procedure used in a workplace organization to evaluate the character and contribution of group members.
- Performance reviews are regular, formal assessments of how well staff have performed their duties over a period of time.
- Performance evaluation (also known as performance evaluation, efficiency evaluation, or service evaluation) is the process of reviewing individual performance and professional progress and assessing potential.

Purpose of Evaluation
- May serve as a basis for career change or promotion. Determining whether a nurse can contribute further in another or higher position helps in appropriate promotion or placement.
- Identifying employee strengths and weaknesses will serve as a guide for developing appropriate training and development programs to improve the quality of their performance in their current jobs.
- Acts as feedback to employees. Knowing how well they are doing or where they stand compared to their managers helps employees know what they can do to improve their current performance and move up the management hierarchy.
- This represents an important incentive for all employees whose appraisal system ensures continued attention from management and continued opportunities for further growth. Employees find that not only are they constantly being watched, they are not being forgotten.
- Implementing a periodic evaluation system encourages superiors and managers to pay more attention to their subordinates as they are expected to fill out evaluation forms on a regular basis and justify their estimates.
- Performance reviews are often the rational basis for payments such as performance bonuses. Estimates of relative contributions to employee traits help determine rewards and privileges.
- Performance appraisals serve as a means of assessing the effectiveness of employee selection and classification

measures. Alternatively, knowing the characteristics of superiors and subordinates is useful for selecting and assigning personnel.
- Maintaining performance appraisal records for permanent employees helps management stop relying solely on the personal knowledge of potentially moving bosses.

Purpose of Judgment

- The purpose of setting salary standards for the purpose of evaluation, raising wages, and granting performance improvement.
- Selection of qualified individuals for promotion, termination or termination of employees for poor performance.
- Performance appraisals that are not for appraisal purposes occupy the highest position and are for development purposes.

They are primarily educational and may involve guiding employees to achieve professional progress by working within organizational goals.
- Identify the people in your organization.
- Identify individual or group training and development needs.
- Improve relationships between groups.
- Set performance standards and achieve acceptance of those standards.
- Recognize your employees.
- Discover employee ambitions.
- Align these with your organization's goals.
- Ensure team building.
- To provide feedback to employees.

Principles of Performance Evaluation

- Evaluations should include content that relates to the people being evaluated in the specific environment.
- It should provide criteria for evaluating performance and specify the criteria whenever possible.
- Performance evaluation should be able to distinguish between good, and bad performance.
- Any performance evaluation must be practical or metrological. I am sure there must be a way.

Performance Evaluation Tactics

Irancerich Donnelely and Gibson identified five possible parties. Who can rate? Or rate others.
1. Supervisor
2. Peers
3. Rates
4. Subordinates of the vertee
5. Raters outside of the organizational environment.

In most of the cases employees should be rated by their immediate supervisors.

In most cases, employees should be evaluated by their immediate supervisor.

When should evaluations occur?

- Most organizations evaluate senior or tenured employees once or twice a year.
- New hires are evaluated approximately six weeks to two months after hire. Also, an employee at different developmental stages may be evaluated more or less than twice a year, depending on the goals set in the previous evaluation.
- The progressive disciplinary process is an example of an evaluation that is often conducted every two weeks.

Reviews must include progress notes made by the reviewer at the bottom. Goals should be set for the timing of the evaluation and the period leading up to that date.

Basics of a Good Rating System

- It should be easy to understand. If the system is too complicated or takes too long, it can be selfmassively grounded and complicated, but no one but the experts will understand.
- It must have the support of all line personnel who manage it. If people think the line is too theoretical, too ambitious, too unrealistic, or pushed by a dumb recruiter who doesn't understand, then their requirements are the line operator's time. I will send. There must be similar goodwill and understanding between the appraiser and the customs officer.
- The system should fit into the organization's processes and structures. That is, a system that works very well in companies whose activities are compact. Similarly, when events are interdependent and interrelated, an individual's performance data cannot be considered sufficiently discrete or reliable to assess that individual's performance.
- The system must be valid and reliable. Evaluation effectiveness is the degree to which the evaluation actually reflects the employee's intrinsic merit. Rating reliability is the consistency of ratings made by different raters or by her one rater at different times.
- The system should include incentives for satisfactory performance.
- The system should be evaluated periodically to ensure that it continues to achieve its objectives. Not only is there the risk that subjective standards will outweigh the objective ones that were set in the first place, but there is also the added risk that the system will fail. This is done rigorously in complex rules and procedures, many of which are no longer useful.

Performance Evaluation Criteria

The criteria can be divided into her two main categories: Objective criteria and subjective criteria. Examples of objective criteria are production quality ranges, work samples, years of service, training coverage, absenteeism, accidents, etc. Examples of subjective criteria are the evaluation of an employee's ability to work by superiors, peers, and subordinates, the level of communication of ideas to upper management, the level of knowledge of company goals, and the contribution to sociocultural values. All subjective criteria rely on human judgment and opinion and are therefore subject to certain types of errors that can occur in the evaluation process.

Performance Appraisal Method

- **Appraisal method:** Appraisal is the evaluation of one person by another. Evaluation is basically direct observation. Evaluation is a team applied to the expression of opinions or judgments about a particular fact or character. Opinions are usually expressed in terms of scales and values. Valuation techniques are tools that can quantify such judgments. The oldest and easiest way to assess performance is to compare one man to all others and rank them in a simple order. This way, the order of all the individuals that make up the group will be from highest to lowest.
- **Rating scale methods:** As the name suggests, these methods provide a kind of scale for measuring absolute differences between individuals. The scales used are usually his two kinds of:
  1. *Individual:* When two or more categories are provided that represent individual levels of competence or traits, raters can tick the category they believe best describes the person being assessed. For example, expertise can be categorized into five categories on separate scales. Very good, above average, below average and bad.
  2. *Continuous (or graphic):* The notation is displayed as a continuous line directly above the category. Four types of criteria are used in the rating scale. That is, descriptive adjectives and behavioral patterns, either numerically or alphabetically from masculine to masculine.
- **Checklist method:** A list consisting of a series of statements about employees and their behavior may be used to assess performance. Each statement in this list is assigned a value based on its importance. The advantage of this method is that the evaluator only needs to provide the facts. The values assigned to the various utterances are not displayed in the list, so raters do not know how highly they rate a particular person. Nor do you need to distinguish between different categories for different characteristics considered for each of your multiple employees.
- **Forced choice method:** The forced choice evaluation form consists of a series of statements that require an individual's evaluation. These statements are grouped into groups of 2, 3, or 4. A group on the evaluation form may consist of only positive statements, may be all negative statements, or may contain an equal number of positive and negative statements. If all groups on the evaluation form contain positive statements, raters only need to check the one statement in each group that they believe best characterizes the person being rated. If all groups have made unfavorable statements, the rater must check the one statement in each group that he believes is the least representative of the person being rated. If each group has 2 positive statements and 2 negative statements, the evaluator performs her two tests for each group. One is the most descriptive statement about the person and the other is the least descriptive statement.
- **On site review:** In this method, workers are evaluated by individual representatives by obtaining verbal evaluations of workers from workplace supervisors. The HR person later writes a note and prompts the manager for additions or corrections. This method is not commonly used because supervisors usually resent what they perceive as intrusive staff intervention.
- **Critical incident technique:** The first step in this method is to create a list of critical job requirements (requirements that are critical to the success or failure of the job) for each job. The concept of a major incident differs from that of an anecdote. Fivers and Gosnell define a critical incident as an incident that significantly affects the outcome of an activity. It can be a positive factor that contributes to behavior or a negative factor that prevents task completion.
- **Confidential reports:** Confidential reports from direct managers remain an important factor in employee promotions or transfers. This format and pattern varies by organization.

Performance Evaluation Tools

The type of evaluation tool used is less important than how it is used. Formal, documented tools may contain specific guidelines or a more open format. General topics can be treated in an anecdotal or episodic form. A tool or assessment form should enable an accurate assessment of individual performance and provide an opportunity to advance individual and organizational personal goals. There are two main categories of performance evaluation tools: structured tools and fixed tools.

- **Structured (traditional) methods:** Constrained distribution scales are normative tools that prevent raters from rating all individuals in the same way. A schematic is provided to the rater and asked to rate that person against all the people the manager is evaluating. Raters indicated that the individuals evaluated were among the top 10% of employees, but not the top employees. This scale also gives employees a quick visual indication of how this rater rated their performance compared to other raters. Because this type of scale ranks the performance of individuals, it can endlessly affect group cohesion and communication effectiveness.
- **Flexible (collaborative) methodology:** The focus of the assessment can also be performed jointly. A technique that has been used for many years is management by objectives (MBO). The MBO method is similar, but more rigid in structure. The MBO approach requires employees to set clear and measurable goals at the beginning of each evaluation period. These goals are addressed separately and in writing as part of the evaluation by both employees and managers. The approach can be simplified if it is performance based and results oriented. The employee then created a real performance contact and defined future professional performance goals.
- **Performance evaluation in clinical nursing practice:** Although the term "clinical practice" is familiar to those working in nursing practice, perceptions of the term vary widely. It can mean a set of tasks or a collection of tasks, or it can mean a process. Clinical practice can be viewed as a method or medium by which professional physicians deal with clients. Clinical practice can be conceptualized as how nurses use specific counseling skills to meet the medical needs of their clients.

Performance evaluation is the systematic or formal evaluation of an individual's job performance and development potential. It is a rational and continuous process of evaluating an employee's performance on a particular job in relation to the job being sought. Performance appraisals should be distinguished from job evaluations. Job appraisals are about judging the value of different jobs, whereas performance appraisals are about measuring an individual's worth to an organization. Job reviews focus on the job, whereas performance reviews focus on the employee's performance and potential.

SELF-ASSESSMENT

Self-assessment is a way to encourage children to assess and evaluate their own learning. This is similar to peer assessment, but rather than giving feedback to a partner, students give feedback to themselves. The benefit of teaching children to self-evaluate their work is that they need to think about what they did well and what they could do better next time.

Self-assessment is a method by which an individual reflects on past experiences and events, facilitates learning, develops and maintains skills and knowledge, and assesses whether an individual's competencies comply with relevant codes of professional practice.

Benefits of Self-Assessment

Using self-assessment as an additional form of learning assessment is a great way to encourage reflection and initiative in learning. Proper self-assessment helps young people develop into independent learners.

What are the benefits of self-assessment for learners?

Here are six benefits of classroom self-assessment:

1. **Check your understanding:** There is a difference between acquiring knowledge and actually understanding something. By having students measure their reactions to something, you can get a glimpse of their actual understanding. In other words, you can show what you know and what you think you know. You can use these gaps to help your students make better progress.
2. **Fosters autonomy:** Helps young learners become more independent by helping them understand how to improve their responsiveness. Regardless of the level or subject of instruction, students are encouraged to recognize what they have done well and identify areas for improvement.
3. **Synthesize the lesson:** Ask students to evaluate their previous reactions to something in the light of the new information. This helps clear up misunderstandings and uncover new insights.
4. **Develop evaluation skills:** Encourage students to judge what is good and bad. Let them set the success criteria for a particular job. This is a higher order thinking ability that helps us make evaluative judgments.
5. **Increase engagement:** Giving students ownership of their learning gives them the opportunity to become more involved in the learning process.
6. **Greater understanding:** Actively addressing the pros and cons of a particular response forces students to think more deeply about the assessment criteria for the assignment. This will give you a deeper understanding of how to make progress in a particular area.

Benefits

- Helps students reflect and self-correct.
- Immediate feedback so students can start improving immediately.

- Self-assessment helps students develop higher-level assessment skills.
- To be honest, students must reflect honestly.
- The self-assessment itself provides another learning opportunity.
- Students need to have a better understanding of the success criteria, which may enable deeper learning.
- Helps students track their progress.
- Formative self-assessment takes attention away from levels and grades.
- Promotes independent learning.
- Self-assessment can reduce grading time for teachers.

Suggestions on how to get the most out of these nursing self-assessment forms:
- Read and learn about the rating scales used in each self-assessment tool. The basic tool uses a simpler 4-point scale and the advanced care self-assessment tool uses a more complex 5-point scale.
- Start with the competency areas you are most familiar with in clinical nursing practice.
- If you are taking too long or need to think and rest, complete the self-assessment form in one or more sessions.
- If you would like to analyze your learning/professional development needs or track your skill development over time, write down or print the completed self-assessment form.
- If you need a second opinion on your nursing skills assessment, talk to a trusted colleague or supervisor.
- Remember that this is a self-assessment and identifies your learning needs. So be honest and specific. We do not record or track these self-assessments, so your self-assessments are completely anonymous and confidential.

CLINICAL PORTFOLIO

The portfolio assessment asks the student or teacher to collect artifacts that demonstrate growth over a period of time. Examples of work results include student essay collections, artwork, lab reports, and reading records. We use evaluation guides and rubrics to evaluate portfolios.

Definition

- A professional portfolio is a structured collection of carefully selected materials that provide reliable evidence of a nurse's professional education and long-term health professional development. A portfolio demonstrates success, demonstrates professional development, and aids in career planning.
- The definition of portfolio is a flat case used to carry a sheet of roses, a combination of investments, or a sample of a finished work. An example of a portfolio is a briefcase. Examples of portfolios are various personal investments. An example of a portfolio is an exhibition of an artist previous work.

Meaning

Portfolio evaluation is one of the tools widely studied in the educational community for serious evaluation. This form of assessment has the unique ability to capture long-term learning in ways that tests and grades cannot. This article examines how Regent's University, a nontraditional, assessment-based educational institution, created a portfolio clinical assessment option for nursing students. By reflecting on their own educational and professional experiences, students develop a clinical portfolio that comprehensively demonstrates their ability to apply nursing processes and make clinical decisions in practice.

Portfolio Needs

- Portfolio management presents individuals with the optimal investment plan according to their income budget, age and ability to take risks.
- Portfolio management minimizes the risks associated with investments and increases the potential for profit.
- Portfolio managers understand clients' financial needs and propose optimal and unique investment policies that minimize risk.
- Portfolio management enables portfolio managers to offer clients customized investment solutions according to their needs and requirements.

Types of Portfolio Management

Portfolio management further includes the following types:
- **Active portfolio management:** As the name suggests, active portfolio management services allow portfolio managers to buy and sell securities. Be actively involved. To maximize personal gain.
- **Passive portfolio management:** In passive portfolio management, the portfolio manager considers a fixed portfolio adjusted to the current market scenario.
- **Discretionary portfolio management service:** With the discretionary portfolio management service, an individual authorizes a portfolio manager to manage their financial needs on their behalf. The individual hands over the money to the portfolio manager, who handles all investment needs, paperwork, filing, etc. With discretionary portfolio management, the portfolio manager has full rights to make decisions on behalf of the client.

- **Non-discretionary portfolio management services:** With non-discretionary portfolio management services, the portfolio manager can only tell the client what is good or bad, but the client retains the full right to make their own decisions.

Clinical Activity Portfolio

The clinical activity portfolio is a record of faculty activities related to the synthesis and application of knowledge and the dissemination of best clinical practice in clinical practice. One of the objectives of the portfolio of clinical activities is to provide systematic information for academic review, allowing independent reviewers to make an informed assessment of an individual's clinical contribution. All faculty involved in the field of clinician education should have a regularly updated portfolio of clinical activities. Portfolios are owned by the instructor and may contain any information the instructor wishes to document.

The following types of activities will be used to assess your effectiveness and scientific contributions in the field of clinical services.
- Develop a dedicated program to attract referrals and enhance the university's reputation based on clinical best practices.
- Plays a key role in clinical practice development/practice guideline development.
- Development of written, video, audio, or computer assisted educational materials for professional or lay groups specifically designed to improve patient care.
- Dissemination of best practice results through oral presentations such as invited talks, grand rounds, and CME events.
- Written scholarship to advance the field (dissemination of knowledge through the publication of case reports and clinical survey reports, reviews, commentaries and analytical studies in peer reviewed journals and texts that synthesize and convey clinical knowledge in ways that improve medical practice).
- Support and enhance academic patient care and/or education in involved clinical settings (e.g., clinical services program or clinic leader), act as a member or leader.
- Academic conferences, quality assurance committees, etc., related to the candidate's field.
- Other contributions to your specialty or specific areas of interest that have promoted science and excellence in clinical practice.
- Receipt of formal awards/recognition for clinical service excellence.
- All portfolios should also include ongoing self-assessment and efforts to improve clinical skills.

CLINICAL LOG

Logbook provides a collection of learning objectives to ensure consistent educational standards in clinical teaching. A journal is a way to record and track what happens in the classroom. Journals are an important tool for class management and can be used in many ways. Record interactions between students who enter the classroom late and student-parent and student-teacher interviews.

Meaning

- This logbook is based on the syllabus of INC.
- Each semester covers all clinical areas of nursing.
- Link theory and practice in the implementation of care interventions.
- This logbook is based on the hours listed in the INC Syllabus.
- This diary/journal is very useful for nursing educators/teachers as it helps in effective implementation of the curriculum.
- Helps teachers assess students' clinical performance and learning process.

Objectives of Logbook

The student internship diary is a document that:
- Presented to the clinical supervisor/evaluator to record activity each time the student observes, assists, or performs a procedure.
- It is each student's responsibility to present the logbook to the clinical supervisor/examiner whenever the student observes, assists, or performs a procedure.
- The logbook must be completed and signed by both the student and the clinical supervisor/evaluator prior to taking the final exam.
- This log records the frequency with which each intervention was observed, assisted, or performed.
- This log determines how often the clinical supervisor reviews the log.

Purposes of Logbook

The purpose of the diary is to record the student's learning experiences and practices in order to acquire the competencies and skills necessary to fulfill the required range of practice as a registered nurse.

Specific Goals

To complete clinical internships students may do:
- Basic biomedicine, applied medicine, research ethics, and the application of professionalism in the delivery of care.

- Acquire knowledge of practical procedures, diagnosis, treatment, and patient management in a variety of clinical settings.
- Demonstrate that you are aware of your limitations and are willing to refer clients when the time is right.
- Demonstrate ethical practice, empathy and respect for quality care.
- Demonstrate a desire for continued professional development.

Clinical Experience Log

The clinical experience log has several functions:
- Create and maintain accurate and detailed records of direct and indirect work performed by trainees and care received by trainees.
- This can be used to identify experience gaps or areas that need more attention.
- Help with internship planning (e.g., check the progress of current internships, think about future internships).
- May be used as evidence of clinical activity when seeking accreditation from an external agency. This protocol consists of 5 parts:
    1. Work observed by the trainee (e.g., work of a supervisor, another psychologist or other professional).
    2. Work done in collaboration with a supervisor, another psychologist or other professional.
    3. Trainee independent work.
    4. (a) Indirect and service level work and (b) Develop leadership skills.
    5. Portfolio of measures (practice-based evidence).

Nursing Diary

This diary is part of the prerequisites for successful completion of the general nursing study. This provides proof of competency attainment for enrollment with the nursing council. It is the student's responsibility to keep the logbook safe as it is required for training each year of the program. Students must remind the examiner/instructor to fill out the journal. After completing the clinical practicum, the diary will be submitted to the clinical supervisor. Examiners/instructors supervise and ensure that students have acquired the skills necessary for proficiency and enrollment. The examiner/instructor will also comment and sign the appropriate section of the logbook.

Practice Assessment Guidelines

- After the student has performed the steps, ask the examiner/instructor to comment, sign and date the logbook.
- Students are allowed two observations of the procedure. The first time in a skill lab with a mannequin and her first time in a clinical setting observing real patients.
- Learner must complete her three counter demonstrations of the procedure. The first two are signed by either the examiner/trainer and the last one is signed by the examiner (nursing educator).
- At the end of each internship, the logbook must be submitted to the clinical director for review. If desired, the journal will remain in the student's personnel file after the program ends.
- Students must complete all prescribed procedures during the academic year.

CONCLUSION

From this chapter students will be able to understand different kinds of assessment skills and apply them in nursing education and clinical practice.

REVIEW QUESTIONS

Long Essays

1. Define clinical evaluation, describe the clinical evaluation criteria.
2. Define case study/presentation, explain.
3. Describe traditional practical examination advantages and disadvantages.
4. Enlist the observation checklist advantages and disadvantages.
5. Define objective structured clinical examination (OSCE), explain the advantages and disadvantages.
6. Define rating scale, explain the types and advantages of rating scale.
7. Define written communication, explain the skills of competent writing.
8. Define progress notes, explain the items to include in nursing progress notes.
9. Define care plan, explain the types, objectives and goals.
10. Define objectively structured clinical examinations, explain the types of stations and role of teacher.
11. Define performance evaluation in nursing, explain the purposes and principles.
12. Enumerate the performance appraisal method.

Short Essays

1. Concept of clinical assessment.
2. Clinical decision-making.
3. Care interventions.
4. Type of clinical evaluation.
5. Rating scale: Advantages and disadvantages.
6. Principles of observation method.
7. How to create skills observational assessments.
8. Checklists: Checklist procedure.
9. Likert scales.
10. Benefits of video-based grading.
11. Elements of written communication.
12. Components of care plan.
13. Process record: Purposes, goals and objectives.
14. Phases process record.
15. Written assignments.
16. Importance of oral exams.
17. Principles for conducting viva-voce.
18. Types of simulation in nursing education.
19. Benefits of patient simulation in nursing education.
20. Restrictions on the use of simulation in nursing education.
21. OSPE instructions for students.
22. Anecdotal notes: Advantages and disadvantages.
23. Performance evaluation tactics.
24. Benefits of self-assessment.
25. Types of portfolio management.
26. Clinical activity portfolio.
27. Clinical log.

Short Answers

1. Proficiency assessment.
2. Competence evaluation.
3. Professional conduct.
4. Rigolosum/oral exam.
5. Skill observation assessment challenge.
6. Performance observation assessment.
7. Rating scale quality.
8. Numeric rating scale.
9. Video assessment.
10. Tips for writing nursing progress notes.
11. Process record format.
12. Verbatim dialogue.
13. Assignment objectives.
14. Practical exam.
15. Simulation objectives.
16. Virtual reality.
17. Hybrid simulation.
18. Self-report techniques.
19. Performance evaluation criteria.
20. Critical incident technique.
21. Confidential reports.
22. Portfolio needs.

Assessment of Attitude and Higher-Learning

Chapter 16

Learning Objectives
- Attitude Component
- Bogardus Social Distance Scale
- Higher Education Assessment Test
- Interpretive Questions
- Hotspot Questions
- Drag-and-Drop Questions

INTRODUCTION

Attitudes, like our physiological motivations and emotional responses, are neither innate nor learned. Purchased from us. Some of these we built ourselves. We passively and voluntarily accept others from the social environment in which we were born and raised. Many of our attitudes are the result of reflection and purposeful thinking, or training and suggestions from others, especially parents and teachers. Attitude is the evaluation of a person's behavior or events based on the beliefs that determine that person's behavior.

DEFINITION

- Attitudes describe an individual's adaptation to a selected group or organization of people. —**Kupsamy**
- Attitudes are collections of specific beliefs, feelings, and reactive tendencies of individuals toward corresponding objects. —**Kerch et al**
- Attitudes are mental frameworks that include motivations, perceptions, emotions, and cognitive responses. A person's positive or negative reaction to his surroundings, other people, and things is based on his attitude.
- An attitude is a person's persistent attitude toward an object, subject, or idea that makes him or her respond according to their interests.
- Attitudes are manifestations of one's concepts, thoughts, or beliefs that direct one's actions in a particular direction.

ATTITUDE COMPONENT

- **Cognitive component:** The opinion or belief portion of an attitude. It consists of the thoughts and beliefs that people have about the object of the attitude. So that's what we learned about something. That's what we believe to be true, e.g., vegetarian food is healthy.
- **Affective component:** The emotional or sensory part of the attitude. The emotional component is whether you like or dislike something. These are the emotions evoked by the object of the attitude, e.g., I like vegetarian food.

BOGARDUS SOCIAL DISTANCE SCALE

A scale used to define social distance in the social sciences. Also called social distance scale. The name of the scale goes back to its founder, the American sociologist Emory Bogardus (1882-1973). The Bogardus Social Distance Scale was developed by Emory S Bogardus to empirically measure peoples willingness to socialize with varying degrees of intimacy with members of various social groups, including racial and ethnic groups is a psychological test scale.

Purpose

Main purposes of the Bogardus social distancing scale are:
- The scale is designed to measure attitudes towards specific racial groups.
- This scale measures the closeness of the relationship that the respondent is willing to accept.

- The Bogardus scale is commonly used in the study of ethnic relations, social class and social values.

Features

- **Social distance:** For Bogardus, social distance is a way of understanding the distance between members of two different groups. This indicates how much or how little each group member sympathizes with each other.
- **Cumulative nature:** The social distance scale according to Bogardus is also a cumulative or Guttmann scale. This means that the agreement with the statement specified as an option is the agreement with the preceding statement in the list of options, e.g., if you agree with the statement with a rating of 1.0, you also agree with the statement below.
- **Seven-point scale:** The 7-point scale is a good choice for measuring the degree of sympathy or hostility between members of two social groups. Combining the traits of both scales results in simpler question patterns that are better answered by the audience.

Benefits

Bogardus social distancing scale benefits include:
- **Ease of use:** Creating and managing scales is very easy. Complications can arise only when formulating each option of the distance scale.
- **Measuring prejudice:** Bogardus' Social Distance Scale measures the prejudice, or underlying thoughts and feelings, between two different groups of people in her who may belong to different social groups.
- **Reliability:** This scale is reliable because it measures each respondent's feelings about the question. The question type also ensures that each respondent selects an option.
- **Ordinal measurement level:** This scale collects ordinal data from each respondent. This helps establish priorities for problem groups.

Disadvantages

- **Order of options:** The order of options has different meanings for different people within a group community or family. This is done based on each member's preferences. Therefore, the validity of the distances in the Bogardus social distancing scale options does not apply to all respondents.
- **Equal distance in quantitative social distance:** The distance between two options is subjective. The distance between 3 and 4 or 6 and 7 must not be equal. Also, it is impossible to prove that option 6 has twice the distance of 3.

- **One-dimensional:** Its nature is one-dimensional and the data is recorded accordingly. I don't have room to elaborate on the rationale for the answer.
- **Validity cannot be measured:** Each member of a social group can choose an answer based on their perception of the problem to other groups. However, this rating does not allow for further investigation as to why the rating was chosen, and therefore cannot measure relevance.

Difference between the Guttman Scale and the Likert Scale

- The Guttman scale accepts what the data represent without applying superficial weighting to the observed variables. Likert scales, however, have a scale that sums the scores of respondents, assuming equal weight for all variables.
- Likert scales focus on the level of respondents' agreement or disagreement with a set of statements following a symmetric scale. The Gutman scale, on the other hand, focuses on the respondent's total score and predicts a perfect response to the statements in the item.
- The Likert scale is a psychometric scale and the Guttman scale is a cumulative scale.

Difference Between Guttman Scale and Thurstone Scale

- Researchers determine the statements used in the Thurstone Scale survey by assigning values to questions. On the Guttman scale, the average level of support for a statement determines what questions are asked. Therefore, if a statement has little support, it is excluded from the survey questions.
- The scale used in determining the outcome of the Thurstone scale ranges from least desirable to most desirable, whereas the outcome of the Guttman scale is determined on a yes or no basis.
- You can apply the median or mode Thurstone scale for analysis. For the Guttman scale, average opinions are used for analysis.
- The comparative value of the Thurstone scale is determined on the basis of the judge's understanding without regard to whether the mathematical calculator is wrong. Judges also decide score match on the Guttman scale, but unlike the Thurstone scale, this is difficult to do.

HIGHER EDUCATION ASSESSMENT TEST

Assessment in higher education is important in measuring the educational effectiveness and quality of an institution's teaching. Assessments are useful to a variety of stakeholders, including students, faculty, and administrators, and can answer a variety of questions about student development, the value of particular courses, and institutional credibility.

Type

- **Formative:** Used to monitor student learning and plan subsequent lessons. Data collected from formative assessments provide insight into a student's strengths, weaknesses and developmental progress.
- **Abstract:** Used to collect data on knowledge acquisition and skill development. Stakeholders can measure how well students are achieving their learning goals, gaining insight into the effectiveness of materials and curriculum design.

Level

Level 1

Assessing the individual learning success of individual students within a course.

- The first level is concerned with assessing the individual learning success of individual students within a course.
- The purpose is to measure a student's learning progress in a particular course.
- The assessment tools you use should provide data that highlights your students' strengths and weaknesses and guide their progress with actionable recommendations for improvement.
- Miller and Leskes found that teachers minimize the awarding of overall grades (A through F) because they do not provide the coordinated, actionable feedback necessary to encourage meaningful student development. We encourage the use of formative and summative assessments.
- These grades "represent an average estimate of overall quality and tell us little about a student's strengths, weaknesses, or room for improvement."

Level 2

Assessing individual student's individualized learning across multiple courses.

The second level is the assessment of individual student's individualized learning across multiple courses. This level of assessment allows stakeholders to measure student progress as they progress through the curriculum of a particular major or program.

Crosscourse assessment of individual student learning achieves the following objectives:

- Provides students with evidence of progress throughout the course
- Provides actionable feedback to students over time
- Provides stakeholders with insight into student performance against program learning objectives.
- Provide information on corrective efforts needed to close developmental gaps and improve the quality of education.

To collect meaningful data, Miller and Leskes suggest that formative and summative assessments at this level consider the following three questions:

1. During the program or has the student improved and/or met standards since entering college?
2. To what extent has the student achieved the main program disciplinary results?
3. To what extent did the student achieve the institution wide learning outcomes over the four years?

Level 3

Course assessment requires programs and institutions to prepare for courses and evaluate the effectiveness of courses in helping to acquire expected knowledge levels and skills.

- Like her previous two levels, course assessment can use both formative and summative assessment.
- Examples of available assessment tools include embedded coursework (exams and projects), commercially developed tests, and course portfolios.
- Course evaluation allows stakeholders to identify areas of the curriculum that need modification to improve educational relevance.
- As Miller and Lesquez put it, faculty and committees "understand how courses fit into coherent learning pathways and use evidence analysis to improve teaching and course design" Responsible. The assessment level involves an evaluation of the program aimed at measuring correspondence with curriculum design and learning objectives. The data collected at this level of assessment reflects how well the program is preparing students to achieve their learning outcomes and also highlights educational gaps within the curriculum.

According to Miller and Leskes, most program evaluations require a summative evaluation that answers her six questions.

- Do the courses in the program, individually or collectively, contribute to the outcomes as designed?
- How well does the program fulfill its purposes in the entire curriculum?
- To what extent do program subcategories contribute to overall goals? Do you do?
- Are the courses organized in a consistent manner that allows for cumulative learning?
- Does the program support the organizational goals as planned? Data must be collected during program entry and exit.

Level 4

The fourth level of assessment involves the assessment of programs with the goal of measuring the alignment between curriculum designs and learning objectives. The data gathered at this level of assessment demonstrates how well a program prepares students to meet learning objectives and further highlights educational gaps within the curriculum. According to Miller and Leskes, the assessment of programs mostly requires the implementation of summative assessments that address the following six questions:

1. Do the program's courses, individually and collectively, contribute to its outcomes as planned?
2. How well does the program fulfill its purposes in the entire curriculum?
3. How well do the program's sub-categories contribute to the overall purposes?
4. Does the program's design resonate with its expected outcomes?
5. Are the courses organized in a coherent manner to allow for cumulative learning?
6. Does the program advance institution-wide goals as planned?

Level 5: Institutional Assessment

Fifth level of assessment in higher education includes measuring the effectiveness of institutions in education. Preparing students for success after graduation. Results collected from institution level assessments are used to improve curriculum design and meet both internal and external educational quality requirements.

- Several stakeholders, including administrators and educators, are responsible for this assessment level.
- Their collaboration is essential to establish a systematic process across the institute to continuously improve the quality of education.
- These processes also allow stakeholders to close the loop between the analysis of assessment data and the resulting remediation work.
- Assessment tools that provide valid data to measure how well an institution is preparing students for educational and professional learning outcomes include preprogram level assessments, level and graduation levels, and individual or cohort level assessments conducted in courses. Required general knowledge and core subject level assessment.

Preliminary or Diagnostic Evaluation

- Before creating a lesson, you need to know what type of student you are creating the lesson for.
- The goal is to know the student's strengths, weaknesses, skills and knowledge before they attend class. Guides can be created based on the data collected.

Formative Assessment

- Formative assessment is used in the first attempt at instructional development. The purpose is to monitor student learning and provide feedback.
- Helps identify gaps at the beginning of the lesson. This feedback will help us know what to focus on as we continue to expand our teaching.

Summative Assessment

- The summative assessment is intended to assess how well the main outcomes at the end of the lesson have been achieved. However, it does not measure the effectiveness and long-term usefulness of learning responses to instruction.
- Long-term benefits can be determined by tracking students taking courses or exams. See if and how they are applying the knowledge, skills and attitudes they have learned.

Confirmation Assessment

Even if instruction is given in the classroom, it must be assessed. The purpose of a positive evaluation is to see if the teaching is still successful after, say, one year and whether the teaching methods are still up-to-date. A positive appraisal can be said to be a broad form of summative appraisal.

Norm-related Assessment

Compares student performance to average norms. For example, this could be a national average standard for history. Another example is when a teacher compares the average performance of a student to the average performance of the school as a whole.

Criteria-based Assessment

Measures student performance against fixed, predetermined criteria or learning standards. It tests what a student should know and be able to do at a particular stage of education. Criteria-based tests are used to assess specific knowledge and skills. This is the syllabus assessment test that is taken in the course.

Ipsative Assessment

Measures a student's performance relative to the student's previous performance. This method attempts to improve upon previous results. Self-confidence can be damaged by not comparing yourself to other students.

INTERPRETIVE QUESTIONS

Interpretive questions have answers that are supported by textual evidence. Sometimes people give different answers, but as long as the evidence supports the question, the question can still be correct. Interpretive level questions examine meaning and patterns of meaning based on objective data and reflections of internal reactions to that data.

Meaning

Interpretation questions have answers that are supported by textual evidence. Sometimes people may give different answers, but as long as the evidence supports the question, the question can still be correct.

Question Type

- **Fact:** Fact questions have only one correct answer.
- **Interpretation:** Interpretation questions have multiple answers supported by textual evidence. Interpretation questions keep the discussion moving and force the reader to refer back to the text.
- **Evaluative:** Evaluative questions prompt readers to decide whether they agree with the author's ideas or points of view. The answers to the evaluation questions depend on the reader's previous knowledge, experience and opinions.

Format

- Related series
- Based on a common data set
- Many

Uses

- Conclusion recognition
- Recognition of just/unjust generalizations
- Recognition of premises
- Recognition of information relevance
- Application of principles
- Use of visuals

Benefits

- Interpretive skills are important in everyday life
- Can measure more complex learning than a single isolated item
- As a set of related items can reveal a broader depth of skill
- Can provide necessary background information
- Can provide measurements and objective assessments of specific mental processes (as opposed to unstructured performance tasks)

Limitations

- Difficulty of construction
  - Introduction materials (general data) are difficult to obtain
  - If found, post-processing is usually required
- Heavy read requirements
- Limited when measuring complex performance
  - Elements of problem-solving skills, but not integrated
  - Awareness not productive skills.

Steps

- Selection of introductory materials
- Building a series of dependent problems
- Confirming introductory materials require a complex mental process.

Suggestions

Introductory material

- Relevance to learning objectives and correct complexity
- Appropriate to student's proficiency
- Basic reading level (no complex words or sentence structures)
- Short but meaningful
- Revised content clarity, conciseness, purpose
- As you create your question, amend the content as needed.

For questions

- Analysis and interpretation of the introductory material is required.
  - Do not ask for answers given directly in the introduction.
  - Do not ask questions that do not require introductory material.
- The number should be proportional to or greater than the length of the insert.
- Please follow the relevant suggestions regarding the objective element.
- For key elements, keep key categories uniform and mutually exclusive.
- Optionally create default key categories for key elements.

Use these sample interpretation questions as a guide to derive some customized questions to help the group understand a situation or problem and reach a decision or agreement.

- What is the positive side of this situation?
- What could have caused this situation?
- Why did this happen?
- What impact does this situation have?
- What do you think is the reason for this impasse?

- What value should be represented to solve this problem?
- What options are valid? Is not it?
- What are your insights?
- What do you think works best? Why?
- What are the alternatives?
- What does it look like in everyday life?
- What are the main differences and similarities between these options?
- How does this relate to your overall goals? Will you do?
- What is most relevant to you?
- What patterns do you hear throughout this discussion? These books increase understanding and provide templates for conversations on various topics.

HOTSPOT QUESTIONS

Hotspot questions are a cool type of question that allow candidates to highlight specific areas of an image. When creating a question, you can specify which part of the image is used as the answer and adjust the size.

Definition

Spot questions are informal tests that are run without much preparation to get a quick sample answer.

Classroom Spot Questions

- **Close reading:** Hotspots are a great tool for close reading activities. Scrutiny is observing the details of a work and extracting evidence. You can set up hotspots to hold the evidence you need to answer specific questions while reading. Students should read and select the part that justifies their answer. These types of questions are the reason hotspot questions exist. Therefore, they will certainly show up in standardized tests.
- **Cards:** Hotspot questions are suitable for any questions about cards. Map questions often ask students to select a specific area related to the question. This is useful for general location learning. (So get to know all the countries in Asia) Or it can be a question that brings in a thematic map or data. Hotspots let students analyze important images that show large amounts of data.
- **Figures:** Figures are used on a variety of subjects. Take anatomy and physiology for example. Suppose you are examining a leg bone. Have students identify each part of the leg. You can also test more theoretical injury-related questions. Combining realworld scenarios with visual elements, this type of application is common in standardized tests.
- **Art analysis:** The patterns of doctrine in art and history can be complex. After teaching students the main components of Renaissance art, ask them to identify those components from images of authentic art. Have them highlight parts that are relevant to topics already discussed in class. This handson application expands student knowledge.
- **Statistical analysis:** The stats page is useless if students don't know how to use it. Guides analysis of statistics using the hotspots tool. Select middle income countries and do not display country names. Include a list of statistics as a worksheet in teacher made. Have students click on the statistic that represents the more developed countries and then the statistic that represents the developing countries. Middle income countries have both elements. This activity is useful both economically and geographically.
- **Photos:** Have students analyze photos using the hotspots tool. See human geography for an example of this. Part of the curriculum is understanding the differences between cities around the world. You can display a picture of a city and let students select the part that supports typical features. This process helps students connect images to concepts.
- **Foreign languages:** Assessing foreign language vocabulary can be difficult. Show the word and have the students choose the correct picture. A similar way to assess this is to use an audio recording to pronounce the word and have the student select the correct image.
- **Evidence:** The best place to use the hotspot feature is where students are required to provide evidence. Let your students show off their work with teacher made. Evidence-based questions encourage students to think more deeply.

Survey Hotspot Questions

- Survey hotspot questions present respondents with one or more selected regions. Clicking on this area allows respondents to express their opinion both graphically and textually.
- A popup window will appear over the survey, showing a 'thumbs up' button and a 'thumbs down' button to indicate whether you like or dislike it.
- Respondents can also leave comments in the text box. This allows researchers to better understand their opinions about the images.
- Hotspot quizzes let you choose whether to force respondents to answer a question or to require an answer. You can also customize the border color of selected areas that require attendee feedback.

Hotspot Questions Data Analysis

The hotspots report provides market researchers with the following insights.

- **Responses:** The number of times each region was selected.
- **Percent of responses:** The number of times each region was selected out of the total number of responses.
- **Comments:** Respondent's comments for each region.
- **Export as XLS:** Exports results in Excel format.
- **Sharing options:** Share your hotspot report by sharing a web link or embedding code.

Using the Hotspot Test in Online Research

- **Concept testing:** Researchers use the hotspot test to experiment with different ideas. Researchers can go to the images with the most likes.
- **Usability testing:** Developers conduct usability testing of websites using hotspot questions. You can view different variations of your website's design and ask respondents if they like certain elements of a particular design.
- **Feedback poll:** If you need to collect feedback on a visual element, the hotspot quiz can be used in any feedback poll. Sometimes people are completely ignoring the background image section. Researchers use this question type to get clear feedback.

Benefits of Hotspot Image Testing

- **Collect feedback early:** Hotspot poll questions allow you to collect feedback from your audience early in the process.
- **Know exactly what your respondents like:** Instead of guessing what your customers like, you can collect data on exactly what your customers want. It is always better to get specific feedback than general feedback.
- **Save time:** Once you know the likes and dislikes of your respondents, you only need to work on specific elements. This saves time compared to revising the entire design.
- **Increase respondent engagement:** Hotspot questions save respondents the trouble of answering many multiple-choice questions. They can be a nice change of pace, and respondents only have to click a button.

DRAG-AND-DROP QUESTIONS

A drag-and-drop question is the dragging of a set of two or more possible answers onto an answer target. A target is a block, table, or other location on the screen. Drag-and-drop questions include instructions on how to answer. For example, you may be asked to select only certain answer types for a goal, use one answer for multiple goals, drag multiple answers to the same goal, or place the answers in a specific order may be the steps are given in the question above.

Definition

A drag-and-drop question type that requires dragging missing words into the gaps of paragraphs of text.

How to Create a Drag-and-Drop Question

- Select the drag-and-drop text question in the left pane and add it to the section.
- Add the question title and statement.
- Upload a background image (recommended width is 880 pixels; the image will be scaled in the learner's view to fit the placeholder).
- Create a text element. Drag-and-drop the text element to set its correct position on the background image. Each element should correspond to a unique position.
- Add feedback for correct and incorrect answers.

Tips for Writing Good Drag-and-Drop Questions

- The question text should be directly descriptive and identify a specific problem that focuses on your learning goals.
- Make sure each element is in a certain unique position on the image.
- Limit the number of text items to 6. More than 6 items can be confusing.
- Keep elements parallel and of similar length, and use consistent grammar.

Benefits of the Drag-and-Drop Question Type

Drag-and-drop ranking questions are most useful for researchers when making decisions to rank items. Here the researcher can keep the text of the question very short. It has the following advantages:

- **Very attractive:** This question is very attractive as it requires the respondent to physically drag-and-drop the answer image into the list.
- **Easy to understand:** This kind of question is very simple and easy. Respondents must rank the photos in order of "most liked/preferred" and "least liked/less liked".
- **Easy to create:** Creating questions is relatively easy. All researchers have to do is upload images of possible answers in the space provided.
- **Clear answers:** This type of question is very easy to answer and gives clear answers, as the respondent can simply drag and drop the images and rearrange them as desired.

REVIEW QUESTIONS

Long Essays
1. Define attitude, explain Bogardus social distance scale.
2. Define higher education assessment test, explain the purposes and levels.
3. Define hotspot questions, explain the classroom spot questions.
4. Define drag-and-drop questions, explain writing good drag-and-drop questions.

Short Essays
1. Difference between Guttman scale and Likert scale.
2. Bogardus social distancing scale benefits.
3. Difference between Guttman scale and Thurstone scale.
4. Interpretive questions: Types and benefits.
5. Using the hotspot test in online research.
6. Benefits of hotspot image testing.
7. Benefits of the drag-and-drop question type.

Short Answers
1. Attitude component.
2. Social distance.
3. Norm-related assessment.
4. Criteria-based assessment.
5. Ipsative assessment.
6. Drag-and-drop question.
7. Feedback poll.
8. Cognitive component.
9. Affective component.

Unit 7
Guidance/Academic Advising, Counseling and Discipline Guidance

Chapters

17. Guidance and Counseling
18. Counseling
19. Guidance/Academic Advising
20. Discipline and Grievance

KEYWORDS

Guidance: Guidance is an assistance given to the individual in making intelligence choices and adjustments.

Counseling: Counseling is a technique of guidance—any type of guidance where individual help is given to students. Personal guidance assists the individual to adjust with psychological and social environment.

Advising: In this stage, the counselor suggests appropriate courses of action. Here the counselor will offer you several options and recommends one according to your aim or interest.

Informing: Here the role of the counselor is to give appropriate and correct information to the clients. For example, you are a student and you need counseling to select your course for the future.

Directive counseling: BG Williamson is the chief, exponent of the directive counseling. It is counselor-oriented counselee is passive.

Non-directive counseling: Carl Rogers is the chief exponent of non-directive counseling. Counselor is role is passive. Counselee is active.

Counter will: People experience difficulty in asking for help and accepting it, because they are reluctant to face the consequences of change or an admission of inadequacy of failure.

Case history: Case history is a systematic collection of facts about the counselee's past and present life.

Rapport: It is a warm-friendly and understanding atmosphere created by the counselor, which is catalytical in the formation of an effective counseling relationship.

Counter transference: This occurs when counselor project their unresolved conflicts upon the counselee. When counselor feels uncomfortable and experience felling of anger, resentment or become overemotional. This is unhealthy.

Resistance: It refers to counselee's move to oppose the counselor's to work towards set goals. This influences counseling outcome positively.

Clarification: To get definite information through this to help clarify the client's thinking without pressurizing.

Concreteness: Using clear language to describe the client's life situation. It promotes clear insight in client's life and provides counselor with a fuller sense of the uniqueness of the client's experiences.

Restatement: Enables the counselor to let the counselee realize that he is being fully understood and accepted. Counselor exactly repeats as said by the client. Client thus gets a rest and a chance to collect his thoughts before going forward.

Paraphrasing: The counselor summarizes. He chooses/selects those ideas and feelings which seem most important and relevant and feeds them back of the client in a more organized form.

Communicating: Exchange of ideas and opinions between two or more people through speech, writing or signs. It involves some factors.

Pre-admission and admission services: Provided for students seeking admission to preuniversity (junior college) courses and degree programs.

Orientation service: Aims to facilitate adjustment to school or college life.

Student information service: Provides the student with sufficient educational, social, and occupational data to guide his choices and decisions.

Counseling service: Aims to assist student to achieve self-knowledge for decision-making and responsible studentship.

Placement service: Designed to give information about the student to aid him/her toward self-knowledge and self-actualization.

Remedial service: The most important service of the guidance program designed to help student towards maximum self-realization and development to become fully integrated, mature, and responsible individual.

Follow-up services: Provides career counseling, systematic contacts with alumni, and provision for continuing education, occupation and involvement in citizenship.

Chapter 17

Guidance and Counseling

Learning Objectives

- Guidance and Advice Objectives
- Need for Guidance and Advice
- Difference Between Accompany and Advice
- Scope of Guidance and Advice in Education
- Principles of Leadership and Counseling
- Effective Leadership and the Benefits of Effective Leadership Advice
- Leadership and Leadership Role Advice
- Instructions and Instructions Advisory: Program Component
- Comprehensive Instruction and Counseling Plan
- Guidance Counselor Responsibilities
- Guidance and Advice for Nurses
- Nurse Manager's Role in Guidance and Guidance Consult

TERMINOLOGY

- **Active listening:** This is a process that involves the use of encouragers to paraphrase and summarize.
- **Empathic understanding:** Observing behavior in combination with observation is the basis for a functioning alliance born from it. Empathic understanding requires warmth, respect, and compassion.

Encouragement

Verbal and non-verbal, including nods, gestures, phrases such as "Uh huh," or simply repeating one, two, or three of her keywords that the patient used.

- **Goal:** A specific achievement or action. These are clearly operational so the observer can determine whether the goals have been achieved.
- **Research:** The basic process of gathering and providing information to advise patients and suggest viable alternative solutions to resolve their concerns.
- **Observation:** Focus on specific non-verbal and verbal behaviors of the patient.
- **Openended questions:** Allows the issue to be explored more deeply, but usually she cannot answer in a few words. Openended questions usually start with what, how, or why.
- **Paraphrasing:** Telling the patient what was said. Paraphrasing is short and used to clarify comments using your own words and the exact keywords the patient said.
- **Emotion reflection:** Involves identifying the patient's emotions and reflecting them to clarify emotional experiences.
- **Summary:** Similar to paraphrasing, except it covers what the patient said over a period of time. An important part of the summary is the final consultation with the patient about accuracy. A summary includes facts, thoughts, and feelings.
- **Unconditional positive gratitude:** Refers to acceptance of the patient for what they are, even when the patient knows their shortcomings. Accepting the patient does not mean accepting the thoughts and actions you are discussing with the patient.
- **Validation:** The concept of validation is to tell the patient what you think is normal. They validate feelings, not actions.
- **Values:** Freedom to choose life orientations or behavioral qualities that are meaningful or important to an individual. They can be instantiated at any time and are

not necessarily bound by cultural norms. For example, spending time with family and being kind to them are values.
- **Grievances:** Employees care about everything, whether or not their grievances are verbalized.
- **Complaint:** A verbal or written complaint is brought to the attention of a supervisor or clerk.
- **Informal complaint:** An informal complaint is defined as an academic or non-academic problem that a student has with a college faculty member, staff member, administrator, department or program.
- **Respondent:** A respondent is a person to whom a complaint or potential complaint is made.
- **Appellant:** The person filing the appeal.
- **Appeal:** You may appeal the resolution of an academic or nonacademic complaint. Appeals must be based on issues of material or procedural error undermining impartial prosecution of the case.
- **Confidentiality:** Committee members, faculty, and administrators involved in complaints and discussion of complaints are expected to adhere to professional standards of confidentiality.

INTRODUCTION

Guidance counseling, also called counseling and guidance, helps individuals discover and develop their own educational, vocational, and psychological potential, thereby achieving optimal levels of personal well-being and social benefit. It is a process that helps guidance and counseling help individuals discover and develop their own capacities to nurture their educational, professional and psychological potential and to achieve optimal levels of personal well-being and social benefit.

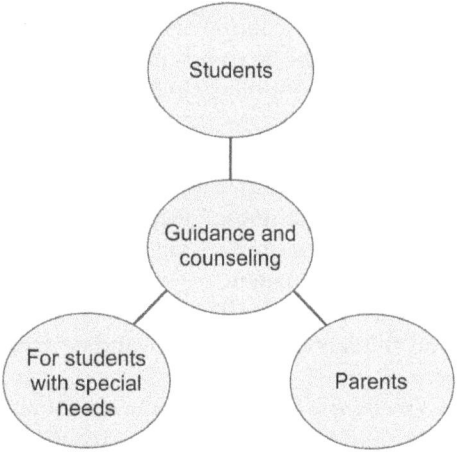

Fig. 17.1: Guidance and counseling needs.

DEFINITION

Leadership

- "To lead means to direct, show, show the way". —**Jones**
- "Counseling includes all activities that enhance a person's self-actualization". —**Bernard and Fulmer**
- Emphasized the goals of counseling 'targeted activities'. —**DV Teideman**
- "Leadership is about helping John see through himself". —**Honalins**
- "Systematic focus on learning and views counseling as educational and developmental". —**RH Mathewson**

Counseling

- "Counseling is a personal relationship in which both counselor and counselor grow". —**Ruth Strang**
- "Counseling means consultation, mutual exchange, joint counseling". —**Humphrey and Traxler**

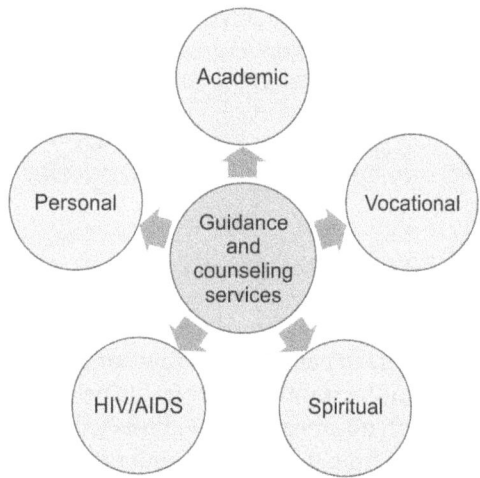

Fig. 17.2: Guidance and counseling areas.

GUIDANCE AND ADVICE OBJECTIVES

- Best personal development.
- Helping students develop self-leadership and personal maturity.
- Helping maximize student well-being and social productivity.
- Helping students live better lives.

Educational institutions guidance and counseling program goals in:

- A clear understanding and acceptance of yourself—your strengths, limitations, interests, abilities, skills, abilities, attitudes and motivations.
- Develop his skills and interests as much as possible by providing relevant experiences.

- To understand the options he faces, the opportunities available to him and the skills needed to achieve the goals he has set.
- Makes own decisions and plans based on self-understanding and knowledge of available options.
- To carry out his plans and adapt to new situations.
- Take responsibility for your decisions.

NEED FOR GUIDANCE AND ADVICE

Students' problems should be properly approached with the intention of solving them. Unresolved issues can affect not only a student's academic performance, but also their personal growth. Teaching and mentoring helps teachers solve student problems through active participation. It also supports teachers in creating a healthy environment within their institution by ensuring the harmonious and holistic personal growth of their students.

Guidance and the need for guidance can be summarized as follows:
- To support the overall development of the student.
- Help students live healthy lives by avoiding things that are harmful to their health.
- Assist in the selection of appropriate educational programs.
- Help you choose a career based on your interests and skills.
- Support student professional development.
- Develop a willingness to change and meet challenges.
- We minimize the mismatch between education and employment and support efficient utilization of human resources.
- Assist with identity verification of new students.
- Identify and motivate students from disadvantaged backgrounds.
- Help students navigate through times of turmoil and confusion.
- Identify and provide assistance to students with special needs.
- To ensure that time spent outside the classroom is used appropriately.
- Help address the challenges posed by student explosion and co-education.
- To minimize the occurrence of disciplinary violations.
- Encourage young people to become independent.
- Assist students in need to obtain financial assistance from appropriate organizations.

DIFFERENCE BETWEEN ACCOMPANY AND ADVICE

The main difference between advice and counseling is shown here.

- Guidance is advice and related information from management to help you solve problems or overcome difficulties. Counseling is professional advice given by a counselor to an individual to help them deal with personal or psychological problems.
- Counseling is preventive in nature whereas counseling is curative, curative or curative in nature.
- Counseling helps the person choose the best options. But in counseling he tends to shift his perspective so that he can find the solution himself.
- Counseling is a comprehensive process. It is an external approach. Counseling, on the other hand, focuses on a thorough internal analysis of the problem until the client understands and fully addresses it.
- Counseling is provided for educational and work-related issues, but counseling is sought when the issue is related to personal and psychosocial problems.
- Guidance is provided by leaders who are managers or experts in a particular field. Unlike counseling, highly qualified counselors who have completed specialized training are in charge.

Basis for comparison	Guidance	Counseling
Meaning	Guidance refers to an advice or a relevant piece of information provided by a superior, to resolve a problem or overcome from difficulty	Counseling refers to a professional advice given by a counselor to an individual to help him in overcoming from personal or psychological problems
Nature	Preventive	Remedial and curative
Approach	Comprehensive and extroverted	In-depth and introverted
What it does?	It assists the person in choosing the best alternative	It tends to change the perspective, to help him get the solution by himself or herself
Deals with	Education and career related issues	Personal and socio-phychological issues
Provided by	Any person superior or expert	A person who possesses high level of skill and professional training
Privacy	Open and less private	Confidential
Mode	One to one or one to many	One to one
Decision-making	By guide	By the client

- The tour can be open, so the degree of privacy is low. Absolute secrecy is maintained as opposed to advice.
- Counseling can be individual or group at a time. On the contrary, advice is always one-on-one.
- Guides make decisions on behalf of clients during counseling. This is in contrast to counseling, where the counselor empowers the client to make their own decisions.

Advice and related information that administrators give to solve problems or overcome difficulties is called guidance. Counseling is professional advice given by a counselor to an individual to deal with personal or psychological problems.

Counseling is preventive in nature, but counseling is more curative, or curative in nature.

Counseling helps the person choose the best option. However, counseling tends to shift perspective so that the person can find their own solution.

Consulting is a comprehensive process with an external approach. Hand counseling, on the other hand, focuses on a thorough internal analysis of the problem until the client fully understands and addresses it.

Counseling is provided for educational and professional problems, but counseling is sought when problems are related to personal and psychosocial problems.

Guides are provided by guides who are supervisors or experts in a particular field. In contrast to counseling, it is performed by highly qualified consultants who have completed specialized training.

Guides open for less privacy. Contrast with advice where absolute confidentiality is maintained.

Counseling can be done individually or in groups at a time.

SCOPE OF GUIDANCE AND ADVICE IN EDUCATION

The scope of guidance and advice in education is as follows:
- **Educational areas:** Education is important for the proper and comprehensive development of the individual. People can get confused when choosing a topic. Guidance and advice help children consider their interests and abilities and choose subjects in which they can progress.
- **Overall personal development:** Instruction and advice focuses on all areas of development. It supports an individual's psychological, emotional and educational development. This will help you understand the problems facing each area.
- **Career advancement:** Guidance and counseling enable individuals to discover their skills and potential. That way, they can work on those skills and turn them into skills that will help them advance their careers.
- **Career needs:** At different stages of life, people may have different interests and preferences in different things. Guidance and advice help individuals discover and advance their professional interests.
- **Help:** Guidance and counseling are ways of providing support to people facing situational problems in their lives and helping them solve those problems.

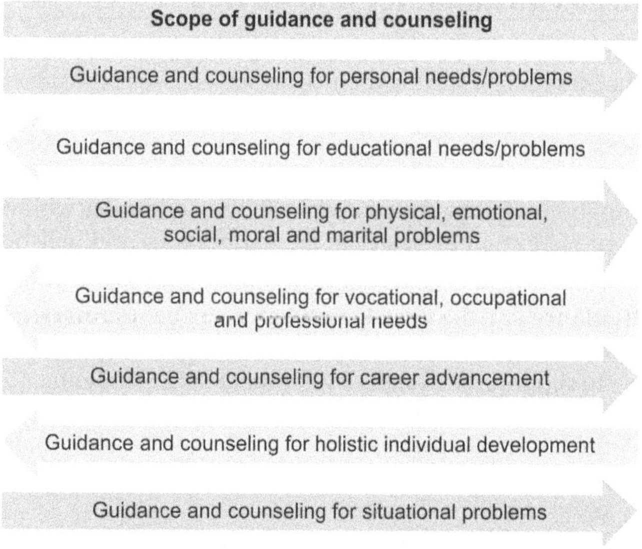

Scope of guidance and counseling

Guidance and counseling for personal needs/problems

Guidance and counseling for educational needs/problems

Guidance and counseling for physical, emotional, social, moral and marital problems

Guidance and counseling for vocational, occupational and professional needs

Guidance and counseling for career advancement

Guidance and counseling for holistic individual development

Guidance and counseling for situational problems

Fig. 17.3: Scope of guidance and counseling.

- **Adaptation:** In life, one has to go through many changes and experience many changing atmospheres. Guidance and counseling help individuals adjust to these changes.
- **Decision-making:** Guidance and counseling help individuals develop the ability to make effective decisions about important issues.

PRINCIPLES OF LEADERSHIP AND COUNSELING

- **Leadership and counseling are unique to each individual:** Each individual is unique. We know that no two people are the same. They differ in skills, interests, talents, personality traits, values, attitudes, etc.
- Leadership and consulting are about the 'whole person' and should focus on the overall growth of the individual, not just one part of the personality. This means that any situation or problem faced by an individual should always be viewed from a holistic perspective and lead to holistic personality development.
- **Guidance and advice is always goal oriented:** Goal setting is an important task of guidance and advice. Setting realistic goals and working towards them is a fundamental requirement of any counseling.

- Advice and advice is a professional service. Only professionally trained personnel may provide advice or advice. When performed by an untrained individual, it causes even greater harm to the client.
- Guidance and advice should be based on a good knowledge of the characteristics of stages of human growth and development. Each stage of human life has its own characteristics and developmental tasks to accomplish.
- The accomplishment of these tasks and the impact of their interaction with the environment are decisive factors that shape the overall character of people at a certain stage of life.
- Guidance and advice is available to all who need it: All individuals, regardless of age, caste, gender, occupational status, etc., need guidance and advice at all stages of development. It is well known that this should be given to all people who need help at any point in their lives.
- Guidance and counseling are not developmentally specific. Necessary at all stages of life. At every stage of life, humans need guidance on a variety of issues. Guidance and advice is an ongoing process. I understand that guidance and advice are not limited to problem solving only.
- The primary focus is on helping students achieve holistic growth. If these services are for the express purpose of helping an individual deal with a problem, we may need to terminate them after a solution has been found.
- Orientation and counseling should be based on reliable data. Information about the person/student forms the basis for orientation and counseling suggestions. Therefore, the counselor must have reliable data/information about the person. Counselors should seek to gather information from appropriate sources (parents, teachers, peers, etc.) using validated and credible psychological tests and tools.
- A flexible approach to teaching and counseling is required. Flexibility means flexibility in using data selection tools, methods/strategies to guide the approach to monitoring, etc. An approach tested for one student will be a learning experience for another. Gives insight into other students' similar problems.

EFFECTIVE LEADERSHIP AND THE BENEFITS OF EFFECTIVE LEADERSHIP ADVICE

- Students receive appropriate guidance on how to deal with mental health issues that can negatively affect their academic performance. Through these sessions, students develop specific problemsolving skills that help them to some extent deal with specific problems in their lives.
- Students are advised on how to deal with various situations they encounter in their daily school life. For example, how should you speak politely and treat your colleagues? This advice gives perspective on how to act in certain scenarios.
- It helps shape the behavior of the students and also instills good discipline in them. With proper guidance and support, students can achieve their goals. Students were advised to know what to do and how best to get things done.
- Students learn to live in peace and harmony with others in the school community. It also teaches you to appreciate others in your class.
- Helps bridge the gap between students and school administrators by allowing them to resolve issues through appropriate counseling channels within the office.
- Students receive comprehensive guidance on career paths and opportunities to help them make informed choices and understand what they can do after school.
- Students can talk to teachers about different experiences they have had. You can talk openly about issues that you cannot share with your parents.
- It is acceptable to speak openly about alcohol, drugs, personal feelings, or any form of abuse. Teaching and guidance also help students become better people because they receive instruction on how to act and behave in specific situations.
- Students facing special challenges in life are able to ask questions, solve problems and clarify advice through instruction. Therefore, in counseling, the person in charge will be empathetic and will give you a consultation, so you can consult with peace of mind.

LEADERSHIP AND LEADERSHIP ROLE ADVICE

Guidance and advice has his three functions: Coordination oriented and development-oriented. It also helps teachers understand their students and helps them identify particularly gifted and underperforming children. This helps teachers understand personal differences between students and the community.

Adjustmental

- Guidance and counseling are adjustmental in the sense that they help the students in making the best possible adjustment to the current situations in the educational institution, in the home and the community.
- Expert and individual assistance is provided to quickly adapt problem areas as needed.
- In the words of Leonardo, instruction and counseling must enable students to accept the things they cannot

change in life in order to modify or change the things they can change. You have to be successful in life and be able to discern what you should be doing. What can and cannot be changed in life.

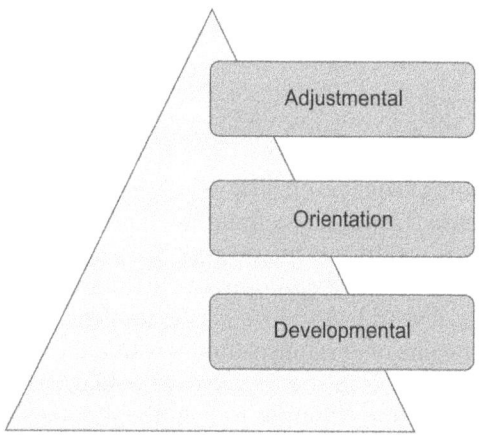

Fig. 17.4: Leadership role of advice.

Orientation

- Orientation and advice also has orientation function. They guide students toward career planning, educational programs, and issues of alignment with long-term personal goals and values.
- This orientation serves as the basis for realistic planning for future education and post-education careers.

Development Assistance

Counseling is development oriented as it assists students in their growth and self-actualization. Helping you achieve selfdevelopment and self-actualization prevents problems and maladjustments, rather than healing the damage caused by them.

INSTRUCTIONS AND INSTRUCTIONS ADVISORY: PROGRAM COMPONENT

- **Response services component:** The purpose of the response services component is interventions, or alternative interventions, for students in preschool through 12th grade who are at risk of being affected/or educational development.
- **System support:** The system support component describes administrative activities that ensure the delivery of quality counseling programs and services that students benefit indirectly through the support of other programs.
- **Counseling curriculum:** The counseling curriculum component consists of competency-based lessons and units designed to help all students in grades K-12 develop competencies in essential life skills.
- **Individual planning:** The individual planning component guides students in how to plan, monitor and manage their personal and social development throughout the learning process. Each student is taught the steps necessary to achieve the set goals.

COMPREHENSIVE INSTRUCTION AND COUNSELING PLAN

An effective counseling/counseling program includes programs and activities planned based on student needs, knowledge in the areas of personal/social education and lead career development, gain student outcomes related to skills, attitudes. It should engage meaningfully with key stakeholders such as the student's family, school staff, and the community. A comprehensive instruction and counseling program and service plan should include:
- Statement of vision and mission
- Identification of priorities or key target areas
- Statement of expected outcomes
- Strategies and activities for achieving outcomes
- Measurable success indicators (strategies to assess effectiveness of activities).

The plan should pay particular attention to the role of mentors and advisors in supporting and contributing to her six priorities for education and youth in Manitoba.
1. Improving outcomes for particularly underperforming learners.
2. Communities strengthening links between school families and schools.
3. Strengthening school planning and reporting.
4. Improving professional learning opportunities for educators.
5. Strengthening inter-secondary pathways for post-secondary education and work.
6. Researching policy and practice and evidence.

GUIDANCE COUNSELOR RESPONSIBILITIES

- Conduct oneonone and group counseling sessions to advise and support students on their academic and professional development.
- Assess student characteristics and help students achieve their goals.
- Develop and implement consulting strategies using modern mentoring techniques.
- Identify problem behaviors and take appropriate action to correct them.
- Consider social and cultural differences in all student affairs.

- Evaluate student progress and highlight a sense of accomplishment.
- Conduct assessments, analyze results, and provide targeted feedback.
- Cooperation with parent education staff and external partners.
- Organization and planning of orientation programs and internships.
- Advertisement of educational institutions and study programs to prospective students.
- Conduct and facilitate teaching and training workshops for teachers.

GUIDANCE AND ADVICE FOR NURSES

- Supports young people with normal developmental disabilities.
- To assist individuals in temporary crisis.
- Identify early signs of behavioral disorder.
- Refer cases that require professional attention.
- Supports tutors who are helping individuals but also want guidance and validation themselves.

Student Counseling Issues

- The main issue with the counseling process is its nature. It requires certain personal qualities such as spontaneity, honesty, nonpossessive warmth, and sensitivity to the faint signals of students. Counselors must not only possess these qualities, but must convince students that they possess them.
- Counseling also requires advanced skills. knowledge of information gathering and analysis techniques; understanding and familiarity with youth culture in general. different social environments.
- Success requires patience and perseverance. In Roger's words, it is necessary to create a nonthreatening, non-judgmental environment that is characterized by an attitude of empathy and respect towards students.
- More than a cursory knowledge of psychotherapy principles may be required.
- The university's impressive list of desirable qualities is both a hint and a warning to the swamp that well-meaning but ill-equipped amateurs can fall into.
- A further problem may arise from the potential conflict of goals and beliefs in the interview process inherent in counseling. How does a strong-willed adviser with morals rooted in deepseated ethical principles react when confronted with "nihilistic values"? How do professional teachers respond to "countercultural" statements that deny the legitimacy of their beliefs? In other words, how do consultants achieve the necessary "neutrality of understanding" in the consulting process?

- The complexity of counseling relationships is made clear by Munroe in enumerating the prerequisites of such relationships. These terms have been described as "ethical in nature" and contain claims of a higher level of confidentiality than would normally be expected of a teacher and of the nature of the relationship being inherently voluntary. Claim responsibility for the client's own actions.
- Some teachers who acted as consultants reported feeling inadequate when the complex realities of the deviation problem were exposed in the classroom.
- Family background, financial difficulties, health concerns, and emotional entanglements may be woven together, and only through a lengthy adaptation process that requires support wholly beyond the counselor's strengths and resources. You can free your students. This increases frustration on both sides. A counselor's diagnosis revealed a situation in which escape seemed nearly impossible.
- Confidentiality issues often arise early in the counseling process. In some cases, the interview may occur at the first meeting, which provokes criticism of the counselor's colleagues.

NURSE MANAGER'S ROLE IN GUIDANCE AND GUIDANCE CONSULT

Modern care managers face many challenges in today's competitive environment, but the fundamental challenge for managers is to make management work is. No matter how good the plan, no matter how flexible the policies and procedures of the laboratory organization. In any case, "working through people" is a big challenge for nursing administrators. Human resources are considered the most important organizational capital. Leading people in an organization consists of two tasks he has become one. One is the task of dealing with each employee as an individual with very different needs and behaviors.

All managers experience disruption when working with employees or workgroups, but lower level managers are most likely to experience work interruptions, stress due to the situation and low levels of job satisfaction, money lack of information, inadequate material and human resources contributes to the development of conflict.

Conflict Sources

- Unclear work boundaries and responsibilities
- Communication disorders are flawed and can lead to misunderstandings and conflicts between people and groups.
- Personality conflicts

- Differences in power and status
- Differences in goals.

Avoid inconvenience, make people happy with a good working environment and maintain employee morale. Counseling (individual or group) and guidance are provided whenever and wherever needed. Organizations that mentor and advise individuals must continually work to help individuals grow within their capabilities in directions that are most beneficial to them and their organizations.

Care managers can take the following steps to improve employee morale while advising and mentoring:
- Keep your employees informed of your organization's policies.
- Provide adequate work incentives related to job security, working conditions, opportunities for advancement and social standing.
- Provision of social facilities such as recreational accommodation and medical facilities.
- Encourage employee participation in management.
- Analyze and eliminate the causes of employee dissatisfaction within the organization.
- Encouraging employee group activities such as social gatherings and picnics.

CONCLUSION

Counseling in this sense is a ubiquitous activity in which many people and organizations participate. This information is provided to individuals by parents, relatives and friends, and by communities at large, through various educational, industrial, social, religious and political institutions, especially news and broadcasting services. Part of such guidance may be the provision of information that enables others to broaden their exploratory behavior. A career counselor can, for example, provide information about an individual's abilities and interests as determined by psychological tests, or information about training opportunities and the requirements of various occupations. But effective counselors do not try to solve people's problems for them. Instead, the counselor tries to clarify the person's own thoughts.

REVIEW QUESTIONS

Long Essays
1. Define counseling, explain the objectives of guidance and advice.
2. Enumerate the scope of guidance and advice in education.
3. Discuss the principles of leadership and counseling.
4. Describe comprehensive instruction and counseling plan.
5. Explain the nurse manager's role in guidance and guidance consult.

Short Essays
1. Need for guidance and advice.
2. Difference between accompany and advice.
3. Effective leadership and the benefits of effective leadership advice.
4. Leadership and leadership role advice.
5. Guidance counselor responsibilities.
6. Student counseling issues.

Short Answers
1. Development assistance.
2. Response services component.
3. Counseling curriculum.
4. Guidance and advice for nurses.
5. Conflict sources.

Chapter 18

Counseling

Learning Objectives

- Counseling Meaning, Counseling Objectives, Goals and Purposes
- Need Advice/Counseling
- Scope of Counseling
- Advisory Staff
- Consultation Procedure
- Counseling Features
- Core Principles of Counseling
- Consulting Skills
- Counseling Ethics
- Types of Advice
- Benefits of Counseling
- Organization of Counseling Services
- Counseling Rules and Roles
- Counseling Approach
- Counseling Techniques
- Policy Counseling
- Non-Policy Consulting
- Eclectic Counseling
- Counselor Qualities
- Counselor Duties
- Advisor Characteristics or Qualifications Objectives of Student Counseling

INTRODUCTION

Counseling is an interactive process between a counselor and a client or counselor to meet the client's needs. Counseling may be educational, personal, social and/or professional in nature. Educational counseling helps students make the right decisions about educational choices. Tell us about the courses you want to take and the interests and skills you want to develop. Some schools call this academic counseling. Student counseling helps students improve their academic performance, and counselors attempt to investigate various factors behind a student's poor or better performance. Career selection, on the other hand, is considered in career advice or career orientation.

COUNSELING MEANING

- Counseling refers to the advancement of people to a personal level. He seeks help in educational, professional or psychological areas only if he has a problem.
- Counseling addresses the student's needs, abilities, goals, aspirations, plans, decisions, behaviors and limitations.
- Counseling is a type of specialized and personalized service that effectively uses information collected about an individual.

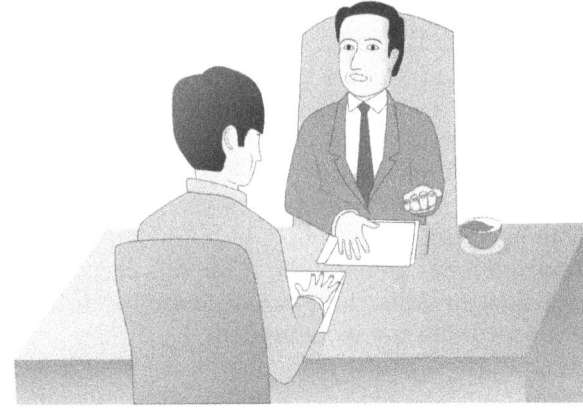

Fig. 18.1: Counseling process.

- This information provides self-insight, self-analysis, and self-orientation. This self-orientation helps individuals maximize their professional and psychological alignment.

DEFINITION OF COUNSELING

- In Bernard and Fulmer's view, counseling is essentially about understanding and working with the individual to discover and address their unique needs, motivations and opportunities. To help you understand.
- Counseling is defined by Biswa Road as the process by which a person accepts and utilizes information and advice to help solve or successfully manage current problems.

COUNSELING OBJECTIVES

- Psychological, emotional and intellectual actions are required to help the client accept actual or imminent changes resulting from stress.
- Encourage the client to consider the alternatives offered and decide which option is appropriate and will help solve the problem.
- Relieves suffering for people dealing with difficult situations.
- Change behavior by reducing stress and risk.
- Helps counselors gain autonomy and independence.
- Helping clients explore and maximize their potential and self-fulfillment.
- Develop special skills and correct attitudes for publicity.
- Assist in the planning of student education and professional development programs.
- Help students develop plans to solve their problems.
- Help students progress in exploration and discovery. To maintain or further develop the whole personality.
- Help students control waste and stagnation.
- To minimize the occurrence of disciplinary violations.
- Motivate students to become independent.

COUNSELING GOALS

- **Developmental goals** are those that help clients achieve or promote the expected human growth and development (i.e., social, personal, emotional, cognitive, physical well-being, etc.).
- **Prevention goals:** Counselors help clients avoid undesirable outcomes.
- **Improvement goals:** If the client has certain competencies or skills, these can be identified or further developed with counselor support.
- **Remediation goals:** Remediation is about helping clients overcome and/or treat undesirable developments in their lives.
- **Exploratory goals:** This involves exploring options for assessing skills and trying out new and different activities, relationships with the environment, etc.
- **Reinforcement goals:** Reinforcement is used to identify states in which the client relies on the appropriate way of thinking and feeling.
- **Cognitive goals:** Cognition involves mastering the basic foundations of learning and cognitive skills.
- **Physiological goals:** Physiological goals ensure a basic understanding and habit of living for physical health.
- **Psychological goals:** This means developing good social interaction skills, learning emotional regulation, developing a positive self-concept, etc.

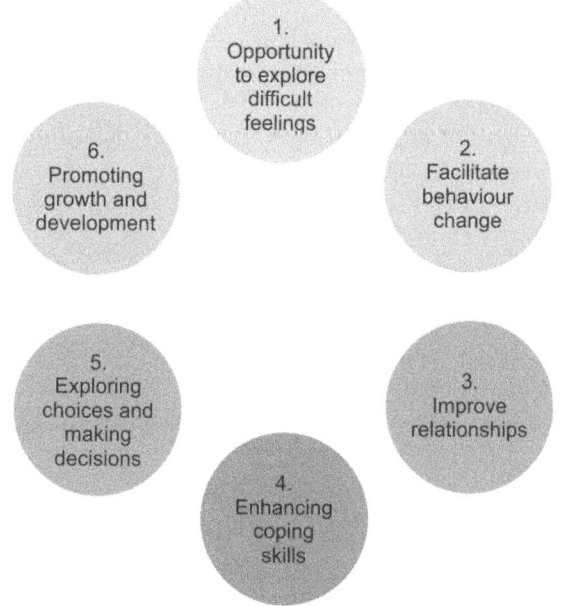

Fig. 18.2: Goals of counseling.

PURPOSE OF COUNSELING

- **Achieving positive mental health:** Positive mental health is the state in which a person is able to form meaningful relationships with others and lead a fulfilling life. One of the purposes of counseling is to help individuals achieve positive mental health.
- **Problem solving:** Another purpose of counseling is to help individuals get out of difficult situations and problems. It must be remembered that individuals can only be assisted in finding solutions to their problems on their own.
- **Decision-making:** Another important purpose of counseling is to enable individuals to make decisions independently. Counselors can help individuals by providing necessary information and clarifying

counselor goals, but decisions must be made by counselors themselves.
- **Increased personal effectiveness:** A competent person is one who has the ability to control impulses, think creatively, and identify, define, and solve problems. The purpose of consulting is to improve individual performance.
- **Change attitudes and perceptions:** Growth requires constant change. Counseling can help change an individual's attitudes and perceptions.
- **Behavior change:** Another purpose of counseling is to assist with behavior change. Weeding out unwanted behaviors and learning desirable behaviors are considered necessary to achieve efficacy and appropriate adaptation.

NEED ADVICE/COUNSELING

- To support the student's overall development.
- To support the correct choice of courses.
- To support the correct choice of sculptor.
- To support the student's professional development.
- Prepare for development decisions and changes to face new challenges.
- Minimize the mismatch between education and employment and support the efficient use of human resources.
- Encourage young people to become independent.
- To help new students find their correct identity. Guidance and counseling services are needed to help students effectively deal with the normal developmental challenges of adolescence and to face life situations with courage.
- Identify and motivate vulnerable students in society.
- To help students in times of turmoil.
- Helps control waste and stagnation.
- Identify and support students with special needs.
- Some students have special needs, such as gifted, disadvantaged, or disabled students. They need special attention and opportunities.
- Ensure appropriate use of time spent outside the classroom.
- To solve the problem of the exploding number of students speaking.
- Control immigration to prevent brain drain.
- To make up for the shortcomings of the house.
- To minimize the occurrence of disciplinary violations.

SCOPE OF COUNSELING

Individual Counseling

- Adolescent identity relates to relationships with teenagers, parents and peers
- Anxiety
- Anger management
- Child concerns in the family, siblings, school experiences, peer relationships
- Depression
- Family of origin dynamics and issues
- **Gender:** Identity, sexuality, homosexuality
- Grief and grief
- **Relationships:** Personal and interpersonal dynamics
- Recovery from sexual abuse
- **Older adults:** Challenges, limitations, transitions
- **Singles:** Single, newly single, single through divorce or being widowed
- Spirituality
- Stress management
- Workplace stress and relationships
- **Young adults:** Identity, relationships, and occupation.

Marriage and Premarital Counseling

- Marriage and relationship dynamics
- Extended family relationships
- Infertility issues.

Family Counseling

- Youth and child behavior in family relationships
- Adult children
- Divorce and separation issues and reconciliation
- **Family dynamics:** Communicating about conflicts of alienation
- Family of origin/extended family issues
- Life stages and transitions
- **Parenting patterns:** Patchwork single parent homes
- Problems relationship counseling remarriage

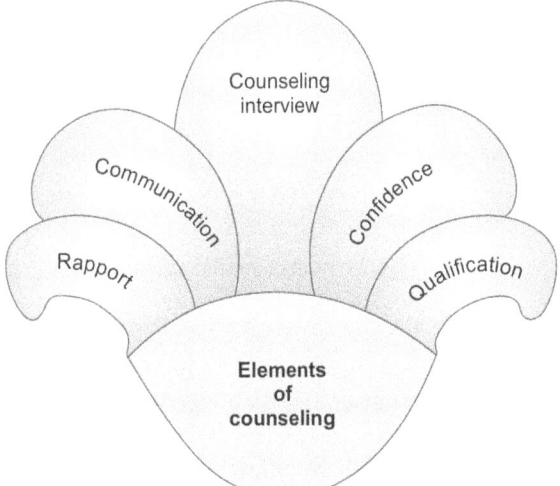

Fig. 18.3: Elements of counseling.

ADVISORY STAFF

- **Supervisor/principals/tutors/medical supervisors:** Support from these individuals is essential to the success of your counseling program. They recognize the need to provide program facilities, coordinate with other staff, promote programs, and evaluate counseling programs.
- Teachers are the most important professionals in the school/university environment.
- **Parents:** Counseling programs extend beyond nursing schools, so parents should be made aware of their needs. Range of counseling programs.
- **Counselors:** Nursing schools may agree to be told that they have their own counselors.

CONSULTATION PROCEDURE

In the consultation process, goals are determined by the client. He is encouraged and supported by his advisors to formulate goals as specific as possible. The more specific the goal, the easier the process. People are generally thought to be goal-oriented, so the more specific the goal, the more likely the client and counselor will be on track toward it. Clients share their experiences and problems, focus on their fears and goals, and support their hearts to help them. Helping a counselor identify their own fears and anxieties can also help. In the process of identifying fears, the counselor will suggest some alternatives while not interfering with the client's decisions.

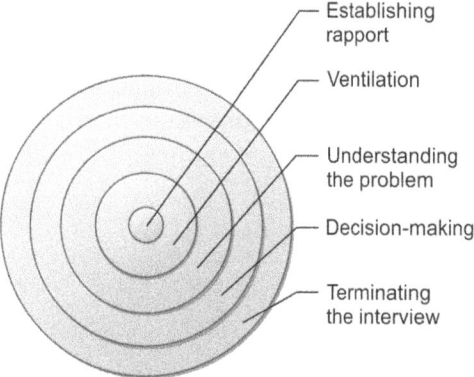

Fig. 18.4: Steps in counseling process.

How to Navigate the Consultation Process

- Create a safe and trusting environment.
- Help the person articulate their concerns.
- **Active listening:**
  - Explore customer intent, paraphrase, summarize, reflect, interpret
  - Focus on feelings, not events.
- Convert the problem statement into a goal statement.
- Consider possible approaches to goals
- Help people choose the path towards their goals.
- Sign contract to implement plan (or take next step). proposed to the consultation process. Basic consulting model. This model consists of five stages.

The Counseling Process

Procedures and procedures techniques counselor's tools

- **Relationship building:** This is the first step in building relationships through mutual understanding between counselors. This stage helps the counselor relax and talk openly about their problems. This is facilitated by the consultant's friendly and straightforward demeanor. Building a relationship does not happen suddenly and it can take time to get to know each other and relax. Counselors build relationships with counselors and strive to create a friendly atmosphere where conversation flows naturally. Advisors can sit in chairs next to their advisors. Anything that suggests an authoritative relationship between the two is avoided. Interviews require both sides to be open and to use words that are appropriate for the situation. Counselors need to understand the importance of body language and how it is interpreted by students.
- **Ventilation:** The counselor's role at this stage is to actively listen to the counselor and observe nonverbal cues such as posture, gestures, and eye contact. You can encourage the counselor to continue the conversation by saying "Yes" or "Continue".
- **Problem understanding:** The purpose is to make the person seeking advice fully aware of their problem. As counseling progresses, the counselor's anxiety begins to decrease and she gains insight into her problem.
- **Decision:** This phase consists of considering different possible solutions to the problem and choosing the best solution and how to implement it. Counselors do not make decisions for the person seeking advice. Rather, he guides the decision-making process.
- **End of interview:** This is a summary phase to review progress and consolidate agreed solutions. Please note that the conversation during counseling cannot be completed by the end of one session. The consultation process can take many months to reach its final stage. However, this model describes the consultation process and course of action to follow.

Thorne's Mode

Brian J Thorne suggested this his 9 step model:
1. Advisor seeking help
2. Advisor trying to contact advisor

3. Define a helpful situation
4. Encourage counselor to speak up
5. Counselor agrees to help
6. Increase insight into problem
7. Establish new goals
8. Decision-making
9. Completion of consultation process.

Seven Steps of the Counseling Process

Critical steps for clients: To be successful in counseling, clients must take the following four steps:
1. **Willingness:** This includes recognizing that change needs to happen and that help is needed. Your next move often requires overcoming your fear of stepping out of your comfort zone and engaging with new thought patterns and behaviors.
2. **Motivation:** The willingness to make and embrace change requires maintaining and maintaining motivation. Without these, the counseling process fails when the real work begins.
3. **Commitment:** Customers may be ready and motivated, but change will not happen without continued perseverance and commitment. A commitment is a series of repetitive decisions to endure and move forward.
4. **Beliefs:** Counseling is unlikely to be successful unless the client trusts himself, the counselor, and the process. The steps of initiating and continuing a consultation require belief that the consultation will be successful.

Counselor's key steps: Each step of the counseling process is critical to establishing and maintaining an effective relationship between counselor and client. Together they support what Carl Rogers (1957) describes as the basic requirements for successful therapy.
- **Unconditional positive concern:** Through acceptance and nonjudgmental behavior, the therapist creates space for the client's needs and treats them with dignity.
- **Empathy:** Counselors show true understanding even when they disagree with the client's point of view.
- **Consistency:** Counselor words, feelings, and actions embody consistency.

COUNSELING FEATURES

- Counseling is based on personal relationships.
- These two of her, one is asking for help and another of her is professionally trained and can help the first one.
- The primary goal is to help counselors independently discover and resolve their own personal problems.
- Counselors must develop a relationship of mutual respect, cooperation, and tenderness between two people in order to provide appropriate help and support.
- Counselors help clients discover problems, set goals, and guide them through challenges and problems.
- The focus of the counseling process is on the counselor's self-management and self-acceptance.
- Counseling is democratic, and counselors establish democratic patterns that leave counselors free to do whatever they want, working together rather than under their guidance.

Counselor Characteristics

Interpersonal

- Listen carefully
- Fairness
- Confidentiality
- Patience
- Sensitivity to people's attitudes
- Kindness
- Sympathetic understanding
- Integrity
- Speak the customer's language
- Resistant performance
- Carefully, listen to customer complaints.

Personal Customization

- Recognize your own limits
- Flexibility and adaptability
- I can accept criticism
- Maintains emotional stability
- Allow for ambiguity. Show confidence.

Health and Grooming

- Free yourself from annoying mannerisms
- Pleasant voice
- During vitality and vitality periods
- Pleasant appearance.

Leadership

- Ability to inspire and inspire, guide others.
- I have high ethical standards.
- Amplifies important information.
- Show the consultant the path to problem resolution. Guides him to make the right choices in his own decisions (spontaneous).

CORE PRINCIPLES OF COUNSELING

According to McDaniel and Shakhtar, the counseling process is based on several basic principles:
- **Principle of acceptance:** According to this principle, all clients are accepted and individual must be treated as Consultants must give due consideration to client rights.

- **Principle of tolerance:** Counseling is a relationship that fosters optimism and shapes the environment for the individual. All thoughts embrace the relativity of counseling.
- **Principle of respect for the individual:** All schools of counseling advocate respect for the individual. Respect for an individual's feelings should be an integral part of the counseling process.
- **Principle of thinking with the individual:** Thinking with the individual is the focus of counseling. For whom is it important to think differently? And "why think"? The counselor's job is to think about all the forces around the client, to be involved in the client›s thought process, and to cooperate with the client's problems.
- **Principle of learning:** All assumptions about counseling assume that there is a learning component in the counseling process.

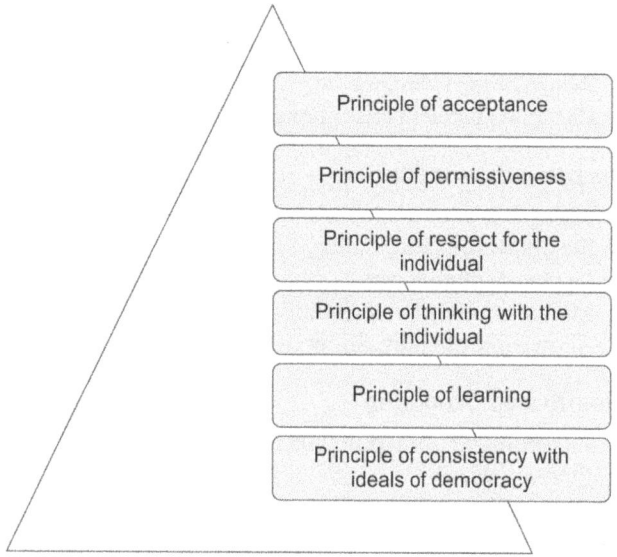

Fig. 18.5: Principles of counseling.

- **Congruence with democratic ideals principle:** All principles are tied to democratic ideals. The ideal of democracy is acceptance of the individual and respect for the rights of others. The counseling process is based on the ideal of respect for the individual. It is a process of accepting individual differences.

CONSULTING SKILLS

As a professional consultant, handling client inquiries and achieving the best possible results for your clients requires a number of core skills. The most important skills a professional counselor must possess are:

- **Effective listening:** Without listening carefully to the problem, we cannot move on to the next step of counseling. Therefore, a counselor should be a good listener and someone who pays close attention to the client and their details.
- **Good communication skills:** A counselor is someone who listens to clients, analyzes their problems, and develops action plans to achieve their goals. In fact, being a good communicator is very important to make the person feel comfortable in the environment and not hesitate when the client talks about their problem in front of them. Building good relationships is very important.
- **Problem solving skills:** This includes distinguishing between symptoms and problems, identifying possible causes and problem triggers, and generating a set of possible solutions to the actual problem.
- **Analytics:** Successful consultants are not only good listeners, they are also great analysts, using their skill and expertise to get to the root of the problem and analyze it. Without analytics, goals cannot be set and clients cannot execute action plans, so the whole process is wasted.
- **Accessibility and accessibility reliability:** Counselors must be accessible to clients in order to gain their trust, but perhaps more importantly, counselors must be able to communicate, listen, and be professional, must be sincere and empathetic.

Attributes and Required Advisor Skills

Pre-training Qualities

- Confidence
- Objectivity
- Good mental health
- Reliability
- Open minded
- Accessibility.

Inter-training Attribute

- Interview setting and interview setting started.
- **Physical arrangement:** Chairs should face each other to provide learning opportunities for both.
- **Greetings:** A warm and friendly greeting facilitates the assistance process.
- Please maintain eye contact.
- Demonstration of correct posture.
- Focus of the problem.
- Identify critical issues.
- Narrow your topic.
- Manage interactions with individuals.
- Restated.
- Interpretation.
- Dealing with pauses and silences.

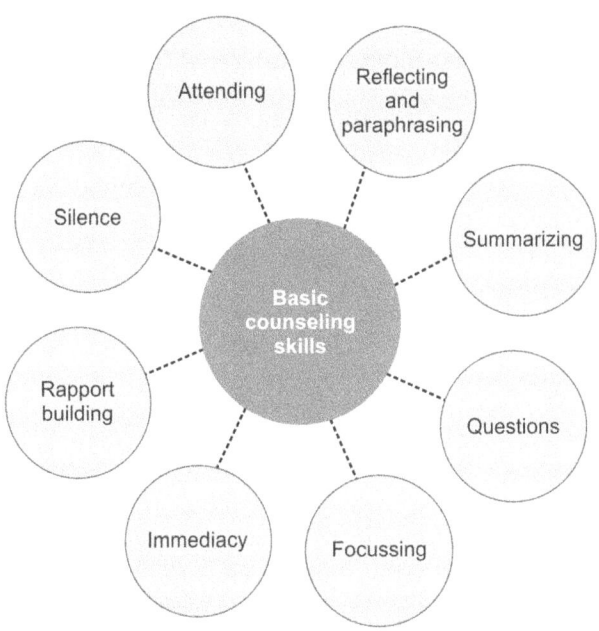

Fig. 18.6: Basic counseling skills.

COUNSELING ETHICS

Counseling ethics is a framework that can be used to resolve ethical dilemmas. All principles are considered equal, and generally no principle has more weight or importance than another. Applying ethical principles provides sufficient scope and information to clarify aspects of a problem and to develop acceptable courses of action for resolving ethical dilemmas. There are ethical principles that are considered relevant to counseling.

Respect for autonomy: Client's freedom to choose their direction—respect for the fact that the client has the opportunity to freely make decisions to deal with the obsession. Others—the counselor's role is to recognize and respect the client's autonomy. Autonomous behavior is behavior that cannot affect the autonomy of another person. Individuals must be aware of the choices they make and their impact and consequences on others. Restrictions on client autonomy apply to clients who are currently unable to understand the consequences of their actions, such as children and mentally ill patients.

Harmless: This term means to do no harm. It is a concept born in the medical field. Autonomy concerns individual clients, nonmalice concerns counselor skills. Counselors have a responsibility to avoid interventions that may or may harm their clients. In practice, counselors are expected to thoroughly assess client concerns and apply appropriately identified and described interventions.

Philanthropy: Represents a responsibility to do good and contribute to the well-being of our clients. Counselors are expected to do what is best for their clients and to offer alternatives where necessary if they cannot help. Werfel also argues that philanthropy "requires consultants to engage in professional activities that are of public interest." Counselors are expected not to have a discriminatory attitude towards any individual or group. Forester Miller and Davis (1996) point out that justice directs counselors to act fairly, but that it is about justice, not that all people are treated equally. I'm here. It is the counselor's ability to recognize inequalities and intervene accordingly.

Loyalty: This principle deals with the relationship of trust between counselor and client. Even if such loyalty (to the client) is uncomfortable or uncomfortable for the counselor, the client's interests take precedence over the counselor's (Welfel 1998). The client must be able to trust the counselor's words and actions to be true and trustworthy. However, counselors do not have to share every momentary thought or reaction.

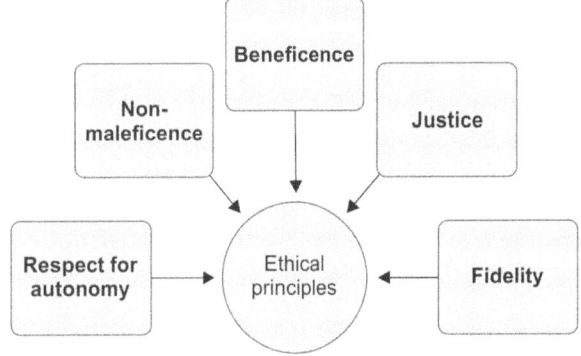

Fig. 18.7: Ethical principles.

TYPES OF ADVICE

- **Instructional advice:** In instructional advice, an advisor gives specific instructions or directs the person seeking advice to do a specific thing, e.g., he is asked to act in a certain way. You are asked to abstain from alcohol and drugs. He is expected to respect his colleagues and superiors.
- **Nondirected advice:** In the case of nondirected advice, the mentor does not give instructions, but observes the recipient's behavior and attitude toward work, peers, superiors and subordinates. If he is wrong, the counselor comes to his aid, realizes he was wrong, and corrects him. He does not direct or guide him in anything.
- **Cooperative counseling:** This is the type of counseling that can be done by working fully with the counselor and

having them identify shortcomings in the counselor's behavior and attitudes so that they can get themselves back on track and improve. Working together to win the hearts and minds of our clients. Advice seekers gain trust, are more willing to cooperate, and develop self-discipline.

- **Mental health counseling:** Mental health counselors are responsible for supporting people experiencing emotional distress such as anxiety, depression, and frustration. There are many reasons why people need psychological counseling. This includes lingering sadness, extreme anger, addictions, family issues, eating disorders, and more. After discussing the problem with the client, the mental health counselor tries to offer ways to overcome the situation and promote well-being.
- **Career counseling:** Slightly different from the traditional counseling process, career counseling provides career guidance to applicants and guides them on the right path to a successful career based on their interests and abilities. I mean the career counseling curriculum is designed to help people make decisions about changing jobs or leaving a career, and can be used at all stages of life. Career counseling specialists will assess your aptitude, personality and interests and suggest the best career options for you.
- **Rehabilitation counseling:** Rehabilitation counseling helps people with disabilities achieve their goals, participate fully in their communities and live independently. It is a systematic way of helping people with emotional, physical, cognitive and intellectual disabilities achieve their life goals and live worthwhile lives. Rehabilitation consultants support affected people in overcoming mental disorders.
- **Relationship counseling:** Also called couples therapy. People seek such counseling if something serious is affecting their love life. People choose relationship counseling for a variety of reasons, including a desire for a stronger relationship with their partner or spouse, problems arising from disagreements, unhealthy abuse, and the rush that has affected their lives. Relationship therapists help couples work through problems they can overcome. They are facing and forming a long-term commitment.

BENEFITS OF COUNSELING

- **Leads to self discovery:** Her one of the main benefits of individual counseling is that it helps you discover yourself. Knowing yourself is one of the most difficult and most important things to achieve in order to live a peaceful and prosperous life.
- **Build confidence, hope and encouragement:** Another important benefit of counseling is to build confidence, hope, encouragement and motivation. Motivation and hope give you the strength to face life's problems and take a step forward to achieve your goals.
- **Helps deal with emotions:** Expressing emotions and feelings can be very difficult. It can be complicated at times. Seeing a therapist can help you control your emotions.
- **Contribute to self acceptance:** You may find yourself in situations where you feel unworthy and unjust. Helpful advice here.
- **Give direction to your point of view:** Another benefit of one-on-one counseling is to give direction to your point of view. It presents you with different sides and points your perspective in the right direction.
- **Provides peace of mind:** Peace of mind is something that everyone wants to advocate these days. We try to have peace in our lives, but when we have peace of mind, we have peace. This is one of the benefits of consulting.
- **Develop skills:** Counseling can also help improve skills. Skills such as decision-making and communication are improved through participation in counseling sessions. Personal skill development is also important as it enhances individuality.
- **Help improve your lifestyle:** As everything has evolved, so has our lifestyle. This is also one of the most important jobs of counseling. Along with lifestyle changes comes many other changes.
- **Gain insight into the problem:** Another benefit of counseling is that it provides insight into the problem. It helps you understand and reflect on other people's perspectives. In many cases, we fail to address the problem because we are unable to consider both sides of the problem.
- **Helps overcome drugs and alcohol:** Drug and alcohol addictions are very harmful and difficult to get rid of. Counseling can help overcome alcoholism and drug addiction.
- **Eliminate negative feelings:** Another benefit of counseling is that it clears out all the negativity within you and gives you the strength to fight your problems. You will have a positive attitude towards life and will be able to see things from a completely different perspective.

ORGANIZATION OF COUNSELING SERVICES

Counseling is a form of 'talk therapy'. This is a process where single couples or families meet with a trained professional counselor to discuss the problems and challenges they face in their lives. Expert advice is confidential and non-judgmental.

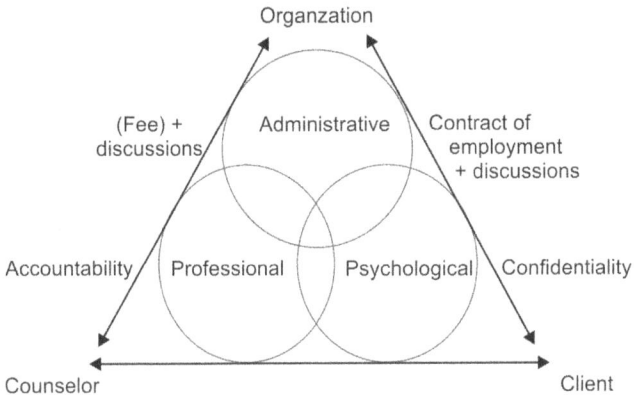

Fig. 18.8: Organization of counseling.

Purpose: Development of cognitive skills and application of skills necessary for everyday life.

Areas of Work

- Confidence building
- Motivation for achievement
- Decision-making, goal setting, planning and problem solving skills
- Interpersonal effectiveness (including social skills)
- Communication skills
- Intercultural effectiveness
- Responsible behavior.

Organizational Structure

- **For universities:** The dean is supported by the dean of psychology and education, an advisory board and an advisory officer.
- **For new universities:** The advisory officer, in conjunction with the deputy director and academic advisor, with the assistance of the advisory board, can plan according to needs and student numbers. Less than 1,000 students require a liaison officer, but over 1,000 students require an assistant supervisor.
- **For formal colleges:** Advisory committee for over 1,000 students.

School Advisory Committee Composition

- **Principal must be the chair or chairman of the school advisory committee.**
- **Counselor or career master or counselor:**
  - The school counselor, career counselor or guidance teacher shall serve as secretary and governor of the school advisory board.
  - If possible, we may appoint a full-time consultant.
  - During his absence, a teacher trained in career guidance will take over the role of master craftsman.
  - Even if the school has a fulltime counselor, it may have teachers who are trained to provide the counselor with the support they need.
- **Faculty representative:** The principal serves on the advisory committee ex-officer.
- **School doctor:** The school doctor serves as a member of the school advisory committee.
- **Chairman or secretary of the board of directors:** Member.
- **Physical education teacher (PET):** Member.
- There are several experts in various fields in the community.

Consulting Services Tools

Non-testing Tools

- Interview
- Second observation
- Anecdotal report
- Cumulative dataset
- Checklist
- Rating scale
- Sociometry
- Autobiography and diary.

Psychological Testing Tools

- Ability testing
- Performance test
- Aptitude test
- Personality test.

Specific requirements for the organization of advisory services:

- Student database.
- Education and education career information service.
- Community service integration and counseling services program.
- Educational programs for teachers, counselors and teachers. Other staff who provide knowledge about current trends in counseling.
- Budget provisions.
- Presence of physical facilities, room furnishings and fittings. Other equipment necessary for teaching and counseling departments.
- Providers of civilian personnel and public consultation rooms.
- Trained counseling and advisory staff.
- Consulting services.
- Evaluation equipment such as psychological tests, inventories.

COUNSELING RULES AND ROLES

- **Helpful roles:**
  - It is about working with individuals or groups to help solve some problem.
  - As noted by Kagan et al (1988), remedial interventions may lead individual couples to seek individualized social and psychotherapy (e.g., marriage counseling)
  - Crisis interventions and various treatment suggestions for students needing help with unresolved life events are also examples of initiatives at the funding level.
- **Role of prevention:**
  - Here the counseling psychologist attempts to "anticipate workarounds and, if possible, prevent possible future difficulties." Preventive interventions can focus on so called psychoeducational programmers aimed at preventing problems and events from occurring.
  Example: Drug prevention/awareness programmer suicide prevention program for high-risk and psychological adoptions that gives orphans a sense of belonging.
- **Education and development role:**
  - Its purpose is to help individuals develop plans to maximize the benefit of experiences that enable them to discover and develop their potential.
  - Examples of this are various workshops and seminars. Another example is a study skills course aimed at helping college students develop bright students more efficiently.
  - A key feature of the development role is that doing it allows you to go beyond prevention and participate in improvement.

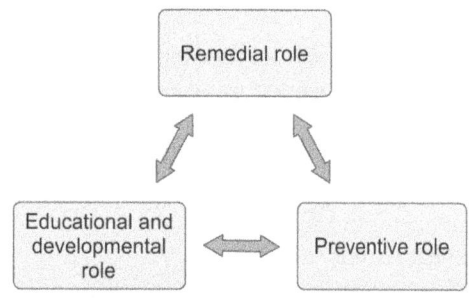

Fig. 18.9: Role of counseling.

Counselor's Role in Schools

- Counseling individual students or small groups to help resolve identified problems.
- Teach the counseling curriculum.
- Talk to your parents about your child's concerns.
- Discuss student needs with teachers and administrators.
- Attend and present workshops for parents, teachers and community members.
- Interpret test results with parents, students and teachers.
- Work with school and community staff to assemble resources for students.

ADVICE COMPARED TO OTHER TERMS

- **Guidance and advice:** Guidance and advice are not synonymous.
- **Consultation and interview:** The interview is part of the consultation. Techniques used in counseling.
- **Counseling and advice:** Advice is not advice. A wise advisor gives advice even when it is not absolutely necessary.
- **Counseling and education:** Counseling does not mean teaching. Teaching is related to academic and instinctive issues, while counseling is related to social and emotional issues.
- **Counseling and psychotherapy:** Counseling is not considered psychotherapy, but is used as a form of therapy by psychotherapists. Counselors work in the educational field and psychotherapists work in the medical field.

COUNSELING APPROACH

Humanistic Counseling Approach

Humanistic counselors assume that problems are caused not by life events themselves, but by the way we experience them. Our experiences influence or affect how we feel about ourselves, affecting self-esteem and self-confidence. A humanistic approach to counseling thus encourages clients to understand how negative reactions to life events can lead to psychological distress. This approach aims at self-acceptance of both the negative and positive aspects of our character and personality.

- Humanistic counseling recognizes the uniqueness of each individual.
- Assume that everyone has an innate capacity to grow emotionally and psychologically towards the goal of self-actualization and personal fulfillment.
- Humanity counselors assume that problems are not caused by life events themselves, but by the way we experience them.
- Our experiences influence and are influenced by how we feel about ourselves, thereby affecting our self-esteem and confidence.
- A humanistic approach to counseling thus encourages clients to understand how negative reactions to life events can lead to psychological distress.

- This approach aims at self-acceptance of both the negative and positive aspects of our character and personality.
- The goal of the humanities counselor, therefore, is to help clients explore their thoughts and feelings and develop their own solutions to problems.
- This is very similar to the coaching approach, except that the coach focuses on the present rather than the past. In essence, coaching aims to address the "how" and counseling aims to address the "why."

Client-Centered Counseling

Client-Centered therapy focuses on the belief that the client, rather than the counselor, is an expert in their own thoughts, feelings, experiences and problems. Therefore, it is the customer who can best find the right solution. Counselors do not suggest or endorse courses of action, ask probing questions, or try to interpret what the client is saying. You are fully responsible for resolving the issue. The goal of the counselor when responding is to reflect and clarify what the client is saying.

Trained, client-centered counselors strive to demonstrate empathy, warmth, and honesty, which they believe promotes self-understanding and psychological development in their clients.

- Empathy means being able to understand a client's problem from within one's own frame of reference. Counselors must be able to accurately communicate this understanding to their clients.
- Warm this up to show the client is valued no matter what happens during the counseling session. Counselors must be open-minded, about what clients say and do, without imposing judgments on them.
- Credibility (also known as consistency) refers to the consultant's ability to be open and honest and not to act superficially or hide behind a "professional" facade.

Behavioral Counseling Approaches

Behavioral counseling approaches are based on the premise that the environment determines a person's behavior. Behavioral therapy focuses on individual behavior and aims to help people change unwanted behaviors. Unwanted behavior is defined as an unwanted reaction to something or someone in the environment. Using this approach, the counselor identifies unwanted behavior in the client and works with them to change or adjust the behavior.

COUNSELING TECHNIQUES

The three main techniques used in the school counseling process. The modalities include directive counseling, nondirective counseling, and eclectic counseling.

- **Directive counseling:** In this counseling, counselors play an active role because they are seen as a means to help people solve their own problems. This type of advice is also called advisor centric advice. This is because, in this consultation, the client himself/herself

Flowchart 18.1: Classifications of organizational counseling.

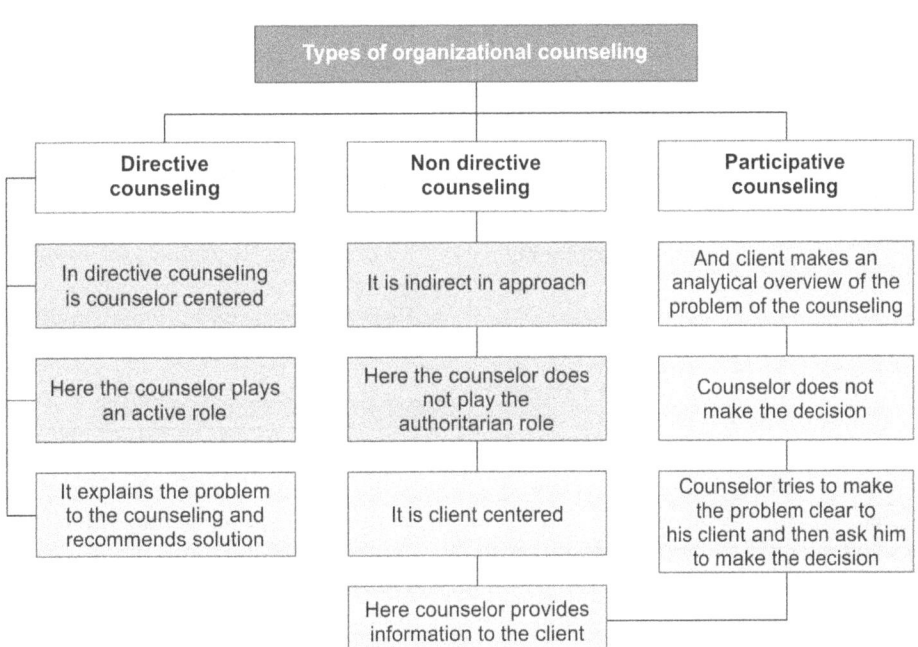

does everything, including analysis, synthesis, diagnosis, prognostic prescription, and aftercare.
- **Nondirective counseling:** In this type of counseling, the counselor, client, or student, rather than the counselor, is the focus of the counseling process. He plays an active role and this kind of advice is a process of growing up. The purpose of this consulting is client independence and integration, not problem solving. In this counseling, the client comes to the counselor with a problem. Counselors establish relationships with counselors based on mutual trust, acceptance, and understanding.
- **Eclectic counseling:** Eclectic counseling combines directive and nondirective techniques depending on situational factors. This approach to counseling is best characterized by the counselor's freedom to use whatever procedures and techniques they deem most appropriate for a particular point in time and for a particular client. This consultant is someone who is willing to use any method that shows promise, even if the theoretical underpinnings are very different.

POLICY COUNSELING

Directional counseling is also called prescriptive counseling because the counselor prescribes a solution or course of action to the student.

Characteristics of Directive Counseling

It has the following characteristics:
- During the interview, attention is focused on a specific problem and its solution.
- During the interview, the counselor takes a more active role than the client or student.
- Although it is the student or client who makes the decision, the counselor will do everything possible to force the counselor or client to make a decision consistent with the diagnosis.
- The counselor seeks to direct the thoughts of the counselor or client by providing information, explanation, interpretation, and counseling.

Instructions Consulting Procedures

- **Analysis:** Data collection is done from a variety of sources using a variety of tools and techniques.
- **Aggregate:** Data should be summarized and organized to reveal reconciliations and discrepancies in customer assets and liabilities.
- **Diagnosis:** This phase attempts to identify the root cause of the problem you are experiencing.
- **Prognosis:** At this stage, it is necessary to predict the future development of the client's problem.

- **Action:** This includes setting up a report consultant or plan programmer.
- **Follow-up:** Here, the counselor attempts to solve the client's new problem, or a new problem of the original problem, and judges the effectiveness of the counseling provided to the client.

Benefits of Direct Consultation

- Economical in terms of time.
- The focus was primarily on the problem rather than the individual.
- Referential counseling focuses more on the intellectual rather than the emotional aspects of a person's personality, but less on the emotional level.
- The direct counseling methods used were directly persuasive and descriptive.

Instructional Advice Restrictions

- Advisors are never independent of advisors.
- Advice bound by instructions does not prevent the recipient of the advice from making future mistakes.

Advisor's Role in Directed Advice

- Advisors play a critical role in this advice process. He is the linchpin of the process and the leader of the situation.
- Counselors solve most conversation problems, but the focus is not on the individual. Counselors do not actually work with counselors, but under them.
- Counselors seek to guide the thinking of counselors and clients by providing information, explanations, interpretations and, in some cases, advice.
- Counselors will collect any information about students or counselors and analyze it for proper understanding.
- Summarize and organize data to understand student capabilities and limitations, adaptations and inconsistencies.
- He draws conclusions about the nature and causes of his problems. He predicts the future development of his own problems.
- He prescribes what students should do to solve problems and tracks the consequences and impact of his lessons.

NON-POLICY CONSULTING

Carl Rogers is the principal architect of this school.
- Also called permissive advice or client-focused advice.
- In this type of counseling, the client is the linchpin or central counselor. Consultants play a central role.
- Those who actively participate in the process use consultants to gain insight into their problems and make decisions for action.

Taking Over Nondirective Advice

- Customer independence and integrity were more important than customers themselves
- Emotional aspects were more important than intellectual aspects.
- Creating an atmosphere of understanding for the client was more important than facilitating self-understanding.
- Counseling leads to the subject's voluntary choice and conscious choice of action options.

Nondirective Counseling Steps

- The client recognizes the need for counseling and can seek help. Help is sought, but not given.
- Counselors can define situations and create innate atmospheres.
- The counselor's demeanor was friendly, compassionate and loving. He cares about children and encourages individual freedom of expression on this issue.
- Counselors try to understand the feelings of the individual.
- Counselors accept and recognize both positive and negative emotions.
- The counselor pays attention to the client's or child's negative feelings about self and gradually transforms them from negative self-feelings to positive self-feelings, from emotional release to insight.
- The counselor asks the client to act on the insight.
- It is desired to reduce the need for assistance and it is the client's decision whether or not to contact you.
- Positive action to resolve the problem situation begins to take hold.

Benefits of Nondirective Counseling

- This is a slow but sure process that empowers individuals to make adjustments.
- It does not use tests, so it is tedious and difficult.
- It can remove emotional blockages and bring an individual's repressed thoughts to the level of consciousness, thereby reducing intention.

Restrictions on Nondirective Consultation

- This is a very slow and lengthy process. This is not possible in schools because counselors have to look after many students.
- The child, client, student, or counselor cannot make decisions on their own. Therefore, we do not rely on God's judgment or wisdom.
- There are many people who can guide you from stage to stage. The counselor's passive demeanor can make the counselor very frustrated and reluctant to express their feelings.

ECLECTIC COUNSELING

Eclectic counseling can be defined as the integration and combination of directive and nondirective counseling. In this consultation, the consultant was neither too aggressive as in the directive consultation nor too passive as in the nondirective consultation. In choice counseling, the counselor first considers the counselor's personality and needs, and then selects the directive or nondirective technique that best suits the purpose.

Thorne is a principal architect at a multi-purpose consulting firm.

Multifaceted Consultation Procedures

- Diagnosing causes
- Analyzing problems
- Pre-planning for changing factors
- Ensuring effective negotiation terms
- Encourage clients to ask questions, develop their own resources, and responsibly try new fitting models
- Appropriately address related issues that may assist in coordination.

Generalization

- In general, passive methods should be used whenever possible.
- In the early stages when the client is telling their story, passive techniques are preferred. This allows for emotional release.
- Active methods are used when there are certain indications.
- Complex methods should not be tried until the simpler methods fail.
- All counseling must be client-centered.
- Every child should be given the opportunity to solve problems indirectly.
- Referential methods generally involve conflicting situations in which a solution cannot be reached without the cooperation of others.
- Even when the decision is made to use passive methods, some degree of direction is inevitable in counseling.

Limitations of Eclectic Consultation

- Eclectic consultation is not possible because the referential and non-referential concepts cannot be integrated.
- According to some authors, eclecticism is vague, superficial, and opportunistic.

Eclectic Counseling Consultant Competence

- Eclectic counseling presupposes a high level of competence and is used by consultants as a basis for indiscriminate use or ignorance of certain practices advocated by other philosophies.
- Competent and multifaceted counselors are familiar with all other major philosophical theories in counseling and apply this knowledge in choosing techniques and establishing positive working relationships with clients.
- Rejection of a philosophical framework is justified if the consultant can come up with a better way to solve the problem at hand.
- Counselors must recognize the fact that problems differ from person to person.
- Seekers and students must be accepted for what they are and efforts must be made to understand them. Each issue must be treated as unique.
- Any prejudice that all counselors' personal problems should be treated the same way should be discarded.
- A consultant's job is very difficult. He must alter and interpret everything that is available about that individual.
- Staff should be careful to be warm, cooperative, friendly, responsive and understanding when dealing with students, but at the same time be impersonal and objective.
- But to be impersonal and objective you don't have to be indifferent.

COUNSELOR QUALITIES

Counselor qualities and skills can be summarized as follows:
- Good and active listener.
- **Good observer:** Observes the nonverbal behavior of the person seeking advice and explores its meaning and possible stress.
- **Attention:** Give the counselor full attention through posture, nonverbal cues, eye contact, etc.
- Warm, friendly and sincere personality.
- Maintaining confidentiality.
- Introspective, creative, imaginative—paraphrases the words of the advice-seeker and expresses his or her own thoughts on the feelings of the advice-seeker.
- Uses appropriate questioning techniques use open-ended rather than closed-ended questions to allow advice-seekers to expand.
- Maintain silence when needed.
- Do not panic if the counselor is silent for too long, interrupt if necessary.
- Give your counselor the autonomy to solve your own problems through the right questions.

Counsel or counselor relationships can be very rewarding, but they can also be very demanding. Counselors/tutors may be assisted by a counselor/counselor to discuss issues related to counseling, if necessary. For example, when a teacher assumes the role of student counselor, she may feel inadequate in certain aspects of counseling.

Counselors and co-tutors can be very helpful in addressing these shortcomings. If a consultant requires such assistance, the principles of confidentiality must be respected. Guidance and counseling services should be established in all higher education institutions. It is important to have a counseling department at an institution where the services of trained counselors are available.

COUNSELOR DUTIES

- **Counseling programs and their organization:** This includes, for example, career information services, self-inventory and personal data collection services, counseling services, career preparation services, referral services and employment services. Up or adaptation service.
- Orientation includes preparation such as gathering data on career sources, distributing information to students, and planning activities.
- Data collection should be about the person conducting and analyzing the test.
- An interview and individual counseling should be conducted.
- You will need to contact them through an external agency such as parents' counseling center or employment security office.
- Requires placement and follow-up work.

Counselor Responsibilities

Counselor responsibilities are specifically:
- **Student assessment:** Use appropriate test and non-test equipment.
- Student orientation involving tutors, principals, librarians, physicians and other resources.
- Use counseling techniques to help emotionally troubled students.
- Help students overcome academic and social deficiencies.
- Help students overcome financial, health, sexual, domestic and confusion issues.
- Collaborate with other teachers to develop a better understanding of students.
- Engage parents and others involved in the counseling process.
- Maintain current student records regarding counseling.

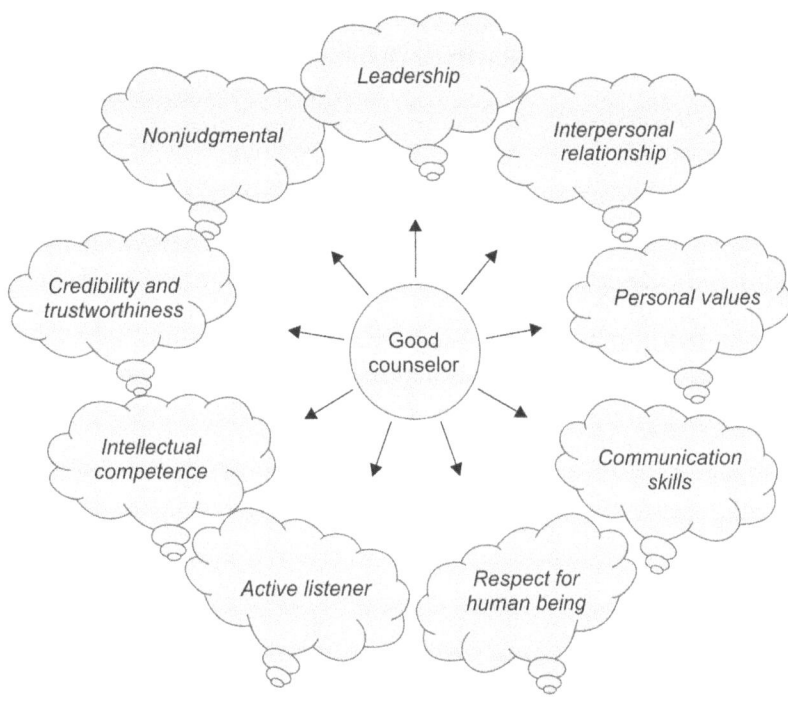

Fig. 18.10: Qualities of good counselor.

- Arrange money transfer services for those in need.
- Evaluation and implementation of rework.
- Implementation of career courses for those who wish to work in the nursing profession.
- Disseminate information on employment, leisure and career opportunities.

ADVISOR CHARACTERISTICS OR QUALIFICATIONS

Personality Traits

- **Broad interests:** Consultants should be interested in a wide variety of professions and organizations.
- **Collaboration:** Consultants should enjoy working with all employees.
- **Refinement:** Counselors should not be overconfident, but they should be humble and humble with students.
- **Magnetism:** Counselors should give others confidence and reassurance.
- **Observations:** Counselors should understand difficulties and teachers should show human understanding and genuine love for those around them.

Education and Preparation

Excellent education including knowledge of the humanities such as sociology, psychology, economics, history and geography.

- Know the principles of counseling.
- Learn about secondary school goals, curricula and methods.
- Know your professional activities.
- Knows how to communicate professional information.
- Learn about psychological tests in counseling services.
- Know the organization of counseling services.

Testimonials

- Competence as a programmed counseling leader
- Competence as a counselor
- Competence in interpreting and using information
- Competence in mediation and follow-up services
- Competence in using community resources
- Ability to evaluate consulting services themselves.

OBJECTIVES OF STUDENT COUNSELING

Dansmoore and Miller believe that the core of student counseling is for students to help themselves. From this perspective, they describe the following goals of student counseling:

- Provide students with information on topics related to success.
- Would you like to receive information about students that will help you solve problems
- Create a sense of mutual understanding between students and teachers.

- Help students develop plans to solve their own problems.
- Help students better understand themselves (interests, skills, abilities, opportunities).
- Promoting and developing special skills and right attitudes.
- Inspires commitment to success towards achievement.
- Assist students in planning their educational and career choices.

It is clear that the purpose of counseling is to clarify problems and meet voluntary needs. Counselors help students understand their problems and help them solve them on their own. In this process, the student's role is to objectively self-evaluate the situation, and the counselor's role is to formulate the decision-making process and stimulate the student's insight and sensitivity. Counseling does not solve problems, but it can help solve problems and, when solutions are not possible, help you overcome challenges and live with them. In short, counseling aims to develop self-understanding, self-acceptance, and self-confidence in students.

CONCLUSION

Counseling helps clients make better decisions. It helps individuals improve their skills, increase their confidence in their academic and professional achievements, set career direction, and increase their awareness and awareness of the needs of their clients and others. Through counseling, clients can improve communication with special people, develop more meaningful relationships, and effectively deal with feelings of depression and anxiety. Personal academic or professional concerns can be discussed in a consultation.

REVIEW QUESTIONS

Long Essays

1. Define counseling, explain the objectives, purposes and goals of counseling.
2. Discuss the scope of counseling.
3. Explain the core principles of counseling.
4. Describe counseling ethics.
5. Enumerate the organization of counseling services.
6. Define counseling approach, explain in detail about humanistic counseling.
7. Approach and client-centered counseling.
8. Define eclectic counseling, explain eclectic counseling consultant competence.
9. Describe the counselor qualities and duties.

Short Essays

1. Consultation procedure.
2. Counseling process: Procedures techniques counselor's tools.
3. Seven steps of the counseling process.
4. Counseling features.
5. Counselor characteristics.
6. Consulting skills.
7. Attributes and required advisor skills.
8. Benefits of counseling.
9. Counseling rules and roles.
10. Behavioral counseling approaches.
11. Counseling techniques.
12. Characteristics of directive counseling.
13. Advisor's role in directed advice.
14. Counselor responsibilities.
15. Nondirective counseling steps.
16. Advisor characteristics or qualifications.
17. Objectives of student counseling.

Short Answers
1. Need advice/counseling.
2. Elements of counseling.
3. Individual counseling.
4. Advisory staff.
5. Thorne's mode.
6. Philanthropy.
7. Loyalty.
8. Types of advice.
9. Consulting services tools.
10. Counselor's role in schools.
11. Directive counseling.
12. Eclectic counseling.
13. Benefits of direct consultation.
14. Non-policy consulting.

Chapter 19

Guidance/Academic Advising

Learning Objectives
- Leadership Concepts
- Objectives of Instruction
- Leadership Principles
- Pipe Element
- Leadership Characteristics
- Basic Assumptions of the Guide
- Organizing Counseling Services
- Individual Counseling Services
- Personal Counseling Needs
- Individual Counseling Procedures
- Educational Counseling

INTRODUCTION

Counseling is one of the main uses of psychology. It enables or supports individuals in solving educational and psychological problems. "Guide" means any guidance or suggestion for progress. In the fields of psychology and pedagogy, the word "instruction" has a specific meaning. It refers to the process that helps individuals discover themselves.

LEADERSHIP CONCEPTS

- Leadership is the process of assisting an individual in developing his/her body, mind, personality and character, and helping him or her to achieve maximum educational, professional, personal or psychological alignment.
- Counseling is considered a type of professional service provided to individuals to resolve serious problems.
- Counseling is any form of support given to children so that they can develop their individuality to the fullest.
- Counseling is not confined to a professional setting as it is a continuous process from early childhood through to old age.
- Counseling in education means helping students choose courses that meet their needs and interests, for example, to achieve the best possible academic performance.
- Leading is not just about imposing your opinions on others or making decisions for those who carry the burdens of other people's lives.

DEFINITION OF LEADERSHIP

- **Jones** (1951) states that "leadership" includes personal assistance from someone who can best accomplish where a person goes, what to do, or a goal. We believe it is intended to help you decide how. It helps solve problems that arise in life.
- **Crows and Crows:** The basis of all leadership is the assistance that competent people give individuals to develop their personal perspective, to make their own decisions, and to direct their lives by implementing those decisions or support.
- **Fowlers** strongly believes that the purpose of counseling is to help students make more favorable adjustments.

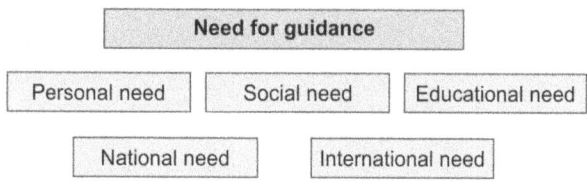

Fig. 19.1: Need of guidance.

OBJECTIVES OF INSTRUCTION

- Your child should be informed in detail about the subjects and courses offered by the schools in which they may attend.
- To help him familiarize himself with the curriculum.
- Assist your child in obtaining information about the possibilities and desirability of further education.
- Help your child learn about the purpose and function of different types of schools.
- Help your child understand the requirements for admission to the school of their choice.
- Help the child become familiar with school rules, regulations and related social life.
- Help students to understand themselves: their potential, strengths and weaknesses.
- Help your child develop good study habits.
- To help him choose a hobby.
- Help children choose subjects according to their needs, abilities and interests.

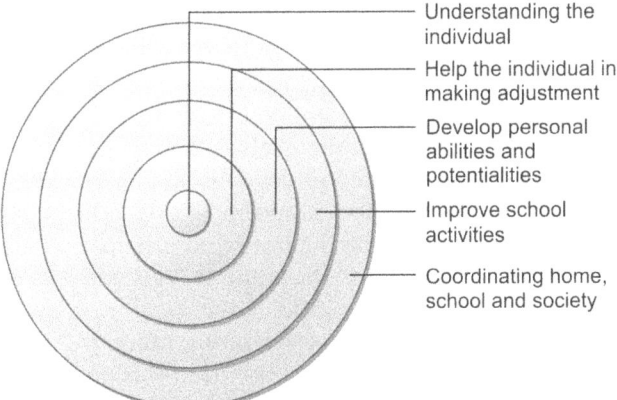

Fig. 19.2: Objectives of instruction.

- **Understanding the individual:** The main objectives of counseling are to discover and understand the abilities and potential of the individual, to assess oneself in relation to personal and social experiences, and to it is about making more efficient use of the self in everyday life.
- **Help individuals adjust:** Another goal of counseling is to assist individuals in making the most satisfactory adjustments to their families, schools, teachers, students and society.
- **Develop individual skills and opportunities:** Another purpose of counseling is to help individuals develop skills, opportunities and perspectives to develop their body, mind, character and personality traits. That's it.

- **Improving school activities:** Advisory programmers help school officials solve problems and improve all school activities.
- **Coordinating homeschool and community:** Erikson correctly stated that one of his key purposes of counseling was to coordinate the influence of homeschool and community on the child.

LEADERSHIP PRINCIPLES

- Personal weakness comes first.
- All people are different.
- Counseling is primarily concerned with people in social settings.
- Personal attitudes and personal perceptions form the basis of behavior.
- Individuals generally act to improve their perceived self.
- Individuals have an innate ability to learn and can assist in making decisions that lead to realistic self-determination.
- The person needs an ongoing counseling process from an early age.
- Every person may need information and personal support from qualified professionals.

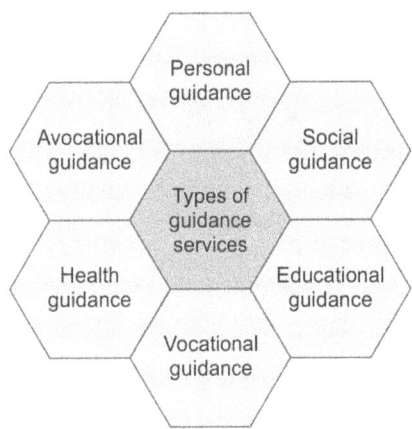

Fig. 19.3: Types/areas of guidance services.

PIPE ELEMENT

- Counseling focuses attention on the individual rather than the problem.
- Counseling helps individuals discover their abilities.
- Counseling is based on the individual's interests, abilities, assets, needs and limitations.
- Leadership leads to self-development and self-orientation.
- Leadership encourages individuals to plan wisely for the present and the future.

- Guidance helps individuals adapt to their new environment.
- Counseling can help you be successful and happy.

LEADERSHIP CHARACTERISTICS

- Leadership is based on individual differences. It is a wellknown fact that no two people are the same. Individual abilities, potential, tendencies, abilities, aptitudes, and intraindividual variability vary.
- Counseling is the basis of the revised Code of Ethics. It is important to follow a strict code of ethics when providing programmed advice.
- Counseling is based on educational and professional goals. This means that counseling can help you achieve your educational and professional goals and objectives.
- Counseling can increase personal insight. Counselors help individuals gain insight to make their own choices and decisions.
- The guidelines consider most people to be average normal people. All students should be made aware that counselor services are available to everyone.
- Counseling is a slow but continuous process. Individuals need a lot of time to make the right adjustments and cannot make wise choices, decisions and adjustments in a day or so.
- Counseling is universal and essential for all students at all levels. Recommended for those who are looking for it and those who are not looking for it.
- Counseling is the planning of counseling staff to review the overall situation and to plan for the future in educational, professional and social fields.
- Counseling is developmental and comprehensive, counseling is developmental as it addresses month by month, year by year and stage by stage.
- Counseling is the practical part of the training. Education sets goals and leadership ensures the realization of those goals.
- Counseling is primarily childfocused. Counselors and counselee do not impose anything on the individual, but only explore the child's needs and offer suggestions.
- Advice is considered an organizational service and not an ancillary activity. It is a service that serves a specific purpose.
- Counseling is a professional and general service to many people, including teachers, parents and principals. Counselors and career ladders do their part.

BASIC ASSUMPTIONS OF THE GUIDE

- Individual differences in innate abilities, skills, and interests are enormous.
- Changes within individuals themselves are very important.
- Native skills are usually not specialized.
- Abilities and talents are not dependent on race, color or gender.
- Help is needed in certain critical situations.
- Schools are strategically positioned to provide the support they need.
- Counseling is progressive and voluntary, but not prescriptive.

NEED ADVICE

- **Educational needs:** Students should be able to choose topics for counseling, choose books, choose hobbies, choose activities within the curriculum, develop study habits, plan time and work, focus on learning, and build social relationships, and on building social relationships when satisfactory progress and adjustment were obtained.
- **Psychological needs:** Psychological and social counseling is required. Young people in the 20th century face great emotional strain in their homes and communities. Our schools have a growing number of problem children, delinquents, laggards and misfits.
- **Occupational needs:** Vocational guidance helps individuals to get to know themselves, learn appropriate information about their professional skills and opportunities in the world of work, and find the right career path according to their skills, interests and to help you make a choice. A person with the aptitude finds and gets the right job in their chosen field.
- **Social needs:** Society is becoming more and more complex. The first changes occurred throughout the fabric of our economic, social and political systems.

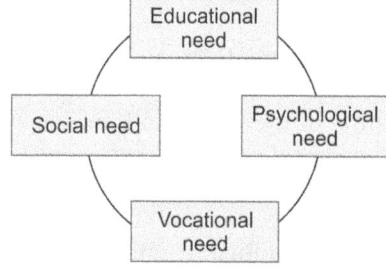

Fig. 19.4: Need of advice.

TYPES OF COUNSELING

- Educational counseling
- Vocational counseling
- Religious counseling

- Family counseling
- Guide to citizenship
- Guide to leisure and recreation
- Guide to personal health
- Guide to right behavior
- Guide to care and cooperation
- Health and cultural a guide to action.

ORGANIZING COUNSELING SERVICES

Needs for Organizing Counseling Services

- Helps teachers focus on opportunities for each student at different levels and in different directions.
- Helps students and their parents to make appropriate and appropriate future career plans.
- Helps to understand the physical, social, emotional and intellectual characteristics and needs of the student.
- Efficiently provide critical and reliable scientific data about students.
- Provide children with the knowledge to successfully adjust in school and in the community.
- A well-organized counseling program saves time, money and effort.
- Help students find suitable careers and jobs.
- Helps teachers understand children's individual differences in different areas.
- Appropriately utilize skills training opportunities and interests of school personnel.
- Coordinates the work of everyone involved in the counseling program.
- Make appropriate use of community resources to facilitate the counseling program.
- Help students achieve self-development, self-orientation, and self-actualization.
- Consider the activities and functions of staff engaged in school counseling.
- Helps build good relationships.

Principles for the Organization of Guidance Services

The principles for the organization of guidance services in schools are:
- Counseling services should target all categories of students.
- The organization of educational, professional and personal counseling programs of all kinds should be responsive to the interests, needs and goals of the student.
- Counseling services should consider the child's overall environment when organizing counseling programs for children.
- Counseling programs may differ between industrial and agricultural schools.
- Counseling services must consider the student as a whole.
- It also needs to address student-specific needs and issues.
- Must maintain adequate information regarding work and school requirements and opportunities.
- Instruction services must work with all education authorities to provide instruction.
- Students' problems should be addressed before they become serious.
- It should be aimed at enhancing the student's self-awareness and self-orientation.
- Counseling services should be adequately prepared for the testing tools used in the process.
- Individual interests and commitments should be paramount in organizing counseling services.
- Should be as simple as possible.

Restrictions on Organization of Counseling Services

- Psychologists, counselors and career counselors are required to organize counseling services and programs in schools. But in reality, most schools do not have such staff. As a result, counseling programs can become systematically dysfunctional.
- Counseling services programs require a number of infrastructural facilities, such as adequate accommodation and seating arrangements. These are considered very important for implementing counseling programs in schools.
- Government policy regarding the organization of counseling programs in secondary schools is not particularly favorable and clear. This makes it difficult for school administrators to implement counseling programs aimed at improving students.
- Most secondary schools do not have organized counseling programs.
- In the organization of school counseling services, psychological tests such as personality tests, interest surveys, aptitude tests, attitude scales, and standardized achievement tests suitable for students are rarely available in most schools. Also, some schools do not have these psychological tests or records at all.
- Teachers on whom the success of school counseling depends do not have sufficient knowledge efficiency and competence to provide appropriate instruction to students.
- In most schools, teachers are not trained in counseling or counseling her program.

- Counseling services and programs are not included in the scope of student assessment or testing. In other words, it is not an exam subject, so naturally teachers are not interested in unpaid work.
- Secondary school teachers are so overburdened with teaching duties that they do not devote the time they need for this purpose.

INDIVIDUAL COUNSELING SERVICES

Individual counseling services are a form of assistance provided to help individuals understand their potential, develop their potential, maximize their potential and solve problems. Personal issues include physical health, home issues, school issues, leisure issues, sexual issues, other emotional and psychological issues, and work-related issues.

Individual Counseling Stages

Primary School

- Early childhood refers to the stage of growth and development.
- This stage lays the basic foundation for physical, mental, emotional, social and other personality development.
- It is considered the most striking period of life in which character traits, attitudes, values and habits develop.
- Individual counseling tasks or goals at this stage include getting off to a good start in school, building a good physique, and regulating emotions.

Second Stage

The most important stage of personal development as this is the stage of stress and tension, storms and quarrels, heightened emotions and oversuggestion, fear and worry, conflict and frustration. It is believed that the main objectives of individual counseling at this stage are to:
- Guide individuals in solving physical health problems.
- Involving individuals to resolve issues related to gender, emotional and mental health.
- Help the person adjust with family.
- Provide individual counseling on social adjustments, including school adjustments.
- Help individuals progress reasonably in school.

University Level

The main purposes or functions of individual counseling during the university level are:
- Counseling is important for helping individuals work through all kinds of emotional, sexual, and other personal problems.
- Counseling is also necessary to help individuals adjust to their new environment.
- Counseling is also necessary to help individuals develop sound thoughts and build new philosophies of life.
- Counseling is also important to help you participate in social activities.
- Counseling is also important to assist individuals in making appropriate educational progress.
- Counseling is also important for individuals to find suitable employment opportunities.

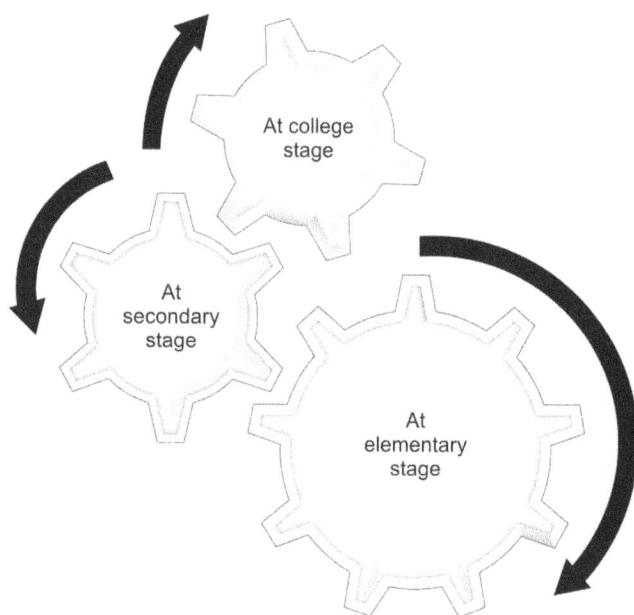

Fig. 19.5: Stages of individual counseling.

PERSONAL COUNSELING NEEDS

- **Physical health issues:** You may need professional advice and treatment to heal physical ailments and strengthen your body.
- **Family problems:** There are many family problems such as strained relationships between children and parents, between husband and wife, between siblings, constant quarrels between father and mother, presence of stepfather or stepmother in the house. Jealousy between different siblings within a family is another factor in home environment that can be a powerful source of maladaptation.
- **Use of free time:** Instruction may be required for the beneficial and individual use of free time. You may need guidance on sports games and hobbies.
- **Personal problems:** Personality problems can be the main cause of disagreements such as bullying, teasing,

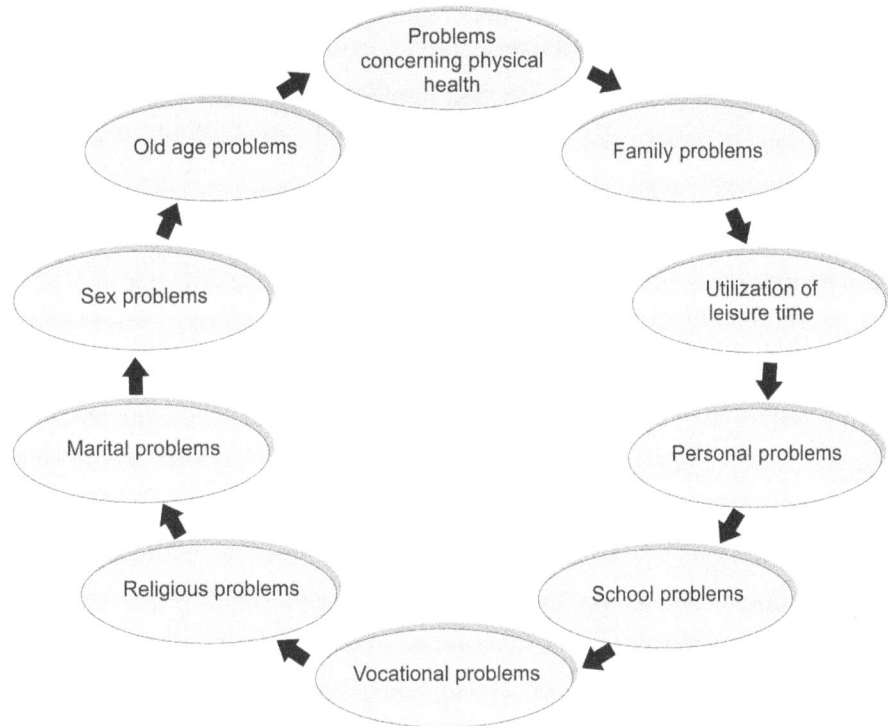

Fig. 19.6: Personal needs of counseling.

fear, anxiety, nail biting, thumb sucking, bruxism, inferiority complex. These issues require competent support.
- **Difficulty in school:** The person may not progress in a variety of academic, physical, social, and recreational activities and needs guidance.
- **Career issues:** You may need advice on choosing a career, obtaining training for a particular job, or changing careers.
- **Religious issues:** Individuals may have certain religious doubts or wrong philosophies of life and may need advice.
- **Marital issues:** Happy people are those who have a good life partner. You may need guidance in making the right mate choice.
- **Sexual problems:** Menstrual nightmares, excessive sexual curiosity, and heterosexual interests and activities can lead to sexual problems. Individual counseling is essential in helping individuals resolve sexual problems and lead healthy sex lives.
- **Age issues:** Being older brings its own issues. At this age, various organs of the body become weaker, and various senses such as sight, hearing, and smell become weaker day by day. These age groups need guidance on proper use of time and maintaining physical strength.

INDIVIDUAL COUNSELING PROCEDURES

Fact Finding

- Record all physical information such as age, gender, physical health, visual impairments, hearing impairments, and deficiencies such as nose and throat impairments.
- Family details such as family background, height, education, parents' income, family and other family birth order, domestic discipline, interrelationships between different families are then considered.
- Then details about classmates, teachers, subjects, extracurricular activities, exam success, sports and attitudes towards extracurricular activities. Watch out for failures, promotion status, class differences, and major difficulties in school or college subjects.
- You should pay attention to information about your career choice, special skills, professional interests and ambitions, previous jobs, job satisfaction or dissatisfaction, job dissatisfaction, etc. Parents, siblings, other relatives, playmates, classmates, teachers, friends, neighbors, etc.
- Next, information about mental abilities, such as intelligence and other mental abilities, should be collected using various tests and examinations designed for this purpose.

- Finally, we look at details of other personality traits, such as the individual's emotional maturity, interests, motivations, ambitions, and ideals.

Source

- **Parents:** Parents can provide very useful information about their child. This information can be obtained by inviting parents to school for specific jobs or by contacting parents at home.
- **Teachers:** Teachers can also provide a lot of information about their students. This information is based on observations of personal records obtained during examinations, job interviews, and home visits.
- **Students:** Students (individual) the primary sources of data were the students themselves and others within the school. Their friends and associates will also provide a lot of useful information about them.
- **Advisors:** Advisors can obtain information about students from a variety of sources. This information may be obtained from your general practitioner, social worker, or community member.

Diagnosing the Problem

- After collecting relevant information about the person, the counselor wants to analyze that information to find ways and means to solve the problem.
- This process, which involves analyzing information and finding ways or means to solve the problem, is called diagnosing the problem.
- A counselor cannot provide individual counseling to an individual without properly diagnosing the problem.

Prediction

- The purpose is to visualize how successful the consultant is in solving individual problems.
- The counselor visualizes the results of the guidance provided to the individual to solve the problem.
- For example, observing a person's past performance in mathematics and measuring their intellectual ability can provide a preliminary assessment of what the person will achieve after counseling.

Therapy

- Here the counselor provides a satisfactory solution to the problem. He excites the person about his problems.
- Various techniques used in treatment include sublimation of suggestion by substitution, rational persuasion, reeducation, play therapy and environmental modification, psychoanalysis, group therapy, occupational therapy, and instructional therapy.

Follow-up

It is important to know to what extent the issue has been resolved after consultation. Follow-up is therefore essential. Individual consultations are more or less incomplete without follow-up. Follow-up uses the following methods:

- **Index method:** This method displays the details of the interview, e.g., interview name, age, gender, address, purpose of interview, content of problem.
- **Questionnaire method:** The consultant conducts a questionnaire to the consultants. The questionnaire contains items addressing various aspects of the progress of the issue for which advice was provided.
- **Letter contact:** In this method, the counselor is contacted by letter and can also counsel the person.

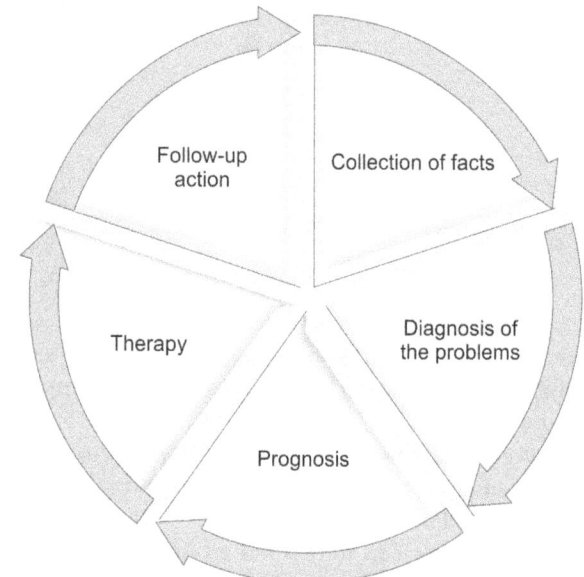

Fig. 19.7: Individual counseling process steps.

EDUCATIONAL COUNSELING

Counseling services are designed to help students adapt appropriately to the environment in which they live and to make the best possible contribution according to their strengths and limitations. Educational counseling is the counseling of students in all aspects of education.

- Focuses on helping students achieve academic satisfaction. Choosing the right degree according to author Jones, teaching is about helping students make decisions and adjustments about school curricula and school life.
- Aims educational counseling to provide a favorable environment for personal development and training through the special characteristics of the student on the one hand and the various possibilities and requirements of the student on the other.

Educational Counseling Purposes

- To supervise a student's academic program.
- Identification of special learners. Academically retarded gifted, creative people.
- Support for incoming students.
- Consider and support the educational needs of special learners.
- Diagnose student learning difficulties in a variety of subjects.
- Assist students in adapting to the curriculum and curriculum requirements of the educational program.
- Providing employment information.

Basic Principles of Educational Instruction

- Instruction should be available to all
- Common tests should be used
- You must select a curriculum
- Corrective action should be taken first
- Relevant information should be obtained
- Follow-up should be available
- Relationships between the school and parents should be established.

Elements that Play a Role in Educational Counseling

- Secondary schools are less selective
- Emphasize individual differences
- Increasing complexity of society
- Expansion of school provision
- Concepts of child growth and development
- Positive effects of group testing
- Effects of social and economic conditions.

Educational Advice Need

- **Waste and stagnation:** Waste and stagnation are common in education. The number of failed exams is a great loss to the nation.

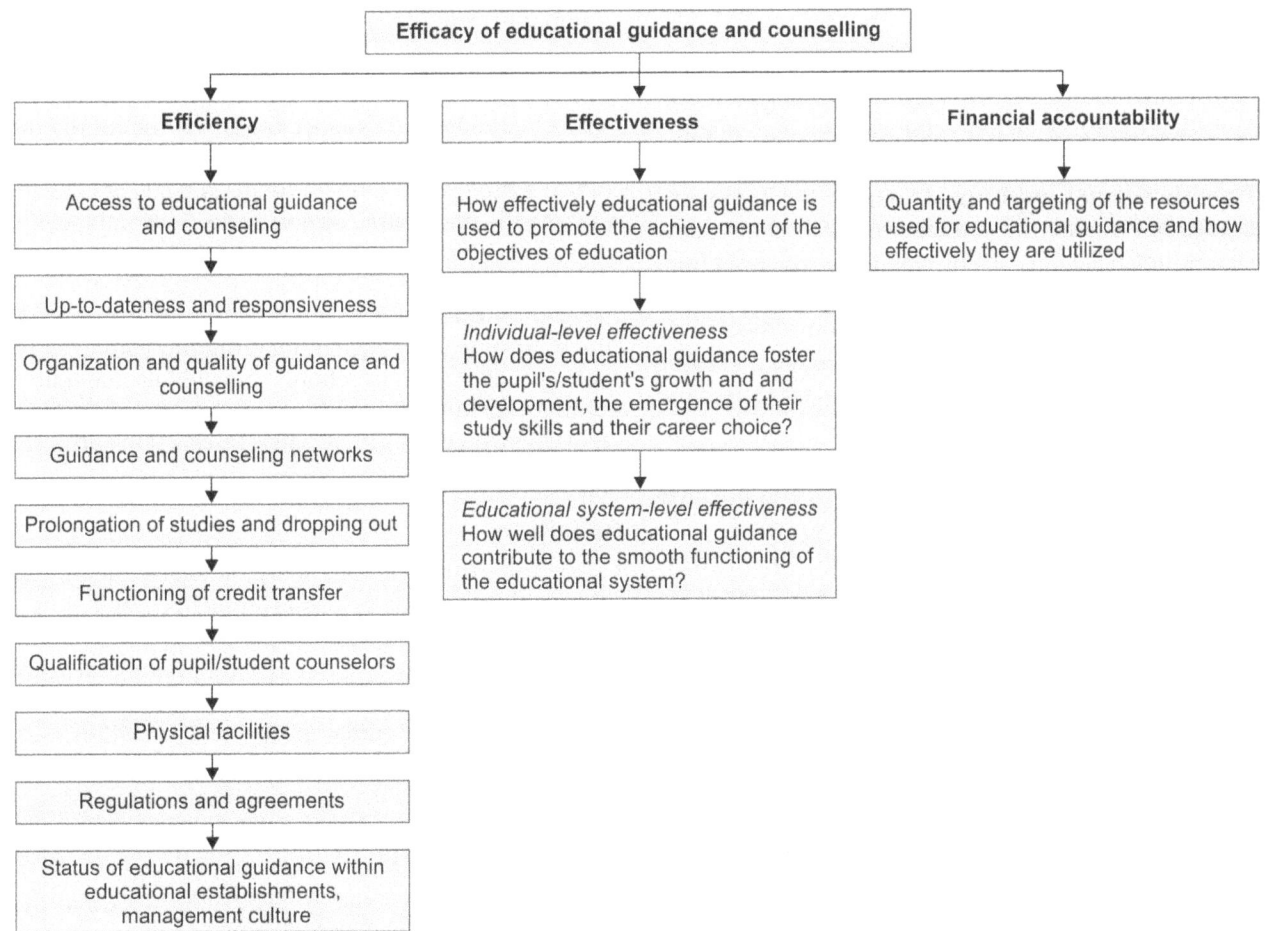

Flowchart 19.1: Efficacy of guidance and counseling.

- **Curriculum diversification:** Curriculum diversification in high schools and multipurpose schools. Therefore, you will almost certainly need advice when choosing a subject to study.
- **Further education decisions:** Students need educational counseling to help them maximize their potential and resources.

Future Career Preparation

There is an urgent need to help students prepare for their future careers, keeping in mind their potential interests and abilities and the demands of society.

Simple vocational training is not enough to lead a balanced life. Children need to be raised to live together and help each other.

Educational Counseling Goals

- **Wise curriculum selection:** It is well known that success in a student's education depends on wise selection of the curriculum. Therefore, a key objective of education is to select a curriculum according to abilities, inclinations and interests.
- **Improving learning methods:** Another goal of educational counseling is to improve learning methods. Learning methods include elements such as reading mode, note-taking, memorizing, and summarizing.
- **Provide special teaching strategies for backward students:** Primarily for students who fail exams, show signs of misbehavior, lack discipline, or run away from class. Advice on developing. Educational methods for backward children that take into account the causes of backwardness will be further developed, including special schools and specialists, special curricula and special teaching methods.
- **Special arrangements for gifted students:** Another specific purpose of educational guidance is to organize special educational programs for gifted students.
- Considering audit errors, a large number of audit errors cause a lot of waste and stagnation. Many students become emotionally unbalanced through failure.
- Educational counseling is designed to help students obtain information about the possibilities and desirability of further schooling.
- Educational counseling helps students know the requirements for admission to the school of their choice.
- Educational counseling is designed to help students understand the purpose and function of different types of schools.
- Educational counseling should support career choices.

Educational Counseling Level

Elementary

- Help students develop good habits, correct attitudes and basic skills.
- Give your students a good start.
- Help your students plan smarter.
- Help students get the most out of their education.

Secondary Education

- Helping children know themselves
- Helping children understand the world around them
- Help your child make correct subject choices
- Help your child adjust to college education.

On the University Stage

- Provide library facilities for students to broaden their intellectual horizons.
- Provides specific instruction and exam preparation for specific subjects.
- Provide specific advice on book and reference selection.
- Teach individuals how to read books, take notes, summarize and organize material, and use citations.

CAREER ADVICE

In this technological age, occupation is one of the most important aspects of human life. That's why we have to choose a profession. One of the main goals of education is to provide maximum support in professional life. If the goals of vocational training are not achieved, the training becomes worthless.

Career guidance is essentially an effort to preserve young people's valuable natural skills and young people's expensive education in schools. Individuals maintain the wealth of all human resources by investing and utilizing them where they bring the greatest satisfaction and success to themselves and society.

Definition

- According to the international labor organization, career guidance is to assist in solving problems related to career choice and career progression, taking due account of the relationship between individual characteristics and career opportunities.
- According to the career guidance association, career guidance is the process of helping individuals choose a career, prepare for it, start a career, and move forward.

Career Guidance Needs

- To increase the number of occupations
- Career guidance to maintain good health

- To promote personal and social values
- Discover and harness human potential
- Respond to the individual and complex needs of society
- Promote economic growth of individuals and societies.

Table 19.1: Difference between educational and vocational guidance.

Aspects of guidance service	Educational guidance	Vocational guidance
Principles	Americans philosophy on educational and vocational guidance	To aid economy to cover its workforce demand
Task	Helping in vertical and horizontal permeability of educational career	Assisting people to realize a free occupational choice
Field	School career, individualized guidance and counseling, parent counseling, innovation in educational system	Vocational orientation, vocational counseling, obtaining apprenticeship, promoting professional training
Governmental body	Under jurisdiction of the individual states	Subordinate to the federal employment office
Professional and assistant staff	School counselors, school psychologists, and student advisors	Vocational counselors, rehabilitation counselors, apprenticeship officer
Organizational structure	At school and university level clearly differ	Centralized and authorized by the federal authorities

Career Guidance Specific Goals

- Help students develop a thorough understanding of the characteristics and functions of the profession, roles and rewards.
- To identify the general and specific skills, competencies, etc., required for the position.
- Provides many insights into working conditions and provides opportunities for school experiences that help individuals discover their abilities and develop broader interests.
- Help individuals develop the view that all honest work has value and is the most important basis for career choices.
- We help individuals master the art of analyzing job listings and develop the habit of analyzing information before making final decisions.
- To assist him in gathering information about himself, his general and special abilities, interests and abilities that he may need to make wise decisions.
- Support financially disabled children over legal age to obtain scholarships and other financial assistance from public and private sources.
- Assist students in gaining knowledge of the facilities offered by various educational institutions for vocational training, admission requirements, duration of training offered, participation fees, etc.
- Adapt workers to the work they do. It helps him understand his relationship with workers in his own related industries and with society at large.
- So that students can get reliable information about the dangers of tempting shortcuts to happiness.

Career Counseling Features

- Helps children reach their full potential.
- This is a process that helps provide professional information that broadens an individual's professional horizons and attracts interest in professional self-development.
- This is the process that helps individuals choose and prepare for a career in life and find suitable employment. You can also observe his work progress.
- It is the process that helps people develop and accept an integrated and correct image of themselves and their role in the economy of the society to which they belong.
- This is a process that helps individuals assess their role in terms of reality or practicality.
- This is a process that helps individuals achieve their career goals. The process of achieving professional goals should serve society.
- This is the process of helping individuals make adjustments related to their profession and work.
- This is the process of helping individuals make adjustments related to their profession and work.

Career Guidance Level

Elementary Level

- Habits, skills, and attitudes develop during this time.
- Develop basic skills and attitudes.
- Get into the habit of planning your work.
- To build good relationships.

Secondary Education

- Help students assess or recognize professional support and responsibility.
- Bring students closer to different professions and their requirements.

- Help students make the right choices.
- Help prepare students for their desired career.
- Help students find suitable jobs in their chosen field.
- Help students think seriously about going to college or not.

Inside University Stadium

- To enable people to conduct comprehensive cancer research that they want.

- Help students combine their studies with the careers open to them.
- Help students become familiar with different fields of work.
- Help students find out about higher education opportunities and various programs such as financial aid and scholarships.
- Help students develop contacts to help them successfully execute their plans.

REVIEW QUESTIONS

Long Essays

1. Define leadership, explain the principles of leadership.
2. Describe the needs for organizing counseling services.
3. Enumerate the individual counseling procedures.
4. Define educational counseling, explain the purposes, principles and elements.
5. Define career advice, explain career guidance specific goals and features.

Short Essays

1. Objectives of instruction.
2. Pipe element.
3. Leadership characteristics.
4. Principles for the organization of guidance services.
5. Restrictions on organization of counseling services.
6. Individual counseling services.
7. Educational counseling goals.
8. Difference between educational and vocational guidance.
9. Career guidance level.

Short Answers

1. Assumptions of the guide.
2. Types of counseling.
3. Need advice.
4. Individual counseling stages.
5. Personal counseling needs.
6. Educational counseling level.

Chapter 20

Discipline and Grievance

Learning Objectives
- Discipline Meaning and Purpose
- Nature of Discipline
- Discipline Components
- Disciplinary Characteristics
- Principles for Maintaining Discipline
- Disciplinary Matters
- Disciplinary Matters Management
- Complaints Committee

INTRODUCTION

The etymology of the word "discipline" is believed to be the Latin word "disciplina" which means control, rule, education, practice, instruction, state of being trained. The English word "discipline" is thought to derive from the Latin word "discipulum" which means student. Students are expected to respectfully follow their teachers and, in their opinion, to develop in themselves the qualities necessary for a successful life.

The use of the word "control" is appropriate where a person is required to work under certain rules, where "regulation" is used. When children obey their elders with courtesy and respect, the word "courtesy" is appropriate. But "discipline" is a word that encompasses all of the above.

DEFINITION

Discipline is defined as the practice of teaching others to follow rules and norms by correcting undesirable behavior through punishment. In the classroom, teachers are disciplined to ensure that rules are followed. School rules are enforced and students are in a safe learning environment. Although the word discipline seems negative, the purpose of using discipline is to teach students boundaries and limits so that they can achieve their personal and academic life goals.

DISCIPLINE MEANS

Discipline means the following rules, acts, regulations, orders, controls and powers. It can also refer to punishment. Discipline is used to create automatic mechanisms like habits, routines, and blind obedience. It can affect others and yourself.

Self-discipline refers to the practice of restraining yourself, controlling your emotions, and ignoring your impulses.

Disciplinary action is any action taken against a student (or group of students) when a student's behavior interferes with continuing educational activities or violates predetermined rules by a teacher, school board, or body in general. It is a measure that teachers are required to take.

Discipline that guides behavior and sets boundaries helps children learn how to care for themselves, others, and the world around them.

DISCIPLINE PURPOSE

The purpose of this discipline is also to develop attitudes, habits, ideas and codes of conduct throughout the social life of the school. These should be organized on a cooperative basis and inspired by the higher ethical teachings of the school. Recognizing that the school must consciously pursue common goals in the spirit of development and cooperation, and rebuild the school in the spirit of each member contributing to the common good according to their unique talents. School life organized in this way becomes as continuous as life in a democratic society, and discipline permeates the whole school life.

NATURE OF DISCIPLINE

- Discipline is more than strict technical adherence to rigid and inflexible rules and regulations.
- Discipline simply means working cooperatively and acting in an appropriate and normal manner, as a responsible person would expect of an employee.
- Discipline requires punishment.
- Discipline is training to correct or perfect strengths.
- Discipline means order: Opposite of chaos and chaos.
- Discipline is control gained by enforcing obedience.

DISCIPLINE COMPONENTS

Some of the main discipline components used in educational institutions are:
- **Institution leaders:** An institution's success or failure depends on the personality of its leader. He must have some kind of philosophy about discipline. He must have some sound ground rules to guide him in his dealings with teachers and students.
- **Teachers:** Teachers are the source of discipline and character building. A good teacher solves half the problem of discipline in a school. All teachers, in addition to being clever and original, must themselves be good disciplinarians. This depends on his keen insight, perseverance, compassion, love, justice and fairness.
- **Extracurricular activities:** Sports scouting NCC. This type of community service and community activity develops the self-discipline and self-confidence that are the foundations of the discipline. Through these activities, students are able to conduct practical lessons based on their own will. Social cooperation, respect for authority, and leadership training can pave the way for teaching them the foundations of true discipline.
- **Building traditions:** It is already known that the higher and nobler the traditions established by a school, the greater the effort of students and teachers to maintain these traditions. I am here. Traditions are passed down from disciple to generation, and when properly guided disciples will never attempt to weaken the noble traditions established by their predecessors.
- **Teaching methods:** When good teaching methods are employed, students are much less likely to be disengaged or deviated from the course. Educational methods need to be designed to develop well-adjusted, self-disciplined individuals and build high morale.
- **Autonomy in schools:** In any middle school, students should participate appropriately in discipline administration, health sports drama and other school activities. Such connections make them follow rules and regulations much more meaningfully and easily than if they were imposed from above.
- **Good school environment:** Every institution or school should create a calendar at the start of a new class with a clear understanding of goals, program management rules and regulations, curriculum and collaboration plans.
- **Appropriate rewards and punishments:** Students' achievements and successful efforts should be recognized and rewarded. However, rewards must not promote unhealthy competition among students. These are very small and need to be managed in a way that appeals to the students' higher motivations.
- **Effective team workers:** The cohesiveness, collaboration and caring that exists within school staff has a positive impact on students. Young students at school carefully observe the activities of their teachers and try to imitate them for better or worse. Therefore, in order to promote discipline among students, it must first be established and maintained among school personnel.

DISCIPLINARY CHARACTERISTICS

The basic characteristics of discipline can be summarized as follows:
- Disciplinary action concerns an individual's self-discipline to comply with organizational rules and regulations.
- This is an important preparation to encourage individuals and groups to carry out instructions and suggestions that the organization has identified as acceptable behavior.
- This is a passive approach in the sense that it encourages individuals to take certain behaviors that distinguish them from others.
- We are proactive in imposing penalties for violations of the values and norms established by the organization.
- About the most effective time management.
- Discipline means completing all tasks within the given time frame.
- Balances the three units of our being: body, soul and spirit.
- It is the ability to stay focused and stay on course.
- Discipline means always honoring the promises you make to yourself and others.
- Determination to keep going even in difficult situations.
- Always on time.

PRINCIPLES FOR MAINTAINING DISCIPLINE

- Discipline based on fear or suspicion is very temporary or transitory, so the basis of discipline must be love, trust and charity. To maintain true discipline, principals, like students, need to feel love for one another. Love creates trust and lays the foundation for discipline.
- Good discipline must be based on cooperation. It is very important to maintain and maintain collaboration between school leaders and teachers, teachers and students, teachers and parents and students. Without cooperation, it is very difficult to maintain good discipline. To do this, it is essential that everyone builds good relationships.
- No penalties should be imposed to maintain discipline. If you do not quit a bad habit in some way, you need to apply that habit. When punishment is repeated over and over again, various complexes arise in the student's brain. As a result, your personality may be out of balance. Punishment should therefore be avoided whenever possible.
- The atmosphere throughout the school should be beautiful and harmonious. This responsibility should not lie solely with teachers or authorities. Rather, parents and society at large must take responsibility for creating such an atmosphere.
- Schools and educational institutions should provide a variety of creative activities so that children can be physically and mentally satisfied by engaging in various activities according to their own interests. By doing so, there is no chance of any disciplinary issues arising.
- Children should learn the importance of discipline. A mere discourse based on the examples of various greats is not enough for this. Rather, knowledge about it should be passed on to the children, and examples should be presented in front of the children by the principal himself and the teachers.
- Students and teachers should be given sufficient freedom and opportunity to carry out their duties at an institution or school.
- Since children spend most of their time at home, parents should be encouraged to make home life enjoyable and comfortable. Good school efforts can fail when home life is inappropriate and tainted. Legal guardians should therefore be motivated by a variety of means to make family life healthy and accommodating.

DISCIPLINARY MATTERS

- Disorder and lack of discipline in students affect society.
- The use of abusive language, disrespect to teachers, freedom struggles in educational institutions, coercion of copies in exams, and violent strikes by students are common among students.
- There are many other causes of disciplinary violations. Lack of parental attention, peer and peer pressure, lack of values-based education, lack of good role models, and a flawed education system that places too much emphasis on finishing textbooks on time.
- Under pressure to complete textbooks, teachers can easily stop providing moral education to their students. For this reason, character development comes second and last, but excessive use of electronic devices, especially the use of mobile phones and laptops all day just for games and unnecessary work, can be medically harmful to students.
- The worst thing about this issue is that it is often misunderstood by political leaders who use it as a tool to create anarchy.

Reason for Discipline Violation

- **Favoritism:** Teacher favors some students, while others see this favoritism as an insult to them, leading to rebellion.
- **Rules are not enforced:** If students are not punished for their crimes, they will commit other crimes.
- **Teacher-student relationship:** The teacher-student relationship is integral to any learning process. Any rift in this relationship will result in a discipline violation.
- **Lack of motivation:** If students lack motivation, they will want to work without discipline.
- **Bad habits:** Some students have developed bad habits from previous classroom experiences. For example, if a student develops a habit of arriving late for school, it can be difficult to change that behavior.

Types of Discipline in Schools

School and student disruption is a serious problem, as aggression and disruption among students can lead to violent student-teacher relationships. This is a major concern for policy makers. This includes behavioral disturbances such as theft, insults, dishonesty and lying, which can cause physical damage to school and home property and can also cause psychological and emotional distress. The main types of disciplinary violations in schools are:

- **Being late to school:** This is the most common form of discipline violation in school. Many students come to school late, and they are not punctual. Some of them are not interested in regularly attending morning assemblies in the evening.
- **Talking in class:** It is quite difficult for teachers to maintain silence in class. Sometimes in a teacher's lesson, the

lesson is inadequate and the students seem upset. They may show disinterest in lessons due to rigid and outdated teaching methods and strategies.
- **Homework neglect:** Pedagogical intuition often observes students neglecting homework. It is clear that you have enough time to write them 100 friendly punishment sentences, but it shows that they are not interested in doing their homework every day.
- **Lying:** Students often lie on a variety of occasions, leading to disciplinary problems in class. They lie because they lack the confidence and coverage to face reality.
- **Disrespectful behavior towards teachers:** This form of discipline usually occurs in students entering puberty. They are mostly disrespectful towards teachers in various cases. They refuse to follow the teacher's instructions.
- **Stealing:** It is commonly observed that some students steal pencils, books, pens, copies, and other items from their classmates. This is a kind of disciplinary violation and requires the serious attention of the teacher to solve it in time.

DISCIPLINARY MATTERS MANAGEMENT

Teachers today are expected to play several constructive roles. They must not only teach the subject, but also take on the role of advisor and take the moral responsibility of shaping the character of their students. Counseling trained teachers can make students feel heard when they talk about their learning needs and know how to handle different situations. Such teachers know the importance of treating students with dignity.

Another step is to establish an active parent-teacher association (PTA) in each school to make parents aware of the importance of taking responsibility for their children's learning and behavior, and keeping close contact and watching your child's progress. Parents should have a say in disciplinary action taken in the event of disciplinary violations. A healthy working relationship between teachers and parents definitely has a positive impact on students.
- Appropriate arrangements should be made to establish personal contact between teachers and students.
- School authorities need to understand students' problems.
- Eliminate deficiencies in the education system. The university education commission, secondary education commission and Kothari Commission have made very important proposals on which work may be carried out.
- The examination system should be improved.
- In order to enable students to earn a living, the importance of work experience and professional training should be emphasized to avoid disappointment and dissatisfaction in future life.
- Schools need to build close relationships with families and society. Parents of students and leaders of society must also take responsibility for solving this problem.
- Employment opportunities must be easily accessible.

COMPLAINTS

An individual complaint is a complaint that management's actions violated an individual's rights through collective bargaining agreements, laws, or unfair practices. Examples of this type of complaint include disciplinary disputes, demotions, classifications, denial of benefits, etc.

Definitions

- A complaint is a formal dispute between an employee and management regarding terms and conditions of employment.
- Complaints are complaints duly recorded under the complaints procedure.
- Complaints are dissatisfaction or feelings of unfairness about your employment situation that are reported to management.

Complaint Characteristics

- Complaint refers to any form of dissatisfaction or dissatisfaction with any aspect of an organization.
- The complaint must be employmentrelated and not a personal or family matter.
- Dissatisfaction can arise for real or imagined reasons. File a complaint if you feel you have been treated unfairly. The reasons for such feelings may be valid or invalid, valid or irrational, valid or absurd.
- Complaints are not expressed or spoken. But it has to be expressed somehow. However, dissatisfaction itself is not resentment. First, employees can make oral or written complaints. If this is not addressed promptly, workers will feel unfair. Now that dissatisfaction has grown and has taken the form of complaints.
- Broadly speaking, complaints stem from failure to meet expectations of the organization.

Forms of Complaints

Complaints can take one of the following forms:
- **Fact:** Substantial complaints occur when legitimate employee needs are not met. For example, a salary increase was agreed but not implemented for various reasons.
- **Imaginary:** Employee dissatisfaction is due to employee misunderstandings, attitudes, or information rather than legitimate reasons. Such situations can cause imaginary complaints. Management cannot be held responsible in such cases, but must clear the 'fog' immediately.

- **Veiled:** Employees may be dissatisfied for unknown reasons. When we are under pressure from family, friends, relatives, or neighbors, we may go to work with a heavy heart. A new employee gets a new table and almirah can be a nuisance to other employees who have not been treated equally before.

Reasons for Complaints

Complaints can arise for several reasons:
- **Economy:** Fixed wages, overtime premiums, wage revisions, etc. Employees may feel that their salaries are lower than others.
- **Working conditions:** Poor physical conditions at work, strict production standards, defective tools and equipment, poor quality materials, unfair regulations, lack of awareness, etc.
- **Supervision:** Refers to the supervisor's attitude towards the employee.
- **Workgroups:** Employees cannot adapt to their colleagues. They suffer from neglect, victimhood, and are subject to ridicule and humiliation.
- **Miscellaneous:** This includes promotions, security measures, transfers, disciplinary rules, fines, leave entitlement, medical facilities, etc.
- To investigate complaints and assess their merits. The Complaints Bureau also has the authority to investigate harassment cases. Anyone with a serious complaint may contact the principal or lodge a complaint with the Student Complaints Office. If the person does not wish to file a complaint, they may write to the complaints office letterbox/suggestion box located at school administration block.

The purpose of the complaints room is to: The mission of the complaints room is to foster responsiveness and responsible attitudes among all stakeholders in order to maintain a harmonious and educational atmosphere in the institute.
- Maintain the integrity of the school by ensuring a conflict-free atmosphere within the school, including promoting warm student-student and student-teacher relationships.
- Encourage students to express their grievances and problems freely and openly without fear of becoming victims.
- We have set up an opinion/complaint box in front of the administrative building so that students who wish to remain anonymous can submit written complaints and suggestions regarding the improvement of their studies and school management.
- We advise our students to respect each other's rights and dignity and to show the utmost restraint and patience whenever disagreements arise.
- We advise all students not to instigate other students' teachers or school administrators.
- Instruct staff to be affectionate towards students and not to take revenge on students for any reason.
- Any form of vandalism on or off the premises is strictly prohibited. Any violation of school rules or disciplinary rules must be reported immediately to the principal.

GRC Scope

- **Academic matters:** Relating to the timely issuance of transcripts, transfer certificates, transcripts, or other examination-related matters.
- **Financial matters:** Payment of donations and various items from library dormitories, etc.
- **Other matters:** Specific concerns regarding sanitary conditions, food preparation, transportation availability, teacher harm, etc.

Functions on Matter

- Upon receipt of a written complaint from the student, the case will be dealt with immediately.
- The cell will formally review all cases and act in accordance with administrative policies.
- The cell will inform the authorities of the cases that have been processed and the number, if any, of pending cases that require direction and direction from higher authorities.

Student and Faculty Grievance Mechanisms

Students are the protagonists of any educational institution providing education and we aim to make every effort to ensure transparency in all our activities at various stages. With this spirit in mind, the school has established the following mechanisms for students to seek grievance relief. Complaints may broadly include the following complaints from affected students:
- Academic
- Non-academic
- Review complaints

Fourth Complaints About Harm

- Complaints about attendance
- Complaints about billing exam fees
- Complaints about exam administration
- Harassment by classmates, teachers, etc.

Procedures for Submitting Complaints

- Students are free to submit complaints in writing or in any format available to the administration and put it in the box.

- The complaints department handles cases forwarded with the required documentation.
- The complaints department shall ensure that the complaint is properly resolved within the time limit set by the department in charge.

Responsibility for Correction

- Ultimate responsibility for correcting complaints rests with the principal.
- The school expects complaints to be resolved in a timely and results-oriented manner. Any complaints are expected to be resolved within a reasonable time.
- The school complaints department monitors the status and progress of complaints resolution and reports to the principal on the status of the complaint.

COMPLAINTS COMMITTEE

As part of an ongoing effort to ensure transparency of all activities at various stages, the university provides students with appropriate mechanisms to resolve complaints. This committee will directly deal with all complaints related to common problems at both academic and administrative laboratory level. Aggrieved members must submit a petition to the complaints committee in an envelope marked "confidential". Upon receipt of the petition, the complaints resolution panel will endeavor to provide the principal with recommendations on how to proceed. In the event of a false and frivolous complaint (provided), the Complaints Correction Board shall recommend the chief/disciplinary authority to take appropriate action against the complainant. We also respond to "suggestion boxes" and verbal complaints from students and parents. All complaints are investigated by management and the complaints desk.

Objectives of the Grievance Committee

- To ensure a conflict-free atmosphere within the university, including promoting warm student-student and student-teacher relations, and to maintain the integrity of the university.
- Responsive and explanatory to resolve student grievances in a timely manner and to take action in the operation of the university to maintain a harmonious educational atmosphere within the university.
- Manipulates complex situations to reduce perceived distress and frustration.
- Encourage students to express their grievances and problems freely and openly without fear of becoming victims.
- We advise college students to respect each other's rights and dignity and to show the utmost restraint and patience whenever disagreements arise.
- We advise all students not to provoke students to other student's teachers or to university authorities.
- We advise all staff to be kind to students and not to take revenge on them for any reason.
- To assist students who have been denied eligible services offered by the college.
- Hold university staff accountable and courteous in their dealings with students.
- Resolve student complaints effectively with a fair and just approach.

Complaints Resolution Committee Duties

- The function of this cell is to investigate complaints submitted by students and evaluate their merits. The complaints office is also empowered to investigate harassment cases.
- If you have a serious complaint, please contact a member of the department personally or discuss it with your class teacher.
- If the person does not wish to lodge a complaint, he or she may submit a complaint in writing to the letter box/suggestion box of the complaints cell in the administration block.
- Complaints may also be emailed to the email address principal@srsect.edu.in or to the student complaints officer.
- After receiving a written complaint from the student, the case will be dealt with promptly. The complaints bureau will process cases forwarded along with the required documentation.
- The complaints department verifies that the complaint has been properly resolved within the deadlines set by the responsible department.
- This cell formally investigates all cases and produces a statistical report on the number of cases received. This cell provides the authorities with reports on the cases that have been processed and the number of pending cases, if any, that require direction and guidance from higher authorities.

Composition of the Appeals Committee

- The principal shall determine the composition and term of the Appeals Committee for her two years.
- The Quorum Committee shall consist of members from the education and non-educational divisions.
- All complaints referred to the complaints committee/director/director shall be recorded in a register maintained for that purpose by the secretary of the complaints

committee the number of resolved or pending complaints is reported to clients monthly.

Student Complaints and Responsibility for Complaints Disciplinary Committee

- Set up a complaint box to record complaints and actions taken.
- Hold biweekly or monthly meetings to discuss issues raised by complainants.
- If the complaint in question is trivial in nature, promptly resolve the complaint.
- By the end of the academic year, meeting reports and resolved complaints will be submitted to IQAC.

REVIEW QUESTIONS

Long Essays
1. Define discipline, explain the purposes and nature of discipline.
2. Describe the principles for maintaining discipline.
3. Explain managing disciplinary matters in nursing schools.
4. Define compliant, explain the characteristics, forms and reasons for complaint.
5. Define complaints committee, explain objectives of the grievance committee.

Short Essays
1. Components of discipline.
2. Characteristics of discipline.
3. Types of discipline in schools.
4. Student and faculty grievance mechanisms.
5. Procedures for submitting complaints.
6. Complaints resolution committee duties.
7. Composition of the appeals committee.
8. Student complaints and responsibility for complaints disciplinary committee.

Short Answers
1. Reason for discipline violation.
2. Favoritism.
3. Teacher-student relationship.
4. School complaints department.
5. Grievance.

Unit 8
Teaching (EBT) in Nursing Education

Chapter

21. Teaching (EBT) in Nursing Education

KEYWORDS

Evidence-based learning: Evidence-based learning describes a set of strategies and tools that are empirically proven to demonstrate learning outcomes. More literally, the term refers to a process that shows evidence of learning taking place.

Evidence-based intervention/instruction: Instructional techniques or strategies which have been demonstrated through experimental research or large-scale field studies to be effective.

Evidence-based practices: Practices for teaching reading grounded and proven in research.

Active learning: A teaching and learning approach that "engages students in the process of learning through activities and/or discussion in class, as opposed to passively listening to an expert.

Asynchronous instruction: Asynchronous instruction is the idea that students learn similar material at different times and locations.

Authentic assessment: Assessments in which student learners demonstrate learning by applying their knowledge to authentic, complex, real-world tasks or simulations.

Blended or hybrid course: Blended or hybrid courses are classes in which some percentage of seat time has been reduced and replaced with online content and activities.

Bloom's taxonomy: Bloom's taxonomy is a cognitive framework of learning behaviors organized hierarchically in six categories: Knowledge, comprehension, application, analysis, evaluation, and synthesis.

Classroom climate: The intellectual, social, emotional, and physical environments in which our students learn.

Collaborative learning: An umbrella term that covers many different methods in which students work together to solve a problem, complete a task, or create a product.

Experiential learning: Experiential learning is a process by which students develop knowledge and skills from direct experience, usually outside a traditional academic setting.

Fixed mindset: Mindset refers to the beliefs and attitudes held by a person and can affect their learning outcomes and achievement.

Flipped classroom: A flipped classroom is a teaching approach where students a first exposed to content before coming to a class session and then spend class time engaging more deeply with the ideas and concepts.

Inquiry-based learning: Inquiry-based learning is an umbrella term that includes pedagogical strategies such as problem-based learning and case-based learning that prioritize students exploring, thinking, asking, and answering content questions with peers to acquire new knowledge through a carefully designed activity.

Learning management system (LMS): A learning management system is a platform that enables instructors to organize and distribute course materials in a digital format.

Object-based learning (OBL): OBL is a teaching method whereby students engage with authentic or replica material objects in their learning in order to gain discipline-specific knowledge or to practice observational or practical skills that can be applied in various fields.

Problem-based learning: A form of student-centered teaching that focuses on having students work through open-ended problems to explore course material.

Project-based learning: A form of student-centered teaching that engages students with course content as they work through a complex project.

Retrieval practice: Retrieval practice involves retrieving new knowledge from memory in order for durable retention in long-term memory.

Scaffolding: A process by which Instructors build on a student's previous experience or knowledge by adding in specific timely support structures in the form of activities or assignments for students to master new knowledge or skills and achieve learning goals.

Student-centered teaching: Instructor-center teaching refers to instructors teaching content solely through a passive approach such as lecturing while students listen and take notes with minimal interaction with other students.

Teaching development plan (TDP): A written document that helps instructors focus on teaching specific career goals.

Teaching (EBT) in Nursing Education

Chapter 21

Learning Objectives

- Value-Based Practice-Meaning and Purpose
- Ethics Review
- Important for Values-Based Education
- Values Education
- Values Education in Schools
- Values-Based Nursing Education
- Value Development Strategies
- Approaches to Values Education
- Ethical Decision-Making
- Student Ethical Standards
- Student-Faculty Relationship
- Evidence-Based Teaching
- Evidence-Based Teaching Strategies
- Using Evidence-Based Instruction in the Classroom
- Care Education Applications

TERMINOLOGY

- **Ethics (or morality):** A code of conduct (or code of conduct) that distinguishes between right and wrong, etc.
- **Applied ethics:** The study of ethics in specific situations, professions and organizations, e.g., medical ethics and research ethics, etc.
- **Honesty:** The quality of a person's trustworthiness that "does not lie, cheat, or steal".
- **Value:** Individual relative value attached to intrinsic or extrinsic object experience or person.
- **Validity:** A measure of sound thinking in which consistent, fair and reflected logic is the norm.
- **Virtue:** Quality of life according to proclaimed moral values. People are virtuous when they are fair, honest, responsible, and charitable.
- **Discipline:** The key to success in student life is to be disciplined and punctual in whatever you do.
- **Ethical standards:** Honesty, reliability, justice, respect, responsibility, observance of the law, confidentiality, personal responsibility practices.
- **Student achievement:** Positive student achievement as a result of participating in a multicultural curriculum and contributing to a psychologically safe environment.
- **Autonomy:** The ability of the group and each member of the group to act according to a set of shared moral values rather than under the influence of desires and socially imposed expectations.
- **Authenticity:** The degree to which an individual and a group exhibit behaviors that are congruent with shared beliefs and values despite external pressures to conform to traditional practices that are often based in colonialist values.

INTRODUCTION

Nursing faculty members are challenged to teach core nursing values. Clinical evaluation of senior nursing students reveals that the approach to values integration espoused in this paper is actualized through application of value based caring behavior in the capstone clinical experience. The revised curriculum provides the conceptual moral and practical learning necessary to assure that the future nursing workforce is grounded in the concept of caring. Values-based practice (VBP) is an approach to working with complex and conflicting values in healthcare that is: Complementary to other approaches to working with values (such as ethics) in focusing on individual values.

A partner to evidence-based practice in supporting clinical judgment in individual cases.

DEFINITION

- Ethics is the science of judging specifically human ends and the relationship of means to those ends. In a sense, it is also the art of controlling the means to human ends
—**Thomas Garret**
- Value-based practice (VBP) is a clinical skills-based approach to addressing complex and conflicting values in the healthcare system. Here are his two frameworks for evidence-based practice (EBP).

VBE MEANING

Value-based practice (VBP) is a clinical skills-based approach to addressing complex and conflicting values in healthcare. These are two frameworks of evidence-based practice (EBP).

Value-based practice (VBP) is an approach to addressing complex and conflicting values in healthcare by: A focus on personal values complements other approaches that address values (such as ethics).

Evidence-based practice partners to support clinical practice case by case assessment Through this personal focus, the VBP applies science to the specifics of individuals (clinicians, patients, caregivers, etc.) involved in specific clinical decisions values).

Values-based education is essential to human development and helps us in many ways throughout our lives.

VBE PURPOSE

Value-based education aims to train students to face the outside world with the right attitudes and values. It is the process of holistic character building of the student. These include personality development, citizenship development, and spiritual development. Some believe that personality

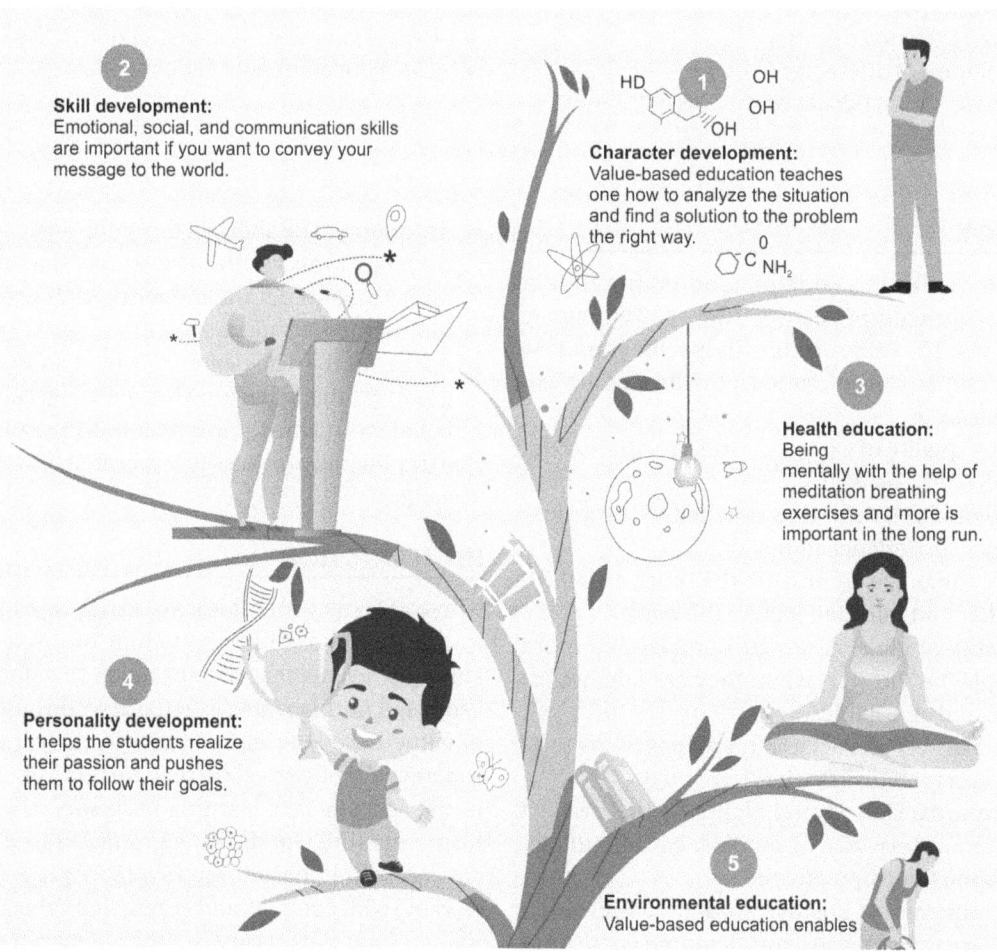

Fig. 21.1: Five important pillars of value-based education.

is a child's innate character and can never be developed or strengthened. But this is not true. Self-development sessions and proper school selection can radically change a child's personality.
- Gives students a positive direction in shaping their future and also helps them find meaning in life.
- Teach the best way of life that benefits both you and those around you.
- Values education also helps students become more responsible and rational.
- Helps you better understand your outlook on life and live a richer life as a responsible citizen.
- It also helps students build strong relationships with family and friends.
- Develop character and individuality in students.
- Values education develops in students a positive outlook on life.

ETHICS REVIEW

Ethics plays a very important role in education. Ethics is interpreted as a discipline that deals with good and evil with responsibility and moral obligation. Ethics is a well-established level of judging whether an action is right or wrong. Not just honesty, but unique values such as honesty and discipline are categorized and applied to our daily lives. Ethics influence behavior and help people make the right decisions. Without ethics, it is very difficult to master life and act responsibly. The importance of ethics cannot be ignored at any level of life. It is important to put it into practice in the classroom.

Ethics

Ethics are moral principles that govern the conduct and behavior of individuals and groups. The focus is on the right and wrong of actions and includes the decision-making process to determine the ultimate consequences of those philosopher WD. He lists six basic human duties.
1. Loyalty—do no harm to others
2. Reparations—making amends to those we have hurt
3. Gratitude—retribution for those who have helped us
4. Justice—treating people as they deserve
5. Charity—as much as we can helping others
6. Self-improvement—improve yourself but not at the expense of others.

ICN Code of Ethics

The International Council on Nursing (ICN) code of nursing (1973) states: Similar to ANA code base. It is about the nurse's responsibility to other people, society, colleagues, and the profession as a whole. The nurse's primary responsibilities in ethics in nursing consist of her four parts: Promoting health, preventing disease, restoring health, and alleviating suffering.

NURSES AND PEOPLE

- A nurse's primary responsibility is to care for people who need care.
- Caregivers promote a care environment that respects individual values, customs and spiritual beliefs.
- Nurses will keep personal information confidential and use good judgment when sharing this information.
- The former term "patient" has been replaced with the term "people" and these responsibilities are broader.
- This code provides guidance to nurses on two general areas of ethical behavior in nursing. First, individual values, customs and religious beliefs must be respected.
- Secondary personal information about this person must be kept confidential or disclosed only on discretion.

Nurses and Practice

- Nurses are personally responsible for maintaining competence through nursing practice and continuing learning.
- Caregivers will maintain the highest standard of care reasonably possible under the realities of the particular situation.
- When assuming and delegating responsibilities, nurses use personal judgment.
- Nurses must follow professional standards of conduct that reflect professional perceptions at all times when acting in a professional capacity.

Nurses and Society

- Nurses share responsibility with other citizens to initiate and support action to meet public health and social needs.
- This code establishes the responsibility of nurses to actively promote public health by initiating and supporting actions to meet health and social needs.
- Social needs are important because they are often narrowly related to people's health. Poor housing conditions, unemployment, poor sanitation, malnutrition and illiteracy are only considered social needs.

Nurses and Staff

- Nurses maintain collaborative relationships with colleagues in nursing and other areas.
- Caregivers will take appropriate action to protect individuals when caregiving is endangered by co-workers or others.

Nursing and Professionals

- Nurses play a key role in setting and enforcing desirable standards of nursing practice and education.
- Nurses are actively involved in developing core competencies. Nurses, through professional organizations, participate in the creation and maintenance of just social and economic working conditions in nursing.

Articles of the Nursing Code of Ethics

Currently, the nursing code of ethics contains nine major provisions.

1. Nurses practice with compassion and respect for the inherent dignity and unique qualities of all human beings.
2. The nurse's primary work is with patients, including individual families, groups, communities and groups.
3. Nurses are committed to and protect the health and safety of their patients.
4. Nurses have authority and responsibility for nursing practice. We act in line with our commitment to providing the best patient care.
5. Nurses are responsible for themselves and others, including the responsibility to promote health and safety, maintain character and integrity, maintain competence, and pursue personal and professional development. We have the same obligations to others.
6. Through individual and collective efforts, nurses create, maintain, and improve an ethical environment of work and employment conditions conducive to safe, quality care.
7. Nurses, in all roles and settings, advance the profession through research and academic inquiry, professional standards development, and nursing and health policy development.
8. Nurses work with other health professionals and the public to uphold human rights, promote health diplomacy and reduce health disparities.
9. The nursing profession, collectively through its professional organizations, must articulate nursing values, uphold professional integrity, and integrate principles of social justice into nursing and health policy.

IMPORTANT FOR VALUES-BASED EDUCATION

- Values are goals and beliefs that guide behavior and provide a basis for decision-making. In the workplace, values are standards of behavior favored by professionals and professional groups and form a framework for evaluating behavior.
- Nursing is a profession based on professional ethics and ethical values, and nursing performance is based on these values. The core values of nursing include altruism, autonomy, human dignity, honesty, integrity and social justice.
- Fundamental ethical values are commonly shared in the global community and reflect the human and spiritual approach of the nursing profession.
- Our professional values are expressed in our code of ethics. In fact, the code of ethics defines the practice of the nursing profession, the quality of professional nursing, and professional norms.
- Advances in technology and the expanding role of caregivers create complex ethical dilemmas for caregivers.
- Values can be communicated, changed and promoted through education, directly or indirectly. Each student enters nursing school with a set of values that can change during the process of socialization.
- The targeted integration of professional values into nursing education is critical to securing the future of nursing.
- One of the main results of teaching ethics and professional values to students is enhancing their ability to make autonomous ethical decisions.
- Nursing students first acquire professional values through a process of mentoring and socialization by school teachers. Professional socialization is a way of developing professional values, beliefs and behaviors.

VALUES EDUCATION

Values

Education is an exciting process of teaching values based education. The idea is about an educational process that instills moral guidelines for building a more civilized, majority-governed society. Values education along these lines promotes resilience and understanding well beyond our political and social conflicts and stark contrasts, human rights barriers with guaranteed protection, very minority and most minority groups. Emphasize the gathering of vulnerable people and the protection of nature.

Values Education Objectives

- To provide a realistic and comprehensive understanding of human values and to educate students to be responsible citizens in their personal and social lives.
- Foster and promote values such as truth, humility, honesty, perseverance, cooperation, compassion and love.
- To enable students to understand, appreciate, support, protect and promote the sovereignty, unity and integrity of India.

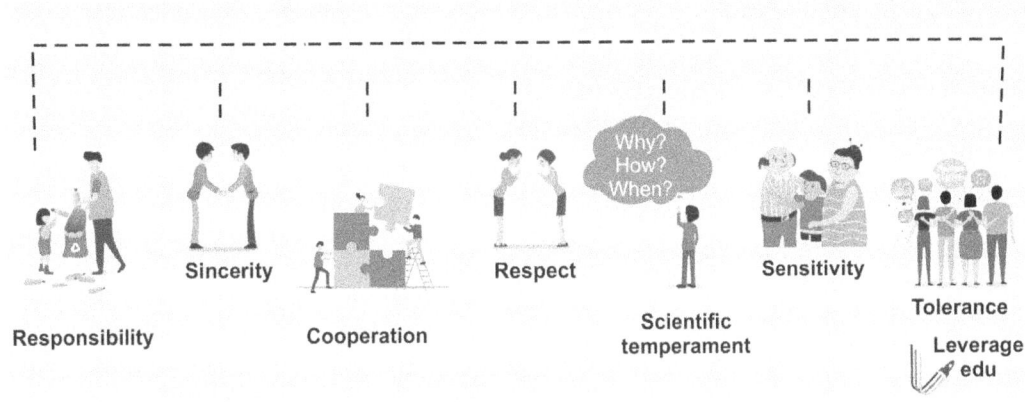

Fig. 21.2: Importance of value education.

- Cultivate a spirit of scientific research and a scientific temperament, and foster the ability to think creatively and independently.
- To provide scientific education for the development of the physical, mental, moral, social, spiritual and economic aspects of life.
- Help students distinguish between good and bad, right and wrong.
- Respect the dignity of individuals and society.

Types of Values

- **Personal values:** Personal values mean everything a person needs in social relationships. Personal values include beauty, morality, selfconfidence, initiative, regularity, ambition, courage, vision, and imagination.
- **Social values:** People cannot live without communication with others. People seek social values such as love, affection, friendship, noble group, reference group, impurity, hospitality, courage, service, justice, freedom, patience, forgiveness, adjustment, sympathy, tolerance, etc. Social values are more important to a healthy and benign environment for any organization.
- **Moral values:** Ethical values are about taking care of yourself and others, respecting the authority of others, keeping your promises, avoiding unnecessary problems with others, and avoiding cheating and dishonesty, avoid appreciate others, and let them work encouraged.
- **Spiritual values:** The ultimate moral values are called spiritual values. Spiritual values include purity, meditation, yoga, discipline, control, clarity, and devotion to God. Spiritual values education emphasizes the principle of self-discipline. Freedom from self-discipline, contentment, lack of needs, general greed, and integrity.
- **Universal values:** Universal values determine the meaning of human existence. Through universal values, we connect with humanity and the universe. Universal values can be experienced as fraternity, love, compassion, service, heaven, truth and eternity.
- **Cultural values:** Cultural values are about right and wrong, good and bad habits and behaviors. Cultural values are reflected in language, ethics, social hierarchies, aesthetics, education, law, economics, philosophy and all kinds of social organization. After categorizing the values, we need to decide which of the above values makes the most sense. Universal values are the foundation for us to enjoy a prosperous and fulfilling life.

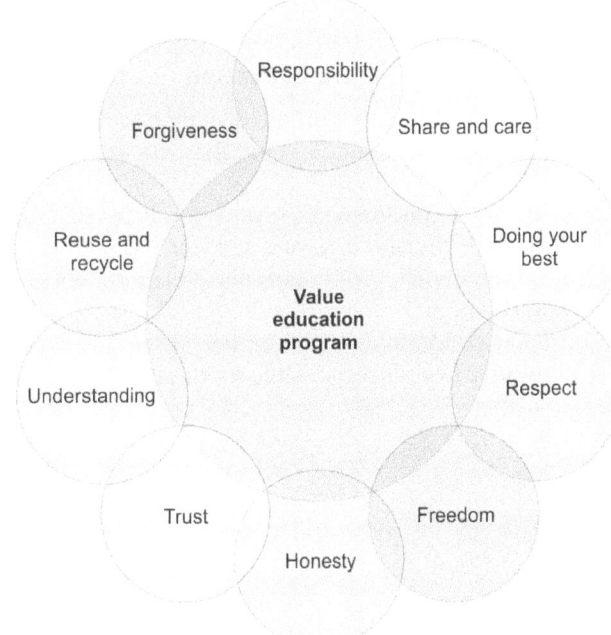

Fig. 21.3: Value-based education program.

VALUES EDUCATION IN SCHOOLS

Values education can in other words be described as character building or good education. In human life where religion has no meaning, it is an education in which students take in values from teachers and put them into practice in the future. Which one is the most valuable for your character? Values education starts at home and continues throughout life, but values education in schools has a significant impact on people's lives.
- Participation in educator inquiries.
- Show that you are committed to completing school assignments.
- Enhances the ability to work independently.
- Apply common sense to life learning.
- Mindfulness in the classroom.
- Allow students to make their own decisions.
- Builds a healthy brain.

The Importance of Values Education

- Provides students with a progressive path to the future and also helps them understand the true meaning of their lives.
- This helps you understand how best to live a life that benefits both you and those around you.
- Values education helps students become more sensitive and practical.
- This helps children have a better perception of life and lead positive lives as responsible residents.
- It also helps build strong relationships with family and friends.
- It changes the character and character of the student.
- Values education changes positive attitudes towards life in the minds of students.
- It can be argued that in the current political climate this is more important than ever.
- Values education is the teaching and learning of ideals that society considers important.
- The objective of the student is not only to recognize values, but to reflect them in their actions and attitudes.

Introduction to Values Education

Values education is the study of understanding what is important for human happiness. In order to meet all the requirements of the values education seminar, the attached rules for course content are relevant:
- **Universal:** Must be suitable for all people on all occasions and in all regions, regardless of faith, nationality, religion, etc.
- **Rationale:** Must appeal to human thought. It should be fun to think about, not based on authoritative opinions or the beliefs of the blind.
- **Natural and undeniable:** Usually it must be appropriate for the person experiencing the course, and when we live by such values it triggers our bliss. It should be clear from experience and not based on belief, belief or speculation.
- **Comprehensive:** Values education is designed to change our consciousness and our lives. Therefore, it must cover all aspects (thinking, behavior, work, cognition) and levels (identity and existence of family society) of human life and occupation.
- **Leading to kindness:** Values education ultimately aims to promote harmony among humans and with nature.

Components of Values Education

Values education can be described in other words as character education or good education. Below are some of the key elements of values education:
- **Character education:** Character education or moral education is a very important part of values education. It helps a person to be well behaved and socially acceptable welfare.
- **Health education:** This type of education is designed to give individuals the knowledge and skills to keep themselves and others healthy.
- **Environmental education:** This education enables individuals to explore environmental problems and take essential actions to solve them. This helps us make responsible decisions to maintain the quality of our environment.

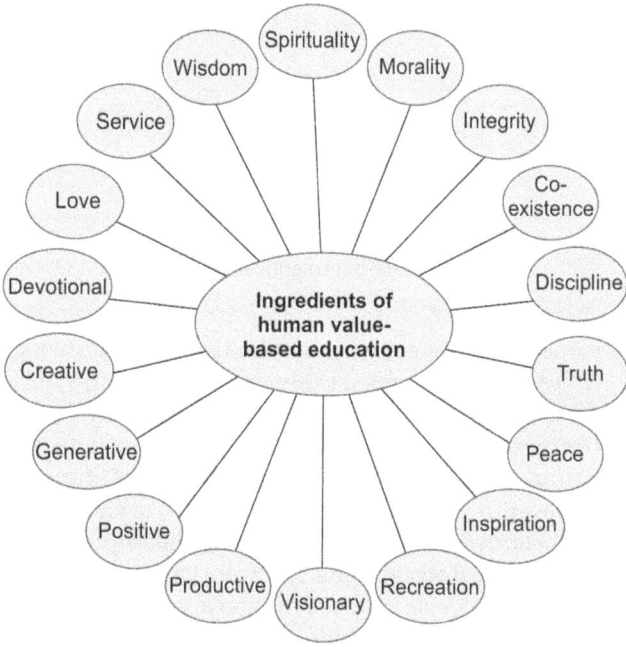

Fig. 21.4: Value-based education components.

VALUES-BASED NURSING EDUCATION

Nursing values are the foundation of nursing practice. They guide behavioral standards, provide a framework for evaluating behavior, and influence practical decisions. By developing an educational system centered on values, students become good global citizens. Someone who is caring and compassionate, who works together to solve problems, and who has the resilience to face whatever uncertainties life can throw at them.

- Incorporating values into the curriculum should not be restricted to specific classes. Values education should form the background of all academic and non-academic activities.
- To instill in students values such as loyalty, kindness, honesty, compassion and selflessness, it is important to integrate learning modules taken from real-life situations.
- Research shows that values-based education creates an environment that may promote academic learning and achievement while developing social and relationship-building skills.
- Children who learn the values from an early age become more confident, capable, smarter, more effective learners, and better citizens.
- Professional values relate to a person's professional beliefs about the suitability and desirability of something. Moreover, values are an important factor in determining caregiver motivation and reward.

The Need for Values Education

Values-based education is fundamental to developing and deeply helping people in many ways.

- Provide positive guidance and guide students in creating their own futures. Even discovering the motives behind their lives.
- It represents the most ideal attitude towards life, serving both people and those around them.
- Values education encourages students to become progressively more careful and rational.
- Encourage a deeper understanding of life's perspective and a successful life as a competent resident.
- We also encourage students to build strong relationships with their loved ones.
- Build student character
- Values education creates a positive outlook on life in the second student's brain.

Personality Building

Personality building is important in shaping a child into a winning personality. It can lead to many changes in the child's attitudes and perceptions of behavior. Some of its benefits are described below:

- Students become more responsible for their actions towards teachers and colleagues.
- Students become more regular with their homework and lessons.
- Learn to cooperate with teachers and classmates in all situations.
- Learn how to handle all classroom situations with maturity.
- Students pay attention during class.
- Helps students make their own decisions without hesitation.
- It fosters a positive mind and good attitude.
- Values education creates strong relationships between students and teachers.

VALUE DEVELOPMENT STRATEGIES

Value Development Goals

- Develop awareness of attitudes.
- Encourage students to develop positive attitudes towards the following values:
  - Active and healthy lifestyles through regular participation in various forms of physical activity and recognition of the contribution of the learning domain to physical, mental, emotional and social health.
  - Personal responsibility through responsibility for health and physical activity.
  - Social justice through inclusion and respect for the rights of others.
  - Recognizing excellence and achievements of others.
  - Cooperation and teamwork by working coherently within a group.
  - Fair play by following the rules and respecting the decisions of referees.
  - Prevention and safety through the development of a safe classroom environment.
  - Environment through the demonstration of conservation activities and the use of techniques to minimize impact.

Strategy 1: Embed Values into Existing Curriculum

No wonder values are so important and need to be projected. But what is needed is that they be filtered and installed so that they are not preaching or moral preaching itself. Therefore, it should be noted that the activities that can be performed under each statistic are different.

- **Prayer:** Prayers are held in almost all schools before regular school hours begin. Prayers should be given in a native language spoken by both the teacher and the student in an appropriate and quiet atmosphere.

- **Geography (social studies):** Geography is a subject that can easily contribute to the value debate. Teachers may pause at key points during the lesson, ask students or groups of students to make choices, and then indicate that individual choices matter.
- **Literature:** All values are attributes of a good life and these are easily achieved by having children read good literature. In language lessons, teachers can choose reading material that is relevant to the values being studied.
- **Drama:** Drama is a great medium for communicating values. Therefore, teachers must choose works that teach values.
- **Science:** Science subjects can be very well addressed by science teachers to instill values in their students.

Strategy 2: Values through Extracurricular Activities

The main purpose of education is to develop all aspects of the human intelligence so that students can make our country a more democratic, coherent and social, to be responsible and able to contribute to cultural enrichment, environmentally sustainable and internationally competitive. All of this is truly achievable if the right values are taught in schools.

Activities

- Visit and observe a nearby planetarium
- Take students to a nearby forest to observe different types of trees and animals
- Visit fields where various food crops are grown
- Promotion of stamp collection
- Organize seminars, discussions and workshops
- Write a diary
- A special meeting at school
- Stories
- Celebration of national festivals of different religions
- Prayer and meditation
- Shramadhan
- Annual trip
- Competition in sports and games
- Cultural program
- Silence.

Values

- Striving for knowledge, inquisitiveness, scientific temperament.
- Love of nature, responsibility and environmental protection.
- Nutritional value.
- Curiosity can increase the value of collecting new and old items.
- Participation to improve communication skills.
- Self-discipline.
- Cooperation, time, awareness, good behavior, nationalism, obedience, regularity, integrity.
- Antisocial, equality, loyalty, gentle behavior, justice, kindness, non-violence, responsibility.
- Unity of diversity.
- Devotion to God, self-discipline, self-actualization, mastery of the senses.
- Hard work, gratitude, service, friendship and a sense of duty.
- The exchange of ideas, warmth, love of nature and creativity.
- Sports team spirit and generosity.
- Cultural and moral values.
- Control of language.

Strategy 3: Cultivating Values through Stories

- Teachers can tell stories or ask students to give specific points and develop stories.
- Interacting with stories gives students the opportunity to reason about the causes and consequences of actions and to consider moral choices.
- Exploring values through narrative responses allows students to explore issues and potentially despised issues without necessarily being emotionally charged.

Strategy 4: Communicate Values through Discussion of Slogans

- The main aim or goal here is to help students analyze slogans and find out the values hidden in them so that they can apply them in their own lives.
- The slogans will be written on the blackboard by the teacher or at least he will distribute papers with the five slogans printed on them to the students.
- Each slogan is presented individually for discussion and students are asked to analyze each other's answers.
- Students are also asked to share their opinions and feelings, and then encouraged to interact in groups. A group can consist of 10 of her students or up to 12 students.

Strategy 5: Teach Values through Games

- Games are another approach to teaching values among the different types of activities in the curriculum.
- The main purpose or goal here is to help students focus on the values they hold dear and share them with each other.

- Techniques used are housie games brainstorming and discussion.
- Before the Howie game begins, the students begin to pray. The teacher then introduces the value housie game to the students and distributes the value housie game slips to the class.

APPROACHES TO VALUES EDUCATION

Douglas Supreka outlines his eight different approaches to values education. These can be briefly explained as follows:

1. **Arousal approach:** Students are encouraged to make spontaneous, free and irrational decisions without thinking. Do you hesitate them? We give students maximum freedom and provide an environment that creates provocative situations that provoke spontaneous reactions. For example, the reaction to pictures of starving children.
2. **Approach to admission to school:** Students are forced to act according to certain desired values. Positive and negative reinforcement by teachers contributes to the education of values. This can be achieved through the teacher›s natural actions and reactions. This tried and tested method proved to be very unsuccessful.
3. **Awareness approach:** This approach helps students become aware and aware of their own values. Students are encouraged to share their experiences. Teachers present valuable situations and dilemmas through readings, movies, roleplays, small group discussions, and simulations. Students engage in the process of drawing conclusions about values from their own and others' thoughts, feelings, beliefs, and actions.
4. **The moral reasoning approach:** Kohlberg's theory of the six stages of moral development is the most commonly used framework for this approach. Teachers create learning experiences that foster moral development. These experiences fall into the general category of what Kohlberg calls role acquisition. Empathy is a key factor in taking on the role.
5. **Analytical approach:** Groups or individuals are encouraged to consider issues of social value. Clarification of values questions and identification of value conflicts are required. They are encouraged to arrive at value determinations by ascertaining the truth and evidence of the facts purported and by applying analogous cases in estimating and testing the value principles underlying the determination.
6. **Values clarification approach:** Helps students use both rational thinking and emotional awareness to explore individual behavioral patterns, classify and update values. This approach was used by Raths et al (1966) and Simon et al (1972) in which children are asked to write down a self-analysis and response worksheet consisting of drawing questions and activities.
7. **Commitment approach:** This allows students to see themselves not merely as passive reactants or free individuals, but as internally relative members of social groups and systems. Action projects can help you clarify and restructure your own values and determine how deeply you bond with them.
8. **The union approach:** The purpose is to enable students to perceive and act upon themselves not as individual egos, but as part of a larger, interconnected whole: Humanity, the world, and the universe.

ETHICAL DECISION-MAKING

The ethical decision-making process should recognize these situations, consider all available options, eliminate unethical views, and select the best ethical alternative. Ethical decisions create trust, and with it comes fairness, responsibility, and consideration for others. An ethical decision-making process should recognize these situations, consider all available options, eliminate unethical beliefs, and select the best ethical alternative.

Ethical Decision-Making Framework

If ethics is not based on religion, sentiment, law, social practice, or science, what is it based on? Countless philosophers and ethicists have explored this important I have tried to answer the question. At least five different ethical codes or standards have been proposed. The most important ones are described below.

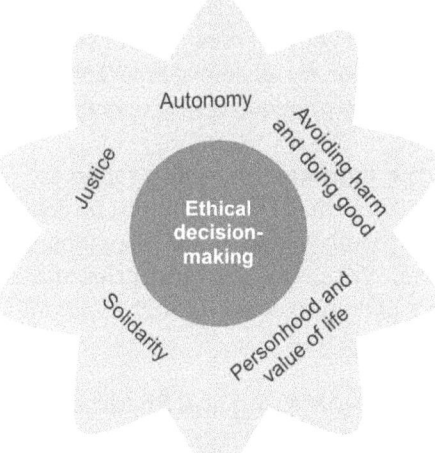

Fig. 21.5: Ethical decision-making.

- **Utilitarian approach:** This approach stipulates that the most ethical actions are those that yield the greatest

benefit and cause the least harm. In other words, a choice that is as balanced as possible between good and bad.
- **The right approach:** The right approach suggests that the most ethical decisions are those that best protect and respect the moral rights of all involved. This approach argues that people have dignity based on their humanity, or their ability to freely choose what they want to do with their lives.
- **Fairness or fairness approach:** All equals should be treated equally. Greek philosopher Aristotle and others contributed to this idea. Today, this idea is used to show that ethical decisions treat everyone equally. If not, it should be based on explainable criteria.

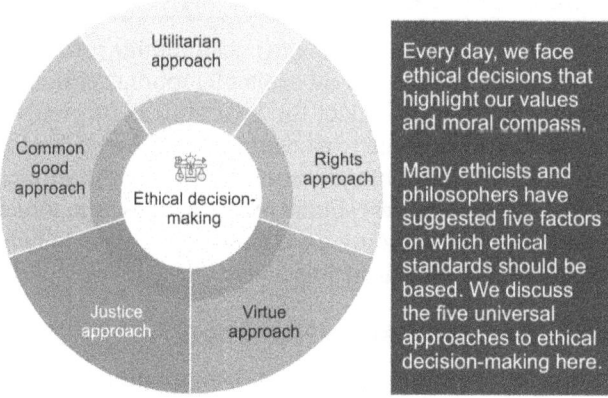

Fig. 21.6: Approaches to ethical decision-making.

- **The common good approach:** Greek philosophers also contributed to the idea that living in community is a good thing. People's actions must contribute to this. This approach suggests that relationships within society are fundamental to ethical thinking and behavior. Respect and compassion for all others, especially those who are vulnerable, are prerequisites for maintaining an ethical way of life.
- **The virtue approach:** The ancient approach to ethics is the belief that ethical behavior must be consistent with certain virtues that ensure the development of humanity in general. Virtues are the tendencies and habits that enable a person to act to the fullest potential of their human nature.

Ethical Decision-Making and Roadmap

Below is an overview of the ethical decision-making roadmap.
- **Gather facts:** Do not jump to conclusions until the facts are on the table. Ask yourself questions about the issue at hand, such as the 5 whys law. Facts are not always easy to find, especially in situations where ethics matter. Some facts are unavailable or cannot be definitively proven. Also indicate what assumptions are being made.
- **Define ethical issues:** Clearly define ethical issues before considering solutions or new plans. If there are multiple ethical focuses, only the most important should be addressed first.
- **Stakeholder identification:** Identify all stakeholders. Who are these key actors? And who are the secondary stakeholders? Why are you interested in this topic? Consider the possible positive and negative consequences. How big are these episodes? And what are the odds of these outcomes actually happening? We distinguish between short-term and long-term effects.
- **Consider honesty and character:** Consider what the community thinks is good judgment in this situation. How would you feel if a national newspaper wrote about your decision? What is public opinion?
- **Think creatively about possible actions:** There are other possibilities and alternatives not yet considered mosquito? Try to find additional solutions and alternatives when considering small numbers.
- **Determine appropriate ethical behavior:** Consider options based on the consequences, obligations, and character aspects of each option. What is the best argument to justify that choice.

HBS ethical decision-making framework	
Step	**Important criteria**
Define the ethical issue	• Describe the situation and context • List facts and assumptions • Identify conflicts of interest
Reflect on personal values	• Consider your personal ethics statement • Consider major ethical theories • Reflect on your ethical lens (ELI) • Consider discipline specific ethics (e.g., CPA)
Consider stakeholder perspectives	• Identify relevant stakeholders and positions • Consider positions of other ethical lenses (ELI) • Consider entity's ethical standards
Analyze alternatives	• Develop and analyse multiple alternatives • Consider strengths and weaknesses of each • Consider mitigating options • Seek advice—discuss with key stakeholders
Decide and support	• Disclose decision and rationale • Support decision and acknowledge criticisms • Reflect on results

STUDENT ETHICAL STANDARDS

Student development theory reflects the typical developmental challenges young people often face at the point in life when most students decide to pursue higher education.

Most people make decisions and invest in relationships that will affect them for years to come. Student development theory provides a framework for enabling students to tackle these life challenges.

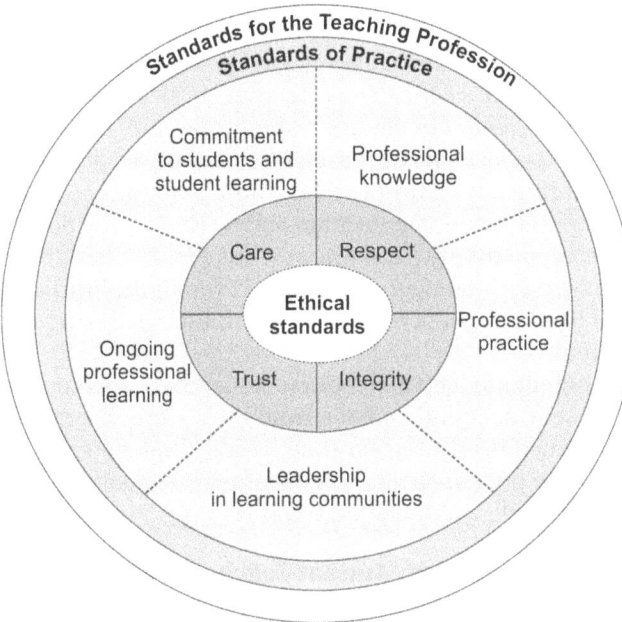

Fig. 21.7: Standards for teaching practice.

College life can present ethical challenges that are difficult to plan for when the unexpected comes your way.

By making the right and ethical choices, you can ensure an environment of respect for all and get the most out of your LSE experience. The school's code of ethics establishes her six ethical principles:

1. **Responsibility and accountability:** We take responsibility for our actions and decisions and raise concerns when they are not right.
2. **Integrity:** We act with honesty and integrity within the limits of the law.
3. **Freedom of thought:** We protect freedom of thought and expression.
4. **Respect and equal opportunity:** We treat everyone with dignity and respect.
5. **Collectiveness:** We are inclusive. We work together, support each other, and act appropriately.
6. **Sustainability:** We minimize our negative impact on the natural and built environment.

Necessity and Importance of Ethics for Students

- To ensure that people with exceptions have the best possible learning outcomes and quality of life in a manner that respects their dignity, culture, language and origin maintain high expectations of increasing the potential.
- Maintain a high level of professional competence and integrity and exercise professional judgment for the benefit of people with special needs and their families.
- Promote the meaningful and inclusive participation of people with special needs in schools and communities.
- Collaborative practices with others serving people with special needs.
- Build relationships with families based on mutual respect and actively involve families and individuals with special needs in educational decision-making.
- Examining evidence, educational data, and using expertise to inform practice.
- Protect and support the physical and psychological safety of people in exceptional circumstances.
- In exceptional circumstances, we will not engage in or condone any conduct that causes harm to any individual.
- Enforcement of CEC professional ethics standards and policies, compliance with laws, regulations and policies affecting professional practice. Advocate for better laws, regulations and policies.
- Advocate for professional conditions and resources that enhance learning outcomes for people of exceptional ability.
- We strive to improve our professional skills through active participation in professional associations.
- Participation in the expansion and dissemination of professional knowledge and skills.

STUDENT-FACULTY RELATIONSHIP

The importance of the student-faculty relationship lies in the idea of facilitating student learning. It is the basis for a successful academic relationship with your boss at work, and even in social development. Student-teacher relationships in schools need more attention as they can act as catalysts for improved academic performance. Meeting a teacher can be a little intimidating at first, but the simple truth is that most teachers admire when students take initiative. Here we detail the importance of connecting with your professor and tips for building a lasting relationship.

- **Achieve academic success:** Students who get to know their teachers are more likely to do well in school. Good teacher-student relationships have improved nearly every measurable aspect of academic success. Students are more likely to attend classes, get higher grades, and graduate when they know and care about their professors.
- **Fostering a sense of teaching and community:** Building good relationships between professors and students is a

major focus. Campus network members are encouraged to network at a deeper level than just grade level.

- **Secure good references:** Students who are connected to professors enjoy another benefit. Your relationship with your professor increases your chances of receiving a good letter of recommendation. An average letter of recommendation speaks to professional skill. However, a good letter will let colleges and potential employers know your strengths, character, and disposition.
- **Seek personal and professional growth:** Getting to know professors is also a great way to develop your interpersonal and professional skills. For example, if you are shy, making an appointment with a professor can help you gain confidence and overcome your fears. Your further contribution to the course will help you improve your speaking skills and better absorb the theories and concepts related to your major.

Characteristics of a Positive Teacher-Student Relationship

- Mutual respect—treating each other with respect
- Open communication
- Teachers are supportive but encourage autonomy
- Each student's individuality is respected
- Friendly and respectful interactions
- Students are given honest and friendly feedback
- Teachers learn about their students and know their differences
- Teachers believe in all students
- Simple sharing gestures (hello, goodbye, smile, pat on the back)
- Respectful communication between two people.

Building Positive Relationships with Students

Improving relationships has a significant positive and long-term impact on the academic and social development of both students. Improving student-teacher relationships alone does not lead to higher grades. However, students who have close, positive, and supportive relationships with their teachers achieve higher levels of performance than those whose relationships are more conflicting.

- Show your students joy and joy.
- Respect and treat students with respect.
- Provide support to students in achieving academic and social goals (e.g., by answering questions in a timely manner and providing support appropriate to the needs of students).
- Help students reflect on their thinking and study skills.
- Know each student's background, interests, emotional strength and academic level to demonstrate your knowledge.
- Avoid getting irritated or annoyed with your students.
- Recognize the importance of peers in school by encouraging students to care and respect each other.

Responsibilities for Student-Teacher Relationships

- **Changes in lecture times and locations:** In general, faculty members are discouraged from changing lecture times and/or locations. In special circumstances, arrangements to change the location and/or time of lessons can be made through the relevant faculty office.
- **Student attendance:** Classroom attendance is an important part of education and teachers are expected to hold students accountable for regular classroom attendance. Students are required to notify the instructor if they are absent from class for an extended period of time.
- **Student advice office hours:** Students are encouraged to seek academic advice from their supervisors and instructors on a regular basis. Faculty members will be able to participate in this guidance from the first day of New Student Orientation Week.

The Importance of Student-Teacher Relationships

- Teachers can start learning more about their students by asking them to write and share about themselves, or by talking to them or asking them questions.
- **Listen to your students:** Stopping and listening to your students is very important for building and maintaining social connections.
- **Create a positive classroom environment:** A reward system can encourage class participation and build positive relationships. Try to be calm and speak with an appropriate tone and pace. Encouraging kindness also goes a long way toward creating a healthy environment.
- Develop a strategy for dealing with stress and frustration by incorporating occasional music or relaxation techniques into the class, or beginning the class with simple breathing exercises.
- **Involve parents:** Maintaining good relationships with parents also helps communication between students and teachers. Share student good points with parents and give advice on how to correct mistakes.
- **Self-exchange:** Teachers are more relatable by sharing (appropriate) stories from their lives.
- Teach children more values such as kindness, respect, empathy, sharing and humanity.

EVIDENCE-BASED TEACHING

Evidence-based teaching is a teaching practice that has proven effective in every classroom. A lot of research has been done on strategies that work in any classroom setting, whether it's an online classroom or a hybrid model. Teachers should invest in each student and get to know them as best they can. This type of educational practice is a hallmark of successful education and includes the belief that all students can succeed.

Meaning

Evidence-based education uses evidence to:
- Determine where the student is in learning.
- Determine appropriate educational strategies and interventions.
- Monitor student progress and assess teaching effectiveness.

Key Evidence

- **Purpose:** Data that each reviewer can identify and interpret in a similar manner.
- **Validity:** Data adequately representing the task required for success.
- **Reliability:** Essential data remaining in the library will not change if collected on a different day or by a different person.
- **Systematic:** Data collected according to a rigorous experimental or observational design.
- **Peer-reviewed:** Approved data.

Benefits

Benefits of implementing EBP for educators and students include:
- Increased likelihood of positive outcomes for children.
- Having data to support practice and program choices enhances accountability and, as a result, encourages managers, parents and others.
- Less wasted time and less wasted resources because educators start with effective teaching. No need to practice or program, trial and error works. No need to find stuff.
- More likely to meet learner needs.
- Evidence that it works makes students more likely to persuade students to try it.

Evidence-Based Practice Steps

According to Cleveland clinic, there are five steps in health science. These steps are also known as evidence-based practice":
1. **Ask:** Formulate clinical questions that can be answered about a patient's problem, intervention, or treatment.
2. **Collect:** Find relevant evidence to answer your question.
3. **Evaluation:** Determine if the evidence is of high quality and worth.
4. **Application:** Use the best available evidence to make clinical decisions.
5. **Evaluate:** Evaluate the results of applying the evidence to the patient's situation.

EVIDENCE-BASED TEACHING STRATEGIES

- Reiterate clear learning goals so that students have a clear understanding of where they are going and what will happen when they get there. This is a practice that brings transparency to learning and teaching.
- Share and model and explain concepts to show students how to complete physical or intellectual tasks. Sharing and modeling vary by discipline. For some, this may mean "thinking it out loud" to show students how an expert does it, or it may be a physical demonstration.
- Regularly solicit student feedback in a variety of ways to check student understanding. Research shows that the habit of asking students for feedback has a greater impact on learning than giving feedback to students. Ask students what they understand and how courses and lessons are structured to help them learn. Resources are available for a Clemson teacher to import into her Canvas. Look for "Clemson's Teachings" in the House of Commons.

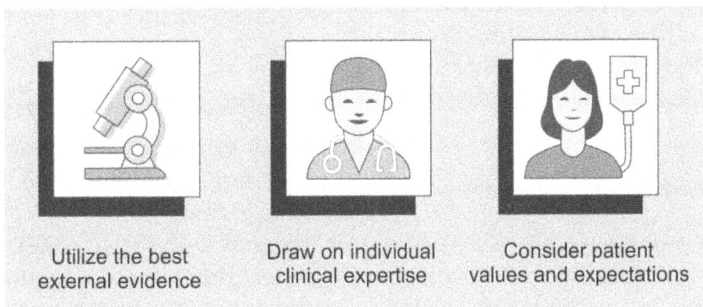

Fig. 21.8: Three main components of evidence-based practice.

- Provide regular feedback to students. Low-risk work is done in a feedback loop. Think "homework," tests, and quizzes. Encourage students to evaluate their own exam results.
- Graphically records information from both teachers and students for visual learning and deeper processing. This area includes adding meaningful and clear visuals to your PowerPoint presentations (visuals are easy to remember), creating graphs, charts and diagrams, and allowing students to create their own diagrams.
- Outside of classes and lessons, you can do repetitions and spatial practice through assigned assignments. Provide opportunities for feedback and exchange of opinions during class. See her 4th above. Repeated practice over a period of time (for example, having students remember information from earlier sections of the course) helps cement learning.
- Create peer-to-peer learning opportunities. This allows students to support each other in understanding concepts. The foundation of good "group work" is meaningful work for students where everyone contributes to each other's learning. In large classes, this can be accomplished by discussing questions in "pair shares" with the person next to you.
- Allow time for success. Set different times for each session to help you learn particularly difficult concepts. Accomplishing anything "on the fly" is difficult, but an instructor who already teaches content can give students more time to explore difficult concepts. Consider exploring the "concept of thresholds" in the content area.
- **Teach learning strategies:** Use common resources and techniques specific to your discipline. Encourage students to take advantage of academic success center and library resources, and provide information about learning opportunities for the specific content areas you teach. Today's students often have gaps in their knowledge of study techniques such as effective note taking, time management, and exam preparation.
- **Encourage metacognition:** Ask students how they think about the topic. This field is currently receiving a great deal of attention in higher education. When students are encouraged to assess their own learning through activities and homework, they are able to take ownership of their own learning and balance the responsibilities of teaching and learning.

USING EVIDENCE-BASED INSTRUCTION IN THE CLASSROOM

- **Using questioning techniques:** Initiate discussion and instruction. Examples of this are questions like "What do you think you will actually use?" and "What do you expect to learn from this lesson?" This helps teachers assess where to start retraining or repeating lessons.
- Built-in quiz questions and pretests enhance student learning and maximize time spent teaching and planning. This includes using games and online quizzes.
- Include conclusion and review questions. "What would you say is the most important thing you learned today?" Asking students when they have questions is not a good way to spark discussion. This type of question is too vague and doesn't take learning styles or preferences into account. All of these techniques test questions and are an effective way to check for comprehension.
- Use the graphic organizer to make connections and build meaningful relationships with your learning. This is also suitable for online graphic organizers. For this type of strategy, it's important to provide relevant examples and link the examples to the content. Examples include asking students to relate what they are learning to real life or other content areas.
- Scaffolding is a process that builds on the skills and information gained in previous lessons, and summarizing information is a valuable technique for maintaining and improving memory. Both techniques are highly effective in helping students learn and retain content.
- **Use in-depth questions and topics in discussions:** A good idea for this type of approach is to start discussions about controversial topics. This is a great way to keep all students aware and engaged. A little stress in the learning environment promotes learning and provides optimal learning opportunities.

CARE EDUCATION APPLICATIONS

Evidence-based practice (EBP) in medicine has become essential to patient safety. EBP involves the conscious use and application of diverse knowledge sources, including the use of published research combined with clinical expertise and patient values and preferences. In the EBP process, healthcare professionals formulate structured queries and search databases to obtain reliable evidence. Nursing students need an education that integrates evidence-based practical knowledge (EBP) into the classroom and clinical practice.

Examples of Evidence-Based Practice in Nursing

Through evidence-based practice, nurses have improved patient care. Key examples of evidence-based practice in nursing include:

- **Oxygen delivery to COPD patients:** Use evidence to determine how to adequately administer oxygen to patients with chronic obstructive pulmonary disease (COPD).

- **Pediatric non-invasive blood pressure measurement:** Use auscultation as suggested by the evidence and compare measurements with data obtained by oscillometric methods.
- **Use the correct size intravenous catheter:** Recognize the benefits of using smaller catheters to improve patient comfort.
- **Recognizing the role of family members:** Families can have a significant impact on how patients present their symptoms to healthcare providers, so acknowledging family involvement is more efficient and effective. I know it can lead to care.
- **Improve infection control practices:** Understand that wearing personal protective equipment and handwashing practices are key to infection control.
- **Recognizing alarm fatigue:** Reflecting current practice, caregivers can develop effective procedures to enable caregivers desensitized to sound by alarm fatigue to adequately monitor patients.

Benefits for the Nursing Community

- Prioritize patient needs. Evidence-based care is research based but also considers individual patient preferences. Since one of the key tenets of nursing is to focus on the patient's needs, evidence-based practice is the key to continuously improving patient outcomes while balancing each patient's preferences and experiences.
- Make better patient care decisions and save caregivers time. Evidence-based practice saves time by eliminating the need to engage in activities that may or may not benefit the patient. For example, nurses should spend up to 20 minutes a day bathing and changing bandages for each patient until studies find that some bandages are better left on longer, and that daily bathing does not affect results. was spending (of course, in certain circumstances it may be appropriate to perform these exercises daily or even more frequently, depending on the individual patient case).

REVIEW QUESTIONS

Long Essays

1. Define ethics, explain ICN code of ethics.
2. Define value-based practice (VBP), explain the meaning and purpose.
3. Define values, explain the types of values.
4. Explain values-based nursing education, describe.
5. Enumerate the approaches to values education.
6. Define student-faculty relationship, explain characteristics of a positive teacher-student relationship.
7. Define evidence-based teaching, explain evidence-based teaching strategies.
8. Discuss using evidence-based instruction in the classroom.

Short Essays

1. Important pillars of value-based education.
2. Important for values-based education.
3. Values education in schools.
4. Importance of values education.
5. Value-based education components.
6. Need for values education.
7. Value development goals.
8. Ethical decision-making framework.
9. Ethical decision-making and roadmap.
10. Student ethical standards.
11. Importance of ethics for students.
12. Building positive relationships with students.
13. Evidence-based practice in nursing.

Short Answers
1. Ethical standards.
2. Student achievement.
3. Authenticity.
4. Nurses and practice.
5. Nursing and professionals.
6. Values.
7. Values education objectives.
8. Universal values.
9. Personality building.
10. Utilitarian approach.
11. Importance of student-teacher relationships.
12. Evidence-based practice steps.
13. Components of evidence-based practice.

Multiple Choice Questions (MCQs)

1. Every system of education is based on:
   a. Ideology of nation
   b. Social development
   c. Intellectual development
   d. Skill development

2. Word philosophy is derived from:
   a. Alpha and Amphia
   b. Phila and Sophia
   c. Sila and Sophia
   d. Neo and Latvia

3. Expected life outcomes from education are referred as:
   a. Learning
   b. Evaluation
   c. Aims
   d. Pedagogy

4. Being the science of wisdom philosophy aims at:
   a. Search for activity
   b. Search for reality
   c. Search for probability
   d. Search for utility

5. Types of education include all *except*:
   a. Formal   b. Informal
   c. Nonformal   d. None of the above

6. It comes from the Greek word "techne" which means an art or craft?
   a. Technique   b. Technology
   c. Technician   d. Telepathy

7. The use of technology to enhance learning process is called _____ in education.
   a. IT
   b. ICT
   c. Information technology
   d. Communication technology

8. Information technology (IT) Act 2000 came into force on:
   a. 17 October
   b. 9 June
   c. 1 June
   d. 1 October

9. Who is known as the father of modern media education?
   a. Edgar Dale
   b. Flanders
   c. Erikson
   d. Charles Babbage

10. Which of these is not a component of a computer network?
    a. Sender
    b. Protocol
    c. Speakers
    d. Data

11. The literal meaning of philosophy is:
    a. Love of wisdom
    b. Love of knowledge
    c. Love of truth
    d. Love of God

12. The word philosophy comes from the word philo-sophia which is?
    a. Latin
    b. Greek
    c. Celtic
    d. Roman

13. Education is the dynamic side of:
    a. Psychology
    b. Sociology
    c. Philosophy
    d. Literature

14. Method of teaching is to fulfill the aims of education and life. This is determined by:
    a. Humanities
    b. Literature
    c. Social sciences
    d. Philosophy

15. Philosophy sets the goal of life and who provides the means for its achievements?
    a. Management
    b. Education
    c. Theology
    d. Cosmology

16. Which is the process of imparting knowledge and guiding the pupils to learn through their own activities?
    a. Learning
    b. Teaching
    c. Both (a) and (b)
    d. None

17. Teaching is a process _____.
    a. Multipolar process
    b. Tripolar process
    c. Bipolar process
    d. All of the above

18. According to modern concept, teaching is a process _____.
    a. Bipolar
    b. Tripolar
    c. Multipolar
    d. None

19. Teaching is an important element in the process of _____.
    a. Learning
    b. Skills
    c. Education
    d. Both (a) and (b)

20. Teaching is communication between ____ persons.
    a. One or more
    b. Two or more
    c. Three or more
    d. Both (a) and (b)

21. Select the valid reasons for using simulation.
    a. Relationship between the variables is nonlinear
    b. Optimized solutions are obtained
    c. Conduct experiments without disrupting the real system
    d. Both (a) and (c)

22. The rules of presenting the contents to make them easy are called _____.
    a. Methods of teaching
    b. Maxims of teaching
    c. Techniques of teaching
    d. Teaching strategies

23. SOLO stands for:
    a. System of the observed learning outcome
    b. structure of the observed learning output
    c. Structure of the observed learning outcome
    d. None of these

24. Formative assessment is assessment _____ learning:
    a. to
    b. of
    c. by
    d. for

25. Summative assessment is assessment _____ learning:
    a. to
    b. of
    c. by
    d. for

26. What act of teacher foster a sense of autonomy in the learning process?
    a. Instructor
    b. Facilitator
    c. Delegator
    d. Formal authority

27. A process of looking at what is being assessed is called:
    a. Assessment
    b. Evaluation
    c. Measurement
    d. Rubrics

28. Validity of an assessment relates to the _____ of an assessment.
    a. Usefulness
    b. Quality
    c. Consistency
    d. Relevance

29. The term emoting refers to:
    a. Emotional intelligence
    b. The universal experience of emotion
    c. The cultural specific experience of emotion
    d. The embeddedness of emotions and social relationships

30. **Appropriate order of four stages of creative thinking:**
    a. Illumination, incubation, verification and preparation
    b. Verification, incubation, illumination and preparation
    c. Preparation, incubation, illumination and verification
    d. Preparation, illumination, incubation and verification

31. **What is the origin of the word education?**
    a. 'E' and 'Catum'
    b. Edu and 'Catum'
    c. Word 'Educate'
    d. None of these

32. **Which of the following statements is correct?**
    a. Education is an art
    b. Education is a science
    c. It is neither art nor science
    d. To some extent it is art and to some extent it is science

33. **What is called education acquired without any specific purpose fixed period and place?**
    a. Indirect education
    b. Individual education
    c. Informal education
    d. Formal education

34. **Which one of the following sentences is correct about the nature of teaching?**
    a. It is diagnostic
    b. It is remedial
    c. It is diagnostic as well as remedial
    d. All the above statements are correct

35. **What is the compulsory element of learning?**
    a. Ability to read
    b. Bright mind
    c. Tendency to know
    d. None of these

36. **What is the place of principal in an educational institute?**
    a. Overall head of the school
    b. Manager of the school
    c. Owner of the school
    d. Founder of the school

37. **If a student failed in any class, what should be done to him?**
    a. He should be given a chance to improve and sent to the next class after he improves
    b. He should be kept in the same class
    c. He should be advised to leave studies
    d. All the above methods are right

38. **Why are curriculum activities used in teaching?**
    a. Make teaching easy
    b. To make teaching interesting, easy to understand and effective
    c. To make teaching attractive
    d. To assist the teacher

39. **What are the three components of the educational process?**
    a. Education, teacher and books
    b. Teacher, student and education
    c. Teaching, learning and practice
    d. Direction, instruction and skill

40. **What is teaching through deductive method?**
    a. From general to specific
    b. From specific to general
    c. From macro to micro
    d. From easy to difficult

41. **What is the main center of informal education?**
    a. Society
    b. Family
    c. Radio and television
    d. All of the above

42. **Which is the first school for a child's education?**
    a. Society
    b. Friends
    c. Family
    d. School

43. **Which one of the following education systems supports scientific progress?**
    a. Realistic education
    b. Idealistic education
    c. Naturalistic education
    d. None of these

44. **What is the meaning of lesson plan?**
    a. To read the lesson before teaching it
    b. To prepare all that the teacher wants to teach in a limited period
    c. To prepare detailed answers of all the questions to be asked in the class
    d. To prepare the list of questions to be asked

45. **On what depend the values of an educational experience in the eyes of the idealist?**
    a. Whether or not the pupil has been properly motivated
    b. Whether or not it preserves accepted institutions
    c. The extent to which it satisfies pupil desires
    d. The manner in which it affects future experience

46. Which educational activity is most desirable to the pragmatist?
    a. Approximates the goals which educational scientists have set up
    b. Results from the indiscrimination of the pupil in democratic theory
    c. That is beneficial effect upon the future experiences of the pupil
    d. That characterizes by spontaneous, active, continuously pleasurable and practical for the pupil

47. What is the viewpoint of progressive educators regarding the issue of liberal vs vocational education?
    a. Vocational ends load one to degrade learning
    b. Liberal arts subject should proceed vocational training
    c. Vocational and liberal education should not be separated
    d. All subjects should have a vocational orientation

48. Who was the supporter of Naturalism in Education?
    a. Froebel
    b. Armstrong
    c. John Locke
    d. Rousseau

49. What do you mean by curriculum?
    a. A child learns through curriculum
    b. Sum total of the annual study
    c. Sum total of the activities of a school
    d. Indicates the course to be taught by the teachers to the students throughout the year

50. Which system of education was propounded by Mahatma Gandhi?
    a. Teaching by activities
    b. Teaching through music
    c. Teaching through listening, meditation, etc.
    d. All of the these

51. Who raised the slogan "Back to Nature"?
    a. Realism
    b. Pragmatism
    c. Naturalism
    d. Existentialism

52. Practice is made in:
    a. Inductive method
    b. Deductive method
    c. Drill method
    d. Discussion method

53. Who said, "reverse the usual practice and you will almost always do right"?
    a. Mahatma Gandhi
    b. Rousseau
    c. Dewey
    d. Plato

54. "Human institutions are one mass of folly and contradiction." Whose statement is this?
    a. Bernard Shaw
    b. Rousseau
    c. Dewey
    d. Ravinder Nath Tagore

55. According to which school of philosophy of education, exaltation of individual's personality is a function of education?
    a. Pragmatism
    b. Idealism
    c. Marxism
    d. Both (b) and (c)

56. Which is not "naturalism's aim of education"?
    a. Education is the notion of man's evolution from lower forms of life
    b. To equip the individual or the nation for the struggle for existence to ensure survival
    c. To help the pupils to learn to be in harmony with and well-adapted to their surroundings
    d. To inculcate ethical and moral values in the pupils

57. Which school held the view, "God makes all things good, man meddles with and they become evil"?
    a. Marxism   b. Existentialism
    c. Naturalism d. Pragmatism

58. Which school maintained self-expression with the accompanying cries of "no interference", "no restraints"?
    a. Extreme form of naturalism
    b. Most widely accepted form of naturalism
    c. Truest form of naturalism
    d. Most valid form of naturalism

59. Which is not the nature of philosophy?
    a. It is a science of knowledge
    b. It is a collective ensemble of various viewpoints
    c. It is a planned attempt on search for the truth
    d. It is the totality of man's creative ideas

60. Which branch of philosophy deals with knowledge, its structure, method and validity?
    a. Logic   b. Aesthetics
    c. Epistemology d. Metaphysics

61. Which school maintained, "natural impulses of the child are of great importance and are good in themselves"?
    a. Biological naturalism
    b. Mechanical naturalism
    c. Naturalism of physical science
    d. Romantic naturalism

62. Which branch of philosophy examines issues pertaining to the nature of "reality"?
    a. Ontology
    b. Metaphysics
    c. Axiology
    d. Epistemology

63. On what is based the need for teaching philosophy of education?
    a. All pupils are not alike
    b. Different systems of education found in different countries
    c. Different philosophies expressed different points of view on every aspect of education
    d. Different ways of teaching-learning

64. What is the goal of education according to idealism?
    a. Perfect adaptation to the environment
    b. Realization of moral values
    c. Satisfaction of human wants
    d. Cultivation of dynamic, adaptable mind which will be resourceful and enterprising in all situations

65. Aim of education according to the existentialists is:
    a. Humanitarian and humanist self-realization
    b. Adaptation to practical life
    c. Objective knowledge
    d. A good understanding of the world outside

66. The realist's aim of education is:
    a. Self-realization
    b. Spiritual and moral development
    c. Happy and moral development
    d. Total development of personality

67. Naturalist's conception of man is:
    a. Man's very essence of being is his spiritual nature
    b. It is spirit rather than animality that is most truly man
    c. There exists in the nature of things a perfect pattern of each individual
    d. Nature would have them children before they are men

68. Which philosophy of education considers psychology as an incomplete study of and an inadequate basis of educational theory?
    a. Realism
    b. Pragmatism
    c. Idealism
    d. Naturalism

69. Which among the following does not fit into the scheme of educational goals of the idealists?
    a. Care of body
    b. Moral values
    c. Skills
    d. Self-expression

70. Religious education is strongly advocated by:
    a. Pragmatists
    b. Idealists
    c. Realist
    d. Existentialists

71. Which of the following is said about the idealists?
    a. They are content with "briars"
    b. They like "roses"
    c. They are satisfied neither with "briars" nor with "roses"
    d. They want "roses" and "briars" both

72. Which school of philosophy of education advocated project method of teaching?
    a. Realism
    b. Pragmatism
    c. Idealism
    d. Naturalism

73. Playway method of teaching has been emphasized in the scheme of the education of:
    a. Naturalists
    b. Realists
    c. Pragmatists
    d. Existentialists

74. Which is the most widely accepted method of education, according to the pragmatists?
    a. Lecturing by the teacher
    b. Leaving the child free to learn
    c. Learning by doing
    d. Heuristic method

75. The pragmatists are against:
    a. The external examinations
    b. The specialist teachers
    c. Breakdown of knowledge into separate subjects
    d. Eternal spiritual values

76. **Pragmatism has a greater sense of responsibility than naturalism with regard to moral training because:**
    a. The free activity which pragmatic-system of education entails does not mean licence, rather it means a guided activity
    b. They emphasize teaching of values
    c. They consider education, basically, a social process
    d. They do not want the teacher to abdicate from the scene

77. **Which of the following claims of the pragmatists is not acceptable?**
    a. The free activity of the pupil is likely to result in permanent attitudes of initiative and independence and moral discipline
    b. Training in citizenship is possible through school and community activities
    c. Training in character through school's co-curricular activities is possible
    d. Child's own experience is valuable for adequate development of child's personality

78. **Project method of teaching is an outstanding contribution of:**
    a. Realism
    b. Pragmatism
    c. Naturalism
    d. Idealism

79. **Which is the characteristic of the project method?**
    a. Problematic act
    b. Carried in its natural setting
    c. Used for all-round-development of child's personality
    d. A voluntary undertaking

80. **Which among the following is not essentially desirable in the project method?**
    a. The task of the project is as real as the task of the life outside the walls of the school
    b. The task of the project involves constructive effort or thought yielding objective results
    c. The task of the project should be full of message for the children
    d. The task of the project should be interesting enough so that the pupil is genuinely eager to carry it out

81. **Which is a great disadvantage of the project method?**
    a. It consumes much of the time of the child
    b. It leaves gaps in the knowledge of the child
    c. Children are generally not interested in it
    d. Teachers, generally, do not like to teach through it

82. **Learning by project method is technically known as:**
    a. Incidental learning
    b. Efficient learning
    c. Systematic learning
    d. Adequate learning

83. **Education, according to the pragmatist is:**
    a. Wholly pupil-oriented
    b. Wholly society-oriented
    c. Wholly purposive
    d. Wholly interdisciplinary

84. **Who among the following is not a follower of pragmatic philosophy?**
    a. William James
    b. Pestalozzi
    c. John Dewey
    d. Kilpatrick

85. **What is not associated with pragmatism?**
    a. Purposive education
    b. Experience-based education
    c. Freedom-based education
    d. Education for self-realization

86. **Who emphasized realization of truth, beauty and goodness as the aims of education?**
    a. Idealists
    b. Pragmatists
    c. Realists
    d. Naturalists

87. **Which statement about truth is not correct according to the philosophy of pragmatism?**
    a. It is made by man
    b. It is everchanging
    c. It is eternal
    d. It is what emerges to be true in actual practice

88. **In whose methodology of teaching "experimentation" is the key-note of?**
    a. Idealism
    b. Existentialism
    c. Realism
    d. Pragmatism

89. **The term "progressive education" related to:**
    a. Realism
    b. Pragmatism
    c. Idealism
    d. Existentialism

90. **Who said, "no fixed aims of education and no values in advance"?**
    a. Progressive educators
    b. Idealists
    c. Realists
    d. Marxists

91. **Which school of philosophy of education stresses the direct study of men and things through tours and travels?**
    a. Social realism
    b. Idealism
    c. Existentialism
    d. Marxism

92. **Which school believes that all knowledge comes through the senses?**
    a. Idealism
    b. Sense realism
    c. Pragmatism
    d. Existentialism

93. **Which school raised the slogan "things as they are and as they are likely to be encountered in life rather than words?"**
    a. Pragmatist
    b. Realists
    c. Idealists
    d. Existentialists

94. **As Huxley pleaded for the introduction of "a complete and thorough scientific culture" into schools, he is claimed to be:**
    a. An idealist
    b. A realist
    c. A pragmatist
    d. A naturalist

95. **Realism in education was born out of:**
    a. The enthusiasm of the renaissance
    b. The great religious movement of the 17th century
    c. A cleavage between the work of the schools and the life of the world outside that occurred during the 19th century
    d. The degeneration of humanism after renaissance

96. **Behavior is a function of:**
    a. Performance and education
    b. Performance and environment
    c. Personality and education
    d. Personality and environment

97. **In the light of relevant past events, contemporary events and their understanding should find a place in the teaching of history. Who maintained this principle?**
    a. Naturalists
    b. Idealists
    c. Realists
    d. Marxists

98. **The most important thing to keep in mind for a teacher according to realism in education is:**
    a. The method of teaching
    b. The value and significance of what is taught
    c. The nature of the child
    d. Organization of the content to be taught

99. **Which school of philosophy very strongly advocates that education should be vocational in character?**
    a. Existentialism
    b. Naturalism
    c. Realism
    d. Pragmatism

100. **Which is not an aspect of mind according to the realists' theory of knowing?**
    a. Awareness
    b. Consciousness
    c. Behavior
    d. Processing of awareness

101. **Who believe that "objects have a reality independent of mental phenomena"?**
    a. Idealists
    b. Realists
    c. Naturalists
    d. Existentialists

102. **Marxist educational philosophy is closer to:**
    a. Idealism
    b. Realism
    c. Naturalism
    d. Pragmatism

103. **Which among the following statements is not a characteristic of Marxism?**
    a. It presupposes a reality independent of man's mind
    b. Its educational philosophy is essentially materialistic
    c. Its major objective is the development of child's personality
    d. It asserts that physical environment can definitely change the nature of the child

104. **Which school of philosophy of education regrets dualism between cultural, and vocational curriculum?**
    a. Marxism
    b. Idealism
    c. Existentialism
    d. Naturalism

105. According to which educational philosophy, socially useful labor must form the central pivot of the entire school?
    a. Idealism   b. Marxism
    c. Existentialism d. Naturalism

106. Which of the following has been asserted about schools by Marxist educational philosophy?
    a. They should stand above politics
    b. They should disinterestedly serve society as a whole
    c. They should function as deliberate instruments of state policy
    d. They should not be mere weapons in the hands of the ruling class

107. Which of the following characteristics is common to pragmatism, naturalism and existentialism?
    a. Emphasis on spiritual aims of education
    b. Emphasis on the individual
    c. Emphasis on physical environment
    d. Emphasis on value education

108. Whose is the ultimate concern "what is existence"?
    a. Idealists only
    b. Realists only
    c. Existentialists and idealists both
    d. Existentialists only

109. Which of the following philosophies held that 'men in the world feel lonely and anxious, being unsure of their meaning and fearful of their annihilation'?
    a. Existentialism b. Idealism
    c. Marxism   d. Pragmatism

110. According to existentialists, the essence of existence means:
    a. Unity with the ultimate reality
    b. Spiritual good and happiness
    c. Tensions and contradictions which condition loneliness and anxiety
    d. Continuous growth and development

111. Who was nineteenth century founder of existentialism?
    a. Hegel
    b. Soren Kierkegaard
    c. Rousseau
    d. DJ O'Connor

112. Who was twentieth century existentialist?
    a. Soren Kierkegaard b. DJ O'Connor
    c. Jean Paul Sartre   d. Hegel

113. Which of the following is more generally acceptable by modern educationists?
    a. There should be one single aim of education unchangeable over time and space
    b. There is one grand objective of education and that is the development of the inner nature of the child
    c. Contribution to the welfare of the society should be the only aim of education
    d. Education is bound to have several aims since its concerns are several such as the individual, the society, the family, the nation and so on

114. What is development of human potentialities in education?
    a. Individual aim
    b. Social aim
    c. Individual as well as social aim
    d. Specific aim

115. What is development of social sense and cooperation among the individuals through education?
    a. Individual aim
    b. Social aim
    c. National aim
    d. Constitutional aim

116. Which among the following is not an acceptable criticism of social aims of education?
    a. They are anti-individual
    b. They are unpsychological as they do not take into account the capacities and interests of the individual
    c. They hinder the growth and development of art and literature
    d. Man, in them, becomes only a means to an end

117. Which among the following is not emphasized by the individual aims of education?
    a. Individual freedom
    b. Self-expression
    c. Development of inner potentialities
    d. Development of values of tolerance and non-violence

118. Which of the following statements does not go in favor of the individual aims of education?
    a. The individual is an asset to the society his development and growth are necessary
    b. The society is strong if the individual is strong
    c. Every individual is unique; development of his potentialities is essential
    d. Society is supreme and all individuals are only parts of it

119. Which among the following is the most correct view about social and individual aims of education?
    a. Individual aims should be given preference to social aims
    b. Social aims should be preferred to individual aims
    c. Individual aims are implied in the social aims of education
    d. Individual and social aims are only two sides of the same coin

120. Which statement is most acceptable to the academicians about "bread and butter aim" of education?
    a. It is the most important aim and should be given top priority by educationists
    b. It is equally important along with other aims of education
    c. It is only partly acceptable
    d. It is important for only a section of the society

121. Which of the following does not pertain to intellectual development aim of education?
    a. Cultivation of intelligence
    b. Spiritual development
    c. Development of cognitive powers
    d. Training and "formation" of mind

122. Preparing the child for future life as an aim of education is preparing child for:
    a. Some suitable vocation
    b. Some particular course of study
    c. Facing all kinds of emergencies and situations of future life
    d. A happy married life

123. The most effective method of character-formation is:
    a. Teaching virtues through religious books
    b. Organizing specialists' lectures on importance of values in life
    c. Teaching by high character teachers
    d. Rewarding virtuous behaviors and presenting high character models in the schools

124. Harmonious development of the child aim of education means:
    a. Development of all the qualities of the mind to the maximum possible extent
    b. Development of a sound mind in a sound body
    c. Development of physical, mental, moral and spiritual potentialities of the child in a balanced manner
    d. Development of the adjustment capacities of the child

125. The social aims of education imply that:
    a. The state is an idealized metaphysical entity
    b. The state is above the individual citizen
    c. The state is superior to the individual transcending all his desires and aspirations
    d. The state has to give not to take anything from the individual

126. Rigid system of state-education is justified on the basis that the state:
    a. Is supreme to dictate what shall be taught and how shall be taught
    b. Has absolute control over the lives and destinies of its individual members
    c. Has a right and a bounden duty to mould the citizen to a pattern which makes for its own preservation and enhancement
    d. Has better resources to manage education

127. Social aims of education imply the training of:
    a. The individuals for the purpose of serving the needs of the society
    b. Individuals according to their needs
    c. The individuals according to their capacities
    d. The individuals according to the facilities

128. What does the individual aim of education imply?
    a. Education must secure for everyone the conditions under which the individuality is most completely developed
    b. It must contribute to the peace and happiness of the whole society
    c. It should have more and more institutions every year
    d. It should be by and large the concern of the private sector

129. According to which philosophy of education, childhood is something desirable for its own sake and children should be children?
    a. Idealism   b. Pragmatism
    c. Naturalism   d. Realism

130. Who emphasized that education should be a social process?
    a. Vivekananda   b. Rousseau
    c. Dewey   d. Pestalozzi

131. Which of the following is a type of counseling service?
    a. Orientation
    b. Developmental
    c. Termination
    d. Informal

132. Counseling is _____ centered process.
    a. Time
    b. Individually
    c. Money
    d. Counselor

133. Which of the following is an organized service to identify and develop the potentialities of pupils?
    a. Problem solving
    b. Guidance
    c. Counseling
    d. None of them

134. _____ counseling services meant to gather record maintain and use adequate information about each pupil.
    a. Orientation
    b. Counseling
    c. Information
    d. Appraisal

135. Education is the creation of a sound mind in a sound body is stated by aristotle:
    a. Mahatma Gandhi
    b. Aristotle
    c. Rigveda
    d. Pestalozzi

136. One of the principles of health education is participation:
    a. Description
    b. Narration
    c. Participation
    d. Comprehension

137. The cognitive domain in educational objectives refers to knowledge:
    a. Knowledge
    b. Attitude
    c. Skills
    d. Behavior

138. According to _____ evaluation is the process of determining to what extent educational objectives are being realized?
    a. Dr Sudha Rao
    b. Stevenson
    c. Plato
    d. Ralph Tyler

139. Which of the following is an organized clinical instruction in the presence of the patient?
    a. Bedside clinic
    b. Nursing rounds
    c. Individual conference
    d. Group conference

140. Which type of method provides an opportunity for observational learning?
    a. Lecture
    b. Project
    c. Seminar
    d. Demonstration

141. The person who formulates, processes and convey the message is called:
    a. Receiver
    b. Recorder
    c. Sender
    d. All the above

142. Is considered as planned learning activity dealing with original (or) raw data in the solution of the problems?
    a. Laboratory procedures
    b. Demonstration
    c. Discussion
    d. Lecture method

143. "Education" word derived from Latin word "educate" means:
    a. Lead
    b. Stop
    c. Communicate
    d. Transmit

144. These are the factual description of meaningful incidents and events that the teacher has observed in students lives anecdotal.
    a. Cumulative
    b. Anecdotal
    c. Attitude scale
    d. Rating scale

145. Following are the members of the panel discussion *except*:
    a. Audience
    b. Instructor
    c. Moderator
    d. Chairperson

146. The term lecture was derived from the Latin word lecture which means?
    a. To read
    b. To explain
    c. To speak
    d. To read aloud

147. It is the exact written report of the conversation between the nurse and patient:
    a. Process recording
    b. Case analysis
    c. Anecdotal
    d. Nurse record

148. The person who guides the seminar is the:
    a. Speaker
    b. Chairperson
    c. Organizer
    d. Instructor

149. It is one type of teaching method, which we use in the form of drama?
    a. Puppet shows
    b. Roleplay
    c. Fancy dress
    d. None of these

150. The panel discussion teaching was developed in the year:
    a. 1955
    b. 1929
    c. 1973
    d. 1992

151. The ideal duration of nursing round in a ward is:
    a. 20 mm
    b. 30 mm
    c. 15 mm
    d. 45 mm

152. Which of the following is visual form of communication?
    a. Charts
    b. Tables
    c. Posters
    d. All the above

153. Which of the following is last stage in the communication?
    a. Encoding
    b. Response
    c. Decoding
    d. None of the above example for upward

154. Given communication:
    a. Business proposals
    b. Suggestion box
    c. Exit interviews
    d. All the above

155. Voice mails are which form of communication?
    a. Downward
    b. Upward
    c. Horizontal
    d. Diagonal

156. Video conferencing is which form of communication?
    a. Downward
    b. Upward
    c. Horizontal
    d. Diagonal

157. Which type of communication is important to effective interpersonal interaction?
    a. Meta communication
    b. Symbolic communication
    c. Nonverbal communication
    d. None of the above

158. Good communication requires awareness of:
    a. Symbolic communication
    b. Meta communication
    c. Verbal communication
    d. Nonverbal communication

159. Which of the following is the basis of a therapeutic relationship?
    a. Trust
    b. Passion
    c. Intimacy
    d. Empathy

160. Trust is the described by initial developmental task:
    a. Taylor
    b. Andrew
    c. Eriksson
    d. Fayol

161. Interpersonal relations based on:
    a. Mistrust
    b. Intimacy
    c. Mutual trust
    d. Empathy

162. Which is not an advantage of short answer type tests?
    a. Easy to score
    b. Costly
    c. Response is quick
    d. Reliability of score is improved

163. Advantages of objective test are *except:*
    a. Precise, brief and clear
    b. Reliable, valid, objective and practicable
    c. More stationary is required
    d. A large number of students can be tested

164. The advantage of rating scale is:
    a. Easy to score
    b. Easy to administer
    c. Used for a large group
    d. All of the above

165. Rating scale may all *except:*
    a. Descriptive rating scale
    b. Algebraic rating scale
    c. Graphic rating scale
    d. Numerical rating scale

166. Purposes of bulletin board are:
    a. Motivates the learner
    b. Gives the correct initial information
    c. Supplements and correlates the instruction and save time
    d. All of the above

167. Advantage of bulletin board *except*:
    a. Not effective for illiterate group
    b. Explain important events
    c. Summarize and high lights events
    d. Serve as an introduction to a particular topic

168. Features of a good chart is:
    a. Clear, simple and not overcrowded
    b. Should highlight the main points
    c. Should be sufficiently large to be seen easily
    d. All of the above

169. Disadvantages of charts are *except*:
    a. Charts cannot be used for large group
    b. It cannot be used for illiterate people
    c. It is portable
    d. None of the above

170. Maturity-immaturity theory of motivation was propounded by:
    a. McGregor
    b. Maslow
    c. Federick Hertzberg
    d. Chris Argyris

171. Formal education is given *except*:
    a. School
    b. Colleges
    c. Educational institutes
    d. Home

172. Education process is:
    a. Bipolar
    b. Tripolar
    c. Both (a) and (b)
    d. None of the above

173. Motivation is an:
    a. External feeling
    b. Internal feeling
    c. Both (a) and (b)
    d. None

174. Commercial agencies of education are:
    a. Press
    b. Cinema
    c. Radio and TV
    d. All of the above

175. Philosophies of education are:
    a. Idealism
    b. Pragmatism
    c. Naturalism
    d. All of the above

176. Principle of counseling *except*:
    a. It is concerned with developing student's self-understanding and self-determination
    b. It is not concerned with "whole" individual
    c. It is more than activity of specialists
    d. It is a continuous and slow process

177. Areas of counseling are:
    a. Educational
    b. Health and living conditions
    c. Vocational
    d. All of the above

178. Types of counseling services are:
    a. Orientation service
    b. Appraisal
    c. Information service
    d. All of the above

179. Nontesting tool for collecting information *except*:
    a. Observation
    b. Interview
    c. Aptitude
    d. Commutative record card

180. Demonstration and return demonstration are essential for acquisition of:
    a. Knowledge
    b. Skill
    c. Attitude
    d. Aptitude

181. Phases of counseling are:
    a. Assessment
    b. Setting goals
    c. Intervention and termination
    d. All of the above

182. Purposes of flash cards are:
    a. Give health education
    b. Narrate a story
    c. To teach students
    d. All of the above

183. Advantages of essay type test are *except*:
    a. Test the ability to communicate in writing
    b. Take comparatively short time for the teacher to prepare the test
    c. Lack of objectivity
    d. Test depth of knowledge and understanding

184. **Types of objective tests commonly used in nursing are:**
    a. Multiple choice tests
    b. Matching type tests
    c. True and false items
    d. All of the above

185. **The number of members the panel has is:**
    a. 4-8
    b. 10-12
    c. 12-15
    d. 15-20

186. **Territoriality means _____.**
    a. It is a concept of the space and things that an individual considers as belonging to the self
    b. It is a concept of relating irrelevant messages into meaningful form
    c. A process of coping mechanism
    d. All of the above

187. **Which stage of curriculum lays foundation of all other stages?**
    a. Directive
    b. Formative
    c. Functional
    d. Evaluative

188. **The stage that design the curriculum is:**
    a. Formative
    b. Evaluative
    c. Directive
    d. Functional

189. **Name the step of curriculum in which committee for curriculum preparation is constituted:**
    a. Assessment
    b. Planning
    c. Implementation
    d. Development

190. **Features of good unit planning are:**
    a. It should be comprehensive
    b. Its aim should be clear and well defined
    c. A good unit plan provides place for beginning and ending
    d. All of the above

191. **Tones and Stanton explain what stages of curriculum?**
    a. Directive
    b. Evaluative
    c. Formative
    d. Creative

192. **Post Basic BSc Nursing is an example of curriculum:**
    a. Correlated curriculum
    b. Integrated curriculum
    c. Both (a) and (b)
    d. None of the above

193. **Principles of curriculum are:**
    a. Principle of leisure
    b. Principle of conservation
    c. Principle of linking with life
    d. All of the above

194. **A plan showing the placement of students in theory and practical area is called:**
    a. Master rotation plan
    b. Curriculum
    c. Clinical rotation plan
    d. Lesson plan

195. **Course planned must have:**
    a. Objectives of the course
    b. Resource material
    c. Brief course description
    d. All of the above

Answer Key

1. (a)	2. (b)	3. (c)	4. (b)	5. (b)	6. (b)	7. (b)	8. (a)	9. (a)	10. (c)
11. (b)	12. (b)	13. (c)	14. (d)	15. (b)	16. (b)	17. (c)	18. (b)	19. (c)	20. (b)
21. (d)	22. (b)	23. (c)	24. (d)	25. (b)	26. (c)	27. (b)	28. (d)	29. (d)	30. (c)
31. (a)	32. (d)	33. (c)	34. (d)	35. (c)	36. (b)	37. (a)	38. (d)	39. (b)	40. (a)
41. (d)	42. (c)	43. (a)	44. (a)	45. (b)	46. (a)	47. (b)	48. (d)	49. (d)	50. (d)
51. (c)	52. (c)	53. (b)	54. (b)	55. (d)	56. (d)	57. (c)	58. (a)	59. (d)	60. (c)
61. (a)	62. (b)	63. (c)	64. (b)	65. (a)	66. (c)	67. (d)	68. (c)	69. (a)	70. (b)
71. (c)	72. (b)	73. (a)	74. (c)	75. (c)	76. (a)	77. (a)	78. (b)	79. (c)	80. (c)
81. (b)	82. (a)	83. (c)	84. (b)	85. (d)	86. (a)	87. (c)	88. (d)	89. (b)	90. (a)
91. (a)	92. (b)	93. (b)	94. (b)	95. (c)	96. (d)	97. (c)	98. (b)	99. (c)	100. (c)
101. (b)	102. (b)	103. (c)	104. (a)	105. (b)	106. (c)	107. (b)	108. (c)	109. (a)	110. (a)
111. (b)	112. (c)	113. (d)	114. (a)	115. (b)	116. (a)	117. (d)	118. (d)	119. (d)	120. (c)
121. (b)	122. (c)	123. (d)	124. (c)	125. (d)	126. (c)	127. (a)	128. (a)	129. (c)	130. (c)
131. (a)	132. (b)	133. (b)	134. (d)	135. (b)	136. (c)	137. (a)	138. (d)	139. (a)	140. (d)
141. (c)	142. (d)	143. (a)	144. (d)	145. (d)	146. (d)	147. (a)	148. (b)	149. (b)	150. (b)
151. (d)	152. (a)	153. (b)	154. (d)	155. (a)	156. (b)	157. (a)	158. (a)	159. (a)	160. (c)
161. (c)	162. (b)	163. (c)	164. (d)	165. (b)	166. (d)	167. (a)	168. (d)	169. (c)	170. (d)
171. (d)	172. (c)	173. (b)	174. (d)	175. (d)	176. (b)	177. (d)	178. (d)	179. (c)	180. (b)
181. (d)	182. (d)	183. (c)	184. (d)	185. (a)	186. (a)	187. (a)	188. (a)	189. (b)	190. (d)
191. (d)	192. (c)	193. (d)	194. (c)	195. (d)					

Index

Page numbers followed by *f* refer to figure, *fc* refer to flowchart, and *t* refer to table.

A

Ability
    observation assessment 332, 332*f*
    testing 305
Academic counseling 371
Academic matters 403
Academic performance 315
Accountability 301, 419
    assessment for 302
    towards team 157
Achieve academic success 419
Achievement test 1, 301, 312, 314
Active agencies 7
Active experimentation 63
Active learning 75, 407
    strategies 156, 156*f*
Active portfolio
    clinical 350
    management 349
Active response principle 175
Active student participation 136
Activity 60, 416
    assessment 301
    principle 92
    principles of 128
    tools 229
Adaptability 78
    principle of 290
Adaptation 366
Admission
    service 362
    to school, approach to 417
Advice
    need of 390*f*
    types of 377
Advisor characteristics 385
Advisor role 382
Advisor skills, required 376
Advisory staff 374

Aesthetics 27
Agency benefits 263
Aids, ineffectiveness of 231
Alternate response items 324
Ambiguity 316
Ambulatory care 192
Amplifiers 289
Analytic scoring 301
Analytical approach 417
Analytical simulation 66
Anchor 301
Anecdotal notes 313, 345
Angry parents 163
Animated explainers 261
Animations 252
Apathy 125
Appeal 364
Appellant 364
Application pedagogical technology,
    fields of 14
Appraisal method 347
Aptitude testing 1
Argument development 311
Arousal approach 417
Art analysis 358
Assessment
    cycle 81
    data 329
    issues 314
    method 310, 311
    motivates learners 309
    purpose of 306
Asynchronous 294
    instruction 407
Atmosphere, controlled 13
Attention 384
Attitude
    and ethics 343
    and perceptions, change 373

    component 353
    scale 313
Attribute properties 183
Audience, role of 140
Audio 127
    aids 231, 258, 272
    material 232
    media 223, 225, 272
    tape recorder 272*f*
Audio technology 294
    advantages of 276
    disadvantages 276
    integration guidelines 276
Audio-visual
    communication tutorial 227
    guidance 281
    materials 232
Audio-visual aid 1, 225, 229
    basic of 227*f*
    classification of 231
    importance of 227, 232
    preparation 201
    types of 232
    use, history of 226
Auditions 272
Authentic assessment 23, 302, 407
Authenticity 409
Automatic configuration 266
Aware silence 188
Awareness approach 417
Axiology 2

B

Backward students, special teaching
    strategies for 396
Bad habits 401
Balanced diet 240*f*
Bar chart 237, 238
Bar graph 239

Basic understanding, lack of 70
Bedside
    clinical teaching 199, 199f
    teaching tips 198
Bedside clinic 196, 199
    goals 197
    preparation for 198
Behavior
    change 373
    feedback on appropriate 118
    guide to right 391
    outcome 74
    patient 205
    risk taking 83
Behavioral counseling approaches 381
Behavioral modification techniques 118
Behavioral objectives 99, 99f
Behavioral reforms 9
Benchmark 73
Best motivator 227
Biological naturalism 31
Blackboard 242
    color of 242
Blended course 179, 407
Blended learning 2, 17, 69, 109
    features 69f
    models 69
Bloom's taxonomy 1, 319f, 407
Bluetooth 298
Blu-ray 264
    advantages of 265
    disadvantages of 265
    properties of 265
Board
    effective use of 242
    games 169, 170
    uses of 242
Bogardus social distance scale 353
Branched programming 176
Broadcast 266
Bulletin board 226, 243, 243f
    details 244
    features 244
    purpose 243
    usage 244
    use 244

C

Cable TV 291
Candidates, movement of 331
Capstone experience 302
Cards 358
Care
    continuity of 338
    education applications 422
    improving access to 295
    intermediate 192
    interventions 329
    long-term 192
    managers 370
    plan 217, 337
    product plan 204
    reduced continuity of 297
Care plan
    benefits 205
    goals 338
    principles of 204
Career
    advancement 366
    advice 396
    counseling 378, 397
    issues 393
    master 379
    needs 366
Career guidance
    level 397
    needs 396
Caregivers connected,
    helps keep 297
Caring 79
Cartoon 241
Case
    analysis method, objectives of 200
    manager responsibilities 192
    presentation format 202
    selection 203
Case study
    analysis model 165f
    analysis, writing 163f
    answers 217
    criteria for good 202
    method 203f
    types of 203
Cause and effort chart 237
Cellular network 298
    types of 298
Central tendency error 335
Chairman, role of 140
Chalk, color of 242
Chalkboard 242
    fixed 242
Chart 236
    types of 237, 237f, 238
Chronic disease
    ability to manage 297
    care 297
Chronic obstructive pulmonary
    disease 422
Chunk 2
Citizenship, guide to 391
Clarification session 158
Class
    co-operation 171
    discussion 131
    performance 122
    period 179
    size 113
Classical conditioning 2, 57f
    concepts of 55
    principles of 55, 56f
Classmates and teachers, student
    interaction with 283
Classroom 121
    activities 311
    barriers 54
    climate 1, 117, 117f, 407
    communication
        facilitator 123
        factors affecting effective 123f
    embedded assessment 302
    environment, positive 420
    flipped 408
    ingenious helpers in 280
    interactions, types of 122
    learning 70f
    lively and active 229
    observation 110
    opaque projectors 255
    operations goals 115
    preparation 116
    spot questions 358
    take back control of 120
    teaching method 128
    tests 315
        types of 316
    used in 279
Classroom management 110, 114f, 115,
    117
    factors affecting 118
    factors influencing 119f
    techniques of 118
Clear goals 94
Clemson's teachings 421
Client-centered
    counseling 381
    therapy 381
Clients, critical steps for 375
Clinical assessment, concepts of 328
Clinical education
    objectives of 182
    use of 182
Clinical evaluation, types of 330
Clinical incident, phases of 200f
Clinical instructor
    functions 186
    qualities 187

Clinical learning
  environment 182
  experience selection, factors
    influences 183
  outcomes 185
Clinical meeting, phases of 194f
Clinical nursing practice 348
Clinical portfolio 349
Clinical supervisor 179, 181
Clinical teaching 189
  challenges 188
  chart of process of 182f
  domains of 181f
  meaning of 182
  method 181
    use 187
  skills 188
  strategies 188f, 189
  unit 179
    director 179
Clinical test 328
Clinical training 62
Clinician educator 181
Cognitive component 353
Cognitive domains, categories of 100
Cognitive psychology 2
Collaborative practice 173f
Color 240
  coding, use 236
Column graph 239
Commitment 375
Communication 52, 78, 83, 84, 86, 121, 128, 196, 281f, 329, 362
  and response, high speed 281
  barriers 125, 126f
  different formats 288
  effective 77
  facilitate 124
    instant 70
  factors affecting 122
  implementation of satellite-based 293
  national and region-specific 293
  non-verbal 122
  one-way 272
  satellite-based 293
  targeted 184
  types of 121
  verbal 122
Communication skills 20, 162, 189, 343
  good 376
  interpersonal 122f
Communicator 123
Community excursions 150
Community-based
  learning 19, 110
  research 62

Compact disk 273
  accessories 273
  use of 273
Compatriots, obligations of 37
Competency
  objectives of 23
  test 302
Competency-based education 17, 21, 22, 24, 112
  benefits of 24
  characteristics of 22
  mastery framework 23f
  pros and cons of 24
Competent writing, skills of 336
Competition 212
  regulated 171
Complaint 364
  forms of 402
  reasons for 403
  resolution committee duties 404
Completion task 324
Complex open reactions 102
Computer 280, 289
  applications of 280
  boosted distance learning 280
  education, benefits of 280
  importance of 154
  instruction, benefits of 279
  literacy 70
  nonjudgmental nature 279
  role of 280
  simulation 66
  software helps 280
Computer-aided educational programs, types of 154, 154f
Computer-assisted
  education 154
  instruction 279
  learning 153
Computer-based
  instruction 224
  training 2
Computing devices 290
Concept mapping 207, 208f
  benefits of 209
  tips 209
Concept testing 359
Conference, types of 195
Confidence 168
  hope and encouragement, build 378
Confidential reports 347
Conflict resolution 19
Cons care plan 205
Consistency 79
Constructive combat 17

Consultation procedure 374
Content
  maps, types of 208
  personalization and timeliness 128
  type of 114
Cooperative counseling 377
Cooperative practices 112
Core concept, elements of 94
Core curriculum 93, 179
  concepts 94
Correction task 324
Corruption 266
Cosmology 27
Counseling 179, 364, 365, 366f, 371, 372
  and advice 380
  and education 380
  and psychotherapy 380
  approach 380
  benefits of 378
    nondirective 383
  core principles of 375
  curriculum 368
  elements of 373f
  ethics 377
  goals of 372f
  meaning 371
  objectives 372
  organization of 379f
  personal needs of 393f
  prescriptive 382
  principles of 366, 376f
  process 371f, 374
    steps of 375
  program 384
    goals 364
  purpose of 372
  role of 380f
  rules and roles 380
  scope of 373
  service 362
    organization of 378, 391
    restrictions of 391
  skills, basic 377f
  techniques 381
  types of 390
Counselor 374, 379
  characteristics 375
  duties 384
  key steps 375
  qualities 384, 385f
  responsibilities 384
    guidance 368
  role 380
  tools, procedures techniques 374
Course embedded assessment 73

Course plan elements 105
Course planning 103, 105
  principles 103
Course-embedded assessment 302
Creative students, positive environment for 228
Creativity 84, 168
Critical correction 188
Critical incident technique 200, 347
Critical reflection 19
Critical thinking 75, 83, 84, 168, 211, 343
  and judgment 311
  and reflection 339
Criticism 129
Cross-age peer tutoring 162
Cross-section model 269
Cultural awareness 84
Cultural connections 28
Cultural factors 6
Cultural heritage, transmission of 9
Cultural values 413
Cumulative nature 354
Curiosity 168, 233
Current issue 189
Current knowledge base 83
Curriculum 37, 41, 217
  alignment 179
  assessment 98, 309
  booklet 217
  diversification 396
  domains, categories of 101f
  factors affecting 90f
  hidden 109
  knowledge 77
  principles of 91, 91t
  process stages 98, 99f
  structure 86
  types 89, 92, 93t
Curriculum design 94f
  principles of 95, 95f
  problem-centered 95
  tips 95
  types of 94
Curriculum development 98f
  competency-based 23
  factors influences 90
Curriculum planning 89, 95, 96f, 97, 98, 110, 302
  level of 97
  stages of 96, 97t
Curriculum-embedded assessment 302
Customer's willingness 329
Cutoff score 302

D

Data
  collection 203, 204
  processing 281
  security 264
Database, incomplete 205
Daydreaming 125
Debate 167, 211
  benefits of 211
  method of learning 168f
  preparation for 168
  structure for 168
Decision-making 67, 343, 366
  clinical 329
Delayed treatment 295
Delegator 80
Delhi Agricultural Television Project 294
Demand learning, enables on 262
Demerits 140
Democratic action, principles of 118
Democratic ideals 43
  principle 376
Demonstrate growth 253
Demonstration 109, 111, 136
  disadvantages of 139
  methods 137
    applications of 138
  phases of 137f
  types of 137
Demonstrator 79
Design curriculum 95
Detection method 113
Device selection criteria 307
Dewey's educational philosophy
  criticism of 48
  fundamentals of 47, 47f
Dewey's philosophy 47
  of education, principles of 48, 48f
Dewey's practical philosophy 47
Dewey's theory of education 48
Dialpad meetings 285
Digital
  audio 275
  content assessment 24
  daily 223
  games 170
  learning 180
  literacy 84
  media 223
  photography 294
  resources authentic and age appropriate 70
  transmission 296
  video disk 264

Digital versatile disk 264, 264f, 289
  advantages 264
  disadvantages 264
Dignity 79
Diorama 271
  type 271
Direct consultation, benefits of 382
Directive counseling 381
  characteristics of 382
Discipline 37, 399, 409
  components 400
  nature of 400
  types of 401
  violation, reasons for 401
Discourage cramming 229
Discrimination tests 305
Discuss 306
Discussion and evaluation, post-debate 169
Discussion filmstrip 251
Discussion forums 217
Discussion methods 111
Display boards 231
Distance education 2
Diversity 16, 18, 227
  principle 291
Document camera 289
Documentation 310, 338
Drag-and-drop question 359
  type, benefits of 359
Drama 416
Dramaturgical participation 232
Drop method, benefits of 200
Drugs and alcohol, helps overcome 378
Dunn and Dunn learning styles 83
Durability overtime 40

E

Early public address systems 274
Eclectic consultation, limitations of 383
Eclectic counseling 382, 383
  consultant competence 384
Eclectic tendency 29
Eclectic trends, key elements of 38
Eclecticism 29, 38
E-commerce 282
Economics 8
Economy 281, 283
Education 3, 4, 8, 11, 27f, 28, 40, 47, 111, 154, 160, 282, 282f, 385
  access to 228
  aims of 42f
  and development role 380
  character 42, 414
  characteristics of 4, 4f

classification of 5f
comparative 8
competency-based 22, 22f
conveys values 9
decisions 396
digital media in 224
etymological meaning of 3f
features of 8
forms of 4f
functions of 9f
history of 8
ideals of 42f
importance of 3
informal 5
meaning of 46
nature of 7f
non-formal 5
outcome-based 24
people with disabilities 280
personalized 17
progressive goals in 35
relationship-based 21
research areas of 8
role of 38
scope of 8
system 124
team 124
technology 13
types of 4, 6, 35, 43
underground 16
Educational areas 366
Educational benefits 250
Educational communication 232
Educational counseling 390, 394
    goals 395, 396
    level 396
    purposes 395
Educational environment 118
Educational goal 6, 6f, 7
    benefits of 6
    importance of 6
    types of 100, 100f
Educational guidance 397, 397t
Educational impact 38
Educational institutions 7, 160
    guidance 364
Educational instruction,
    basic principles of 395
Educational learning process 50
Educational management 8
    strategies 120
Educational media 223, 225
    categories of 227
    role of 233

Educational method 37
    importance of 112
Educational model 14
Educational needs 390
Educational objectives 302
Educational philosophy 26
    principles of 44, 45f
Educational psychology 8, 90
Educational purpose 100
Educational support services 124
Educational technology 8, 11, 13, 14
    goals 12
    importance of 11
    objectives of 12f
    scope of 13f
Educational television programs 292
    types of 292
E-education, types of 287
Effective leadership advice, benefits
    of 367
E-learning 112, 286, 342
    benefits of 288
    function 287
    importance of 287
    meaning 287
    restrictions 289
    strategies 287
    types of 287
Electronic media 223, 225, 278, 279f
Electronic medical record documents
    217
Eliminate negative feelings 378
Emotional barriers 55
Emotional domain, categories of 101
Emotional impact 272
Emotional intelligence 85f, 86
    components of 85, 85f
    symptoms 85
Emotional reaction 339
Emotionally intelligent, characteristics
    of 85
Emotions
    perceive 85
    reflection 363
    understanding 85
Empathic understanding 363
Empathy 78
Emphasize theory 13
Encounter, methods of 113
Encourage metacognition 422
Encourage self-evaluation 166
Energy 293
Engagement 54, 233
Enhanced virtual models 69
Entertainment 282

Environment 31
Environmental education 414
Environmental orientation 230
Environmental studies 8
Epistemology 27
Equality 309
Erotic realism 32
Error experiment 58
Essay type test 318
    disadvantages 320
Ethical behavior, determine
    appropriate 418
Ethical decision-making 417, 417f, 418,
    418f
Ethical issue 418
    clarify 333
Ethical principles 377f
Ethical standards 409
Ethics 79, 409
    applied 409
    ICN code of 411
    influence behavior 411
Evaluation tool 307
    characteristics 309
    selection of 310
Evidence-based
    instruction 407
    intervention 407
    learning 407
    physical examination 189
    practical knowledge 422
Evidence-based practice 407, 422
    components of 421f
    frameworks of 410
    steps 421
Evidence-based teaching 420
    strategies 421
Evolution chart 237
Exam structure 113
Examine problem 159
Examine solution 160
Excursion 150
    organization 150
    types 150
Execution 149
Exercise
    advanced 158
    hidden 171
    preliminary 146
    reflective 75
Exhibition 144
    disadvantages 145
    planning 145
    property 144
    purpose 144
Existential harmony 41

Existentialism 29, , 40-42
   features of 40
Experience
   centrality of 20
   cone of 232, 233*f*
   reconstruction of 47
Experiential learning 19, 61, 407
   styles 62
Experimentalism 29, 47
Expert-led explainer videos 261
Extracurricular activities 400

F

Facebook live 285
Face-to-face
   delivery 109
   driver model 69
Faculty and staff, evaluation of 302
Faculty representative 379
Fair mindset 24
False experience 232
Familiar education mode 293
Family counseling 373, 391
Family dynamics 373
Family members, recognizing role of 423
Family problems 86, 392
Faster grading 335
Favoritism 401
Fear 125
Feedback 66, 75, 157, 171, 185
   immediate 293
   individualized 335
   instant 280
   poll 359
   positive and negative 188
   providing 134
Fichte's view 27
Fieldwork 62, 109
Film, educational role of 259
Filmstrip
   principles 251
   types 251
   using 251
Financial matters 403
Financial obstacles 231
First hand experience, best substitute for 230
First practice session, configure 136
Flannel board 226
   benefits of 245
Flannel box, use of 245
Flannel sheet 245
   preparation 245*f*
   purpose 245
   selection tool 245
Flash cards 226, 247, 247*f*
Flex model 69
Flexible methodology 348
Flexible system 293
Flipchart 238, 239, 245
   benefits 246
   different types of 245*f*
   instructions for use 246
   steps of preparation 246
Flowchart 208, 238
Forced choice method 347
Foreign languages 358
Foresight principle 129
Formal teaching 51*f*, 311
Formation stage 96
Formative assessment 23, 75, 80, 112, 302
Fosters autonomy 348
Framing questions 319*f*
Free writing, use 166
Freedom 37, 44, 227
Functional nursing 191

G

G network 298
Game elements, audio driven scenarios with 65
Game-based learning
   elements of 212
   theory 170*f*, 173*f*, 213*f*
   types of 170, 170*f*
Game-based teaching methods
   benefits of 171
   disadvantages of 171
Gamification 2, 17
   model 213*f*
Gaming, purpose 170
Gandhi's educational philosophy 42
Gandhi's pedagogical experiment 43
General guidelines 339
General instructions 142
General philosophical concepts 29
Generous mistake 335
Genetics 31
Gentile view 27
Gifted students, special arrangements for 396
Gloves 267
Goal type test 324
Good projects, fundamentals of 210
Good rating system, basics of 346
Google hangouts 284
Grading system 316
   advantages of 316
Grammar 336

Graph 239
   types of 240*f*
   use 239
Graphic aids 231
Graphic board 242
Graphic rating scale 334
Graphically records information 422
Grievance 364, 399
   committee, objectives of 404
Grooming 375
Group activities 119
Group conference 194, 195*f*
Group discussion 130, 132
   disadvantages of 132
   rules 130, 131*f*
   techniques 131
Group education 17
Group formation 136
Group meeting 112
Group project 149
Growth 47
   and development, promote 163
Guidance 280, 365
   and advice 380
   counseling, efficacy of 395*fc*
   need of 388*f*
   scope of 366, 366*f*
Guidance service
   areas of 389*f*
   aspects of 397
   principles for organization of 391
   types of 389*f*
Guide, basic assumptions of 390
Guidelines 196
Guttman scale 354
Gyan Darshan Educational Channel 294

H

Halo mistakes 335
Hand puppet 267
   benefits 268
   prepare 267
Handling and manipulation, opportunities for 227
Handout 249, 249*f*
   preparation 249
   guidelines 249
Hardware approach 14
   characteristics of 15
   fundamentals of 14
Hardware teaching, use of 15
Harmless 377
Health 375
   education 414
   environment 37
   team, members of 204

Healthcare provider
  benefits 295
  disadvantages for 296
Healthy interaction, encouraging 228
Healthy work environment, building 162
Hearing aid 225, 229
Hierarchical map 208
Higher education assessment test 354
Holistic education 19
Home care 192
Homework neglect 402
Hospital, reduce trips to 297
Hotspot image testing, benefits of 359
Hotspot questions 358
  data analysis 358
Human bonds 28
Human learning, sanctity of 19
Human rights 18
Humanism 29
Humanistic counseling approach 380
Humanistic existentialism 29
Humanistic pragmatism 35
Humanistic realism 32
Humanity, universal spirit of 45
Humor 242
Hybrid course 407
Hybrid simulation 342
Hypothesis generation 189

I

Idealism 2, 28, 33
  criticism of 40
  disadvantages of 34
  educational principles of 34
  general characteristics of 34
  importance of 34
  meaning of 33
  philosophical significance of 33, 33f
  principles of 33
  types of 33, 33f
Illness and infections, less susceptible to 295
Illness and recovery, home care during 296
Images, use of 248
Imaginary experiences 234
Independent education 43
Index cards, preparing 247
Index method 394
Indigenous wisdom 19
Individual and social goals, integration of 42
Individual counseling 373
  functions of 392
  procedures 393

process steps 394f
services 395
stages 392
Individual journeys 150
Individual meetings 193
Individual readiness assurance test 158
Individual student
  decisions and reasons 200
  progress 23
Individualism 34
Infection
  reduced risk of 297
  slowing spread of 295
Informal complaint 364
Informal techniques 310
Information 281
  literacy 84
  materials 248
  remember important 208
  technology characteristics 126
Information communication technology 126
  challenges 128
  components 126f
  materials, expensive 128
  stands 126
Inpatient education challenges 189
Inside university stadium 398
Insight learning concepts 59
Inspiration 78
Institution
  leaders 400
  types of 7, 7f
Institutional assessment 356
Institutional curriculum 97
Instruction, objectives of 389, 389f
Instructional advice 377
  restrictions 382
Instructional media 223, 226f
Instructional study 16
Instructor's role 196
Instruments, complicated 316
Insurance coverage 295
Insurance issues 297
Integrity 419
Intelligent classroom principles 290
Intense paraphrasing 188
Interactive process 52
Interactive video 261
Intercampus access control 293
Intercollegiate visits 150
Intercultural understanding, promote 124
Interdisciplinary care 112
Internal reactions, reflections of 357

International Council on Nursing 411
Internet 224, 281
  applications of 281f
  importance of 282, 282f
  role of 283
  usage 281
Internships 61, 62, 112
Interpersonal education, need of 172f
Interprofessional education 172, 173f
  facilitation, key challenges of 172
  importance of 173
  need for 172
  promoting 173
Interprofessional health care 174
Interprofessional learning activities, preparation for 173
Interprofessional nursing 112
Interprofessional research 112
Interprofessional teams 172
Interprofessional teamwork 112
Interschool visits 150
Inter-training attribute 376
Isolation 284
Item analysis procedure 316

J

Job preparation 43
John Dewey's philosophy of education 46
John Watson's conditioning theory 56
Journal organization 166
Journaling 163, 166
  benefits of 167f
  purposes 164
  rules 164
Journals students, types of 166
Judgment, purpose of 346

K

Knowledge 33, 73, 91, 100, 150
  assessment of 318
  storage 14
  tests, multiple tests 342
Kohler's insight learning experiments 59
Kolb's cycle of experimental learning 60f
Kothari commission 402

L

Laboratory
  and internship work 280
  experience 111
  simulations 66
Language 125, 147
  learners 81
  problems 231
  skills 124

Laptop 289
Large venue systems 275
Layout 240
Leadership 86, 168, 364, 367, 375, 388
   characteristics 390
   concepts 388
   effective 367
   principles of 366, 389
   role advice 367, 368*f*
Leading students 16
Learn Thorndike's law 57
Learner
   age 113
   assessment of 75, 80, 82
   auditory 81
   emotional intelligence 84
   empowerment 152
   engagement, improve 262
   feed 90
   imagine things 236
   interpersonal 81
   kinesthetic 81, 278
   life-long 24
   mathematics 81
   musical 81
   natural 81
   performance recording, automatic 154
   problem-based 160
   reinforcement 228
   responsibility and autonomy 152
   rhythmic 81
   self-assessment for 348
   visual 81
   writing 81
Learner-centered 230
   curriculum design 94
Learning
   adaptive 290
   and training, active transitions in 228
   authentic 179
   benefits of
     active 156
     blended 70
     cartoons 241
   brain-based 110
   collaborative 290, 407
   competency-based 16
   components of team-based 157*f*
   constructivist 17, 170
   controlled 154
   cycle, stages of experiential 62
   deeper 180
   determinants of 81
   direct assessment of 302

direct measures of 73
disabilities 83
distance 2, 109, 283
electronic 180
expanding 70
expeditionary 17
experiences 60
flexibility 283
flipped 17
forms of experiential 61
goals for 73
hybrid 2
importance of reflective 63
improve 310
indirect measures of 74
informal 2
inquiry-based 408
internet-based 281*f*
interprofessional 112
lab 109
level of 137*f*
management system 2, 408
materials 113
model of self-directed 152
modify new 227
natural way of 113
object-based 408
objectives 109, 137
pathway 110
peer 162, 164*f*
personalized 2
preferences, adult 153
principles of 52, 53, 376
   experiential 61, 61*f*
projects 149
provide cumulative 104
purposes, simulation for 66
reflective 63
remote 109
scenario-based 65, 65*f*
self-directed 152, 152*f*
simulation 19, 66
skills 84
speed of learners 113
steps of transformative 19*f*
technology-enabled 17
theory 55
to life, roleplay simulations bring 214
traditional 164*f*
transformative 18*f*
types 81
video-assisted 261*f*
video-based 261
Learning barriers 54
   overcoming 55

Learning environment 87
   positive 184
   promote deaffriendly 124
Learning experience
   criteria for selecting 183, 184*f*
   interactive 70
   organizational process 104
   principles for selection of 183, 184*f*
Learning goals 15
   developing specific 15
Learning methods
   diversify 104
   improving 396
Learning needs 82
   procedures for determining 82
Learning outcomes 74, 99*f*
   writing effective 185*f*
Learning process 51, 51*f*
   active participation in 189
   autonomous 153
Learning style 83
   accommodate different 283, 335
   principles of 83
Lecture
   animated 262
   format 111
   projects and presentations 311
   style 79
   times and locations, changes in 420
Lecture method 128
   benefits of 129
   disadvantages of 128*f*, 129*f*
   principles of 128
Leisure and recreation, guide to 391
Lesson
   implementation of 77
   preparation and analysis 64
   programmed 174
Lesson plan 78, 102, 103
   benefits 102
   steps 103
Life
   completion of 48
   philosophy of 42
Lifespan 266
Lifestyle, improve your 378
Lighthearted conservation 82
Likert scale 334, 354
Linear programming 176
Linking with life, principle of 92
Liquid crystal display
   panels 255
     advantages 255
   projector 255*f*

Index

Listening
    active 79, 363
    barriers 125
    effective 376
    skills, good 214
Literacy skills 84
Literature 416
Live classroom 223
Livelihood 42
Liveliness 228
Living activities 91
Local school excursion 150
Logbook 306
    objectives of 350
    purposes of 350
Logical bonds 28
Logical error 335
Low fidelity mannequin 342
Loyalty 377

M

Magazine 250
    use of 167
Magnaboard 242
Malicious takeover 128
Man's highest nature 39
Management techniques 121
Marital issues 393
Marketing 253
Marriage counseling 380
Mass media 224
Materials
    importance of 229
    selection of 230
Maturity, principle of 92
Mechanical damage 266
Mechanistic naturalism 31
Media
    appeal 278
    education 224
    literacy 84
Medical care, accept 82
Medical education, competency-based 179
Medical history 332
Medical information, protecting 295
Meeting
    schedule 195
    types of 195
Memory 227
    stronger 171
Mental health
    achieving positive 372
    care 297
    counseling 378

Mentor 180, 181
Metaphysics 27
Methodology 41
Methods and techniques, use of 154
Microclass settings, create 134
Microlearning 2
    enable 262
Microlesson cycle duration 134
Microlesson plan, create 134
Microphone 289
Microscope
    parts of 252f
    structure of 252f
Microteaching 132, 137f
    advantages of 134
    cycles, repeating 134
    phases 133f
    procedure 133f
    process 134f
    steps 132f
Mindset, fixed 407
Minor illnesses, counseling of 297
Mirror pyramid 332
Misconceptions 320
Mobile
    education 17
    health 294, 296
    learning 298
        issues 299
    radio technology, use of 298
    technology 297
        benefits of 298
        disadvantages of 298
Mobility 283
Mock teaching
    procedures for 67
    process 67f
Model instructions, mass expansion of 14
Model lessons
    criticism of 134
    observation of 134
Modern learning approaches 60
Monitor student comprehension 124
Monologue 292
Monopoly-like games for schools 170
Moral perspective 6
Moral reasoning approach 417
Moral values 413
Morality 409
Motion picture film 258
    applications 258
Motivating approach 171
Motivation 79, 171, 225, 229, 233, 375
    lack of 401
Motivational factors 86

Moulage 270
    preparation 271f
Movie
    educational value of 258
    film, use of 260
    selection 231, 260
    usage 260
Moving visuals 258
    benefits 259
    disadvantages 260
Multimedia 225
    integration 283
    packages 127
    presentations 217
Multisensory activation 138
Multi-touch technology 223

N

Narrative chart 237
National education 37
    philosophy 113
National satellite project 294
Naturalism 28, 30
    characteristics of 30
    criticism of 31, 41
    forms of 31, 31f
    principles of 31
Naturalistic goals 31
Naturalistic perspective 6
Nature
    and humans, positive communication between 44
    ethical in 369
    faith in 30
    protection of 412
Navdanya 16
Navigate consultation process 374
New knowledge, rapid generation of 13
Newspaper 250
Non-academic competencies 180
Nondirective counseling 382
    steps 383
Non-discretionary portfolio management services 350
Non-policy consulting 382
Nonprinted media 225
Non-projected aids 225
Non-projected images
    disadvantages of 236
    use of 236
Non-projection media 225, 236
Non-projective visualization, benefits of 236
Non-testing tools 379
Norm-referenced tests 180

Numeric rating scale 334
Nurse 411
   guidance and advice for 369
   patient interaction record 218
   primary responsibility 411
   role 82, 338
   visits, importance of 206
Nurse-patient interaction
   evaluating 219
   recording 219
Nursing 34, 412
   behavior 205
   code of ethics 412
   community, benefits of 423
   diagnosis 204, 338
   diary 351
   educator 351
   faculty members 409
   plan format 338
   steps for 203
   students, writing advice for 218
Nursing care
   cases, merits of 203
   philosophy, importance of 30
   plans 338
   primary 191
Nursing education 409
   philosophy of 90
   types of simulation in 342
   values-based 415
Nursing philosophy 29, 30
   components, individual 30
Nursing process 203
   notes 336, 337
Nursing rounds 206
   disadvantages 207
Nursing team meeting 195
   benefits 194
   goals 195
Nursing visit
   benefits 207
   procedures for conducting 207
   purpose of 206
Nutrition courses 104

O

Objective data 204
Objective idealism 34
Objective test 303, 323
   benefits of 323
   classification of 324
   disadvantages of 324
Objectives structured clinical examinations 331, 343, 343f
Observation technique decision 136

Obsolescence 316
Occupational needs 390
Occupational values 9
Official agencies 7
One-on-one instruction, concepts of 155
One-to-one lessons 155, 155f
   advantages 155
   concept of 155
   disadvantages 156
One-way peer teaching 162
Online assessments 311
Online course 180
Online learning 70f, 180
   benefits of 283
   convenient 283
   drawbacks of 283
   program 180
Online program, full-time 180
Ontology 27
Opaque projector 254, 254f
   advantages 255
   disadvantages 255
   uses 254
Operant conditioning 56, 57, 57f
Oral examination 331, 340
Oral test 340
Organization 79, 102, 147
   specific instructions for 104
Organizational barriers 174
Organizational counseling, classification of 381fc
Organized information storage 281
Organized system 52
Organizing counseling services, needs for 391
Orientation 133, 136
Outpatient teaching, challenges of 189
Overlay chart 238
Oxygen delivery 422

P

Pain, duration of 334
Panel discussion 132, 140
   concept 141
   members 140f
   privilege 141
   technique 141
Paper and pencil performance 305
Paraphrasing 362, 363
Parents 37, 374
Participation, principle of 118
Passing scores, determining 310
Passion 79
Passive institutions 7
Patient assignment, factors affecting 190

Patient care
   issues, identify 195
   progressive 192
Patient satisfaction 295
Patient-centered care 337
Patient-related challenges 188
Peace education 19
Peace of mind, provides 378
Pedagogy 2, 8, 111, 180
Pedler 64
Peer enthusiasm 171
Peer evaluation 209
Peer learning, importance of 162
Peer relationships 87
Peer review 158
Peer sharing 161, 161f
   examples of 162
Peer teaching 161f, 162
   disadvantages of 163
Peer-to-peer
   learning, features of 162
   model 162f
Perception 102
   barriers 125
Perennial studies, pedagogical application of 39
Perennialism 29, 39, 40
   criticisms of 40
   educational applications of 39f
Performance appraisal method 347
Performance evaluation 345, 348
   criteria 347
   principles of 346
   tactics 346
   tools 347
Performance test 315
   classification 315
Personal advertising 282
Personal care philosophy 30
Personal counseling needs 392
Personal customization 375
Personal development 366
Personal health, guide to 391
Personal problems 365, 392
Personal quality, principle of 118
Personal values 413
Personality building 415
Personality traits 385
Personalization, principles of 291
Philanthropy 377
Philosophical system, construction of 41
Philosophy 5, 8, 26, 27f, 28
   branches of 27
   education 8, 26, 27
   meaning of 27

of science, critique of 41
pedagogical application of 30
Photos, use of 248
Physical education teacher 379
Physical health issues 392
Physical management readiness 229
Physical placement flexibility, principle of 291
Physical preparation 82
Physical set up 201
Physiological processes, denial of 32
Pictorial chart 238
Picture boards 238
Pie chart 237, 238
Pie graph 240
Placement 209
   service 362
Plan care with team members 196
Planning 66, 149, 193, 205
   individual 368
   period 180
   procedure 205
Pluralism 34
Policy counseling 382
Political ideology 6
Political philosophy 27
Politics 8
Population explosion 13
Portfolio 311
   assessment 303
   management 349
      passive 349
      types of 349
   needs 349
Poster 240
   benefits of 241
   components 240
   design rules 241, 241f
   use 240
Postsimulation debriefing 136
Power, lack of 231
PowerPoint
   benefits 253
   slide 252
PowerPoint presentation
   disadvantages of 255
   guide 255
   use 253
Practical exam 341
Practical goal 33
Practical test 328
Practicality 230
Practice and interaction 170
Practice assessment guidelines 351
Practice makes perfect 335

Practice oriented 33
Practice sessions, conducting 67
Pragmatism 28, 34
   experimental 35
   forms of 35
   meaning of 34
   principles of 34, 35f
Pre-admission service 362
Prejudice, measuring 354
Presentation, method of 113
Primary school 392
Print materials 248, 248f
Print media
   classify 248
   disadvantages 249
Private students, benefits for 14
Privilege 141
Problem solving 372
   and creativity 280
   facilitate 65
   skills 376
Problem-based learning 2, 17, 158, 158f, 160, 214, 408
   benefits of 160
   case-based 159
   characteristics 159
   drawbacks of 161
   essential elements of 159f, 215f
   functionality 215
   instructions 215
   principles of 159, 161f, 215f
   problem-stimulated 159
   risks of 160
   stages of 158f
   steps of 215f
   student-centered 159
   types 159
Problem-solving, interested in 189
Process record 338
   format 339
   phases of 219f
   requirements 219
   stages of 219
   steps 339
   teaching 218
Professional conduct 329
Professional development 64, 180
   continuing 112
Professional growth 122
Professional nurse requirements 195
Proficiency tests 315
Program assessment 303
Program education characteristics 176
Program instruction assumptions 176
Program statement characteristics 175

Program teaching
   benefits 176
   principles 175
Progress charts, management of 280
Progressivism 29, 35, 36
   disadvantages of 36
Project 210
   design, use 121
   fundamentals 147
   implementation steps 149
   method features 148
   methodology, effective use of 210
   type 149
Project law 147, 148f
   issues 211
   principles 148
Project-based learning 1, 180, 408
   elements of 148f
Projected aids 225, 231, 250, 251f
   value 250
Projected media 225
Projection techniques 314
Projective aids, types of 251f
Projector 289
   overhead 253, 253f, 289
   types of 210
Projects, types of 210
Psychoeducational programmers 380
Psychological needs 113, 390
Psychological perspective 6
Psychological testing 305
   tools 379
Psychology 8
   uses of 388
Psychomotor domain, categories of 102
Psychomotor skill 189
   demonstration procedures 138
Psychosocial problems 365
Public address system 273, 274f, 275
   components of 275
Public address, long line 274
Pull chart 238
Punctuality 79
Punctuation 336
Puppet 267
   preparation 268f
   principles 268
   types of 267, 267f
Puzzle games 170

Q

Q and A method 46
Qualitative assessment 303
Quality care, better access to 297
Quality education 293

Index

Quality team performance, accountability for 157
Quantitative social distance, equal distance in 354
Question journal 166
Questioning techniques, using 422
Questionnaire method 394
Questions, matching types 325f

R

Random factors, diagnosis of 203
Rating scale 303, 313, 331, 333
    limitations 334
    methods 347
    quality 334
    type 334
Realism
    forms of 32, 32f
    meaning of 31
    principles of 32
Realist belief 32
Real-life game 170
Reasoning ability 124
Recognizing alarm fatigue 423
Reconstructionism 36
    aspects of 37f
    elements of 36f
    forms of 37
Reconstructionist goals 37
Reconstrutionism 29
Record objective information 336
Record your evaluation 337
Recovery and selfcare 192
Re-demonstration 139
Re-feedback sessions 134
Reflective coaching, importance of 63
Reflective cycle phases 63f
Reflective journal 217
Reflective learning
    benefits of 64
    theories of 64
Rehabilitation counseling 378
Reimbursement 297
Reinforcement principle, immediate 175
Relationship building 374
Relationship counseling 378
Religious counseling 390
Religious education 43
Religious factors 5
Religious issues 393
Religious perennialism 40
Religious ties 28
Remedial course student evaluation 78
Remedial service 362
Remote patient monitoring 294, 296
Renewal 171
Replication simulation 66
Rescheduling sessions 134
Research knowledge 160
Research papers 217
Research plan objectives 103
Research posters 217
Resources 157, 171
Responsibility 157, 419
Re-teach session 134
Retrieval practice 1, 408
Revenue sources, additional 295
Reward 79
    and punishments, appropriate 400
Right teaching method, benefits of choosing 115
Rigolosum 331
Rod puppets 267
Role assignment 136
Role model 181
Role play
    advantages of 146f
    benefits of 147
    competencies 214f
    confidence through 214
    disadvantages of 146f
    factors affecting 146
    game 146, 170
    level of 147
    purposes of 146
    skills needed for 146f, 214f
    steps 146

S

Safe learning environment 399
Sampling 303
Sanyasi life 43
Satellite
    characteristics 293
    development and launch 293
    education project 294
    life 293
    transmission 292
    type 293
Save money 297
Save time 297
Saves energy and time 228
Scaffolding 1, 110, 408
Scale model 269
Scenario-based learning strategies, benefits of 66
Scholars and thinkers 26
Scholastic realism 32
School advisory committee composition 379
School doctor 379
School environment, good 400
School management, improvement of 14
School of medicine 181
School performance test 315
School program 309
Science 28, 416
Scientific knowledge, use of 196
Scientific naturalism 31
Scoring answer sheet 316
Scoring task 318
Screen patients, unable to 296
Screencast video 262
Screening 78
Secondary education 396, 397
    television project 294
Security principles 291
Security threats 266
Seek personal growth 420
Seek professional growth 420
Seeking knowledge 6
Selecting project, criteria for 147
Selection tool 245
Self acceptance, contribute to 378
Self discovery, leads to 378
Self efficacy 75
Self-assessment 209, 348
    benefits of 348
Self-awareness 86
Self-control 171
Self-determined pace principle 175
Self-directed learning, benefits of 153
Self-esteem 122
Self-exchange 420
Self-expression, creative 44
Self-paced learning, benefits of 153f
Self-report techniques 345
Self-study, disadvantages of 153
Seminar 141
    benefits 143
    cons 143
    elements 142
    field 142
    method 142f
    paper guide 142
    procedures for conducting 142
Sensations 32
Service 282
    learning 61
Session control 184
Seven-point scale 354
Sexual problems 393
Shadow puppet 267
Shopping 282
Short answer tests, benefits of 321
Simple slides, presenting with 262

Simplified model 269
Simulated class restrictions 137
Simulated instruction minimizes 66
Simulated teaching 66
   definition 135
   special features of 135
Simulated training steps 136
Simulation 135, 341
   and play 154
   concepts 342
   cycle 135f
   education 66
   games 169
   ideas for nursing education 68
   life cycle steps 67f
   objectives 342
   suggestion 68
   type of 66, 342
Sincerity 123
Skill 328
   action-based 330
   and abilities 124
   assessment of 328
   beyond presentation 335
   building interpersonal 162
   categories 84
   clinical 189, 343
   cognitive 83
   develop 378
      advanced 228
      evaluation 348
      individual 389
   different 344
   for practice, selection of 136
   observation
      assessment challenge 332
      test scoring 333
   presentation requires special 129
   procedural 330
   selection and discussion 67
   training 65
   writing 330
Skills-based assessments 24
Skinner's operant experiments 57
Skype 285
Slack video calls 285
Slide
   benefits of 256
   design 252
   layout 252
   projector 256, 256f
Small venue systems 274
Smart class
   basic 289
   benefits of 291
   disadvantages of 291

Smart classroom 289
   components 290
   features 290
   intermediate 289
   suggested features for 290
   targets 289
Smart podiums 289
Social change 90
Social curriculum 97
Social distance 354
Social media 224
   learning 2
Social metrics 305
Social needs 390
Social networking 281
Social personality formation 9
Social realism 32
Social skills 78
Social status 16
Social studies 416
Social ties 28
Social values 413
Socialization process, completion of 8
Society 90
   maintenance of 4
Sociology 8
   of education 8
Sociometric method 334
Sociometry 314
Soft skills assessment 335
Software
   approach of 15
   teaching, use of 15
Sound slide film 251
Speaker 289
   role of 140
Speaking skills 330
Spider card 208
Spiritual goal 38
Spiritual harmony and salvation 45
Spiritual perspective 6
Spiritual values 413
Staff development 180
Stakeholder
   identification 418
   perspectives 418
Standardized test 303, 315
Stanford faculty development
      model 184
Stations, types of 344
Statistical analysis 358
Status conferment 9
Stealing 402
Stem 322
Still image 247
   benefits of 235

Still visuals 235
Stimulation techniques, training with 280
Store-and-forward technology 294
Strategy simulators 171
Stress, reduce 171
String puppet presentation 268f
Stringency errors 335
Strip tease chart 238
Student 90
   achievement 77, 409
   advice office hours 420
   assessment 384
   attendance 420
   centered 290
   classify 280
   collaboration 128
   counseling
      issues 369
      objectives of 385
   development theory 418
   ethical standards 418
   examination principle 176
   guidelines 218
   indifference 231
   information service 362
   interaction and motivation 77
   learning
      outcomes assessment 303
      style 114
   outcomes assessment 74
   ownership and investment 23
   participation, increased 283
   performance 305
   preparation 150, 219, 333
   problems, common 205
   reluctance 163
   respect 38
   responsibilities of 119, 151
   roles 153
   roll 196
   skill development 168
   submissions 166
Student-centered teaching 1, 408
Student-faculty relationship 419
Student-teacher relationships
   building good 116
   importance of 420
   responsibilities of 420
   strengthen 65
Study abroad 62
Study plan contents 104
Subject classification 100
Subject curriculum 75
Subject-centered curriculum design 94
Subjective assessment 304
Subjective data 204

Subjective evidence, collect 336
Subjective idealism 34
Subjective judgment 323
Subtask simulator 342
Summative assessment 1, 75, 80, 304, 356
Supervised nursing internship 111
Supervision 151, 403
    duties 124
    lack of 71
Supervisor, role of 153
Support systems 82
Surface graph plot 240
Surrogate experience 227
Survey hotspot questions 358
Sustainable learning, educational processes for 281
Syllabus 75
    building steps 96, 96f
Symposium 139
    technique, characteristics of 139
Synchronous 294
    instruction 1
Synthesis 73, 101
Synthesize knowledge 212
Synthesize lesson 348
System approach 14f, 15, 16f
    benefits of 16
System support 368

T

Tabular chart 237, 238
Tagore stresses 44
Tagore's educational philosophy 44
    fundamental principles of 44
Tagore's general philosophy 45, 46f
Tagore's philosophy of education 44
    evaluation of 46
Tagore's Shantiniketan 45
Talk therapy 378
Tangible experiences 62
Tape recorder 272
    functions 272
Teach learning strategies 422
Teacher 143, 400
    assess growth and proficiency 23
    assessment of 75
        benefits of 78
    behavior
        desirable 223
        principles of 118
    benefits of 263
    clinician 181
    competence and preference 113
    competent 37
    disrespectful behavior towards 402
    essential characteristics of 78
    good character 43
    indifference 231
    instructions 247
    overload 70
    presentation 201
    relation to 309
    responsibilities of 151
    role 46, 105, 210, 259, 315
        importance of 13
    selection of 67
    training 284
        colleges 14
    value of role plays for 147
Teacher evaluation 76
    conduct 78
    criteria and strategies 77
    methods 76
    techniques 76
Teacher-student
    conference 132
    relationship 401
        characteristics of positive 420
Teaching 8, 46, 181, 409
    and community, sense of 419
    barriers 54
    development plan 408
    effective 118
    facilitate 65
    importance of 51
    learning process, model of 51f
    measurements function 308
    media 225
    models 184
    objectives 112, 113
    principles of 52, 53, 227
    process, reflective 63f
    programmed 176
    session 134
    simulation methods in 136
    students 62
    styles 79
    tools 279
    while walking 46
Teaching aid 226f, 228, 272f
    classification of 229, 231
    issues 230
Teaching and learning
    effective tools for 283
    enhanced 23
    principles of effective 52
    process 50
    nature of 52
    strategies 54
Teaching material 228
    functions 228
    need for 228
Teaching method 3, 36, 43, 86, 111, 113, 400
    characteristics of 114
    classification of 113
    features of 129
    regarding 309
    types of 113
Teaching skills
    integration 134
    selection of specific 133
Teaching technology
    characteristics of 13
    classification 126
Team nursing 191
Team workers, effective 400
Team-based learning 156, 156f, 157t
    concept 157
    pillars of 157
    steps 157, 160f
Technology
    barriers 297
    concerns 296
    issues 283
    literacy 84
    use 19
Technology-based services, types of 296
Telecare services 296
    types of 296
Telecommunication 278
    role of 278
Teleconferencing
    benefits 293
    limitations 294
    systems 293
Telehealth 294
Telemedicine 294
    care
        cons of 297
        types of 294
    nursing benefits 297
    service 295
    technology 294
Telenursing 296
Test 37, 203
    design
        and structure 310
        principles of 310
    form, create 310
    preparation principles, basic type 318
    results, report 310

specification 309
steps in construction of 309
types of 318
Testimonials 385
Theme selection and goal development 149
Theory 170
Therapy 394
Thinking 62
problem-based 160
Thorndike's law of learning 58, 58*f*
Thorndike's trial 58
Thorne's mode 374
Thought
clarify your 212
freedom of 419
organize your 208
Thread puppets 267
Three-D materials, use 267
Three-D tools
advantages of 267
use 267
Thurstone scale 354
Time and place, easy to access 283
Time and space, conquest of 272
Time and transportation 150
Time consuming 171
Timetable preparation 280
Tolerance, principle of 376
Tools 64
Track learner skills 70
Traditional methods 348
Traditional practical examination 330
Traditions, building 400
Training facilities, lack of 231
Training goals, individual 6
Training material 248
Training session organization 136
Training videos 262
Transformation theory, principles of 20, 20*f*
Transformational learning
benefits of 20
theory, essential elements of 19
Transformative education
need for 18
principles 18
Tree
chart 238
diagrams 238
Triage 296
Trial and error learning 58
stages 58*f*
TrueConf online 285
Tutorial videos 262
types of 262

U

Undergraduate research experience 62
Uniform curriculum 104
Unit 304
Unit planning 105
criteria for good 105
essential activities for 106
Universal heart, faith in 33
Universal serial bus 265, 265*f*
flash drive
disadvantages of 266
advantages of 266
Usability testing 359
Using cartoons, techniques for 242
Utilitarian approach 417

V

Validation 363
Validity 74, 304, 305, 309, 409
Value development strategies 415
Value education, importance of 413*f*, 414
Value systems, importance of 18
Value-based education 410
components 414, 414*f*
meaning 410
program 413*f*
Values-based practice 409
Ventilation 374
Verbal captions 240
Verbal rating scale 334
Verbal teaching diseases, antidote to 227
Verbatim dialogue 339
Versatility 293
Video cassettes 262, 262*f*
agency benefits 263
benefits for teachers 263
cons 263
Video compact disk player 289
Video conferencing 286, 293, 296
platforms 284
tips, effective 286
web-based 284
Video learning tools 261
Video-based grading, benefits of 335
Video-based learning
advantages of 262
benefits of 261
Videotape 262, 262*f*, 335
Virtual classroom 2
Virtual reality 2, 342
Vision to reality, transitioning from 20
Visual aids 225, 229
Visual analog scale 334
Visual learning 235
strategies 235

Visual media 225
Visual non-projected
three-dimensional 127
two-dimensional 127
Visual print 126
Visual projected 127
Vitamin 322
Viva voce
benefits 341
drawbacks 341
Vocabulary, increase 229
Vocational counseling 390
Vocational guidance 397, 397*t*
Vocational training 17
Voice, active 336
Vulnerability, type of 266
Vulnerable people, gathering of 412

W

Warning note 171
Waste and stagnation 395
Willingness 375
to learn 79
Window chart 238
Wireless mobile telephony public address system 274
Work plan
create 136
preparing 136
Workgroups 403
Working conditions 403
Workshop
benefits 144
principles 144
Write nursing track notes 336
Writing learning outcomes 99
Writing nursing progress notes 337
tips for 337
Writing prompts, use 166
Writing tasks, types of 340
Written advantages 319
Written assignment 216, 340
purpose of 216
types of 217, 217*f*
Written communication 122, 336
elements of 336
Written exam 315
common drawbacks of 316

Y

YouTube live 285

Z

Zoom 284

EU GSPR Authorised Reprsentative
Logos Europe, 9 rue Nicolas Poussin
1700, La Rochelle, France
Phone: +33 (0) 6 67 93 73 78
E-mail: contact@logoseurope.eu

www.ingramcontent.com/pod-product-compliance
Ingram Content Group UK Ltd.
Pitfield, Milton Keynes, MK11 3LW, UK
UKHW050458150426
5217IPUK00025B/1744